Improving Oral Health for the Elderly

Ira B. Lamster · Mary E. Northridge

Editors

Improving Oral Health for the Elderly

An Interdisciplinary Approach

Foreword by Jeanette C. Takamura

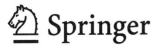 Springer

Editors

Ira B. Lamster
Columbia University College of Dental
Medicine, New York, NY, USA
630 West 168th Street
New York 10032
ibl1@columbia.edu

Mary E. Northridge
Dept. Sociomedical Sciences
Mailman School of Public Health
Columbia University, New York, NY, USA
722 West 168th Street
New York 10032
men11@columbia.edu

ISBN: 978-0-387-74336-3   e-ISBN: 978-0-387-74337-0

Library of Congress Control Number: 2007938326

springer.com

Foreword

Several decades ago, older persons were oftentimes negatively stereotyped, and aging and being older were typically associated with nursing homes, rocking chairs, and dentures. If asked about oral health issues and aging, many Americans would likely have mentioned tooth loss and ill-fitting dentures and would probably have been able to name a popular denture adhesive.

Today, while ageism remains ingrained in our daily lives, there is a growing emphasis on productive, successful, or healthy aging. Older Americans are increasingly presented as individuals who are capable and active by film, broadcast, and print media. This is not to say that older adults are portrayed as free from health concerns. However, the most common contemporary marketing messages pertaining to the health of the older person have focused on physical activity and social engagement, nutrition, and treatments or preventive interventions primarily for chronic conditions such as osteoporosis, arthritis, gastroesophageal reflux disease, erectile dysfunction, and hearing loss. Serious oral health conditions seem to have slipped from view. If asked now about oral health issues that concern older persons, the general public might mention teeth whitening or cosmetic dentistry as often as dental caries or periodontal disease. Yet there is ample evidence that troubling oral diseases and conditions pose significant chronic health problems for many elderly Americans and can affect the overall quality of their lives. Moreover, older persons most likely to have unaddressed needs have limited financial resources and greater difficulty accessing dental care.

The silent epidemic of oral diseases plaguing particularly poor children and poor older adults was brought to light in the final year of the Clinton Administration in *Oral Health in America: A Report of the Surgeon General* (2000). A seminal piece on oral health was issued by the leading spokesperson for the public health of the nation's people; the report generated a range of responses. As with similar reports, the possibility that it would simply grace shelves was always a fear. However, those who understood the importance of its call to action, celebrated it and oral health advocates viewed it appreciatively as the first visible stake placed in the aging policy landscape. Since then, the Centers for Disease Control and Prevention has supported the call for attention to the oral health of older Americans in its annual assessment of the state of aging and health nationwide.

The aging of the population is hardly a phenomenon limited to the United States. The populations of many countries in the developed world are characterized by larger segments of aged persons than in the United States, and developing countries are aging at a significantly more rapid rate than did their developed nation counterparts. Irrespective of the citizenry of the older individual, the oral health disease burden among older persons in the global community is similar in several respects to that observed in the United States. That is, the Global Oral Health Programme in the Department of Chronic Diseases and Health Promotion of the World Health Organization has noted that the elderly poor and disadvantaged worldwide are at increased risk and are least likely to have reliable access to affordable, quality dental care.

Drs. Ira Lamster and Mary Northridge and their colleagues offer *Improving Oral Health for the Elderly: An Interdisciplinary Approach* at an opportune moment in the United States. Last year, the first wave of baby boomers reached age 60, becoming "older Americans," as defined by the Older Americans Act. These boomers will become Medicare beneficiaries in 2011. The last wave of the boomers (those born in 1964) will come of age in 2029 and will join nearly 77 million others as older Americans. In greater numbers than their elders, many more boomers are expected to celebrate birthdays as centenarians and supercentenarians (120 + years).

Dental professionals will need to be well schooled in the risk factors associated with oral health conditions of older persons, specific disorders and diseases, and therapeutic and preventive evidence-based interventions to knowledgeably respond to the imperative presented by the aging demographic revolution. Fortuitously, *Improving Oral Health for the Elderly: An Interdisciplinary Approach* provides precisely this critically important body of information as the nation anticipates an important presidential election and as discussions about health care reform gain momentum. From a policy perspective, the chapters provide a compelling case for attending to oral health disparities and expanding the coverage of dental care beyond surgical interventions via Medicare, the largest health insurance program for older Americans.

Improving Oral Health for the Elderly: An Interdisciplinary Approach offers a significant contribution to the larger discourse about the health of older Americans, filling a gap too long ignored. However, its potential value does not end at our nation's borders. The rapidity of global aging assures that *Improving Oral Health for the Elderly: An Interdisciplinary Approach* will also be an important and welcome resource for dental professionals throughout our graying world.

Jeanette C. Takamura, M.S.W., Ph.D.
Dean and Professor
Columbia University School of Social Work
Immediate Past Assistant Secretary for Aging
U.S. Department of Health and Human Services

Preface

After an intense year of planning, writing, and editing this volume, it is fair to surmise that our devotion to the topic of meeting the oral health care needs of older adults has become a professional obsession. We feared we might be losing perspective on the importance of advancing this objective given our coincident immersion in the ElderSmile program at the Columbia University College of Dental Medicine. And yet, in the April 30, 2007 issue of *The New Yorker*, Atul Gawande, MD, MPH, staff writer for science and medicine and assistant professor of surgery at Harvard Medical School, began his engaging essay titled, "The Way We Age Now" with two full paragraphs devoted to this very topic.

> The hardest substance in the human body is the white enamel of the teeth. With age, it wears away nonetheless, allowing the softer, darker layer underneath to show through. Meanwhile, the blood supply to the pulp and the roots of the teeth atrophies, and the flow of saliva diminishes; the gums tend to become inflamed and pull away from the teeth, exposing the base, making them unstable and elongating their appearance, especially the lower ones. Experts say they can gauge a person's age to within five years from the examination of a single tooth—if the person has any teeth left to examine.
>
> Scrupulous dental care can help avert tooth loss, but growing old gets in the way. Arthritis, tremors, and small strokes, for example, make it difficult to brush and floss, and, because nerves become less sensitive with age, people may not realize that they have cavity and gum problems until it's too late. In the course of a normal lifetime, the muscles of the jaw lose about forty per cent of their mass and the bones of the mandible lose about twenty per cent, becoming porous and weak. The ability to chew declines, and people shift to softer foods, which are generally higher in fermentable carbohydrates and more likely to cause cavities. By the age of sixty, Americans have lost, on average, a third of their teeth. After eight-five, almost forty per cent have no teeth at all.

(Gawande, 2007, p. 50)

Even as Gawande astutely noted how ill prepared the medical profession is to deal with the burgeoning numbers of seniors in the United States, the situation is even more dire in the dental profession. We view this volume as an evolution of an earlier editorial collaboration. The May 2004 issue of the *American Journal of Public Health* (M.E.N., editor-in-chief; I.B.L., guest editor) was designed to focus much needed attention on the egregious dearth of public health attention and public policy interventions in this arena. A "looming crisis" is how one of us characterized the disproportionate impact of oral diseases on seniors and our failure as a society to adequately address this underappreciated health disparity (Lamster, 2004). The vision set forth in that editorial is the basis for our current activities to meet the oral health care needs of older adults, including this book.

Oral Health across the Life Course

In a subsequent editorial for the Swiss journal *Social and Preventive Medicine*, we argued that a life course approach to preventing and treating oral diseases may prove insightful, as it has for understanding the etiology of other chronic diseases (Ben-Shlomo & Kuh, 2002; Northridge & Lamster, 2004). Further, we believe that oral health status may usefully be viewed as a summary statement of many of the important measures of a life experience. Our theory is that oral health in later life results from individuals' lifelong accumulation of advantageous and disadvantageous experiences at the personal, interpersonal, community, and societal levels (Northridge, Sclar, & Biswas, 2003). These experiences differ according to gender, race/ethnicity, and especially socioeconomic factors such as education, income, and occupation. This is true not only for biological and psychological determinants of health but also for social and behavioral determinants, as encompassed in contemporary ecological theories of health and well-being (see, e.g., Krieger, 2001).

Understanding developmental processes of dental diseases and their socioeconomic patterns across the life course is crucial in determining optimal times for interventions to better limit the population health burden and reduce socioeconomic inequalities in oral health and health care. In a recent review in the *Annual Review of Public Health* titled, "A Life Course Approach to Chronic Disease Epidemiology" Lynch and Davey Smith (2005) cogently explained that a life course approach to chronic disease epidemiology explicitly recognizes the importance of time and timing in understanding causal links between exposures and outcomes within an individual life course, across generations, and on population level disease models. They also reviewed empirical evidence linking life course processes to coronary heart disease, hemorrhagic stroke, type-2 diabetes, breast cancer, and chronic obstructive pulmonary disease (Lynch and Davey Smith, 2005).

In arguing for the importance of contemporary and appropriate theoretical frameworks to ensure more effective action for oral health promotion, Watt (2002) highlighted life course analysis among other public health theories concerned with social determinants of health. Nicolau and colleagues have used the life course approach among Brazilian adolescents to examine, e.g., the relationship between social and psychological circumstances and gingival status (Nicolau, Marcenes, Hardy, & Sheiham, 2003) and the association between height and dental caries (Nicolau, Marcenes, Hardy, & Sheiham, 2005).

Another way to conceptualize individual life courses is that they are composed of multiple, simultaneously occurring trajectories through various dimensions of life (work, leisure, home) within specific sociohistorical contexts (see., e.g., Rossi, 1994). While improved nutrition and living standards after World War II have enabled certain populations to enjoy far better health than their forebears did a century ago, not all Americans have achieved the same level of oral health and well-being (Treadwell & Northridge, 2007). According to Allukian and Horowitz (2006), people are much more likely to have poor oral health if they are low-income, uninsured, developmentally disabled, homebound, homeless, medically compromised, and/or members of minority groups or other high-risk populations who do not have access to oral health care services.

Interdisciplinary Engagement

Several societal changes have left many seniors unable to afford any dental services whatsoever, let alone the most appropriate treatments (Lamster, 2004; Northridge & Lamster, 2004). Among the changes responsible for the lack of oral health care for older adults are: (1) rapid population shifts and the resulting larger numbers of older adults in the United States; (2) lack of routine dental service coverage under Medicare; (3) willful neglect; and (4) ageism (Treadwell & Northridge, 2007).

To meet the oral health care needs of older adults, we are convinced that interdisciplinary engagement is essential. Thus, in this volume, contributions were solicited from social workers, policy analysts, physicians, public health researchers and practitioners, demographers, and of course, dentists across different specialties.

We divided this volume into four major sections: (1) population health and well-being; (2) health and medical considerations; (3) oral health and dental considerations; and (4) professional recommendations and future needs. Of particular meaning to us was that several colleagues who hadn't appreciated the connections between oral health and their research specialties before writing their respective chapters became convinced of the linkage after completing their valued contributions. In the frequently invoked and notable words of former Surgeon General David Satcher, we need to reconnect the mouth to the rest of the body in health policies and programs (U.S. Department of Health and Human Services, 2000).

In order to eliminate oral health disparities among the elderly, interdisciplinary collaboration will be key (Pyle & Stoller, 2003). Our hope is that this volume will be used by public health researchers interested in aging, physicians interested in the connections between oral disease burden and a variety of systemic diseases, dentists interested in effectively treating older patients, policymakers interested in reforming access to and reimbursement for prevention and treatment of dental diseases, and those responsible for both large and small health initiatives directed toward improving the quality of life for seniors and their families, friends, and caregivers—that is to say, all of us.

Ira B. Lamster
Mary E. Northridge
New York, USA

References

Allukian, M., & Horowitz, A. M. (2006). Oral health. In B. S. Levy & V. W. Sidel (Eds.), *Social injustice and public health* (pp. 357–377). New York: Oxford University Press.

Ben-Shlomo, Y., & Kuh, D. (2002). A life course approach to chronic disease epidemiology: Conceptual models, empirical challenges, and interdisciplinary perspectives. *International Journal of Epidemiology, 31*, 285–293.

Gawande, A. (2007). The way we age now. *The New Yorker, 30, 2007*, 50–59.

Krieger, N. (2001). Theories for social epidemiology in the 21st century: An ecosocial perspective. *International Journal of Epidemiology, 30*, 668–677.

Lamster, I. B. (2004). Oral health care services for older adults: A looming crisis. *American Journal of Public Health, 94*, 699–702.

Lynch, J., & Davey Smith, G. (2005). A life course approach to chronic disease epidemiology. *Annual Review of Public Health, 26*, 1–35.

Nicolau, B., Marcenes, W., Hardy, R., & Sheiham, A. (2003). A life-course approach to assess the relationship between social and psychological circumstances and gingival status in adolescents. *Journal of Clinical Periodontology, 30*, 1038–1045.

Nicolau, B., Marcenes, W., Hardy, R., & Sheiham, A. (2005). The life course approach: Explaining the association between height and dental caries in Brazilian adolescents. *Community Dentistry and Oral Epidemiology, 33*, 93–98.

Northridge, M. E., & Lamster, I. B. (2004). A lifecourse approach to preventing and treating oral disease. *Social and Preventive Medicine, 49*, 299–300.

Northridge, M. E., Sclar, E., & Biswas P. (2003). Sorting out the connections between the built environment and health: A conceptual framework for navigating pathways and planning healthy cities. *Journal of Urban Health, 80*, 556–590.

Pyle, M. A., & Stoller, E. P. (2003). Oral health disparities among the elderly: Interdisciplinary challenges for the future. *Journal of Dental Education, 67*, 1327–1334.

Rossi, A. (1994). *Sexuality across the life course*. Chicago: University of Chicago Press.

Treadwell, H. M., & Northridge, M. E. (2007). Oral health is the measure of a just society. *Journal of Health Care for the Poor and Underserved, 18*, 12–20.

U.S. Department of Health and Human Services. (2000). *Oral health in America: A report of the surgeon general*. Rockville, MD: Health and Human Services, National Institute of Dental and Craniofacial Research.

Watt, R.G. (2002). Emerging theories into the social determinants of health: Implications for oral health promotion. *Community Dentistry and Oral Epidemiology, 30*, 241–247.

Contents

Contributors

David A. Albert
Director, Division of Community Health and Associate Professor of Clinical Dentistry, Columbia University College of Dental Medicine, 601 W168th Street, Suite 32, New York, 10032, USA; Associate Professor of Public Health, Columbia University Mailman School of Public Health, 601 W168th Street, Suite 32, New York, 10032, USA
daa1@columbia.edu

Steven M. Albert
Professor of Behavioral and Community Health Sciences, Graduate School of Public Health, University of Pittsburgh, A211 Crabtree, 130 DeSoto St., Pittsburgh, PA 15261, USA
smalbert@pitt.edu

Neerja Bhardwaj
Division of Geriatric Medicine and Aging, Department of Medicine, Columbia University Medical Center, New York, USA

Luisa N. Borrell
Department of Epidemiology, Mailman School of Public Health, and College of Dental Medicine, Columbia University, New York, 10032, USA
lnb2@columbia.edu

Nina M. Browner
Clinical Fellow in Movement Disorders, Department of Neurology, Columbia University Medical Center, New York, USA

Ejvind Budtz-Jørgensen
Professor Emeritus, Division of Gerodontology and Removable Prosthodontics, University of Geneva, Rue Barthélely-Menn, 19, 1205 Geneva, Switzerland
budtz@bluewin.ch

Huai Cheng
Division of Geriatric Medicine and Aging, Department of Medicine, Columbia University Medical Center, New York, USA

Natalie D. Crawford
Department of Epidemiology, Mailman School of Public Health, Columbia University, New York, USA

Shelly Dubin
Division of Geriatric Medicine and Aging, Department of Medicine, Columbia University Medical Center, New York, USA

Steven Frucht
Associate Professor of Clinical Neurology, Columbia University Medical Center, 710 West 168th street, NI3, New York, 10032, USA
sf216@columbia.edu

Evelyn Granieri
Division of Geriatric Medicine and Aging, Department of Medicine, Columbia University Medical Center, New York, USA

L. Jackson Brown
President of L. Jackson Brown Consulting

Jennifer L. Kelsey
University of Massachusetts Medical School, Department of Medicine (Division of Preventive and Behavioral Medicine) and Department of Family Medicine and Community Health, Worcester MA 01655
jennykelsey@comcast.net

Ira B. Lamster
Dean and Professor, Columbia University College of Dental Medicine, New York, NY, USA
ibl1@columbia.edu

Ali Makki
Bureau of Health Professions, Faculty Training Fellow in Geriatric Medicine, David Geffen School of Medicine at UCLA; Lecturer and Clinical Faculty, Section of Oral Medicine and Orofacial Pain, UCLA School of Dentistry, Los Angeles, CA, USA; Associate Professor, Department of Oral Diagnosis, Radiology and Pathology, School of Dentistry, Loma Linda University, Loma Linda, CA, USA; Dr. Makki has a private practice limited to Orofacial Pain in Century City, CA, USA

Louis Mandel
Clinical Professor, Columbia University College of Dental Medicine, New York, NY, USA
lm7@columbia.edu

Mathew S. Maurer
Division of Geriatric Medicine and Aging, Department of Medicine, Columbia University Medical Center, New York, USA

Frauke Müller
Professor and Chairman, Division of Gerodontology and Removable Prosthodontics, University of Geneva, Rue Barthélely Menn, 19, 1205 Geneva, Switzerland

James M. Noble
Gertrude H. Sergievsky Center, Department of Neurology, Columbia University Medical Center, 710 West 168th St., New York, 10032, USA
jn2054@columbia.edu

Mary E. Northridge
Professor of Clinical Sociomedical Sciences, Mailman School of Public Health, Columbia University, New York, NY, USA
men11@columbia.edu

Panos N. Papapanou
Division of Periodontics, Section of Oral and Diagnostic Sciences, Columbia University College of Dental Medicine, New York, USA

Susan Roche
Associate Professor, Department of Oral Diagnosis, Radiology and Pathology, School of Dentistry, Loma Linda University, Loma Linda, CA, USA; Dr. Roche also has a specialty practice in Orofacial Pain at Loma Linda University Faculty Dental Offices as well as in Santa Barbara, CA, USA

Stefanie L. Russell
Assistant Professor, Department of Epidemiology and Health Promotion, New York University College of Dentistry, New York
stefanie.russell@nyu.edu

Brian C. Scanlan
Associate Professor of Clinical Medicine, New York Medical College, St. Vincent's Hospital Manhattan, 153 West 11th Street, NR1218, New York, 10011, USA
bscanlan@svcmcny.org

Nikolaos Scarmeas
Assistant Professor of Neurology, Gertrude H. Sergievsky Center, Taub Institute, Department of Neurology, Columbia University Medical Center, New York, USA

Jonathan A. Ship
Professor, Department of Oral Pathology, Radiology, and Medicine, New York University, New York, USA; Director, Bluestone Center for Clinical Research, New York University College of Dentistry, New York University, New York, USA; Professor, New York University School of Medicine, New York University, New York, USA

Lynn M. Tepper
Columbia University, College of Dental Medicine, and Mailman School of Public Health, 630 West 168 St, New York, 10032, USA
LMT1@columbia.edu

Angus W. G. Walls
Professor of Restorative Dentistry, School of Dental Sciences, Newcastle University, Framlington Place, Newcastle upon Tyne, NE2 4BW, UK
a.w.g.walls@ncl.ac.uk

Hans-Peter Weber
Raymond J. and Elva Pomfret Nagle Professor of Restorative Dentistry and Biomaterials Sciences, Harvard School of Dental Medicine, 188 Longwood Avenue, Boston, MA 02115, USA
hpweber@hsdm.harvard.edu

Dana L. Wolf
Division of Periodontics, Section of Oral and Diagnostic Sciences, Columbia University College of Dental Medicine, New York, USA
delw2004@columbia.edu

Victoria L. Woo
Columbia University College of Dental Medicine, Department of Pathology, 630 West 168th Street, New York, 10032, USA

Janet A. Yellowitz
Director, Geriatric Dentistry, University of Maryland, Baltimore College of Dental Surgery, 650 West Baltimore Street, Suite 3211, Baltimore, MD 21201, USA
jyellowitz@umaryland.edu

Angela J. Yoon
Columbia University College of Dental Medicine, Department of Pathology, 630 West 168th Street, New York, 10032, USA

David J. Zegarelli
Columbia University College of Dental Medicine, Department of Pathology, 630 West 168th Street, New York, 10032, USA
djz1@columbia.edu

List of Figures

List of Tables

Part I
Population Health and Well-Being

Chapter 1
The Aging U.S. Population

Steven M. Albert

In 2000, there were 35 million people aged 65 or older in the United States comprising 12.4% of the U.S. population. Furthermore, over 4 million Americans were aged 85 or older comprising 1.5% of the total population (U.S. Census, 2000). The number of older Americans is 10 times higher now than it was in 1900 when there were only 3 million people aged 65 years and older. At that time, older people accounted for only 4% of the total population (Federal Interagency Forum on Aging Related Statistics, 2000, 2006). By 2030, in the United States the number of older people will double to 70 million and the proportion of people aged 65 or older will approach 20% of the total population. This increase in the proportion of older people represents the continuation of a long-standing trend. For example, life expectancy was 46 years in 1900 and increased to 77 years a century later. In fact, the 2000 U.S. Census reported over 50,000 centenarians in the United States.

What are the implications of this massive increase in the number of older adults? How will it affect delivery of medical and dental care and supportive long-term care? What will be its effect on housing, transportation, and workforce training? Far-seeing government agencies have recognized the significance of this shift in the population, which will affect virtually every domain of life. For example, in 2000 the New York State the Office of Aging Commissioned a report called "Aging 2015", requiring every agency within state government to project the impact of this aging revolution on its operations. Every government function was involved, from such obvious candidates as the state Medicaid program and Department of Health to much less obvious agencies, such as offices overseeing zoning regulations and recreation (New York State Office of the Aging, 2004). This effort represents a proper appraisal of the magnitude of this demographic change and the need for an integrated plan to prepare for the challenges of an increasingly older population. In 2006, the first baby boomers turned 60 years, with great attention from the

S.M. Albert
Professor of Behavioral and Community Health Sciences Graduate School of Public Health, University of Pittsburgh, A211 Crabtree, 130 DeSoto St., Pittsburgh, PA 15261,
Tel: 412-383-8693, Fax: 412-383-5846
e-mail: smalbert@pitt.edu

I.B. Lamster, M.E. Northridge (eds.), *Improving Oral Health for the Elderly*,
© Springer Science+Business Media, LLC 2008

media. Yet this milestone represents only a single element of a continuing, gathering transformation of U.S. population.

Demography of Aging: The United States in the First Decade of the Twenty-First Century

The growing proportion of the elderly is a direct effect not only of declining mortality, but also of declining fertility, which results in a greater number of elderly as well as a greater proportion of the population that is elderly. Between 1960 and 2004, overall mortality declined from about 1400 to 800 deaths per 100,000 Americans per year (Federal Interagency Forum on Aging Related Statistics, 2000). This extraordinary reduction in mortality occurred across the entire lifespan, pushing the mean age of death to older and older ages.

The result of this general decline in mortality has been an impressive gain in life expectancy, which increased from 70 to 76 years over the same period. Increased life expectancy is the product of: first, reductions in perinatal mortality; second, improvements in health and living conditions in the first half of the lifespan; and only most recently, advances in medical and dental care for older people (Albert, 2004). For example, in the nineteenth century, control over infectious diseases in childhood (leading to reductions in perinatal and child mortality) and a shift away from manual labor (resulting in major improvements in health and living conditions in mid-life) had already led to an increase in life expectancy and reduction in disability in later life (Costa, 2000). The life-extending technologies of modern medicine and the more effective adult and geriatric medicines available today have had a more modest impact on life expectancy. Simulation studies suggest that even complete elimination of cancer, cardiovascular disease, and diabetes (an unlikely prospect) would raise life expectancy no higher than 86.4 years for men and 94.1 years for women (Olshansky, Carnes, & Cassel, 1990).

A first result of these changes is the great increase in older Americans, mentioned earlier. As shown in Fig. 1.1, the number of Americans aged 65 years and older will approach 90 million in 2050, and the number of elders aged 85 years and older will approach 20 million.

Setting these numbers in the context of the population as a whole clearly demonstrates "population aging," that is, a growing proportion of the population aged 65 years and older. Population aging is best visualized in a comparison of population pyramids over time. These plots present the number of men and women in particular age groups or bands. A pyramidal shape is obtained when a population consists of a proportionally greater number of people at young ages; these people form the base of the pyramid, which narrows as numbers decrease with advancing age. Today, our population pyramids no longer have a pyramidal shape. They appear more as an emerging rectangle or pillar. Fig. 1.2 shows population pyramids for the United States in 2000 and projections for 2050.

In the 2000 population pyramid, ages 35–54 represent a bulge in the center of the figure and indicate aging baby boomers, i.e., people born in 1946–1965. Lower

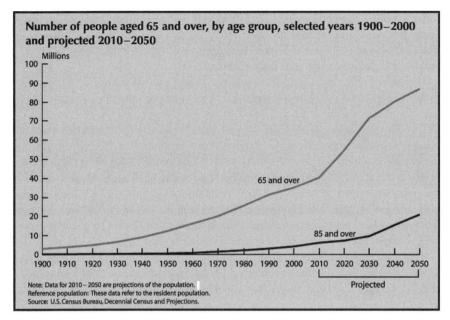

Fig. 1.1 Number of Older Americans, 1900–2050

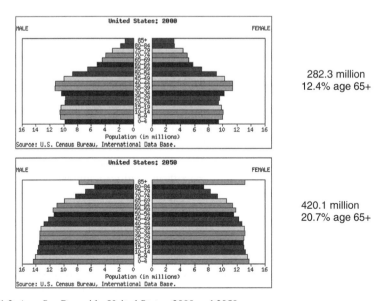

Fig. 1.2 Age–Sex Pyramids, United States, 2000 and 2050

fertility after this period, which continued over the next three decades, has led to fewer people at younger ages and hence the absence of a wide base for the pyramid. The median age in the United States in 2000 was 35 years, again showing absence of a wide base for the pyramid (U.S. Census, 2000).

The age–sex pyramid in 2000 shows the strong preponderance of women over men in later life. Among people aged 65 years and older, the sex ratio (that is, the number of women for each man) is 1.4; for people aged 85 years or older, it is 2.5, and for centenarians, it is 4.0. This asymmetry affects living arrangements and marital status in important ways, leaving older women more likely to live alone, depend upon children when frail, and enter nursing homes at higher rates than men.

By 2050, the U.S. population is projected to reach 420.1 million, with 20.7% of the population aged 65 years or older. The number of people aged 85 years or older will increase to about 9 million men and 14 million women and together account for 5.5% of the U.S. population. This increase in the number of the oldest-old will pose special challenges for medical, dental, and supportive care.

One last feature of the changing demography of old age in the United States deserves mention and is increasingly visible in American cities. With each decade, older Americans are becomingly increasingly diverse in racial and ethnic composition. Over the next half century, the proportion of non-Hispanic White elders will decline from 82% to 61%. African-American elders will increase from 8 to 12%, and Latino elders from 6 to 18% (Federal Interagency Forum on Aging Related Statistics, 2006). The proportion of other groups of ethnic elders, such as Asians, will also increase as a result of new immigration and aging of these immigrant families. These changes will offer new challenges and opportunities for health care delivery. Geriatric assessment and delivery of medical and dental care and social services will increasingly have to take into account a more diverse elderly population (Albert, 2006).

The Health of American Elders

How healthy are American elders? One indicator of general health is whether or not people consider themselves to be in good health. The proportion of older Americans who consider their health to be "good," "very good," or "excellent" is 76% among White elders and 60%–62% among minority elders (Federal Interagency Forum on Aging Related Statistics, 2006). This proportion declines with age. Among White elders, for example, the proportion reporting good to excellent health was 81% among elders aged 65–74 years, 73% among elders aged 75–84 years, and 67% among elders aged 85 years or older. Among the population as a whole, the proportion reporting this degree of satisfaction with health is about 90% (Erickson, Patrick & Shannon 1995). Thus, while old age is associated with decrements in self-rated health, a majority still consider their health to be "good" or better. Although people at different ages may select a different standard or benchmark for "good" or "excellent" health ("response shift"), it is nevertheless impressive that a high proportion of elderly are satisfied with their health.

Another indicator of health is the prevalence of chronic conditions. The U.S. National Health Interview Survey (NHIS) asks respondents if a physician has ever told them they have any of a series of chronic disease conditions. In the NHIS, over a third of elderly report a diagnosis of hypertension, arthritis, or heart disease, 20% of elderly report having diabetes or cancer, and 10% of elderly report having stroke or chronic pulmonary conditions. Other surveys estimate that 5%–10% of elders aged 65 or older meet criteria for Alzheimer's disease. By the time elders reach an age of 85 years and older, the prevalence of these conditions increases dramatically. The impact of these conditions is visible in older adults' high consumption of health services and prescription medication.

A visit to any physician's office, hospital, or pharmacy easily shows that older people are the primary users of these services. For example, in 2004 the volume of office-based physician visits per 100 people was 219 for people aged 18–44 years, 376 for people aged 45–64 years, and 675 for people aged 65 years and older (National Center for Health Statistics 2006, Table 89). Medication prescribing recorded during these physician visits follows the same pattern. The total number of prescribed drugs per 100 people in 2003–2004 was 327 for people aged 18–44 years, 795 for people aged 45–64 years, and 1698 for people aged 65 years and older (National Center for Health Statistics 2006, Table 92). The percentage of the population with at least one prescription medication was 36%, 64%, and 85% in the same age groups, respectively, and 7%, 24%, and 46% for people prescribed three or more medications (National Center for Health Statistics 2006, Table 93). A similar trend is evident in hospital inpatient admissions. The proportion of people with one or more hospital admissions in 2004 was 7.1% for people aged 18–44 years, 8.1% for people aged 45–64 years, and 17.4% for people aged 65 years and older (National Center for Health Statistics 2006, Table 95).

Apart from this medical care burden, chronic disease is perhaps even more important as a source of disability. The prevalence of functional limitation, such as difficulty stooping, reaching over one's head, writing, walking a quarter mile, or lifting 10 pounds is high among American elderly. The ability to lift 10 pounds is important because a bag of groceries weighs approximately this amount. One-third of women and one-fifth of men aged 65 years and older report difficulty in at least one of these five common functions (Freedman, Martin, & Schoeni, 2002). Mobility limitation is the most common impairment, with 24% of women and 14% of men reporting inability to walk a quarter mile. The quarter mile indicator is significant as this is the standard distance elders need to walk in urban areas to obtain such needed services as food shopping, bus transportation, and medical and dental care (Newman, Simonsick, Naydeck et al., 2006). Nearly 14% of women and 7% of men report this functional limitation. These estimates from the NHIS exclude older adults living in nursing homes (some 1.4 million people) or chronic care hospitals; they apply only to community-dwelling elderly and thus underestimate the extent of functional limitation in older Americans. Moreover, the prevalence of functional limitation in community-dwelling elderly appears to have changed little over the past decade.

This stability in functional limitation stands in contrast to declines in the prevalence of disability, defined as long-term inability to perform basic self-maintenance tasks (also known as activities of daily living or ADLs, such as bathing or dressing), ongoing inability to manage a household independently (also known as instrumental activities of daily living or IADLs, such as being able to shop, cook, clean, or use the telephone), or residence in a skilled nursing facility. Over the past 20 years, the prevalence of chronic disability in older adults has declined from 25% to 20% (Manton, 1992; Manton & Gu, 2001; Freedman, Martin, & Schoeni 2002). This decline in aggregate disability has different sources. The largest contribution to the decline comes from a change in the prevalence of disability in household tasks or IADLs. Disability in this domain declined from 6% to 3%. Disability in the more basic self-maintenance ADLs has not shown this degree of decline, while residence in skilled care facilities has declined from about 6% to 5% of the elderly population (Albert, 2004).

Declines in disability are robust in that they have been documented in a variety of national probability-based surveys and persist across different definitions of disability (Freedman, Martin, & Schoeni, 2002; Freedman, Hodgson, Lynn et al., 2006). It is less clear if these declines represent true improvements in health. Between 1984 and 1999, need for help in managing money (8.4% to 3.8%), doing laundry (7.9% to 5.3%), and using the telephone (3.2% to 2.2%) all declined, but over this same period direct deposit banking, microwaves, and adapted telephones were also introduced (Spillman, 2004). At this point, it is difficult to separate how much of this reduction in disability is due to improvements in physical and cognitive ability in later life, and how much is due to improvements in home and community environments (Albert, Bear-Lehman, Burkhardt, Merete-Roa, & Noboa-Lemonier, 2006).

Oral Health and Health Care Delivery in Older Americans

Former Surgeon General C. Everett Koop drew attention to the importance of oral health when he asserted that "you are not healthy without good oral health" (1993). Beyond its immediate effect on the quality of teeth and gums, oral health affects speaking, chewing, and swallowing. Nor is oral health confined to the mouth. Oral bacterial infections are associated with systemic diseases, and loss of teeth and other oral health issues affect mental health. Oral cancer is also a concern, with older adults disproportionately affected among age groups (U.S. Department of Health and Human Services, 2000).

Oral health in old age follows patterns described earlier for general health. Better dental care and nutrition across the lifespan has led to less edentulism, or total tooth loss. In 1993, one-third of non-institutionalized adults aged 65 years and older reported loss of all teeth, which represented a continuing decline over the prior decade (Vargas, Kramarow, & Yellowitz, 2001). In 2002, the proportion of edentulous older adults stood at 27.9% (Federal Interagency Forum on Aging Related Statistics, 2004). Likewise, the proportion of older adults with untreated dental caries has declined, but in both cases, improvements in oral health have been uneven, with minority and low-income elderly less likely to realize benefits. For example, 45.9% of older adults who fall below federally defined poverty levels reported retaining no natural teeth, compared to 27.3% of elders not meeting criteria for poverty (Federal Interagency Forum on Aging Related Statistics, 2004). The incidence of certain oral conditions, including oral cancer and periodontal disease, increases in older age. Also, use of dental prostheses, which are common in old age, poses its own problems. Ill-fitting dentures, for example, can increase the risk of oral candidiasis.

Receipt of dental care among older adults continues to increase over time, although in 2004, only slightly more than half of older adults reported having had a dental visit (*Health, United States, 2006*, Table 91). Here, too, racial disparities are apparent. The proportion of White elders with a dental visit was 58.6%, the proportion among African-American elders was 33.6%, and the proportion among Hispanic elders was 42.5%. These proportions should be compared with the proportions of younger people having had a dental visit in 2004, namely, 76.4% of children and 64% of adults aged 18–64 years (*Health, United States, 2006*, Table 91).

Finally, it is important to note that Medicare does not cover routine dental care and thus only about a quarter of older adults have dental insurance (Vargas, Kramarow, & Yellowitz, 2001). This gap in care is troubling because oral health care for older adults may be more complex than care for younger people. Changes associated with aging (such as changes in salivation or decreased ability to provide adequate self-care) and the cumulative accrual of oral health challenges (missing teeth, failing fillings, periodontal disease) make oral health care more important for elders than younger people, not less important. In addition, providing oral health care may be difficult for older adults with cognitive impairment (which may make cooperation difficult) or mobility limitations. Mouth care in institutional settings is often neglected, although the nursing home minimum data set (MDS) includes a section on resident oral health. The prevalence of dental pain in nursing home residents, especially those with dementia, is high (Cohen-Mansfield & Lipson, 2002).

Residence and Supportive Care

As was already mentioned, American elders are increasingly less likely to live in skilled care settings. Between 1985 and 2000, the number of elderly residing in skilled care facilities declined from 54 to 43 per 1000 (Federal Interagency Forum on Aging Related Statistics, 2006). This decline is evident even for the oldest old. In 1985, 220 of every 1000 elders aged 85 years and older were residing in a nursing home. By 1999, only 183 per 1000 of the oldest old were living in these settings. Again, it is hard to know if this shift away from institutional care represents a true improvement in health at older ages or whether the influence of other factors, such as the availability of new residential arrangements that allow mildly or moderately disabled elders to remain in the community, is a contributor to this trend. The growing number of assisted living facilities, many of which provide Alzheimer's care in less medically intensive settings, now accommodates elderly who at one time might have entered nursing homes. Similarly, the availability of home- and community-based long-term care services offers families new options for maintaining dependent elders in the community. Caregiver support delays institutionalization of elders with dementia (Mittelman, Ferris, Shulman, Steinberg, & Levin, 1996) and improves caregiver ability to manage challenging behaviors and threats to mental health (Belle, Burgio, Burns, Coon, Czaja et al., 2006). Finally, the shift to a more ethnically heterogeneous elder population may also play a role in the decline of the nursing home as a long-term care destination for elders. Minority families appear to be more reluctant to rely on institutional care, although this too may change over the next decades (Federal Interagency Forum on Aging Related Statistics, 2006).

In concert with the expanding range of home- and community-based services available to families, the typical caregiving arrangement for home care will likely become a combination of informal (family) and formal (paid) care. While family care continues to be the modal arrangement, the prevalence of joint family–paid care arrangements is increasing. This trend, however, is highly sensitive to the availability of Medicare- and Medicaid-funded home care. Between 1994 and 1999 the trend toward increasing joint caregiving arrangements ended because of new strictures on the Medicare home care benefit (Murtaugh, McCall, Moore, Meadow, 2003).

A Demographic Portrait of the Oldest Old in America

We conclude this chapter with a brief demographic portrait of the oldest old in the United States. How will the oldest old differ from other elderly? Will they retain their teeth in high numbers? What other oral health conditions will they suffer from over and above the prevalence experienced by younger age groups?

The oldest old are typically defined as people aged 85 years and older (Taeuber & Rosenwaike, 1992). Characteristics of this group include the following:

- They are high consumers of supportive care. Nearly 25% reside in nursing homes and another 25% receive formal (paid) home care. Yet even in this age group, 50% live in the community and report no need for help in daily personal care activities (ADLs).
- They are the fastest growing segment of older population in the United States. In fact, the United States will have the largest number of oldest old of any country in the next 50 years. This is a paradox because the United States will *not* have the most elderly aged 65 years and older of any country.
- They are largely female: the sex ratio (number of men per 100 women) is expected to decline from 75.4 (1930) to 59.9 (2050). Men are more likely to live in family setting (59%) than women (37%).
- They are largely White (2.8 million White of 3.0 million overall in 1990). Nonetheless, people aged 65 years and older are becoming increasingly more diverse, as described earlier.

- They are less likely now than in the past to have family caregivers. Familial-aged dependency ratios (persons aged 85 years and older per persons aged 65–69 years) are increasing (from 12 in 1950 to 88 in 2050).
- They are largely widowed. For instance, in 1980, 82% of women aged 85 years and older were widowed compared to 33% among women aged 65–69 years. Half of the men aged 85 years and older are widowed.
- They are largely a low-income group, especially those who are female and living alone (73% of this group met the federal criteria for poverty for 1990–2000). This picture may change with newer cohorts.
- They are increasingly well educated. Educational attainment in this group has increased dramatically from 29.1% having had completed high school in 1985 to an expected 63% having had completed high school by 2015.
- They will have more children if they are female compared to the young-old, although few will also have five or more offspring, which may affect the availability of family caregivers.

Conclusion

The great increase in the number of American elderly will mean a new world of health care, social service delivery, transportation, housing, and much else to meet the needs of increasing numbers of elders who will need services. These services are available and offer great benefit to elders and their families, but careful planning and stewardship will be required to see that they reach elders who need services most. Oral health will figure prominently in this changing picture of better health, but presently there are many challenges for the effective delivery of needed oral health care for older adults.

Given the vast expansion in the population of American elders and the challenges of providing supportive care to growing numbers of disabled elderly, it is worth asking how resources will be marshaled for this effort. Supportive care, that is, help with basic ADLs and household maintenance IADLs, is the greatest expense in elder care (Rice & Fineman, 2004). In this effort, three related and perhaps mutually reinforcing strategies are likely to be important:

1. At the broadest level, government should encourage age-friendly communities (Center for Home Care Policy & Research, 2004). Such communities will likely emerge from the kind of broad rethinking of government services already advanced in New York State and elsewhere.
2. Home- and community-based service provision will likely come to rely more and more on personal assistance care. The bulk of this care is provided by non-medically trained home care paraprofessionals without oral health care expertise. We can anticipate expanded growth in this sector, perhaps augmented by technologies that allow remote care. We can also expect greater consumer direction of such care. Little research is available on the dental health of elders receiving home- and community-based services.

3. Greater support for family caregivers will be required to maintain elders in the community. This support may take the form of greater collaboration with service providers, more hospital-to-home support, tax credits, or any number of other initiatives. Since family caregivers continue to provide the great bulk of care, it is critical to support them in these activities (Albert & Levine, 2005).

With coordinated efforts and continued support from academic research, we can better ensure a more satisfying old age for successive cohorts of Americans by minimizing the impact of diseases and conditions now prevalent in later life and improving the quality of life through better oral health as part of overall health and well-being.

References

Albert SM. Cultural and ethnic influences on aging. *Encyclopedia of Gerontology*, Elsevier Press, 2nd edition, pp. 336–343, 2006.

Albert SM. *Public Health and Aging: An Introduction to Maximizing Function and Well-Being*. New York: Springer Publishing Company, 2004.

Albert SM, Levine C. Family caregiver research and the HIPAA factor. *The Gerontologist*, 45(4): 432–7, 2005.

Albert SM, Bear-Lehman J, Burkhardt A, Merete-Roa B, Noboa-Lemonier R. Variation in sources of clinician- and self-rated IADL disability. *J Gerontol: Med Sci*, 61A: 826–831, 2006.

Belle SH, Burgio L, Burns R, Coon D, Czaja SJ et al., for REACH II Investigators. Enhancing the quality of life of dementia caregivers from different ethnic or racial groups. *Ann Intern Med* 145: 727–738, 2006.

Center for Home Care Policy & Research. *A Tale of Two Older Americas: Community Opportunities and Challenges*. April 2004. http://www.vnsny.org/advantage/AL_NationalSurveyReport.pdf

Cohen-Mansfield J, Lipson S. The underdetection of pain of dental etiology in persons with dementia. *Am J Alzheimers Dis Other Demen*; 17; 249–253, 2002.

Costa D. Understanding the Twentieth Century Decline in Chronic Conditions Among Older Men." *Demography* 37(1): 53–72, 2000.

Federal Interagency Forum on Aging Related Statistics. *Older Americans: Update 2006*. Washington, D.C. U.S. Government Printing Office, 2006.

Federal Interagency Forum on Aging Related Statistics. *Older Americans 2004: Key Indicators of Well-Being*. Washington, D.C. U.S. Government Printing Office, 2004.

Federal Interagency Forum on Aging Related Statistics. *Older Americans 2000: Key Indicators of Well-Being*. Washington, D.C. U.S. Government Printing Office, 2000.

Freedman VA, Hodgson N, Lynn J, Spillman BC, Waidmann T Wilkinson AM Wolf DA Promoting declines in the prevalence of late-life disability: Comparisons of three potentially high-impact interventions. *Milbank Q*; 84(3):493–520, 2006.

Freedman VA, Martin LG, Schoeni RF. Recent trends in disability and functioning among older adults in the United States: A systematic review. *JAMA*; 288(24): 3137–3146, 2002.

Koop CE. *Oral Health 2000*. Second National Consortium Advance Program, 2, 1993.

Manton KG. Mortality and life expectancy changes among the oldest old. In Suzman RM, Willis DP, Manton KG, eds., *The Oldest Old*. New York: Oxford University Press, pp. 157–182, 1992.

Manton KG, Gu X. Changes in the prevalence of chronic disability in the United States black and nonblack population above age 65 from 1982 to 1999. *Proc Natl Acad Sci USA* 98(11): 6354–9, 2001.

Mittelman MS, Ferris SH, Shulman E, Steinberg G, Levin B A family intervention to delay nursing home placement of patients with Alzheimer disease. A randomized controlled trial. *JAMA* 276(21): 1725–31, 1996.

Murtaugh CM, McCall N, Moore S, Meadow A. Trends in Medicare home health care use: 1997–2001. Health Aff (Millwood). 2003 22(5):146–56, 2003.

National Center for Health Statistics. *Health, United States, 2006, With Chartbook on Trends in the Health of Americans.* Hyattsville, MD: 2006

Newman AB Simonsick EM, Naydeck BL, Boudreau RM, Kritchevsky SB, Nevitt MC, Pahor M, Satterfield S, Brach JS, Studenski SA, Harris TB. Association of long-distance corridor walk performance with mortality, cardiovascular disease, mobility limitation, and disability. *JAMA* 3;295(17):2018–26, May 2006.

Olshansky SJ, Carnes BA, Cassel C. In search of Methuselah: estimating the upper limits to human longevity. *Science* 250(4981):634–40, 1990.

New York State Office of the Aging. *Project 2015: White Paper.* 2004. http://www.aging.state.ny.us/explore/project2015/report02/index.htm.

Rice DP, Fineman N. Economic implications of increased longevity in the United States. *Annu Rev Public Health* 25:457–73, 2004.

Spillman BC. Changes in elderly disability rates and the implications for health care utilization and cost. *Milbank Quar* 82(1):157–94, 2004.

Taeuber CM, Rosenwaike I. A demographic portrait of America's oldest old. In Suzman RM, Willis DP, Manton KG, eds., *The Oldest Old.* New York: Oxford University Press, pp. 17–49, 1992.

U.S. Census, 2000. *Gateway to Census 2000.* http://www.census.gov/

U.S. Department of Health and Human Services. *Oral Health in America: A Report from the Surgeon General.* Rockville, MD: National Institute of Dental and Craniofacial Research, NIH, 2000.

Vargas CM, Kramarow EA, Yellowitz JA. *The Oral Health of Older Americans.* Aging Trends, No. 3. Hyattsville, MD: National Center for Health Statistics, 2001.

Chapter 2
The Oral Disease Burden Faced by Older Adults

Ira B. Lamster and Natalie D. Crawford

Introduction

By the year 2030, one in five Americans will be 65 or older, and this age group will require a proportionally larger share of the national health care expenditure than at present. When referring specifically to oral health care services, addressing this challenge begins with an understanding of the patterns of oral disease faced by older adults.

This discussion is important for a number of reasons. First, these developments alert the dental profession to both current levels of disease and anticipated shifts in the future as the population ages. This knowledge will suggest preventive approaches and allow the educational system (dental schools and continuing education programs for dental professionals) to offer appropriate and timely information. Second, increased awareness will prepare the dental profession to address these problems and thereby have a positive impact on the health and well-being of patients. Loss of teeth, oral cancer and reduced mastictory function are just some consequences of oral disease that will affect morbidity, mortality and quality of life. Third, recent interest in the relationship between oral infection/periodontal disease and systemic diseases (cardiovascular/cerebrovascular disease, diabetes mellitus, respiratory diseases) has particular relevance for older individuals since many of these relationships disproportionally affect the elderly. Meurman and Hamalainen (2005) observed that oral infections have a more profound effect upon the elderly compared to other segments of the population. Further, older individuals (at least 85 years of age) needing immediate dental treatment were at nearly four times the risk of death when followed for a 5-year period (Hamalainen et al. 2005). However, few clinical studies examining the relationship of oral infection and systemic diseases have focused solely on older adults. Fourth, this information will provide background for discussion of public and private approaches to address the need for oral health care services in an aging population. Any attempts

I.B. Lamster
Columbia University College of Dental Medicine, New York, USA
e-mail: ibl1@columbia.edu

I.B. Lamster, M.E. Northridge (eds.), *Improving Oral Health for the Elderly*,
© Springer Science+Business Media, LLC 2008

to define national, state or local oral health care policy with a focus on older adults will require information about the disease burden. This is a critical matter since Medicare, which was developed to address the medical care needs of seniors, does not provide dental benefits. Consequently, a significant portion of the population of older adults will not be able to afford appropriate dental services.

A review of the prevalence of oral diseases affecting older adults will provide some insight into the future needs of the population. This concept is relevant here since one of the sentinel measures of oral health status – the number of remaining teeth or the percent of the population who are edentulous – is changing in the United States and other developed countries. Tooth retention is increasing as the population ages. This trend will obviously have an important impact on both the oral disease burden (since there will be a larger number of teeth that are susceptible to dental disease) and the anticipated need for dental services in the future.

This chapter will examine the oral disease burden faced by older adults by focusing on three major oral diseases: dental caries (with discussion of tooth loss and edentulism), periodontal diseases and oral cancer. A more limited discussion of mucosal disorders and candidiasis and myofacial pain/disorders of the temporomandibular joint is also included.

Dental Caries and Tooth Loss

Overview

Dental caries is an infectious disease that requires the presence of bacteria (*Streptococcus mutans, Lactobacillus* species), a substrate (fermentable carbohydrate) and a susceptible host. The byproducts of bacterial metabolism of carbohydrate include lactic acid and uric acid, which can lead to demineralization of the enamel and dentin. When the tooth root is exposed, the cementum covering the root surface is also affected. Dental caries can occur as coronal caries, root caries (Fig. 2.1) and recurrent caries (caries associated with existing dental restorations). When the caries process extends into the root canal system, the result can be necrosis of the pulp tissue. This last phase is frequently accompanied by acute infection and clinical findings of pain and swelling.

The prevalence and extent of dental caries is dependant upon the number of teeth present in the mouth. As the number of teeth increases, the number of susceptible tooth surfaces increases. Further, tooth loss can be a result of caries, periodontal disease, trauma and elective extraction for prosthetic or orthodontic reasons, among other causes.

Prevalence and Incidence

The literature suggests that in many countries with a relatively high standard of living, the percent of the older population that is edentulous is in decline (Surgeon

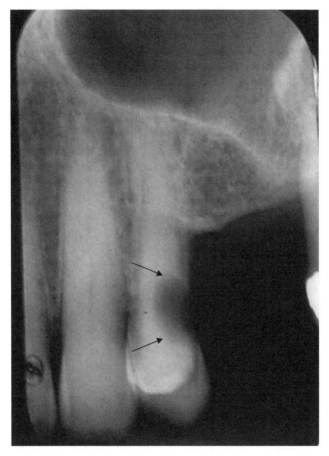

Fig. 2.1 Radiograph illustrating a large carious lesion on the distal root surface of a maxillary first bicuspid tooth (arrows)

General's Report 2000a, Petersen et al. 2004). As a result, a larger percentage of older patients will be susceptible to tooth-related oral diseases. Nevertheless, edentulism is common throughout the world and is generally linked to lower socioeconomic status (Petersen and Yamamoto 2005).

A study from Sweden indicated that between 1971 and 2001, the percentage of 70-year-old individuals who were edentulous decreased from 51% to 7%. Further, the mean number of teeth increased from 14 to 21 (Österberg et al. 2006). Similar but less substantial declines have been reported from the United States, based on a comparison of the First and Third National Health and Nutrition Examination Surveys (NHANES). Between 1971–1974 and 1988–1994, the percent of individuals between 65 and 74 who were edentulous declined from 45.6% to 28.6% (Surgeon General's Report 2000). However, there are distinct geographic differences in edentulism in the United States. Based on data from the Behavioral Risk

Factor Surveillance System survey, the percent of individuals at least 65 years of age who have lost all of their teeth varied from a high of 42.3% in Kentucky to a low of 13.1% in Hawaii (Gooch et al. 2003, see Table 2.1).

Dental diseases (caries, periodontal disease) can be considered cumulative, and a study of the oral health status in China is revealing in regards to the effect of aging on the status of the dentition. The study is noteworthy in that more than 140,000 individuals were examined. The average number of teeth that were present in 12 year olds, 15 year olds, 18 year olds, adults 35–44 years of age and older adults 65–74 years of age were 25.8, 27.9, 27.9, 27.1 and 18.4, respectively. In addition, the caries exposure was much higher for older adults. The Decayed, Missing and Filled Teeth (DMFT) scores were 1.0, 1.4, 1.6, 2.1 and 12.4, respectively, for subjects in each group. Lastly, it was interesting to note that the percent of edentulous individuals in the 65 to 74-year-old group was only 10.5% (Wang et al. 2002). This is a relatively low percentage of edentulism in comparison to other countries, which may be related in part to a lack of dental services to accomplish removal of teeth that should be extracted.

Studies examining tooth loss have reported both the cause of tooth loss and risk factors associated with tooth loss. Fure (2003) reported on tooth loss in an elderly Swedish population. A 10-year follow-up of 55, 65 and 75-year-old individuals demonstrated that an increase in the number of teeth retained occurred with an increase in dental care services received by study participants. Nearly half of the participants had not lost any teeth after 10 years of follow up, and only 13% of participants had lost three or more teeth. Fure also found that while root caries increased with age, coronal caries decreased with age. Further, the main reason for tooth loss was caries.

The available data suggest that when assessed over time, older adults are at high risk for dental caries. At the 10-year follow-up examination, Fure (2004) observed that carious lesions occurred in 95% of the patients and the caries experience increased with age. As an example, for 85-year-old individuals, 25% of root surfaces demonstrated caries, versus 9% for individuals who were 65 years old. Recurrent or secondary caries (associated with existing restorations) were more common than primary lesions.

Table 2.1 Percent of individuals of age 65 and older who reported loss of all teeth (by state). The five highest and lowest states are provided

Highest	Lowest
Kentucky 42.3% ($\pm$3.3)*	Hawaii 13.1% ($\pm$2.9)
West Virginia 41.9% ($\pm$3.7)	California 13.3% ($\pm$2.7)
Tennessee 36.0% ($\pm$4.1)	Utah 14.7% ($\pm$3.3)
Mississippi 35.1% ($\pm$3.7)	Minnesota 14.8% ($\pm$2.5)
Louisiana 33.8% ($\pm$3.5)	Connecticut 16.0% ($\pm$2.5)

*95% confidence interval
Data are from the Behavioral Risk Factor Surveillance System, 2002; From Gooch et al. 2003

Warren and colleagues (2000) reported that among rural Iowans aged 79 years or older, 96% had coronal caries experience and 23% had untreated coronal caries. A history of root caries was found in 64% of individuals and 23% had untreated root caries. This group was unusual in that dental utilization was high. Over 70% reported a dental visit in the last year and most patients paid for their dental services.

A study from Japan confirmed that non-institutionalized elderly populations (70 years of age) are at high risk for caries. Over a 2-year period, almost 36% of adults 70 years and older developed one or more root caries lesions (Takano et al. 2003). Similarly, the oral health component of the Study of Health in Pomerania, Germany (Mack et al. 2004), revealed that in a representative sample of adults 60 years and older, root caries was an important problem. For individuals 60–79 years of age, coronal caries were observed on 2% of all teeth, while restorations on root surfaces were seen in 6% of teeth and root caries lesions were seen on 2% of teeth. For the entire population, 11% had one or more untreated coronal lesions and 27% had one or more untreated root lesions. Imazato and colleagues (2006) examined root caries prevalence among community-dwelling Japanese elderly (mean age was 65.8 years). Nearly 40% had one or more untreated root lesions, and more than 50% had one or more restored or untreated lesions.

While caries appears to be the primary reason for tooth loss experience by older adults living in developed countries, another study indicated that severe attachment loss (a surrogate for periodontitis) was a risk factor for tooth loss (OR = 2.4, p = 0.006). Of interest in this study, the number of remaining teeth had a significant positive effect on the patient's ability to masticate as well as their interest in smiling (Warren et al. 2002).

Evidence suggests that older adults who reside in long-term care facilities are at even greater risk for caries than non-institutionalized individuals of comparable age. Chalmers and colleagues (2005) examined the oral health status of residents of seven nursing homes in Adelaide, Australia. Residents were examined at baseline and 1 year later. All residents demonstrated major medical, mental and/or behavioral impairments. At baseline, the mean age of those examined was 82.3 years, two-thirds of the 224 patients were edentulous, 64% of the residents displayed coronal caries and 49% displayed root caries. In the 1-year interval between examinations, 72% of the residents demonstrated new carious lesions. The investigators noted that compared to community-dwelling older adults in Adelaide, nursing home residents displayed much higher prevalence and incidence of dental caries.

Similar findings have been reported in other studies. Data from a single nursing home in Zagreb, Croatia, revealed that of the 139 residents who were examined, 45% were edentulous. Thirty-one percent of the residents demonstrated untreated caries and an average of nine teeth per resident required treatment (Simonkovic et al. 2005). A study from Finland (Peltola et al. 2004) evaluated the oral health conditions and treatment needs of a group of 260 individuals, 60 years and older, who lived in a long-term care facility. Mean age was 83.3 years, and the average time of residence was 2.2 years. Forty-two percent were edentulous, and denture hygiene was considered 'good' in less than 20% of subjects. Among those with teeth, the mean number was 12.4. In general, oral hygiene was poor, and 37% of individuals required restorations and 42% required tooth extraction. The authors concluded that for individuals unable to care for themselves, there is a significant need to provide assistance with oral hygiene and basic oral health care services.

Determinants and Etiology

Overall, these studies indicate a relationship between tooth loss and caries, and in particular root caries in older individuals. Identification of risk factors for caries in older adults helps to define preventive and treatment strategies for these individuals.

Curzon and Preston (2004) contrasted dental caries affecting the elderly to nursing bottle caries affecting young children. Nursing bottle caries was identified many centuries ago, while dental caries affecting the elderly is a relatively recent problem that relates to increased longevity and retention of teeth for a lifetime. They listed the most important risk factors for recurrent coronal caries and root caries affecting the elderly as increased intake of fermentable carbohydrates, increased plaque accumulation due to the presence of dental restorations and prostheses, reduced dexterity, incapacitation, limited access to professional dental services and reduced salivary flow that is a side effect of a number of medications. Studies have supported the multifunctional nature of caries, and root caries in particular, affecting the elderly. A study of clinical and behavioral risk factors for the development of root caries examined 462 dentate older adults ($\geq$ 65 years of age) who were part of the National Diet and Nutrition Study from Great Britain (Steele et al. 2001). The subject sample was representative of the British population and included 405 individuals who were community dwelling and 57 who were in residential homes and long-term care facilities. The significant risk factors for root caries included the consumption of nine or more intakes of sugar per day (OR = 2.4), the presence of a partial denture which was associated with heavy plaque deposits (OR = 1.6) and less than one daily oral cleaning (OR = 4.7). The authors concluded that these are modifiable risk factors that can be used to develop a preventive strategy for improved oral health of older adults.

In a study of 549 community-dwelling older adults in Thailand (mean age of 66.7 years), root caries lesions were seen in 18.2% of individuals (Nicolau et al. 2000). After adjusting for the effects of other determinants in a multivariate logistic regression model, important risk factors for root caries were more years of education (OR = 2.39, p = 0.002), higher income (OR = 1.85, p = 0.029), being male (OR = 1.76, p = 0.031) and having at least 25 teeth (OR = 1.14, p < 0.001). The association of more years of education and higher income with greater prevalence of root caries may appear counterintuitive. The authors note that the literature is unclear regarding these associations. A number of explanations can be proposed. For example, this finding may be related to increased frequency of tooth brushing and resultant exposure of root surfaces seen in individuals with more years of education and higher income. Imazato et al. (2006) evaluated 287 community-dwelling older adults and identified a high prevalence of root caries.

For those individuals who had at least 20 teeth, there was a strong tendency for root caries to be associated with the report of having a dry mouth ($p = 0.052$) and actual reduced salivary flow ($p = 0.059$). Fewer root caries lesions tended to be associated with increased frequency of brushing ($p = 0.058$).

Periodontitis is associated with loss of periodontal ligament and attachment of the bone to the tooth, which often results in exposure of the vulnerable root surface to plaque accumulation. A study by Saotome et al. (2006) made an important contribution to our understanding of root caries affecting older adults. Studying a large group of 75-year-old individuals, they demonstrated that the presence of periodontitis, as measured by increased clinical attachment loss, was associated with increased levels of lactobacilli, microorganisms that have been associated with the development of root caries lesions. In turn, these individuals were at increased risk for root caries.

Xerostomia is a well-recognized risk factor for dental caries (See Chapters 9 and 15). Saliva has an important protective role, likely related to its buffering capacity. Thomson et al. (2002) followed a group of 528 older adults 60 years of age or older for 5 years. In addition to clinical examinations, the use of medications was recorded at baseline and then at the follow-up examination. Over the course of the trial, the incidence of coronal caries was 67% and root caries was 59%. Data for a total of 20 medication categories were recorded. For coronal caries, use of a β-blocker or antiasthma medication was associated with increased caries risk. For root caries, none of the drug categories were associated with an increased caries risk. The antiasthma drugs were also associated with the sensation of dry mouth. They noted that it is possible that patients using multiple medications will present to the dentist complaining of a dry mouth, unaware of the development of new carious lesions. Therefore, considering the many influential variables, there is a need for more research on the association of polypharmacy and the risk for dental caries in the elderly.

Lastly, much of what has been learned about risk factors for dental caries has been translated into a risk assessment tool that can be used in the clinical management of patients, including elderly patients. A computer-based assessment tool known as the Cariogram has been developed for dental caries (Bratthall 1996; Bratthall and Petersson 2005). The components of the model include: caries experience, related diseases, diet content, frequency of food intake, plaque, infection with *Streptococcus mutans*, fluoride use, rate of saliva secretion, buffering capacity of saliva and clinical judgment. A recent report demonstrated application of this tool for older adults (Alian et al. 2006).

Periodontal Diseases

Overview

The periodontal diseases are a group of inflammatory disorders that affect the supporting non-mineralized and mineralized tissues of the teeth. These disorders begin with bacterial infection and plaque accumulation at the margin of the gingival tissue, which is followed by infection of the gingival crevice, the cuff formed around the teeth by the mucosal tissue. The host responds to this infection by the development of both inflammatory and immune responses to the specific organisms in the plaque. Both the supragingival and subgingival plaques have characteristics of a biofilm.

The initial host response is confined to the soft tissues (gingivitis). Virtually all adults demonstrate some degree of gingivitis. In a smaller number of patients the intensity of the host response leads to loss of soft tissue, the periodontal ligament which connects the tooth root to the alveolus and the alveolar bone surrounding the teeth (Fig. 2.2). When this occurs periodontitis is present. Clinical signs of periodontitis include erythema and edema of the gingival tissues, pocket formation, exposure of the root portion of the tooth, tooth mobility, abscess formation and eventually tooth loss.

A new classification of the periodontal diseases was proposed in 1999 (Armitage 1999). The two major types of periodontitis include chronic periodontitis, a more slowly progressive process that usually correlates with local etiology, and aggressive periodontitis, a more advanced form that may also occur in children and adolescents.

The natural history of periodontitis has been the subject of interest in the 1980s and 1990s. Similar to many chronic diseases, periodontitis is believed to have periods of exacerbation and remission, but with the exception of acute periodontal

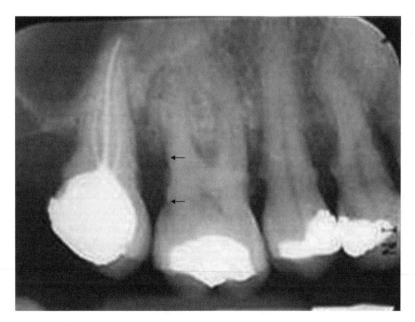

Fig. 2.2 Radiograph illustrating alveolar bone loss associated with chronic periodontitis. For these maxillary posterior teeth, the alveolar crest should be just apical to the crown of the teeth (the lower arrow). The bone loss on the distal surface of the first molar tooth is indicated by the distance between the two arrows. Large calculus deposits are present on all root surfaces

conditions, repair/regeneration of lost tissue is not normally a significant part of that natural history. Therefore, periodontal disease can be considered cumulative and, with retention of teeth (Fig. 2.2), periodontal disease will be more severe in older populations.

A general review of periodontal disease affecting older adults was published in 1998 (Locker et al. 1998). They found that the available literature at that time had a number of deficiencies, which include the lack of agreement on what constitutes periodontitis, as well as the definition of 'advanced' or 'severe' periodontitis, the definition of 'elderly' or 'older adult' and the definition of the primary clinical parameter (probing depth, clinical attachment loss or alveolar bone loss). Nevertheless, Locker et al. (1998) drew a number of conclusions:

1. Evidence of moderate periodontitis is commonly found in a majority of elderly adults. While advanced periodontitis (as assessed by clinical attachment loss or bone loss) is seen in a smaller portion of the population, older subjects demonstrate the highest rate of advanced disease. These authors conclude that approximately 70% of older adults demonstrate evidence of advanced periodontitis, but the number of affected sites/teeth is small.
2. As many as three in four older adults will demonstrate additional loss of attachment when monitored longitudinally over a few years. This progression is not, in general, widespread through the mouth.
3. When monitored longitudinally, patients tend to demonstrate progression of periodontal disease in newly affected sites as opposed to continued loss at previously affected sites.
4. The most important risk factors for periodontal disease include cigarette smoking and the presence of specific periodontal pathogens. In regard to the microbiota associated with periodontal disease, Mombelli (1998) stated that the recognized periodontal pathogen *Porphyromonas gingivalis* assumes greater importance with increasing age; the importance of the pathogen *Prevotella intermedia* is relatively constant throughout the life course, while the importance of *Actinobacillus actinomycetemcomitans* decreases with age, but this pathogen may be important in related cases of 'refractory' periodontitis, even in older adults.

No discussion of the risk for periodontal disease in older adults would be complete without mention of age-associated changes in the inflammatory and immune responses to periodontal pathogens. McArthur (1998) asserts that there are no specific defects in the immune response that could account for periodontitis in older adults. Nevertheless, changes in the immune response with aging do occur (immunosenesence) and further research is needed as the population ages and a larger percentage of the population lives into their seventh, eighth and ninth decades.

It is important to emphasize that loss of periodontal attachment and loss of alveolar bone are not an inevitable consequence of aging (Papapanou et al. 1991; Papapanou & Lindhe 1992). In their studies of more than 500 adults in Japan and Sweden, a subset of older adults maintained an essentially intact periodontium into their seventh and eighth decades of life.

Prevalence and Incidence

A review of data from the Third NHANES (1988–1994) defined periodontal disease as having at least one tooth site with 2 mm, 4 mm or 6 mm of attachment loss (Surgeon General's Report 2000b). Examining the most severe case definition, the percent of population with periodontitis increased from 0.2% at the age of 18–24, up to 23.4% at 65–74 and 29.5% for individuals who were 75 and older. At this case definition, the percent of males with periodontitis was greater than the percent of females. A recent report of older adults in Iowa (mean age of 85 years) indicated that for those individuals with teeth, 45% had at least one site with attachment loss of 6 mm or more and 15% had at least 1 site with 8 mm or more of attachment loss. For the entire cohort ($n = 449$), 26% were edentulous (Levy et al. 2003).

Similar studies have been conducted in other countries. A study of the periodontal status and the need for periodontal treatment has been reported for persons 76–86 years of age in Finland. A total of 364 individuals were examined and 46.2% were edentulous. Of the 175 dentate individuals, the mean number of teeth was 15.1 for men and 14.0 for women. Using the Community Periodontal Index of Treatment Needs (CPITN), 11% of the subjects had one or more sites with a probing depth of 6 mm or more (CPITN $= 4$). The majority of teeth that were missing were molars (Ajwani et al. 2001).

Findings from other developed countries indicate a high prevalence of periodontitis in older adults. The Study of the Health in Pomerania reported on the periodontal status of individuals in Germany who were 60 years of age and older (Mack et al. 2004). Edentulism increased from 16% of individuals who were 60–65 years of age to 30% in those who were 75–79 years of age. They used two definitions of periodontitis: the presence of one or more tooth sites with a probing depth of 4 mm and greater and one or more sites 6 mm and greater. For those 60–69, the prevalence of individuals with at least one site of 4 mm and greater was 85% for males and 71% for females. Using the 6 mm criteria, the prevalence was 44% and 24% for males and females, respectively. For the older adults, 71% of males and 62% of females had at least one site of 4 mm and greater, and 32% of males and 29% of females had at least one site of 6 mm and greater.

Holm-Pedersen and colleagues (2006) from Sweden reported on the periodontal status of community-dwelling individuals who were at least 80 years of age. There were a total of 159 participants, and 30 (19%) were edentulous. Of the remaining 129 subjects, 121 received a periodontal examination. The average number of teeth present was 16.3. The criteria for 'serious' periodontitis were at least four sites with clinical attachment loss of at least 5 mm, with at least one site having a probing depth of 4 mm or more. With that case definition, 50.5% of the population demonstrated severe periodontitis.

As seen for dental caries, the periodontal status of older adults who are institutionalized (in long-term care facilities) tends to be poor, and worse than what is observed for community-dwelling seniors. Lo et al. (2004) examined a large group (3153 individuals) of institutionalized older adults in Hong Kong. The mean age was 79.8 years, and about one-fifth were edentulous. Of the dentate subjects, about one-fifth had severe periodontitis. They also noted that approximately two-thirds reported difficulty chewing.

Longitudinal studies of the progression of periodontal disease have been reported. In a group of healthy older adults in Japan, Hirotomi and colleagues (2002) reported on the progression of periodontal disease over a 2-year period. There were 599 seventy-year olds and 162 eighty-year-old participants at the first examination, and 436 of the younger age group returned for the second examination. In general, periodontal disease in the 70-year-old cohort was pronounced; 47.3% had at least one site with 7 mm or more of clinical attachment loss. Progression of periodontal disease, defined as loss of 3 mm or more of clinical attachment loss, was seen in 75.1% of the participants who reported for the second examination. In contrast, Ajwani and Ainamo (2001) reported on the progression of periodontitis in a group of very old adults (81–91 years old). There were 57 individuals who were seen both at baseline and 5 years later. In this group, the mean number of teeth had decreased from 15.9 to 15.1. In general, there was little change in the periodontal status of these individuals. The authors concluded that periodontal disease is not a consequence of aging. However, considering the overwhelming evidence regarding the prevalence of periodontitis observed in older adults, this small sample may represent a healthy subset of individuals who are resistant to periodontal disease.

As reviewed by Alvares and Johnson (2003) age-related changes in the periodontal tissues have been a subject of interest and investigation. Minor changes in the behavior of keratinocytes in tissue culture from older individuals have been reported (reduced cell division, reduced production of interleukin 1β). Similar differences in gingival fibroblast function in vitro have been demonstrated when comparing cells from younger and older donors. Cells from older adult donors demonstrated reduced protein production, including the vital structural protein, collagen. The conclusion is that periodontal disease is not primarily the result of aging, but may be influenced by changes in cell biology as individuals age. The etiology of periodontal disease in the elderly is considered to be the same as for younger adults, specifically an exuberant host inflammatory/immune response to the subgingival microflora.

In that regard, experimental gingivitis is a model to test the development of clinical inflammation as dental plaque is allowed to accumulate over the course of a few weeks. Fransson et al. (1996) studied the development of gingival inflammation in younger (20–25 years of age) and older (65–80 years of age) adults. All participants had a healthy periodontium at the initiation of the trial and, after 3 weeks of no oral hygiene, the older adults demonstrated a more pronounced clinical and histologic inflammatory response. A subsequent analysis revealed that the older patients had higher levels of both α-2-macroglobin and IgG3 than the younger adults (Fransson et al. 1999). Further, at the conclusion of the experimental period, there was a greater inflammatory cell infiltrate observed in gingival biopsy specimens from the older adults. Confirmatory evidence was provided by Tsalikis et al. (2002). Utilizing the 3-week experimental gingivitis model, as compared to younger adults, older adults demonstrated a significantly greater increase in the gingival fluid levels of the proinflammatory cytokine interleukin 1β.

Determinants and Etiology

Periodontitis is a chronic disorder and is recognized as having a complex etiology and multiple risk factors. As such, these disorders meet the criteria of a 'complex' disease (Rees 2002). While specific microbial pathogens have been associated with periodontitis, the host inflammatory and immune responses are now believed to play a major role in the progression of periodontitis. Further, a variety of other local, systemic, behavioral and social risk factors for periodontitis have been identified in adult populations.

What is quite clear is that the prevalence of periodontitis increases with age (Albandar 2005). A study by Dye and Selwitz (2005) examined the relationship between a number of different periodontitis severity indices and risk factors for periodontitis. Using data from the Third NHANES, the presence of periodontitis was defined by different criteria using the attachment loss extent index (based on the percent of sites with $\geq$ 2 mm of clinical attachment loss), attachment loss (mean attachment loss), derived community periodontal index (based on bleeding, the presence of calculus and probing depth of $\geq$ 4 mm) and the periodontal status measure (which classifies patients as healthy, gingivitis or mild, moderate or severe periodontitis based on bleeding, probing depth, clinical attachment loss and furcation involvement). Data were available from more than 11,000 dentate (> 5 teeth) individuals who received a dental examination and were over 20 years old. For this analysis, age was stratified as 20–39 years, 40–59 years and 60–79 years. For all periodontal indices, older age ($\geq$ 40 years), lower level of education, a history of cigarette smoking, male gender and being a non-Hispanic black were associated with increased severity of periodontitis. This study also identified an interesting interaction between aging and smoking; these two risk factors appeared to act synergistically to increase the risk for periodontitis when measured by clinical attachment loss.

A large body of evidence has been published that indicates that in addition to the systemic disorders attributable to smoking (lung cancer, oral and pharyngeal cancer, cardiovascular and cerebrovascular diseases), the contribution of smoking to periodontitis is enormous. Tomar and Asma (2000) used the Third NHANES database to estimate the number of cases of periodontitis attributable to smoking. They determined that 9.2% of dentate adults met their criteria for periodontitis, and in a fully adjusted model, smoking was associated with an almost fourfold increase in the odds of periodontitis. They determined that nearly 42% of cases of periodontitis in the U.S. population were attributable to currently smoking cigarettes and about 11% of cases were attributable to a history of smoking.

A study of risk factors for periodontitis in a population of older adults from Thailand examined 2005 individuals who ranged in age from 50 to 73 (Torrungruang et al. 2005a). Detailed demographic, medical and dental variables were assessed cross-sectionally. All subjects were classified as having mild, moderate or severe periodontitis based on mean clinical attachment level. Multivariate logistic regression was used to determine the strength of the relationship between different independent variables and periodontitis. In a fully adjusted model, the odds of having severe periodontitis ($\geq$ 4.0 mm of clinical attachment loss) were significantly associated with being 60 years of age or older (OR = 1.6), having diabetes mellitus (OR = 1.6), being a former smoker (OR = 1.7), being a current smoker (OR = 4.4), having 40%–79% plaque-infected surfaces (OR = 3.5), having 80%–100% plaque-infected surfaces (OR = 17.9) and being male (OR = 3.3). Having more than a high school education had an inverse relationship with periodontitis (OR = 0.4). Other potential risk factors for periodontitis such as income, alcohol consumption and obesity were not related to moderate or severe periodontitis.

In another study by the same authors (Torrungruang et al. 2005b) the effect of smoking on periodontitis was investigated. In this group of individuals, 48.7% were non-smokers, 36.9% were former smokers and 14.4% were current smokers. Smokers demonstrated greater supragingival plaque deposits and greater mean probing depth and mean clinical attachment loss than newer smokers or former smokers. Of particular interest, quitting smoking tended to reduce the odds for severe periodontitis.

Diabetes mellitus is a recognized risk factor for periodontitis. As noted in Torrungruang et al. (2005a) persons with diabetes were 1.6 times more likely to have severe periodontitis. A recent meta-analysis of the relationship between periodontitis and diabetes (Khader et al. 2006) indicated that compared to non-diabetics, having diabetes was associated with greater severity but comparable extent of the disease. This analysis included patients of all ages. Khader et al. (2006) noted that they were unable to examine the importance of specific variables, including age, on this relationship. This was due to a lack of specific reporting of variables including age in the original publications.

In summary, cigarette smoking and having diabetes mellitus are the most important environmental determinant and systemic disease, respectively, for periodontitis. These risk factors for periodontitis are observed across all age groups, including older populations.

Oral and Pharyngeal Cancer

Overview, Prevalence and Incidence

In the broadest context, oral and pharyngeal cancers comprise a variety of malignant disorders affecting the cells and tissues in this anatomical region. Nevertheless, discussion of oral and pharyngeal cancer generally refers to carcinoma of the oral cavity and pharynx, and specifically squamous cell carcinoma. As reviewed by Epstein (2003), oral and pharyngeal squamous cell carcinoma is a disease of adults, and older adults in particular. Virtually all cases (95%) are present in individuals 40 years or older, and the average age of diagnosis is 60–65 years of age (Surgeon General's Report 2000). The data indicate that for the United States, oral and pharyngeal cancer is the fourth most common cancer affecting black males and seventh most common cancer affecting white males. In the oral cavity, oral cancer primarily affects the tongue, lip and floor of the mouth (Rhodus 2007). Other areas (i.e., palate and gingiva) are affected, but less commonly. In the United States in 2004, the number of patients diagnosed with oral cancer was estimated to be 28,260. In that year, there were an estimated 7230 deaths from oral cancer (Jemal et al. 2004). It is important to note that differences exist in different countries. For example, in India, after the tongue, the buccal mucosa is the second most common site for development of oral cancer (Lin et al. 2005). This appears to be related to the placement of betel leaves and areca nuts in the cheek area ('betel nut').

Determinants and Etiology

When reviewing the incidence of oral cancer, discussion of the primary risk factors is particularly important. A variety of epidemiologic and animal studies have clearly identified tobacco smoking and alcohol consumption as the two most important risk factors for oral cancer.

While cigarette smoking has been firmly established as a risk factor for oral squamous cell carcinoma (Forastiere et al. 2001), other types of tobacco use including cigar and pipe smoking have also been associated with an increased risk of oral cancer (Garrote et al. 2001). Further, the use of chewing tobacco has more recently been identified as a risk factor (Warnakulasuriya 2004). There are many variations of this product throughout the world, including the combination of tobacco and betel leaves used in Asia (Znaor et al. 2003).

Alcohol consumption is the other major risk factor for oral cancer (Mashberg et al. 1981). While the risk for oral cancer has been associated with the use of spirits, beer and alcohol, a number of studies have suggested that differences occur in the risk with different types of alcohol. In some studies beer and wine have been associated with only moderate effects on oral cancer as compared to consumption of spirits (Huang et al. 2003). Recently, a study from Spain determined that for equal amounts of consumption, use of black tobacco (pipe smoking, cigar smoking) and spirits were associated with a two to fourfold high risk of oral cancer than the use of blond tobacco (cigarette smoking) and wine and beer consumption (Castellsague et al. 2004). This study further emphasized the synergistic effects of alcohol and tobacco use on the development of oral cancer.

Another important risk factor for oral cancer is the use of betel leaves, which is often chewed in combination with areca nuts ('betel nut'). Popular in Asia, the association of betel and areca and oral cancer has been documented in studies published since the 1960s. Recent studies continue to emphasize this linkage. A report from Taiwan indicated that more than 85% of the occurrence of oral cancer could be explained by the use of betel nut (Lin et al. 2005). In another study from Taiwan (Yang et al. 2005), a group of aboriginal patients were followed for 6 years, and the development of oral squamous cell carcinoma and oral precancerous lesions were closely related to the chewing of betel nut.

It has also been observed that certain demographic variables are associated with increased risk for oral cancer. It has long been recognized that being male has been associated with an increased risk for oral squamous cell carcinoma. Morse and Kerr (2006) examined the data from the Surveillance, Epidemiology and End Results (SEER) database. Examining data from 1975 to 2002, both the age-adjusted incidence rates and age-adjusted mortality rates were higher for black males versus white males and were lower and equal for black and white females. The survival rates at 5 years were also higher for whites with oral cancer than blacks, being the lowest for black males. An interesting study on the gender ratio of individuals with oral cancer was reported by Brandizzi and colleagues (2005). Analyzing data from Buenos Aires, Argentina, from 1950 to 2000, they observed a gradual decline in the male-predominant occurrence. From 1950 to 1970, the ratio was 7.1:1 male to female. From 1961 to 1968 the ratio was 4.3:1 and then 2.3:1 for the interval from 1972 to 1984. The most recent data (1992–2000) showed that the ratio had fallen dramatically to 1.24:1. This shift is likely due to increased exposure in women of the primary risk factors of tobacco use and alcohol consumption.

Recent research has begun to focus on genetic risk factors for oral squamous cell carcinoma. Genes controlling matrix metalloproteinase-1 promoter (Cao and Li 2006), CYP 17 (Chen et al. 2005) and epidermal growth factor receptor (Kang et al. 2005) have been implicated as risk factors. These studies have shown a positive association of the gene or specific allele with the development of oral cancer, but this research is still preliminary.

Lastly, viruses have been associated with cancer development, and while no studies have specifically linked viral infection to the risk for oral cancer, Rhodus (2007) notes that several viruses with oncogenic potential can infect the oral tissues. In particular, the human papilloma viruses (HPV), which have been shown to be important risk factors for cervical cancer, are considered potential risk factors for oral squamous cell carcinoma (Miller and Johnstone 2001). While there are many HPV genotypes, a limited number of these have been associated with dysplastic and malignant squamous cell lesions (Furrer et al. 2006). In particular, HPV16 and 18 were found in a much greater percentage of lesion scrapings (100%) versus normal tissue (9%). A recent review of infection with the human papilloma virus as a risk factor for oral cancer suggested that there may be two distinct pathways that account for cancer development: one in which tobacco and alcohol are causative, while in the other HPV infection is causative. Still, these authors state that molecular mechanisms to account for HPV-associated oral cancer are not defined. Nevertheless, this work raises the question of immunization against the HPV16 and HPV18 as a strategy to reduce the occurrence of oral squamous cell carcinoma (Ragin et al. 2007).

In contrast, a number of studies have indicated that the consumption of fruits and vegetables is associated with a reduced risk for oral squamous cell carcinoma. A meta-analysis by Pavia and co-authors (2006) examined 16 studies. Both fruit consumption and vegetable consumption were associated with a significantly reduced risk of oral cancer (OR = 0.51, 95% CI = 0.40 − 0.65, and OR = 0.50, 95% CI = 0.38–0.65, respectively). Both the number of portions of fruits and vegetables consumed each day and the types of fruit consumed had an impact on the magnitude of the reduced risk.

Table 2.2 Trends in 5-year relative survival rates (in percent) for cancer of the oral cavity. For comparison, data for cancer of the colon and larynx are provided

	White			African–American		
	1974–1976	1983–1985	1992–1999	1974–1976	1983–1985	1992–1999
Oral cavity	55	55	60*	36	35	36
Larynx	66	69	67	60	55	53
Colon	51	58	65*	46	49	53*

*Difference between 1974–1976 and 1992–1999 is significant at $p < 0.05$
Adapted from Jemal et al. (2004)

To further extend the relationship of diet to the risk for oral squamous cell cancer, Suzuki et al. (2006) examined the effect of consumption of antioxidants on the risk of oral cancer development in individuals who smoke cigarettes and drink alcohol. Examining 385 patients with oral, pharyngeal and laryngeal cancer and 1925 cancer-free, age- and gender-matched controls, there was an inverse relationship between intake of antioxidants (which included vitamins C, E and carotene) and the risk for oral, pharyngeal and laryngeal cancer. This effect was seen for both men and women and was present for those that smoked cigarettes, drank alcohol and both smoked and drank alcohol.

Trends in the 5-year survival rates of oral cancer are disturbing. As reported by Jemal and colleagues (2004), the survival rate for whites has increased slightly, from 55% in 1974–1976 to 60% in 1992–1999. In contrast, the 5-year survival rate for African-Americans has not changed during this 25-year interval and is significantly below that of whites (see Table 2.2). The same trends are seen when the data for 1992–1999 are analyzed by stage at diagnosis (localized, regional or distant). For whites and African-Americans, the percent diagnosed with localized, regional or distant diseases were 37% vs. 19%, 46% vs. 57% and 9% vs. 15%, respectively. Further, the survival rates differ by race. For localized disease, the survival rates for whites and African-Americans were 83% and 69%, respectively. When examining regional and distant disease, these percentages are 50% and 31% and 27% and 22%, respectively. These data clearly indicate that many oral cancers are not detected at their earliest stages, when prolonged survival or cure is most likely, and that racial differences exist in terms of the outcome of therapy.

Oral Mucosal Lesions and Candidiasis

Caries and periodontal disease are oral disorders that are generally limited to the teeth and tissues (periodontium) in proximity to the teeth. Dysplastic lesions and oral squamous cell carcinoma are disorders of the mucosal tissues that line the oral cavity. In addition, there are a variety of other diseases and disorders that affect the mucosal surfaces that must be mentioned in a review of the oral disease burden affecting older adults.

The Third NHANES database has been analyzed for the occurrence of oral mucosal lesions (Shulman et al. 2004). A total of 17,235 individuals at least 17 years of age received an oral examination and 28% had at least one oral lesion. The chance of a lesion being present increased with age, and the chance of a lesion being present at 70 years of age was almost twice that of individuals who are less than 30 years of age (see Table 2.3). For all individuals, the most common disorders were connected to wearing dentures (8.4% of lesions) and tobacco-related lesions (4.7% of lesions). The palate was the most common location for a lesion (26%), followed by the gingiva (20%), lip (15%) and dorsum of the tongue (14%). This study did not examine the occurrence of specific lesions by age.

Other reports of the distribution of oral lesions in general populations provide some insight into the occurrence of mucosal lesions in older adults. A report by Mumcu and colleagues (2005) examined 765 residents of Istanbul, Turkey, and reported on diseases and disorders of the oral cavity other than caries and periodontal disease. The mean age of the population was 35.6 years, and 21.1% of the population were at least 65 years of age. Though no malignancies were found in this population, older individuals demonstrated the highest percentage of oral lesions, and older age was significantly predictive of the presence of certain lesions (oral pigmentation, OR = 2.2; fissured tongue, OR = 2.9; lingual varices, OR = 8.4; hairy tongue, OR = 3.6; denture stomatitis, OR = 4.5; and petechiae, OR = 25.5). Some of these lesions are considered as variations of normal and do not require treatment (i.e., oral pigmentation) while others indicate problems related to a dental prosthesis (denture stomatitis) where evaluation and treatment are needed. Another study from Turkey examined both oral mucosal lesions and risk factors associated with those lesions in 700 community-dwelling individuals who were 60 years of age and older (Dundar and Kal 2007). A total of 41% of the individuals displayed one or more oral mucosal lesions, with males demonstrating a higher prevalence as compared to females (66% vs. 36%). The most common lesions were fissured

Table 2.3 Prevalence of oral mucosal lesions in the NHANES III survey, as stratified by age

Age	Sample size	With mucosal lesion (%)	Adjusted odds ratio (CI)
17–29	4541	19.0	1.00 (–)
30–39	3244	22.6	1.17 (0.95–1.46)
40–49	2513	28.6	1.34 (1.06–1.70)
50–59	1801	36.4	1.40 (1.08–1.83)
60–69	2236	39.4	1.51 (1.14–2.01)
≧70	2900	42.6	1.92 (1.47–2.51)

Data summarized from Shulman et al. (2004). *Journal of American Dentistry Association* 135 (9), 1279–1286 tongue (9.3% of individuals), lingual varicosities (8.3%), traumatic ulcer (5.7%), denture stomatitis (5.7%) and denture-associated hyperplasia (4.9%). Risk factors for mucosal lesions included being male, the length of time a denture was worn and being either a current or former smoker.

In the United Kingdom, a report on 44,007 biopsy specimens of the oral and maxillofacial areas received over a 30-year period provides some information about the occurrence of oral mucosal lesions in the general population and infers the importance of increased risk of oral lesions with increasing age (Jones and Franklin 2006). For oral lesions, a number of them were found to have a mean age of diagnosis of 55 years and older (suggesting frequent occurrence in older adults). Of these lesions, the most common were squamous cell carcinoma (N = 1559), epithelial dysplasia (N = 1280), non-specific ulceration (N = 919), Sjogren's syndrome (N = 363) and cavernous hemangioma (N = 308). While these data clearly represent a skewed sample, i.e., individuals seen by a dentist, who have an oral lesion that requires a biopsy, the occurrence of certain lesions in older adults is in agreement with other studies.

Other surveys have provided supporting data on the relationship of removable dentures to the development of oral mucosal lesions. Espinoza et al. (2003) reported on a cohort of 889 older adults (65 years and older) living in Santiago, Chile. They observed that 53% of individuals had one or more oral lesions. Twenty-five percent of the cohort was edentulous, and 65% wore dentures (complete or partial). The most common lesions were denture stomatitis (22.3%), followed by irritative hyperplasia (9.4%). Logistic regression indicated that use of a denture was the only variable significantly associated with an increased odds of an oral lesion (OR = 3.26). When specifically examining the variables associated with denture stomatitis, being female, having plaque on the prosthesis and sleeping with the denture in place were significantly associated with lesion occurrence. These data indicate that many dentures are ill-fitting and are frequently associated with erythematous and hyperplastic tissue. A study from Spain (Garcia-Pola Vallejo et al. 2002) emphasized the importance of denture use to the appearance of oral lesions. When compared to those between the ages of 30–49 and 50–69, individuals 70 years and older presented with the highest percentage of oral lesions. Having a complete denture was associated with pseudomembraneous candidiasis, stomatitis and tissue hyperplasia and these lesions were most often seen in the older individuals. The relationship of denture use to oral mucosal lesions was further emphasized in another study from Brazil that evaluated adults who wore partial or complete dentures (Coelho et al. 2004). The lesions, related to both *Candida* infection and inflammatory changes, occurred most commonly in the fifth through seventh decades of life. The highest percentage of lesions was seen in association with a maxillary complete denture.

A large percent of individuals living in long-term care facilities demonstrate oral lesions (Avcu et al. 2005). Xerostomia (59%) and coated tongue (54%) were the most common problems. Another study of institutionalized older patients in France (mean age 82.1 years) revealed that 37% demonstrated candidiasis, and this fungal infection was related to lower protein intake, a vitamin C deficiency and lower serum levels of zinc (Paillaud et al. 2004).

Oral fungal infections are an important problem in the elderly, especially for those individuals who use a removal denture. Lesions classified as 'denture stomatitis' were observed to be fungal infections, primarily *Candida albicans* (Dar-Odeh and Shehabi 2003). While the carriage rate of *Candida albicans* is high even in healthy, dentate individuals (Kleinegger et al. 1996), individuals residing in long-term care facilities are recognized to be at increased risk for *Candida* infection (Fanello et al. 2005; Budtz-Jorgensen et al. 1996). The overgrowth of *Candida* to clinically evident infection is associated with generally mild signs and symptoms and occurs with specific perturbations of the host response or normal oral flora related to the use of inhaled steroids and systemic antibiotics (Kennedy et al. 2000).

These data clearly indicate that older adults, especially those with partial or complete dentures, are at high risk for developing oral mucosal lesions. While a variety of lesions are observed, fungal infections, generally as a result of *C. albicans* infection, are a common occurrence.

Temporomandibular Disorders

Disorders of the temporomandibular joint (TMJ) and associated anatomical structures are important problems that often prove refractory to treatment and can be the cause of significant morbidity for those that are affected. TMJ disorders (TMD) have not always been clearly defined due to a number of factors, including variability in the objective and subjective signs and symptoms, cultural and gender differences and different criteria used for disease classification.

In 1996, the National Institutes of Health sponsored a technology assessment conference on the management of temporomandibular disorders (NIH 1996). Among the conclusions from this conference are that (1) the diagnostic classification of disorders of the TMJ need to be improved and should be based on etiology vs. symptoms, (2) no consensus existed regarding treatment and (3) randomized controlled trials were needed to develop appropriate approaches to clinical care. The lack of a clearly defined diagnostic scheme has prevented a true assessment of the prevalence of TMD. Nevertheless, the prevalence in different age groups has been examined in a number of studies. Österberg and colleagues (1992) evaluated individuals who were 70 years and older. They observed a *decrease* in symptoms of TMD with aging. In a similar sense, Koidis and colleagues (1993) examined patients that ranged from 16 to 70 years of age. They demonstrated that women were affected more than men, yet symptoms of TMD decreased with increasing age.

In later studies, attempts have been made to classify TMJ disorders and to compare prevalence based on pain, with consideration of other variables including age and gender. Huang and colleagues (2002) examined patients who were classified as having myofacial pain, arthralgia or both. Among the most important risk factors for myofacial pain were clenching (OR = 4.8) and female gender (OR = 4.2). Risk factors for myofacial pain with arthralgia included somatization (anxiety associated with physical symptoms; OR = 5.0), female gender (OR = 4.7) and removal of the third molars (OR = 4.0). Age was not a risk factor for any of the disease classifications.

A study has compared objective and subjective measures of TMJ disorders in younger (mean age of 27.5 years) and older (mean age of 83.4 years) subjects (Schmitter et al. 2005). Objective systems were more common in older adults; these individuals rarely complained of pain and rarely sought care for TMD from dentists and physicians. The reverse was true for the younger patients.

These data indicate that older adults are affected by TMD, but at a prevalence that is comparable to, or less than, that experienced by younger adults. Diagnosis and treatment of these disorders in older adults may be complicated by many other systemic or local disorders that affect the elderly, including cognitive impairment, musculoskeletal disorders, the number of teeth that are present and prosthetic replacement of missing teeth.

Conclusions

The three primary measures of oral health status are caries, periodontal disease and oral cancer. In addition, tooth loss is a more global measure of the oral health status of a population. Tooth loss and edentulism are a consequence of caries and periodontal disease, but teeth are removed for a variety of other reasons including lack of restorative dental services, prosthetic reasons, personal choice and lack of resources to pay for dental care. In summary, the preceding review has demonstrated that older adults bear a greater oral disease burden than other age groups.

Dental caries affecting the elderly manifest primarily as root caries (as a result of the exposure of the more vulnerable root surfaces which can occur when periodontitis is present) and recurrent caries affecting dental restorations. The loss of periodontal support for the teeth is cumulative, so when progression of disease occurs on an already compromised dentition, the consequences may be more severe. Lastly, oral cancer is a disease of older adults, with a mean age of diagnosis in the United States of 64 years.

Managing the oral disease burden is complicated by all of the considerations that accompany the care of older adults. First, the physical status of these individuals will vary from those who are community dwelling and capable of caring for their own needs to those who are institutionalized and require help with even the most basic of personal needs, including daily oral health care. The care of older adults is also complicated by illness and the use of medications that can affect the patient's ability to tolerate routine dental care or may have specific adverse effects on the oral cavity such as medication-induced xerostomia. Second, there are important social and structural barriers that limit access to care, including well-recognized risk factors for oral disease such as race, fewer years of education and socioeconomic status (See Chapter 3). In addition, Medicare does not provide benefits for routine and outpatient dental services (www.medicare.gov/coverage) and only 15% of older adults have private dental insurance (Wall and Brown 2003). In addition, benefits provided by these plans often have a limit on the amount of coverage that does not allow for comprehensive dental care. Third, the consequences of untreated oral disease are serious and include severe morbidity and mortality associated with oral cancer; the potential of long-standing, untreated oral disease (primarily periodontitis) contributing to the risk for a number of systemic disorders affecting the elderly including cardiovascular/cerebrovascular diseases; and the effects of tooth loss on mastication and nutritional intake, self-image and comfort with social interactions.

The irony of this situation is that the dental profession and dental care services have advanced in the past two decades to offer new and successful approaches for managing dental diseases and tooth loss. The lack of a coordinated plan to address the oral health care needs of older adults is a great challenge in the United States and in many countries throughout the world (Petersen and Ueda 2006). While solutions can be offered (Lamster 2004), it will take a coordinated effort by government agencies and the profession (including local, state and national professional organizations and dental schools) to provide dental care to the large numbers of older adults who will require these services. Further, these services must be provided by an oral health care workforce that understands the specific needs of older adults. These are daunting challenges at a time when the medical and social needs of the expanding population of older adults will strain the health care system in the United States and other countries.

References

Ajwani, S. & A. Ainamo (2001). Periodontal conditions among the old elderly: five-year longitudinal study. *Special Care in Dentistry* 21 (2), 45–51.

Ajwani, S., Tervonen, T., Närhi, T.O. & A. Ainamo (2001). Periodontal health status and treatment needs among the elderly. *Special Care in Dentistry* 21 (3), 98–103.

Albandar, J.M. (2005). Epidemiology and risk factors of periodontal diseases. *Dental Clinics of North America* 49 (3), 517–532.

Alian, A.Y., McNally, M.E., Fure, S. & D. Birkhel (2006). Assessment of caries risk in elderly patients using the Cariogram model. *Journal of the Canadian Dental Association* 72 (5), 459–463.

Alvares, O.F. & B.D. Johnson (2003). Aging of the periodontium. In Wilson, T. and Kornman, K. (eds). *Fundamentals of Periodontics*, 2nd Edition, Quintessence Publishing Company, Inc., Chicago.

Armitage, G.C. (1999). Development of a classification system for periodontal diseases and conditions. *Annals of Periodontology* 4 (1), 1–6.

Avcu, N., Ozbek, M., Kurtoglu, D., Kurtoglu, E., Kansu, O. & H. Kansu (2005). Oral findings and health status among hospitalized patients with physical disabilities, aged 60 or above. *Archives of Gerontology and Geriatrics* 41 (1), 69–79.

Brandizzi, D., Chuchurra, J.A., Lanfranchi, H.E. & R.L. Cabrini (2005). Analysis of epidemiological features of oral cancer in the city of Buenos Aires. *Acta Odontologica Latinoamerica* 18 (1), 31–35.

Bratthall, D. & G.H. Petersson (2005). Cariogram – a multifunctional risk assessment model for multifunctional disease. *Community Dentistry and Oral Epidemiology* 33 (4), 256–264.

Bratthall, D. (1996). Dental caries: intervened-interrupted-interpreted. Concluding remarks and cariography. *European Journal of Oral Sciences* 104 (4, part 2), 486–491.

Budtz-Jorgensen, E., Mojon, P., Banon-Clement, J.M. & P. Baehni (1996). Oral candidiasis in long-term hospital care: comparison of edentulous and dentate subjects. *Oral Diseases* 2 (4), 285–290.

Cao, Z.G. & C.Z. Li (2006). A single nucleotide polymorphism in the matrix metalloproteinase-1 promoter enhances oral squamous cell carcinoma susceptibility in a Chinese population. *Oral Oncology* 42 (1), 32–38.

Castellsague, X., Quintana, M.J., Martinez, M.C., Nieto, A., Sanchez, M.J., Juan, A., Monner, A., Carrera, M., Agudo, A., Quer, M., Munoz, N., Herrero, R., Franchesi, S. & F.X. Bosch (2004). The role of type of tobacco and type of alcoholic beverage in oral carcinogenesis. *International Journal of Cancer*, 108 (5), 741–749.

Chalmers, J.M., Carter, K.D. & A.J. Spencer (2005) Caries incidence and increments in Adelaide nursing home residents. *Special Care in Dentistry* 25 (2), 96–105.

Chen, W.C., Tsai, M.H., Wan, L., Chen, W.C., Tsai, C.H. & F.J. Tsai (2005). CYP17 and tumor necrosis factor-alpha gene polymorphisms are associated with risk of oral cancer in Chinese patients in Taiwan. *Acta Oto-laryngologica* 125 (1), 96–99.

Coelho, C.M., Sousa, Y.T. & A.M. Dare (2004). Denture-related oral mucosal lesions in a Brazilian school of dentistry. *Journal of Oral Rehabilitation* 31 (2), 135–139.

Curzon, M.E. & A.J. Preston (2004). Risk groups: nursing bottle caries / caries in the elderly. *Caries Research* 38 (Suppl 1), 24–33.

Dar-Odeh, N.S. & A.A. Shehabi (2003). Oral candidiasis in patients with removable dentures. *Mycoses* 46 (5–6), 187–191.

Dundar, N. & B.I. Kal (2007). Oral mucosal conditions and risk factors among elderly in a Turkish School of Dentistry. *Gerontology* 53 (3), 165–172.

Dye, B.A. & R.H. Selwitz (2005). The relationship between selected measures of periodontal status and demographic and behavioral risk factors. *Journal of Clinical Periodontology* 32 (7), 798–808.

Epstein, J.B. (2003). Oral cancer. In *Burket's Oral Medicine, Diagnosis and Treatment*, 10th Edition, B.C. Decker, Inc., Hamilton, Ontario, Canada. pp. 194–234.

Espinoza, I., Rojas, R., Aranda, W. & J. Gamonal (2003). Prevalence of oral mucosal lesions in elderly people in Santiago, Chile. *Journal of Oral Pathology and Medicine* 32 (10), 571–575.

Fanello, S., Bouchara, J.P., Sauteron, M., Delbos, V., Parot, E., Marot-Leblond, A., Moalic, E., Le Flohicc, A.M. & B. Brangerd (2006). Predictive value of oral colonization by *Candida* yeasts for the onset of a nosocomial infection in elderly hospitalized patients. *Journal of Medical Microbiology* 55 (pt 2), 223–228.

Forastiere, A., Koch, W., Trutti, A. & D. Sidransky (2001). Head and neck cancer. *New England Journal of Medicine* 345 (26), 1890–1990.

Fransson, C., Mooney, J., Kinane, D.F. & T. Berglundh (1999). Differences in the inflammatory response in young and old human subjects during the course of experimental gingivitis. *Journal of Clinical Periodontology* 26 (7), 453–460.

Fransson, C., Berglundh, T. & J. Lindhe (1996). The effect of age on the development of gingivitis. Clinical, microbiological and histological findings. *Journal of Clinical Periodontology* 23 (4), 379–385.

Fure, S. (2003). Ten-year incidence of tooth loss and dental caries in elderly Swedish individuals. *Caries Research* 37 (4), 462–469.

Fure, S. (2004). Ten-year cross-sectional and incidence study of coronal and root caries and some related factors in elderly Swedish individuals. *Gerodontology* 21 (3), 130–140.

Furrer, V.E., Benitez, M.B., Furnes, M., Lanfranchi, H.E. & N.M. Modesti (2006). Biopsy vs. superficial scraping: detection of human papilloma virus 6, 11, 16 and 18 in potentially malignant and malignant oral lesions. *Journal of Oral Pathology and Medicine* 35 (6), 338–344.

Garcia-Pola Vallejo, M.J., Martinez Diaz-Canel, A.I., Garcia Martin, J.M. & M. Gonzalez-Garcia (2002). Risk factors for oral soft tissue lesions in an adult Spanish population. *Community Dentistry and Oral Epidemiology* 30 (4), 277–285.

Garrote, L.F., Herrero, R., Ortiz-Reyes, R.M., Vaccarella, S., Lence Anta, J., Ferbeye, L., Munoz, N. & S. Francehesi (2001). Risk factors for cancer of the oral cavity and oro-pharynx in Cuba. *British Journal of Cancer* 85 (1), 46–54.

Gooch, B.F., Eke, P.I. & D.M. Madvitz (2003). Public health and aging: retention of natural teeth among older adults – United States, 2002. *Morbidity and Mortality Weekly Review*, 52 (50), 1226–1229.

Hamalainen, P., Meurman, J.H., Kauppinen, M. & M. Keskinen (2005). Oral infection as predictors of mortality. *Gerodontology* 22 (3), 151–157.

Hirotomi, T., Yoshihara, A., Yano, M., Ando, Y. & H. Miyazaki (2002). Longitudinal study on periodontal conditions in healthy elderly people in Japan. *Community Dentistry and Oral Epidemiology* 30 (6), 409–417.

Holm-Pedersen, P., Russell, S.L., Arlund, K., Viitanen, M., Wimblad, B. & R.V. Katz(2006a). Periodontal disease in the oldest-old living in Kungsholmen, Sweden: findings from the KEDHS project. *Journal of Clinical Periodontology* 33 (6), 376–384.

Huang, G.J., Le Resche, L., Critchlow, C.W., Martin, M.D. & M.T. Drangsholt (2002). Risk factors for diagnostic subgroups of painful temporomandibular disorders (TMD). *Journal of Dental Research* 81 (4), 284–288.

Huang, W.Y., Winn, D.M., Brown, L.M., Gridley, G. Bravo-Otero, E., Diehl, S.R., Fraumeni, J.F. Jr., & R.B. Haves (2003). Alcohol concentration and risk of oral cancer in Puerto Rico. *American Journal of Epidemiology* 157 (10), 881–887.

Imazato, S., Ikebe, K., Nokubi, T., Ebisu, J. & A.W.G. Walls (2006). Prevalence of root caries in a related population of older adults in Japan. *Journal of Oral Rehabilitation* 33 (2), 137–143.

Jemal, A., Tiwari, R.C., Murray, T., Ghafoor, A., Samuels, A., Ward, E., Feurer, E.J. & M.J. Thun (2004). Cancer statistics, 2004. *CA: A Cancer Journal for Clinicians* 54 (1), 8–29.

Jones, A.V. & C.D. Franklin (2006). An analysis of oral and maxillofacial pathology found in adults over a 30 year period. *Journal of Oral Pathology and Medicine* 35 (7), 392–401.

Kang, D., Gridley, G., Huang, W.Y., Engel, L.S., Winn, D.M., Brown, L.M., Bravo-Otero, E., Wu, T., Diehl, S.R. & R.B. Hayes (2005). Microsatellite polymorphisms in the epidermal growth factor receptor (EGFR) gene and the transforming growth factor-alpha (TGFA) gene and risk of oral cancer in Puerto Rico. *Pharmacogenetics and Genomics* 15 (5), 343–347.

Kennedy, W.A., Laurier, C., Gautrin, D., Ghezzo, H., Pare, M., Malo, J.L. & A.P. Contandriopoulos (2000). Occurrence and risk factors of oral candidiasis treated with oral antifungals in seniors using inhaled steroids. *Journal of Clinical Epidemiology* 53 (7), 696–701.

Khader, Y.S., Dauod, A.S., El-Qaderi, S.S., Alkafajei, A. & W.Q. Batayha (2006). Periodontal status of diabetics compared with nondiabetics: a meta analysis. *Journal of Diabetes and its Complications* 20, 59–68.

Kleinegger, C.L., Lockhart, S.R., Vargas, K. & D.R. Soll (1996). Frequency, intensity, species and strains of oral *Candida* vary as a function of host age. *Journal of Clinical Microbiology* 34 (9), 2246–2254.

Koidis, P.T., Zarifi, A., Grigoriadou, E. & P. Garefis(1993). Effect of age and sex on craniomandibular disorders. *Journal of Prosthetic Dentistry* 69 (1), 93–101.

Lamster, I. (2004) Oral health care services for older adults: a looming crisis. *American Journal of Public Health* 94 (5), 699–702.

Levy, S.M., Warren, J.J., Chowdhury, J., DeBus, B., Watkins, C.A., Cowen, H.J., Kirchner, H.L. & J.S. Hand (2003). The prevalence of periodontal disease measures in elderly adults, aged 79 and older. *Special Care in Dentistry* 23 (2), 50–57.

Lin, Y.S., Jen, Y.M., Wang, B.B., Lee, J.C. & B.W. Kang (2005). Epidemiology of oral cavity cancer in Taiwan with emphasis on the role of betel nut chewing. *Journal for Oto-Rhino-Laryngology and its Related Subspecialties* 67 (4), 230–236.

Lo, E.C., Luo, Y. & J.E. Dyson (2004). Oral health status of institutionalized elderly in Hong Kong. *Community Dental Health* 21 (3), 224–226.

Locker, D., Slade, G.D. & H. Murray (1998). Epidemiology of periodontal disease among older adults: a review. *Periodontology 2000* 16, 16–33.

Mack, F., Mojon, P., Budtz-Jorgensen, E., Kocher, T., Splieth, C., Schwahn, C., Bernhardt, O., Gesch, D., Kordab, B., Ulrich, J. & R. Biffar (2004). Caries and periodontal disease of the elderly in Pomerania, Germany: results of the Study of Health in Pomerania. *Gerodontology* 21 (1), 27–36.

Mashberg, A., Garfinkel, L. & S. Harris (1981). Alcohol as a primary risk factor in oral squamous carcinoma. *CA: A Cancer Journal for Clinicians* 31 (3), 146–155.

McArthur, W.P. (1998). Effect of aging on immunocompetent and inflammatory cells. *Periodontology 2000* 16, 53–79.

Meurman, J.H. & P. Hamalainen (2005). Oral health and morbidity – implications of oral infections on the elderly. *Gerodontology* 23 (1), 3–16.

Miller, C.S. & B.M. Johnstone (2001). Human papilloma virus as a risk factor for oral squamous cell carcinoma: a meta-analysis, 1982–1997. *Oral Surgery, Oral Medicine, Oral Pathology, Oral Radiology and Endodontology* 91 (6), 622–635.

Mombelli, A. (1998). Aging and the periodontal and peri-implant microbiota. *Periodontology 2000* 16, 44–52.

Morse, D.E. & Kerr, A.R. (2006). Disparities in oral and pharyngeal cancer incidence, mortality and survival among black and white Americans. *Journal of the American Dental Association* 137 (2), 203–212.

Mumcu, F., Cimilli, H., Sur, H., Hayran, O. & T. Atalay (2005). Prevalence and distribution of oral lesions: a cross-sectional study in Turkey. *Oral Diseases* 11 (2), 81–87.

Nicolau, B., Srisilapanan, P. & W. Marcenes (2000) Number of teeth and risk of root caries. *Gerodontology* 17 (2), 91–96.

NIH (1996) Management of temporomandibular disorders. NIH Technology Assessment Statement, April 29-May 1: 1–25.

Österberg, T., Carlsson, G.E., Wedel, A. & U. Johansson (1992). A cross-sectional and longitudinal study of craniomandibular dysfunction in an elderly population. *Journal of Craniomandibular Disorders* 6 (4), 237–245.

Österberg, T., Johanson, C., Sundh, V., Steen, B. & D. Birkhed (2006). Secular trends of dental status in five 70 year old cohorts between 1971 and 2001. *Community Dentistry and Oral Epidemiology* 34 (6), 446–454.

Paillaud, E., Merlier, I., Dupeyron, C., Scherman, J. & P.N. Bories (2004). Oral candidiasis and nutritional deficiencies in elderly hospitalized patients. *British Journal of Nutrition* 92 (5), 861–867.

Papapanou, P.N. & J. Lindhe (1992). Preservation of probing attachment and alveolar bone levels in 2 random populations. *Journal of Clinical Periodontology* 19 (8), 583–588.

Papapanou, P.N., Lindhe, J., Sterrett, J.D. & L. Eneroth (1991). Considerations on the contribution of ageing to loss of periodontal tissue support. *Journal of Clinical Periodontology* 18 (8), 611–615.

Pavia, M., Pileggi, C., Nobile, C.G. & I.F. Angelillo (2006). Association between fruit and vegetable consumption and oral cancer: a meta-analysis of observational studies. *The American Journal of Clinical Nutrition* 83 (5), 1126–1134.

Peltola, P., Vehkalahti, M.M. & K. Wuolijoki-Saaristo (2004). Oral health and treatment needs of the long-term hospitalized elderly. *Gerodontology* 21 (2), 93–99.

Petersen, P.E., Kjoller, M., Christensen, L.B. & U. Krustrup (2004). Changing dentate status of adults, use of dental health services, and achievement of national dental health goals in Denmark by the year 2000. *Journal of Public Health Dentistry* 64 (3), 127–135.

Petersen, P.E. & H. Ueda (2006). *Oral health in ageing societies: integration of oral health and general health.* World Health Organization, Geneva, Switzerland.

Petersen, P.E. & T. Yamamoto (2005). Improving the oral health of older people: the approach of the WHO Global Oral Health Programme. *Community Dentistry and Oral Epidemiology* 33 (2), 81–92.

Ragin, C.C., Modugno, F. & S.M. Gollin (2007). The epidemiology and risk factors of head and neck cancer: a focus on human papilloma virus. *Journal of Dental Research* 86 (2), 104–114.

Rees, J. (2002). Complex disease and the new clinical sciences. *Science* 296 (5568), 698–701.

Rhodus, N.L. (2007). Oral cancer: early detection and prevention. *Inside Dentistry* (1), 32–42.

Saotome, Y., Tada A., Hanada, N., Yoshihara, A., Uematsu, H., Miyazaki, H. & Senpuku, H. (2006). Relationship of cariogeneic bacteria levels with periodontal status and root surface caries in elderly Japanese. *Gerodontology* 23 (4), 219–225.

Schmitter, M., Rammelsberg, P. & A. Haussel (2005). The prevalence of signs and symptoms of temporomandibular disorders in very old subjects. *Journal of Oral Rehabilitation* 32 (7), 467–473.

Shulman, J.D., Beach, M.M. & F. Rivera-Hidalgo (2004). The prevalence of oral mucosal lesions in U.S. adults: data from the Third National Health and Nutrition Survey, 1988–1994. *Journal of the American Dental Association* 135 (9), 1279–1286.

Simonkovic, S.K., Boras, V.V., Panduric, J. & I. A. Zilic (2005). Oral health among institutionalized elderly in Zagreb, Croatia. *Gerodontology* 22 (4), 238–241.

Steele, J.G., Sheihan, A., Marcenes, W., Fay, N. & A.W.G. Walls (2001). Clinical and behavioral risk indicators for root caries in older people. *Gerodontology* 18 (2), 95–101.

Suzuki, T., Wakai, K., Matsuo, K., Hirose, K., Ito, H., Kuriki, K., Sato, S., Veda, R., Hasegawa, Y. & K. Tajima (2006). Effect of dietary antioxidants and risk of oral, pharyngeal and laryngeal squamous ell carcinoma according to smoking and drinking habits. *Cancer Science* 97 (8), 760–767.

Takano, N., Ando, Y., Yoshihara, A. & H. Miyazaki (2003). Factors associated with root caries incidence in an elderly population. *Community Dental Health* 20 (4), 217–222.

Thomson, W.M., Spencer, A.J., Slade, G.D. & J.M. Chalmers (2002). Is medication a risk factor for dental caries among older people? Evidence from a longitudinal study in South Australia. *Community Dentistry and Oral Epidemiology* 30 (3), 224–232.

Tomar, S.L. & S. Asma (2000). Smoking-attributable periodontitis in the United States: findings from NHANES III. National Health and Nutrition Examination Survey. *Journal of Periodontology* 71 (5), 743–751.

Torrungruang, K., Nisapakultorn, K., Sutdhibhisal, S., Tamsailom, S., Rojanasomith, K., Vanichjakvong, O., Prapakamol, S., Premvirinirund, T., Pusiri, T., Jaratkulangkoon, O., Kusump, S. & R. Rajatanavin (2005a). The effect of cigarette smoking on the severity of periodontal disease among older Thai adults. *Journal of Periodontology* 76 (4), 566–572.

Torrungruang, K., Tamsailom, S., Rojanasomsith, K., Sutdhibhisal, S., Nisapakultorn, K., Vanichjakvong, O., Prapakamol, S., Premsirinirund, T., Pusiri, T., Jaratkulangkoon, O., Unkurapinun, N. & P. Sritara (2005b). Risk indicators of periodontal disease in older Thai adults. *Journal of Periodontology* 76 (4), 558–565.

Tsalikis, L., Parapanisiou, E., Bata-Krykou, A., Polymenides, Z. & A. Konstantinidis (2002). Crevicular fluid levels of interleukin-1 alpha and interleukin-1 beta during experimental gingivitis in young and old adults. *Journal of the International Academy of Periodontology* 4 (1), 5–11.

U.S. Department of Health and Human Services (2000a). *Oral Health in America: A Report of the Surgeon General*. Department of Health and Human Services, National Institute of Dental and Craniofacial Research, National Institutes of Health, Rockville, MD, p. 67.

U.S. Department of Health and Human Services (2000b). *Oral Health in America: A Report of the Surgeon General*. U.S. Department of Health and Human Services, National Institute of Dental and Craniofacial Research, National Institutes of Health, Rockville, MD. p. 65.

Wall, T.P. & L.J. Brown (2003). Recent trends in dental visits and private dental insurance, 1989 and 1999. *Journal of the American Dental Association* 134 (5), 621–627.

Wang, H.Y., Petersen, P.E., Jin-Yon, B. & Z. Bo-Xue(2002). The second national survey of oral health status of children and adults in China. *International Dental Journal* 52 (4), 283–290.

Warnakulasuriya, S. (2004). Smokeless tobacco and oral cancer. *Oral Diseases* 10 (1), 1–4.

Warren, J.J., Cowen, H.J., Watkins, C.M. & J.S. Hand (2000) Dental caries prevalence and dental care utilization among the very old. *Journal of the American Dental Association*, 131 (11), 1571–1579.

Warren, J.J., Watkins, C.A., Cowen, H.J., Hand, J.S., Levy, S.M. & R.A. Kuthy (2002) Tooth loss in the very old: 13–15 year incidence among elderly Iowans. *Community Dentistry and Oral Epidemiology* 30 (1), 29–37.

Yang, Y.H., Chen, C.H., Chang, J.S.F., Lin, C.C., Cheng, T.C. & T.Y. Shieh (2005). Incidence rates of oral cancer and oral pre-cancerous lesions in a 6 year follow-up study of a Taiwanese aboriginal community. *Journal of Oral Pathology & Medicine* 34 (10), 596–601.

Znaor, A., Brennan, P., Gajalakshmi, V., Matthew, A., Shanta, V., Varghese, C. & P. Boffetta (2003). Independent and combined effects of tobacco smoking, chewing and alcohol drinking on the risk of oral, pharyngeal and esophageal cancers in Indian men. *International Journal of Cancer* 105 (5), 681–686.

Chapter 3
Social Disparities in Oral Health and Health Care for Older Adults

Luisa N. Borrell

Introduction

According to the 2000 U.S. Census, approximately 12.4% of the U.S. population or 35 million Americans were 65 years of age or older (Hetzel and Smith, 2001; Gist and Hetzel, 2004). Of these, approximately 17% were minorities (Table 3.1). Even though social security represents the main source of income for many older people (He et al., 2005), 9% of individuals 65 years of age or older live below the poverty level. Blacks (24%) and Hispanics (20%) exhibited the highest percentages among racial/ethnic groups of older adults living below the poverty level (Table 3.1). Finally, although the vast majority of older adults have health insurance coverage, there is variation in their coverage with 63.1% having Medicare and additional private insurance, 7.6% having Medicare and Medicaid, and 26.7% having Medicare only. This is important because oral health services are only covered under Medicaid and private health insurance at additional cost.

These sociodemographic variations within the older population may help shed light on the disparities observed in oral health and health care for older adults that are the subject of this chapter. First, an overview of health disparities is presented. Second, the historical evidence in oral health and health care disparities is highlighted. Third, some of the issues in documenting social disparities in oral health and health care among older adults are discussed. Finally, a research agenda is offered to study social disparities in oral health and health care among older adults.

Health Disparities: An Overview

While some improvements in the health of the U.S. population have occurred over time, the persistence of disparities between groups, notably racial/ethnic and socioeconomic groups, indicates that such improvements have been uneven.

L.N. Borrell
Department of Epidemiology, Mailman School of Public Health, Columbia University, New York 10032, USA, Tel: 212-304-6413, Fax: 212-544-4221
email: lnb2@columbia.edu

I.B. Lamster, M.E. Northridge (eds.), *Improving Oral Health for the Elderly*,
© Springer Science+Business Media, LLC 2008

Table 3.1 Distribution of selected sociodemographic characteristics in persons 65 years of age and older, United States, 2000

Characteristic	Percentage
Age group in years	
65–74	52.4
75–84	35.5
85+	12.1
Female	58.8
Marital status by gender	
Men	
Married, spouse present	71.2
Widowed	14.3
Women	
Married, spouse present	41.1
Widowed	44.3
Foreign-born	10.8
Speak a language other than English	12.6
Race/Ethnicity	
White, non-Hispanic	83.6
Black, non-Hispanic	8.1
American Indian/Alaska Native	0.4
Asian	2.3
Native Hawaiian/Other Pacific Islander	0.1
Hispanic	5.0
High school graduate or more by race/ethnicity	
White, non-Hispanic	76.1
Black, non-Hispanic	51.6
Asian	70.4
Hispanic	36.3
Median household income in US$	23,787
Median net worth, excluding home equity in US$	23,369
Lives below poverty level by race/ethnicity	
White, non-Hispanic	8.0
Black, non-Hispanic	23.7
Hispanic	19.5
Health insurance	
Medicare and private	63.1
Medicare and medicaid	7.6
Medicare only	26.7
Resides in nursing home	4.3

Source: U.S. Census Bureau. Current Population Reports, pp. 23–209, 65+ in the United States: 2005. Washington, DC: U.S. Census Bureau.

Indeed, this improvement differential has actually contributed toward widening the disparities gap (Andersen et al., 1987; Manton et al., 1987; Miller, 1987; Williams and Collins, 1995; Williams, 1999; Lillie-Blanton et al., 1996; U.S. Department of Health and Human Services, 2000b; Freid et al., 2003; Lethbridge-Cejku et al., 2004; National Center for Health Statistics, 2006; Williams and Jackson, 2005).

Furthermore, although the long-standing focus of health comparisons in the United States has been race/ethnicity, the effects of socioeconomic position (SEP) have also been documented. Differences between the "haves" and the "have-nots" have been documented for decades and remain pervasive (Cooper, 1993; Williams and Collins, 1995; Feinstein, 1993; Manton et al., 1987; Navarro, 1990). Lower SEP individuals have worse health outcomes (i.e., premature mortality, morbidity, and life expectancy) than their higher SEP counterparts. Likewise, evidence shows that such differences have been increasing over time, and that these differences are greater within racial/ethnic groups than the racial/ethnic differences across groups (Williams, 1999; Williams and Collins, 1995; Williams and Jackson, 2005). For example, health differences by SEP are greater among African Americans than among whites (Williams, 1999; Williams and Collins, 1995; Williams and Jackson, 2005).

Among these documented health disparities are oral health disparities. More specifically, population health disparities in dental caries and periodontal diseases, the most common oral diseases, have been reported from national and local surveys (Kelly and Van Kirk, 1965; Kelly and Harvey, 1979; Anonymous, 1993; Caplan and Weintraub, 1993; White et al., 1995; U.S. Department of Health and Human Services, 2000b; Beltran-Aguilar et al., 2005; Burt and Eklund, 2005). These studies consistently document that blacks, low-income populations, and those with lower educational attainment exhibited worse oral health conditions than non-Hispanic whites, high-income populations, and those with higher educational attainment.

Similarly, evidence suggests that not only unequal access to care but unequal treatment may be an issue (Smedley et al., 2002; Burt and Eklund, 2005; U.S. Department of Health and Human Services, 2000b). For example, blacks, Hispanics, and Asians are less likely not only to have health insurance than non-Hispanic whites, but also to receive major therapeutic procedures when seeking care. These findings have been reported even when access to care is not an issue, i.e., individuals seeking care at the Veteran Administration Hospital and Medicaid/Medicare recipients. Because dental insurance coverage is not usually part of health insurance packages, it is expected that oral health care disparities are wider than other health disparities, although they are seldom reported. For example, people with dental insurance are more likely to visit the dentist than those without dental insurance. Although race/ethnicity, income, and education are intertwined, blacks, Hispanics, low-income populations, and those with lower educational attainment are less likely to visit the dentist within the past year than non-Hispanic whites, high-income populations, and those with higher educational attainment (Burt and Eklund, 2005). Thus, it is possible that these characteristics act synergistically to increase disparities in access to care, i.e., poor blacks are less likely to access care than poor whites.

Although disparities in oral health and health care have been pervasive in the United States, it is not until recently that interest in health disparities has sparked attention among researchers and policy makers. For example, the 1985 *Secretary's Task Force on Black and Minority Health* (U.S. Department of Health and Human Services, 1985) raised awareness of the health differences between minority groups and the white majority population in the United States. This report was motivated by the release of the Department of Health and Human Services report, "Health, United States 1983" (National Center for Health Statistics, 1983), and underscored the point that although the health of the overall population had significantly improved, blacks and other minority groups were experiencing a disproportionate burden of disease and death. Although this report was the eighth of its kind on the health status of the nation, it was the first report to go beyond the black/white dichotomy by presenting health status information according to ethnicity, namely for Hispanics and non-Hispanics. Moreover, information on Mexican Americans, Puerto Ricans, and Cubans was included whenever the data were available.

Similar to the Secretary's Report, Healthy People 2000 and Healthy People 2010 also documented disparities in disease and death between minority and majority groups (U.S. Department of Health and Human Services, 1991, 2000a). These reviews on health disparities suggest that while the health status of Americans has improved over time, this improvement has been unequal across groups. These findings led to one of the two overarching goals of Healthy People 2010, that is, "to eliminate health disparities among segments of the population, including differences that occur by gender, race or ethnicity, education or income, disability, geographic location, or sexual orientation" (U.S. Department of Health and Human Services, 2000a). Healthy People 2000 and Healthy People 2010 are the continuation of a national health initiative launched in the United States in 1979 with the release of Healthy People: The Surgeon General's Report on Health Promotion and Disease Prevention (U.S. Department of Health and Human Services, 1979).

The Institute of Medicine also called for the elimination of health disparities with a focus on health care in 2002 (Smedley et al., 2002). Although in the United Kingdom and other countries, the terms "inequality" and "inequity" are commonly used when referring to differences in health status among population groups, the United States has adopted the term "health disparities" for government action. Because social conditions shape disparities in health for disadvantaged groups, notably racial/ethnic and socioeconomic groups, the term "social disparities in health" is commonly shortened to "health disparities".

Oral Health, Oral Health Care, and Health Disparities

Despite scientific documentation of oral health disparities by race/ethnicity, SEP, sex/gender, and age group since data have been collected in the United States (U.S. Department of Health and Human Services, 2000b), little attention has been paid to these disparities *within* a growing segment of the U.S. population, namely, adults 65 years of age and older (hereafter referred to as older adults). This lack of scientific attention has been evident before and after the publication of the first *Surgeon General's Report on Oral Health* (U.S. Department of Health and Human Services, 2000b). The publication of this report parallels Healthy People 2010 (U.S. Department of Health and Human Services, 2000a), the first of its kind, and not only underscores the importance of oral health, but also calls attention to the inequities and disparities in oral health status of the American population.

Oral health diseases, including tooth loss, increase with age. An ongoing challenge is to deliver health care to those suffering from systemic diseases associated with oral health diseases. Systemic diseases may exacerbate oral diseases due to medication use (e.g., resulting in xerostomia or dry mouth) or directly (e.g., as occurs with diabetes and musculoskeletal disorders). Findings from the *Surgeon General's Report on Oral Health* suggest that older Americans affected by oral health diseases are more likely to be economically disadvantaged, more likely to be minorities, and more likely to lack dental health insurance than those with good oral health (U.S. Department of Health and Human Services, 2000b). Therefore, social disparities in oral health and health care among older Americans are now present and are likely to increase as racial/ethnic minorities increase in age.

In the decade prior to the release of the *Surgeon General's Report on Oral Health*, several studies investigated dental caries, periodontal diseases, tooth loss, oral cancer, and health care among older adults. Nonetheless, only a few studies explicitly focused on social disparities in oral health and health care (U.S. Department of Health and Human Services, 2000b). For example, previous studies found that periodontal disease using different definitions (i.e., clinical attachment level or CAL, probing depth or PD, or a combination of these outcome measures) is more common among older African American and low-SEP adults than among their white and high-SEP counterparts.

Scientific evidence regarding oral health disparities in periodontal disease among older adults has been consistently reported in both cross-sectional and longitudinal studies (Beck et al., 1990, 1997a,b). Moreover, findings of oral health disparities have also been documented with regard to tooth loss and dental caries in older adults. Finally, these findings of oral health disparities for older adults have been confirmed in both national and international data (Graves et al., 1992; Strubig and Depping, 1992; Galan et al., 1993; Drake et al., 1994; Lawrence et al., 1995; Lawrence et al., 1996; Beck and Drake, 1997; Drake et al., 1997; Marcus et al., 1997; Drake et al., 1995; Hunt et al., 1995). While helpful, this information is limited in scope because it does not represent the racial/ethnic diversity of the American population.

Although the *Surgeon General's Report on Oral Health* (U.S. Department of Health and Human Services, 2000b), together with the oral health objectives set forth in Healthy People 2010 (U.S. Department of Health and Human Services, 2000a), represents landmark documents that strive to measure and report oral health disparities according to sex/gender, race/ethnicity, education, and income, the availability of data to document these disparities represents a major challenge in general, and more so for certain segments of the population such as older adults. For example, to determine the baseline status for selected groups of the population, Healthy People 2010 relies on national surveys and representative local surveys to determine baseline prevalence estimates by race/ethnicity, gender, and education (as an indicator of SEP) for dental caries and periodontal diseases, the most common oral health diseases in children and adults, respectively. However, the lack of a uniform and systematic methodology to document existing disparities across groups between studies at the national and local level, as well as the lack of data for certain groups of the U.S. population, makes comparisons and further documentation of the existing disparities extremely difficult.

Despite the extant body of research in oral health disparities, it is not clear whether or not the findings generated through every study could be used to document or track the magnitude of the increase or decrease in oral disparities across groups of the population over time. For example, a PubMed search was conducted for the period January 1, 2000 to January 25, 2007. Note that PubMed is a service of the U.S. National Library of Medicine that includes over 17 million citations from MEDLINE and other life science journals for biomedical articles back to the 1950s (see www.pubmed.gov). The search was limited to adults aged 65 and older and used a combination of five key words denoting "disparities," i.e., differences, disparities, race, ethnicity, and SEP indicators, along with six key words denoting "oral diseases," i.e., dental caries, periodontal diseases, periodontitis, oral cancer, access to care, and oral health, anywhere in the text of the article.

A total of 237 citations were obtained. Of these, 107 citations were excluded because either the studies were not relevant to social disparities or were literature reviews. The 130 remaining citations included studies in the United States and elsewhere limited to people aged 65 and older or a range of ages, which included adults 65 years and older. Of these 130 studies, 71 (55%) were fully conducted in the United States. Moreover, nearly a quarter (32) of the 130 studies were conducted specifically in adults 60 years and older in the United States and elsewhere. These latter studies will be the focus of this section of the chapter because they examine the oral health needs of the older population. The outcome measures of the identified studies included tooth loss, dental caries (coronal and root), periodontal diseases, treatment need, oral cancer, access to and use of care, self-rated oral health, quality of life, and health attitudes.

Even though a large proportion of the final 32 studies were conducted outside of the United States, the Healthy People 2010 criteria will be applied to all of them in order to define social disparities in oral health and health care. Race/ethnicity is the most commonly used social determinant in the United States. However, other countries use the term "minorities" or "immigrants" to define groups other than the majority population. When the abstracts and articles were examined for these 32 references, several methodological problems were identified: (1) few published studies addressed social disparities in oral health and health care from the viewpoint of the Healthy People 2010 criteria, even for those studies conducted in the United States; (2) no reference group was used in some studies or the analysis was performed in a single racial/ethnic group; (3) the case definition for the outcomes of interest varied across studies, e.g., periodontal diseases was defined using a combination of clinical attachment loss (CAL) and pocket depth (PD), or CAL or PD, separately; and (4) the measure used to assess group differences varied across studies, for example, mean differences and prevalence for dental caries and prevalence, means, and odds ratios (ORs) for periodontal diseases.

These methodological issues are crucial to address if we are to track social disparities across groups and over time to assess progress and setbacks in eliminating social disparities in health in the United States. This following section will cover these issues for older adults in the context of the existing evidence on oral health and health care.

Issues in Documenting Social Disparities in Oral Health and Health Care

Few of the identified published studies presented data on social disparities in oral health and health care according to sex/gender, race/ethnicity, education/income, or geographic location. This pattern held true both for studies conducted in the United States where Healthy People 2010 originated as well as for studies conducted elsewhere. For example, only five of the identified studies presented data according to sex/gender (Lin, et al., 2001; Avlund et al., 2004; Shah, 2003; Avlund et al., 2003; Ikebe et al., 2004), three according to race/ethnicity (Vargas et al., 2001; Persson et al., 2004; Makhija et al., 2006), seven according to socioeconomic indicators such as income and education (Aleksejuniene et al., 2000; Vargas et al., 2001; Ettinger et al., 2004; Ikebe et al., 2004; Shah and Sundaram, 2004; Avlund et al., 2005; Makhija et al., 2006), and eight according to place of residence (Aleksejuniene et al., 2000; Corbet et al., 2001; Lo et al., 2001; Centers for Disease Control and Prevention, 2003; Vargas et al., 2003; Ettinger et al., 2004; Shah, 2004; Makhija et al., 2006).

Using data from a population-based, cross-sectional survey of men and women aged 75 years and older in a suburban area of Copenhagen in Denmark, Avlund et al. (2003) examined social inequalities in oral health as indicated by the number of teeth present in the mouth at examination. This study found that the odds ratio of having a greater number of missing teeth was associated with not owning a house and having no education after adjusting for income in men, while for women, being of low income and having no education were associated with a greater number of missing teeth after adjusting for housing tenure. However, the authors examined the association of education, income, occupation, and housing tenure with number of teeth in women and men, separately. Thus, comparisons between men and women cannot be made to assess significant differences by sex/gender.

Although some of these studies included more than one of the social indicators underscored by Healthy People 2010, the analyses are stratified by a particular indicator ignoring the variation that could be hidden by stratifying one indicator by another, i.e., sex/gender differences within racial/ethnic groups. For example, Makhija et al. (2006) examined oral health-related quality of life according to race, education, income, and transportation difficulties in older adults in Alabama. The analysis was descriptive and failed to adjust for potential confounders. The study found that oral health-related quality of life was decreased in both dentate and edentulous older adults. Moreover, African Americans, those with a sixth grade education or less, those with income less than $16,000 per year, and those with transportation difficulties were more likely to have decrements in oral health-related quality of life compared to dentate elderly only. These findings suggest that oral health-related quality of life may be related to dentate status.

Finally, none of the identified studies compared oral health conditions by age group. The latter could help not only elucidate differences in oral health status, but also to identify the specific needs of subgroups within individuals 60 years of age and older.

Another shortcoming of these studies is the lack of a reference group. The presence and choice of a reference group is important because it helps to not only document differences between groups, but also identify the magnitude of the disparity in question within or between groups (Carter-Pokras and Baquet, 2002; Keppel et al., 2005; Braveman, 2006; Braveman and Cubbin, 2003; Harper and Lynch, 2006; Gakidou et al., 2000). Moreover, the reference group of choice will help to provide continuity for group comparisons over time (Keppel et al., 2005). Among the choices for reference groups are: the total population; the group with the best estimate, i.e., lower prevalence of the outcome; the group with the largest population or most stable estimate; or a fixed estimate, i.e., the target estimates for Healthy People 2010.

Each of these referent group choices has advantages and disadvantages. The estimates for the overall population represent an average of the subgroups, yet this estimate is driven by the larger population subgroup. Using this approach might lead to lower or higher estimates according to the subpopulation with the lowest or highest risk. Further, this approach may overlook the range of risk across subgroups in the population. The use of the best estimates as the reference group would provide a more accurate picture of the magnitude of the problem, yet the best estimate may change over time and therefore will not offer a good reference. The use of the group with the largest population may offer the best choice for group comparisons over time unless there are fast shifts in population size. Finally, the use of a fixed estimate could be problematic due to a secular trend in case definition and population changes. Evidence suggests that the use of these approaches to investigate health disparities in socioeconomic status using multiple socioeconomic indicators has proven useful across different outcomes (Braveman et al., 2005; Krieger et al., 1997; Krieger et al., 2002; Braveman and Gruskin, 2003).

Although differences exist by sex/gender, race/ethnicity, education/income, and geographic location for most oral health conditions among older adults, few of the studies reviewed here chose a reference group a priori or presented data by these indicators (Centers for Disease Control and Prevention, 2003; Shah and Sundaram, 2004; Makhija et al., 2006; Vargas et al., 2003; Vargas et al., 2001). Interestingly, the majority of these studies used multivariable techniques and included multiple covariates in the analyses.

Using data from the Third National Health and Nutrition Examination Survey and the 1995, 1997, and 1998 National Health Interview Surveys in the United States, Vargas et al. (2003) examined trends in access to oral health care utilization (having dental insurance, having a dental visit in the past year, and frequency of dental visits) and oral health conditions (self-rated health, unmet treatment needs, untreated dental caries, decayed, missing, and filled teeth or DMFT, and edentulism) in adults 65 years of age and older by place of residence. The study further presented information by poverty status. When compared to urban older adults, rural older adults were more likely to be uninsured for dental care and were less likely to report dental visits in the past year. Rural older adults also were more likely to be edentulous and report poor dental health than their urban counterparts. There were no differences in unmet dental needs, percentage of people with untreated caries, or mean DMFT by place of residence. Although the differences between poor/near poor and non-poor did not reach statistical significance for any of the indicators, the poor/near poor exhibited worse outcomes than the non-poor regardless of the area of residence.

Although all of these studies examined periodontal diseases, the case definition for the oral health conditions used across studies was different, which makes any further comparisons across studies problematic. For example, three studies examined periodontal diseases (Shah and Sundaram, 2003; Corbet et al., 2001; Borges-Yanez and colleagues, 2006) using different definitions. Corbet et al. (2001) defined periodontal diseases as a combination of the Community Periodontal Index (CPI) and attachment loss. Shah and Sundaram (2003) used the Community Periodontal Index Treatment Needs. Borges-Yanez and colleagues (2006) defined periodontitis as at least one site with loss of attachment greater or equal to 6 mm.

Use of a single clinical measure to identify periodontal diseases is too unspecific for rigorous research. A recommendation would be to use the distribution of clinical attachment loss (CAL) and/or pocket depth (PD) across selected characteristics of the population. For people older than 65 years of age, the case definition of periodontal diseases might meaningfully be based on the mean clinical attachment loss (CAL) and/or pocket depth (PD) at the 90th percentile.

Finally, the type of measure (absolute or relative) to document group differences would facilitate comparisons between study results over time (Keppel et al., 2005). Corbet et al. (2001) and Borges-Yanez and colleagues (2006), while admittedly using different case definitions, nonetheless used odds ratios (a relative measure) to document the likelihood of having periodontal diseases according to sex/gender and place of residence. Shah and Sundaram (2004) and Vargas et al. (2003) used percentage (an absolute measure) to document differences in the presence of untreated caries between groups. Finally, Lin and colleagues (2001) used mean DMFT (an absolute measure) to document these differences. In summary, most studies documenting differences in edentulism and use of care used absolute measures such as the prevalence or mean number of dental visits.

Conclusions and Future Directions

Although social disparities in oral health and health care have been pervasive over the years across different segments of the population defined by sex/gender, race/ethnicity, and socioeconomic position (SEP), a critical review of the scientific evidence to date suggests that little has been done to document social disparities among a growing segment of our population, namely, adults aged 65 years or older. Specifically, few studies have addressed social disparities in oral health and health care among older adults. Those that have are largely descriptive in nature and ignore the social groups defined by society and further complexity obtained by considering the social disparities within and between these groups. Research exploring the intersection of age, sex/gender, racial/ethnicity, and SEP is crucial not only in understanding the existing social disparities in oral health, but in improving access to care and treatment in older adults.

As the older adult population continues to increase in diversity across race/ethnicity and socioeconomic position (SEP), it is our responsibility as committed scientists and practitioners to find ways to embrace this diversity while acknowledging the discrimination experienced by groups defined by society and its hierarchy. This is a daunting task due to the complicated intersections of race/ethnicity, low socioeconomic resources, and dental health insurance coverage. Modifying the dental school curriculum to better prepare future generations of dental providers to take into account the sociodemographic characteristics and needs of the older population may contribute to eliminating current social disparities in oral health and health care.

Changes in Medicare, such as the addition of dental care coverage, are important conceptually, but are far from becoming a viable reality in the current health care climate. One possibility might be to offer Medicare recipients Medicaid coverage so that they obtain access to dental services in those states offering reimbursement for oral health care. Policy solutions are extremely important nowadays given the rising cost of oral health care. The oral health needs of the older population have changed from full dentures to more complex dental treatments such as periodontal and endodontic treatment as they are more likely to retain their teeth. In addition, to improve access to care to this population, the shortage of dental providers in disadvantaged areas that accept the type of insurance this segment of the population is likely to carry (usually Medicaid) will need to be addressed. Such actions may be crucial first steps in eliminating social disparities in oral health and health care for older adults.

References

Aleksejuniene, J., D. Holst, and H. M. Eriksen. 2000. Patterns of dental caries and treatment experience in elderly Lithuanians. *Gerodontology* 17 (2):77–86.

Andersen, R. M., R. M. Mullner, and L. J. Cornelius. 1987. Black-white differences in health status: methods or substance?. [Review] [30 refs]. *Milbank Quarterly* 65 (Suppl 1):72–99.

Anonymous. 1993. Toward improving the oral health of Americans: an overview of oral health status, resources, and care delivery. Oral Health Coordinating Committee, Public Health Service. *Public Health Reports* 108 (6):657–72.

Avlund, K., P. Holm-Pedersen, D. E. Morse, M. Viitanen, and B. Winblad. 2004. Tooth loss and caries prevalence in very old Swedish people: the relationship to cognitive function and functional ability. *Gerodontology* 21 (1):17–26.

———. 2005. The strength of two indicators of social position on oral health among persons over the age of 80 years. *Journal of Public Health Dentistry* 65 (4):231–9.

Avlund, K., B. E. Holstein, M. Osler, M. T. Damsgaard, P. Holm-Pedersen, and N. K. Rasmussen. 2003. Social position and health in old age: the relevance of different indicators of social position. *Scandinavian Journal of Public Health* 31 (2):126–36.

Beck, J. D., and C. W. Drake. 1997. Do root lesions tend to develop in the same people who develop coronal lesions? *Journal of Public Health Dentistry* 57 (2):82–8.

Beck, J. D., G. G. Koch, R. G. Rozier, and G. E. Tudor. 1990. Prevalence and risk indicators for periodontal attachment loss in a population of older community-dwelling blacks and whites. *Journal of Periodontology* 61 (8):521–8.

Beck, J. D., T. Sharp, G. G. Koch, and S. Offenbacher. 1997a. A 5-year study of attachment loss and tooth loss in community-dwelling older adults. *Journal of Periodontology Research* 32 (6):516–23.

——. 1997b. A study of attachment loss patterns in survivor teeth at 18 months, 36 months and 5 years in community-dwelling older adults. *Journal of Periodontology Research* 32 (6): 497–505.

Beltran-Aguilar, E. D., L. K. Barker, M. T. Canto, B. A. Dye, B. F. Gooch, S. O. Griffin, J. Hyman, F. Jaramillo, A. Kingman, R. Nowjack-Raymer, R. H. Selwitz, and T. Wu. 2005. Surveillance for dental caries, dental sealants, tooth retention, edentulism, and enamel fluorosis—United States, 1988–1994 and 1999–2002. *Morbidity and Mortality Weekly Report Surveilancel Summaries* 54 (3):1–43.

Borges-Yanez, S. A., M. E. Irigoyen-Camacho, and G. Maupome. 2006. Risk factors and prevalence of periodontitis in community-dwelling elders in Mexico. *Journal of Clinical Periodontology* 33 (3):184–94.

Braveman, P. 2006. Health disparities and health equity: concepts and measurement. *Annual Review ofPublic Health* 27:167–94.

Braveman, P. A., C. Cubbin, S. Egerter, S. Chideya, K. S. Marchi, M. Metzler, and S. Posner. 2005. Socioeconomic status in health research: one size does not fit all. *Journal of the American Medical Association* 294 (22):2879–88.

Braveman, P., and C. Cubbin. 2003. Optimal SES indicators cannot be prescribed across all outcomes. *American Journal of Public Health* 93 (1):12–13; author reply 13.

Braveman, P., and S. Gruskin. 2003. Defining equity in health. *Journal of Epidemiology and Community Health* 57 (4):254–8.

Burt, B. A., and S. A. Eklund. 2005. *Dentistry, Dental Practice, and the Community*. 6th ed. St. Louis, MO: Elsevier Saunders.

Caplan, D. J., and J. A. Weintraub. 1993. The oral health burden in the United States: a summary of recent epidemiologic studies. *Journal of Dental Education* 57 (12):853–62.

Carter-Pokras, O., and C. Baquet. 2002. What is a "health disparity"? *Public Health Reports* 117 (5):426–34.

Centers for Disease Control and, Prevention. 2003. Public health and aging: retention of natural teeth among older adults—United States, 2002. *Morbidity and Mortality Weekly Report* 52 (50):1226–9.

Cooper, R. S. 1993. Health and the social status of blacks in the United States. *Annals of Epidemiology* 3 (2):137–44.

Corbet, E. F., M. C. Wong, and H. C. Lin. 2001. Periodontal conditions in adult Southern Chinese. *Journal of Dental Research* 80 (5):1480–5.

Drake, C. W., J. D. Beck, H. P. Lawrence, and G. G. Koch. 1997. Three-year coronal caries incidence and risk factors in North Carolina elderly. *Caries Research* 31 (1):1–7.

Drake, C. W., R. J. Hunt, J. D. Beck, and G. G. Koch. 1994. Eighteen-month coronal caries incidence in North Carolina older adults. *Journal of Public Health Dentistry* 54 (1):24–30.

Drake, C. W., R. J. Hunt, and G. G. Koch. 1995. Three-year tooth loss among black and white older adults in North Carolina. *Journal of Dental Research* 74 (2):675–80.

Ettinger, R. L., J. J. Warren, S. M. Levy, J. S. Hand, J. A. Merchant, and A. M. Stromquist. 2004. Oral health: perceptions of need in a rural Iowa county. *Special Care in Dentistry* 24 (1):13–21.

Feinstein, J. S. 1993. The relationship between socioeconomic status and health: a review of the literature. [Review] [74 refs]. *Milbank Quarterly* 71 (2):279–322.

Freid, V.M.., K. Prager, A.P. Mackay, and H. Xia. 2003. Chartbook on Trends in the Health of Americans. Health, United States, 2003. In *Health, United States*. Hyattsville, MD: National Center for Health Statistics.

Gakidou, E. E., C. J. Murray, and J. Frenk. 2000. Defining and measuring health inequality: an approach based on the distribution of health expectancy. *Bulletin of the World Health Organization* 78 (1):42–54.

Galan, D., O. Odlum, and M. Brecx. 1993. Oral health status of a group of elderly Canadian Inuit (Eskimo). *Community Dentistry and Oral Epidemiology* 21 (1):53–6.

Gist, Y.J., and L.I. Hetzel. 2004. We the people: Aging in the United States. U.S. Department of Commerce. Economics and Statistics Administration. Washington, DC: U.S. Census Bureau.

Graves, R. C., J. D. Beck, J. A. Disney, and C. W. Drake. 1992. Root caries prevalence in black and white North Carolina adults over age 65. *Journal of Public Health Dentistry* 52 (2): 94–101.

Harper, S., and J. Lynch. 2006. Measuring health inequalities In *Methods in Social Epidemiology*, edited by M. J. Oakes and J. S. Kaufman. San Francisco, CA: Jossey-Bass.

He, W., M. Sengupta, V.A. Velkoff, and K.A. DeBarros. 2005. U.S. Census Bureau. Current Population Reports, P23-209, 65+ in the United States: 2005. Washington, DC: U.S. Census Bureau.

Hetzel, L., and A. Smith. 2001. The 65 years and over population: 2000. U.S. Department of Commerce. Economics and Statistics Administration. In *Census 2000 Brief*. Washington, DC: U.S. Census Bureau.

Hunt, R. J., C. W. Drake, and J. D. Beck. 1995. Eighteen-month incidence of tooth loss among older adults in North Carolina. *American Journal of Public Health* 85 (4):561–3.

Ikebe, K., C. A. Watkins, R. L. Ettinger, H. Sajima, and T. Nokubi. 2004. Application of short-form oral health impact profile on elderly Japanese. *Gerodontology* 21 (3):167–76.

Kelly, J. E., and C. R. Harvey. 1979. Basic data on dental examination findings of persons 1–74 years. United States, 1971–1974. *Vital and Health Statistics – Series 11: Data From the National Health Survey* 11 (214):1–33.

Kelly, J. E., and L. E. Van Kirk. 1965. Periodontal disease in adults. *Vital and Health Statistics – Series 1: Programs and Collection Procedures* 12:1–30.

Keppel, K., E. Pamuk, J. Lynch, O. Carter-Pokras, Insun Kim, V. Mays, J. Pearcy, V. Schoenbach, and J. S. Weissman. 2005. Methodological issues in measuring health disparities. *Vital and Health Staisticst 2* (141):1–16.

Krieger, N., J. T. Chen, P. D. Waterman, M. J. Soobader, S. V. Subramanian, and R. Carson. 2002. Geocoding and monitoring of US socioeconomic inequalities in mortality and cancer incidence: does the choice of area-based measure and geographic level matter?: the Public Health Disparities Geocoding Project. *American Journal of Epidemiol* 156 (5):471–82.

Krieger, N., D. R. Williams, and N. E. Moss. 1997. Measuring social class in US public health research: concepts, methodologies, and guidelines. [Review] [202 refs]. *Annual Review of Public Health* 18:341–78.

Lawrence, H. P., R. J. Hunt, and J. D. Beck. 1995. Three-year root caries incidence and risk modeling in older adults in North Carolina. *Journal of Public Health Dentistry* 55 (2): 69–78.

Lawrence, H. P., R. J. Hunt, J. D. Beck, and G. M. Davies. 1996. Five-year incidence rates and intraoral distribution of root caries among community-dwelling older adults. *Caries Research* 30 (3):169–79.

Lethbridge-Cejku, M., J.S. Schiller, and L. Bernadel. 2004. Summary health statistics for US Adults: National Health Interview Survey, 2002. *Vital Health Statistics* 10 (222):1–160.

Lillie-Blanton, M., P. E. Parsons, H. Gayle, and A. Dievler. 1996. Racial differences in health: not just black and white, but shades of gray. *Annual Review of Public Health* 17:411–48.

Lin, H. C., M. C. Wong, H. G. Zhang, E. C. Lo, and E. Schwarz. 2001. Coronal and root caries in Southern Chinese adults. *Journal of Dental Research* 80 (5):1475–9.

Lo, E. C., H. C. Lin, Z. J. Wang, M. C. Wong, and E. Schwarz. 2001. Utilization of dental services in Southern China. *Journal of Dental Research* 80 (5):1471–4.

Makhija, S. K., G. H. Gilbert, M. J. Boykin, M. S. Litaker, R. M. Allman, P. S. Baker, J. L. Locher, and C. S. Ritchie. 2006. The relationship between sociodemographic factors and oral health-related quality of life in dentate and edentulous community-dwelling older adults. *Journal of the American Geriatrics Society* 54 (11):1701–12.

Manton, K. G., C. H. Patrick, and K. W. Johnson. 1987. Health differentials between blacks and whites: recent trends in mortality and morbidity. [Review] [55 refs]. *Milbank Quarterly* 65 (Suppl 1):129–99.

Marcus, M., N. M. Reifel, and T. T. Nakazono. 1997. Clinical measure and treatment needs. *Advances in Dental Research* 11 (2):263–71.

Miller, S. M. 1987. Race in the health of America. *Milbank Quarterly* 65 (Suppl 2):500–31.

National Center for Health Statistics. Health, United States, 2006 with Chartbook on Trends in the Health of Americans. Hyattsville, MD.

National Center for Health Statistics: Health, United States, 1983. DHHS Pub. No. (PHS) 84–1232. Public Health Service. Washington. U.S. Government Printing Office.

Navarro, V. 1990. Race or class versus race and class: mortality differential in the United States. *Lancet* 336:1230–1240.

Persson, G. R., R. E. Persson, L. G. Hollender, and H. A. Kiyak. 2004. The impact of ethnicity, gender, and marital status on periodontal and systemic health of older subjects in the Trials to Enhance Elders' Teeth and Oral Health (TEETH). *Journal of Periodontology* 75 (6):817–23.

Shah, N. 2003. Gender issues and oral health in elderly Indians. *International Dental Journal* 53 (6):475–84.

Shah, N., H. Parkash, and K. R. Sunderam. 2004. Edentulousness, denture wear and denture needs of Indian elderly—a community-based study. *Journal of Oral Rehabilitation* 31 (5):467–76.

Shah, N., and K. R. Sundaram. 2003. Impact of socio-demographic variables, oral hygiene practices and oral habits on periodontal health status of Indian elderly: a community-based study. *Indian Journal of Dental Research* 14 (4):289–97.

——. 2004. Impact of socio-demographic variables, oral hygiene practices, oral habits and diet on dental caries experience of Indian elderly: a community-based study. *Gerodontology* 21 (1):43–50.

Smedley, B.D., A.Y. Stith, and A.R. Nelson, eds. 2002. *Institute of Medicine, Committee on understanding and eliminating racial and ethnic disparities in health care. Unequal treatment: Confronting racial and ethnic disparities in health care.* Washington, DC: National Academy Press.

Strubig, W., and M. Depping. 1992. Coronal caries and restorations in an elderly population in Germany. *Community Dentistry and Oral Epidemiology* 20 (4):235–8.

U.S. Department of Health and Human Services. Healthy People: The Surgeon General's Report on Health Promotion and Disease Prevention. 1979. Washington, DC: U.S. Government Printing Office.

U.S. Department of Health and Human Services. Healthy People 2000: National health promotion and disease prevention objectives for the nation. 1991. Washington, DC: Public Health Service.

U.S. Department of Health and Human Services. Healthy People 2010: Understanding and Improving Health. 2000a. 2nd ed. 2000. Washington, DC: U.S. Government Printing Office.

U.S. Department of Health and Human Services. Oral Health in America: A Report of the Surgeon General. 2000b. Rockville, MD: U.S. Department of Health and Human Services, National Institute of Dental and Craniofacial Research, National Institutes of Health.

U.S. Department of Health and Human Services. Report of the Secretary's Task Force on Black and Minority Health. 1985. Washington, DC: U.S. Government Printing Office.

Vargas, C. M., E. A. Kramarow, and J. A. Yellowitz. 2001. The oral health of older Americans. *Aging Trends* 3:1–8.

Vargas, C. M., J. A. Yellowitz, and K. L. Hayes. 2003. Oral health status of older rural adults in the United States. *Journal of the American Dental Association* 134 (4):479–86.

White, B. A., D. J. Caplan, and J. A. Weintraub. 1995. A quarter century of changes in oral health in the United States. *Journal of Dental Education* 59 (1):19–57.

Williams, D. R. 1999. Race, socioeconomic status, and health. The added effects of racism and discrimination. [Review] [54 refs]. *Annals of the New York Academy of Sciences* 896:173–88.

Williams, D. R., and C. Collins. 1995. US Socioeconomic and Racial-Differences in Health – Patterns and Explanations. *Annual Review of Sociology* 21:349–386.

Williams, D. R., and P. B. Jackson. 2005. Social sources of racial disparities in health. *Health Affairs (Millwood)* 24 (2):325–34.

Chapter 4
Access, Place of Residence and Interdisciplinary Opportunities

Healthy People (2000) stated, 'Having adequate access to medical and dental care can reduce morbidity and mortality, preserve function and enhance overall quality of life'.) This statement is particularly relevant to older adults as their oral health has improved over the past 50 years, and their utilization of dental services has increased (Vargas, Kamarow, & Yellowitz, 2001).)Older adults have an increasing need for care; however, barriers to care increase with age, and many elders do not receive care on a routine basis (Stanton and Rutherford 2003). The Surgeon General's report on oral health identified the elderly among the populations most vulnerable to poor dental care (U.S. DHHS, 2000).)

Ensuring that older adults receive routine oral health care is critical, as basic oral health services are essential components of primary health care (Dolan & Atchison, 1993) and having routine preventive care is associated with good oral health. Although there are no studies to support it, the U.S. Public Health Service recommends annual oral examinations for all adults (United States Public Health Service, 1994). Yet many older adults only seek care when they are in pain or discomfort, which predisposes them to poor oral health.

More of the today's elderly are retaining their natural teeth, with fewer adults experiencing total tooth loss (edentulism). In 2003–2004, one-quarter of noninstitutionalized adults 65 years of age and older were edentulous compared to 33 percent in 1993 (Lethbridge-Çejku, Rose, & Vickerie, 2004). Although there was no gender difference in the rate of edentulism, there were large differences in the prevalence of edentulism by socioeconomic status. Persons with family incomes below the poverty line were almost twice as likely to be edentulous as those with incomes at or above the poverty level. In addition, edentulism was higher among Black persons than among White persons (Kramarow, Lentzner, Rooks, Weeks, & Saydah, 1999).

J.A. Yellowitz
University of Maryland, Baltimore College of Dental Surgery, 650 West Baltimore Street Suite 3211, Baltimore MD 21201, Tel: 410-706-7254, Fax: 410-706-7745
e-mail: jyellowitz@umaryland.edu

I.B. Lamster, M.E. Northridge (eds.), *Improving Oral Health for the Elderly*,
© Springer Science+Business Media, LLC 2008

As older adults retain teeth in their later years, they have an increased risk for oral disease and increased need for care.

Portraying older adults as a single cohort misrepresents the diversity of this population, which can span 35+ years. Typically identified as the population 65 years and older, older adults are the most heterogeneous age cohort, having great variability in their physical, functional and cognitive health as well as their health needs and expectations. Compared to those 85 years and older, the population 65–74 years have better general health and oral health, have maintained more teeth and have a more preventive attitude toward health care. It is anticipated that this pattern will continue in the future, when there will be a higher demand for oral health care.

As people age, they are at greater risk of having one or more chronic diseases, multiple medications and cognitive losses which predispose them to oral disease (Hawkins 1999). Studies have reported an increasing number of associations between oral health and systemic conditions such as diabetes, cardiovascular diseases, stroke and aspiration pneumonia (U.S. DHHS 2000; Elter, Champagne, Offenbacher, & Beck, 2004). Although rarely life-threatening, poor oral health can lead to life-threatening conditions, including malnutrition and dehydration (Shay & Ship 1995), cardiovascular disease (Joshipura et al., 1996) and pneumonia (Scannapieco, 1999). Oral health plays an essential role in the quality of life, nutrition and social interaction of the elderly (Gil-Montoya, Ferrerira de Mello, Cardenas, & Lopez, 2006). When oral health is compromised, overall health and quality of life may be diminished (Ettinger, 1987). This is relevant, given that close to 20 percent of older adults report orofacial pain (Riley, Gilbert, & Heft, 1998), and many go without treatment for oral diseases due to the high cost and limited access to dental care.

Providing oral health services to medically compromised and cognitively impaired older adults can present unique challenges, complicated by medical, functional, behavioral and situational factors. Frail, homebound and nursing home residents are at increased risk for oral disease because of comorbid conditions, cognitive impairments, lack of dental care and inadequate oral hygiene. Individuals with diminished mental capacity are often unable to identify pain, provide good daily care or advocate for themselves. These vulnerabilities become the responsibility of family members, caregivers, guardians and health professionals, to advocate and to ensure adequate oral health care is provided to meet the residents' needs (Mouradian, Huebner, & DePaola, 2004).) Oral health maintenance strategies can reduce the morbidity and mortality in long-term care and assist an increasingly frail and dependent population to age successfully (MacEntee, 2000).)

The intent of this chapter is to review older adults' access and barriers to oral health care and the impact of their place of residence. Emphasis is placed on the access issues of nursing home residents and their oral health status. The role of health professionals' knowledge, attitudes and practices is reviewed and their impact on the oral health of older adults. Finally, in an effort to help reduce some of the key access issue to care, guidelines for a proposed curriculum on oral health for primary care providers are presented.

Access to Care

Although independent elders can obtain oral health care from community-based dental practices, many dental offices are not accessible for adults with physical or cognitive impairments; for example, a dental practice may not be accessible to individuals in wheelchairs or staff members may not be prepared to care for those with cognitive impairments. Having limited access to care increases ones' risk of developing dental problems and complex oral disease. Key elements of access to oral health care for older adults include their physical and cognitive abilities and limitations, financial resources, reimbursement issues, availability of dentists as well as the attitudes and practices of the individual and oral health professional. In addition, many older adults have a diminished awareness, capacity and interest in obtaining oral health care. This decline in interest is further complicated by their need to address age-related physiologic changes, systemic disease and dependence upon a caregiver and/or a reduced capacity to pay for care.

As barriers to oral health care accumulate with age, older adults are an increased risk for poor oral health. Avlund, Holm-Pedersen, and Schroll (2001) found over half of those 75 years and older reported limitations due to chronic conditions adversely affecting their ability to effectively care for themselves, and that these conditions often overshadowed their oral health situation. Postponing care until pain develops eliminates the opportunity to diagnose and treat disease in its early stages, and increases ones' risk of developing a serious, disabling and potentially disfiguring disease.

There is a common misconception among many older adults, their family members, caregivers, health professionals, and policymakers that oral health care is not important for older adults. For some older adults, this misinformation is directly related to the accepted dental beliefs of their time. Many older adults were raised during the Depression when dental services were considered a luxury, and learned early in their life that 'teeth do not last a lifetime' and that 'dentures are inevitable'. In addition, many dentists at that time told their patients with a complete set of dentures that they did not have to return for dental care unless they had pain or discomfort. Being aware of these long-held beliefs helps to explain why some older adults' believe that (a) routine oral health care is not necessary; (b) one set of dentures will last a lifetime and (c) if you don't have pain (i.e., no perceived need), you don't need to see a dentist (Strayer, 1995; Locker & Jokovic 1996). Having no perceived need for care is one of the key barriers to access to care for older adults. In addition, perceived need of care is one of the best predictors of utilization (Holm-Pedersen, Vigild, Nitschke, & Berkey, 2005), and helps to explain why older adults have the lowest rate of utilization and the highest prevalence of edentulism of any adult age group (Marvin, 2001).

Financing Oral Health Care

The ability to obtain oral health care is strongly influenced by having adequate financial resources. With more elderly having discretionary income and retaining their teeth, demand for dental services among the elderly has grown. However, as older adults retire, not only do their financial resources decline, but they also lose employer-sponsored dental insurance plans. With less than one-quarter of adults aged 65 years and older covered by private dental insurance (Vargas, Kamarow, & Yellowitz, 2001; Manski, Goodman, Reid, & Macek, 2004), most dental expenses are paid out of pocket (Manski et al., 2004). In addition, older adults without dental insurance are less likely to have had a recent dental visit, less likely to be using preventive dental services or having all their dental needs addressed, and more likely to be making episodic use of the dental care delivery system (Isman & Isman, 1997). Yet having supplemental medical insurance increases older adults' chances of using dental services. This is likely due to the individual being able to divert some of their savings from medical care to their dental expenses. Many patients lack purchasing power to pay for their care. With medical care costs increasing faster than the general inflation rate, personal resources often do not cover individuals' health care needs (Bailit & Beazoglou, 2006).)

Unlike the coverage it provides for medical care for older adults, the Medicare program does not cover the cost of dental care, with the exception of selection of a few oral health services in very specific situations. Medicare will pay for dental services that are an integral part of a covered procedure (e.g., reconstruction of the jaw following accidental injury), or for extractions done in preparation for radiation treatment for neoplastic diseases of the jaw. Medicare will also make payment for oral examinations, but not treatment, preceding kidney transplantation or heart valve replacement, under certain circumstances (Centers for Medicare & Medicaid Services).)

Dental care was excluded from Medicare in the 1960s, when most of our current health care policies for older adults were being initially developed. At that time, the majority of older adults did not have their own teeth; dental care for the elderly was synonymous with denture care (Burt, 1978). Perhaps in fear of losing their independence or becoming a socialized program, organized dentistry chose not to participate in the Medicare program. The lack of oral health care in Medicare compounds the many barriers to oral care for older adults (Meskin, Dillenberg, Heft, Katz, & Martens, 1990; White, 1994).

Dental services under Title XIX of the Social Security Act, the Medicaid program, are an optional service for the adult population, individuals age 21 and older. States may elect to provide dental services to their adult Medicaid-eligible population or elect not to provide dental services at all as part of its

Medicaid program. While many states provide at least emergency dental services for adults, less than half of the states provide comprehensive dental care. There are no minimum requirements for adult dental coverage (Centers for Medicare & Medicaid).

The 2003 Special Grading Project by Oral Health America, entitled A State of Decay reported that not one older American receives routine dental care under Medicare, and under Medicaid, adult dental care is optional and 27 states are failing to meet even the most minimal standards of care. Confounding this situation is that Medicaid pays for the majority of nursing home care in the United States, yet does not cover the cost of dental services provided to Medicaid-eligible nursing home residents. Without a reimbursement mechanism for dental care for nursing home residents, obtaining dental care is often not realistic (Damiano, Brown, Johnson, & Scheetz, 1990).)

Place of Residence

The vast majority of adults 65 years of age and older are independent and reside in the community, with 20 percent in nonmetropolitan or rural areas (Administration on Aging, U.S. DHHS, 2006); close to 5 percent live in long-term care facilities and 5–10 percent are homebound. Poverty status, transportation problems and lack of informal assistance are often reported to be more important than place of residence, when predicting utilization of health services of urban and rural elders. Remote locations and small community sizes that limit sources of assistance, combined with the out migration of younger family members, place rural older adults in a vulnerable position concerning access to formal services and the availability of informal assistance from outside the home.

With increasing age, older adults are more likely to live alone. Compared to those living with a spouse or relative, those who live alone are more likely to be in poverty and experience health problems (Helgeson, Smith, Johnsen, & Ebert, 2002). The living arrangements of older adults in the United States are closely linked to income, health status and availability of caregivers (Fields, 2003.)

Community Dwelling, Homebound and Frail Older Adults

As people age, many want to stay in their homes, surround themselves with loved ones and maintain a level of control over their care. During the past 20 years, there has been a dramatic growth in the availability of community-based personal health services and housing options for older adults, with a growing number of older persons receiving care. Assisted living facilities, Continuing Care Retirement Communities (CCRC) or life-care communities, senior housing, congregate housing and other supportive housing options allow older adults needing assistance with their activities of daily living (ADL) to stay in the community. In addition, many states are funding innovative programs to identify and support caregivers who provide unpaid assistance and support to older adults. A total of 70 to 80 percent of noninstitutionalized older adults receive care from friends and family, with more than 65 percent depending solely on unpaid help (65+ in the United States, 2005). While this arrangement has benefits economically and helps with the shortage of long-term care workers, the use of paid, formal care by community-dwelling older persons has been decreasing, while their sole reliance upon family caregivers has been increasing (AARP, 2006).

Approximately 5–10 percent of the population 65 years and older are identified as homebound or functionally dependent, that is, they are only able to leave their home with great difficulty. The loss of functional independence in older adults is often accompanied by impaired manual dexterity (Kiyak, Grayson, & Crienan, 1993). In addition, homebound elders are often frail, that is, they have multiple chronic diseases and medical problems that complicate their diagnosis, treatment and daily care (Beck & Offenbacher, 1998). Due to both physical limitations and cognitive impairments, most frail adults require some level of assistance to complete their activities of daily living, and are often dependent upon others to ensure they receive daily oral care. Although this group has grown in size, little is known about their health status and utilization of health services.

Nursing Home Residents – Institutionalized Elders

In 2000, a relatively small number (1.56 million) and percentage (4.5 percent) of older adults lived in nursing homes. With increasing age, the percentage of older adults living in nursing homes increases, that is, 1.1 percent of those 65–74 years, 4.7 percent of those 75–84 years and 18.2 percent of those 85 years and older live in nursing homes (AOA, 2006). By 2030, the number of nursing home residents is expected to increase to 3.4 million persons, almost double the current number. This projected increase in nursing home residents will be the result of the dramatic growth expected in the population 65 years and older and not due to a higher percentage of the older population being institutionalized.

Nursing homes are designed to provide care for those with medical needs that require the attention of licensed nurses. Some older adults are admitted to nursing homes for a short stay following a hospitalization, while others require long-term care. Nursing home long-term care is designed for those unable to take care of themselves safely. Long-term care provides a broad range of personal, social and medical services to assist those with functional and/or cognitive limitations, perform self-care and other activities necessary to live independently. Residents of long-term care facilities generally require 24-hour supervision, and have an average length of stay of 2.5 years (CDC, NCHS, 1999).)

Today's nursing home residents are older and more impaired than in the past. In 1985, 45 percent of nursing home residents were 85+ years, compared to 51 percent in 1997 (Sahyoun, Pratt, Lentzner, Dey, & Robinson, 2001). Due to both physical and cognitive impairments, most nursing home residents require assistance with personal care, including oral care. In 1999, 75 percent of all nursing home residents required assistance with three or more activities of daily living (ADL's), and 90 percent required assistance with personal care (Jones, 2002). Activities of Daily Living (ADL) and instrumental activities of daily living (IADL) are the most commonly used measures to assess an individual's ability to provide self-care. Activities of Daily Living include the basic tasks of everyday life, that is, eating, bathing, dressing, toileting and transferring, while instrumental activities of daily living include preparing meals, managing money, shopping for groceries or personal items, performing housework and using a telephone. A limitation in three or more ADL's usually triggers the need for admission to a long-term care facility. In general, White, single persons, and females are more likely to be institutionalized than African Americans, married persons and males (Coughlin, McBride, & Liu, 1990; Wolinsky, Callahan, Fitzgerald, & Johnson, 1992; Murtaugh, Kemper, Spillman, & Carlson, 1997).

One of the primary reasons older adults are admitted to a nursing home is due to dementia, which has been identified in 44–53 percent of the long-term care residents (Magaziner et al., 2000) and in 3–11 percent of community-dwelling older adults (Boustani, Peterson, Hanson, Harris, & Lohr, 2003). Persons with dementia have diminished mental capacities, and as the disease progresses, the loss of cognitive and motor skills reduces the ability to self-care, including oral hygiene procedures (Jones, Lavallee, Alman, Sinclair, & Garcia, 1993; Chalmers, Carter, & Spencer, 2002; Davis Fiske, Scott, & Radford, 2000; Adam & Peston, 2006). Even with the assistance of dedicated caretakers, diminished competency and motor skills can interfere with a patients' ability to provide self-care or to accept assistance from another person (Mouradian et al., 2004).

Oral Health Status

Older adults often present with extensive oral disease, the cumulative effects of oral diseases throughout their lifetime. The National Health and Nutrition Examination Study III data reported that dental caries and periodontal diseases occur with substantial frequency and represent a burden on unmet treatment needs in older adults (Drury et al., 1996). Close to 40 percent of noninstitutionalized adults aged 65 years and older had periodontal disease (Weyant, Newman, & Kritchewvsky, 2004) and 30 percent of those with natural teeth had untreated caries (DHHS, 2000).

The status of ones' oral health can have a significant impact on the quality of life for older adults (Locker, Clarke, & Payne, 2000) as the quality of life is directly related to the presence of oral pain and discomfort. Numerous studies (Kassab, Luloff, Kelsey, & Smith, 1996; Mojon & MacEntee, 1992; Strauss & Hunt, 1993) have shown associations between oral problems and pain, facial esthetics, impaired eating, chewing, and speaking; social interaction and a poor sense of well-being. Yet oral health care can restore oral function, alleviate pain and discomfort and improve one's appearance, which contributes to their well-being, communication and social interactions (Locker, 2004).

Although a few longitudinal studies have examined the relationship between oral health and long-term health outcomes, good oral health is necessary for proper mastication and adequate food intake (Budtz-Jorgensen, Chung, & Rapin, 2001). In addition, edentulism and periodontal disease have been shown to be an independent risk factor for significant weight loss (Ritchie, Joshipura Silliman, Miller, & Douglas, 2000; Weyant et al., 2004). Edentulous individuals are more likely to consume fewer fruits and vegetables, less fiber and higher amounts of fat and calories than their dentate peers (Geissler & Bates, 1984; Norlen, Steen, Birkhed, & Bjorn , 1993), and those with ill-fitting dentures tend to have a lower quality diet (Sahyoun Lin & Krall, 2003) and are at increased risk for malnutrition (Mojon, Budtz-Jorgensen, & Rapin, 1999). In addition, involuntary weight loss in older adults has been associated with poor oral hygiene, xerostomia and the inability to chew (Sullivan, Martin, Flaxman, & Hagen, 1993).

Nursing Homes

Oral Health Care Policy in Nursing Homes

The provision of oral health care in long-term care facilities was promulgated in the 1987 Omnibus Reconciliation Act (OBRA) legislation, and became effective on April 1, 1990. The goal of this legislation was to address the inadequacies of nursing home care. The legislation states that all nursing homes receiving Medicaid and Medicare reimbursements provide routine and emergency oral health care to their residents. The legislation also states that nursing homes are required to provide oral health care internally or from an outside resource for each resident; provide assistance in making dental appointments and arranging transportation; and refer residents with lost or damaged dentures to a dentist. In addition, each resident must receive a comprehensive oral health assessment within 14 days of admission and annually thereafter, as well as a comprehensive oral health care plan. The quality of care standard requires that oral hygiene services be made available to residents unable to carry out their activities of daily living. These federal regulations notwithstanding state regulations concerning oral health care in nursing homes vary widely.

Each state and the federal government share responsibility for oversight of the quality of care provided in nursing homes. The federal government, through the Centers for Medicare & Medicaid Services (CMS), established the requirements that nursing homes must meet to participate in the Medicare and Medicaid programs. CMS contracts with state agencies to check compliance of these standards through onsite surveys at least once every 15 months. Under their shared responsibility for nursing home oversight, state agencies identify and categorize deficiencies and make referrals for proposed sanctions to CMS. For a variety of reasons, the oral health status of nursing homes residents has received limited attention from state surveyors. Surveyors rely heavily on medical records for much of their data collection, which may not provide an accurate assessment of the resident (Fitzpatrick, 2000). Regardless of federal and state regulations, little is known about the quantity or quality of oral health care provided in long-term care facilities.

Oral Health Status of Nursing Home Residents

Despite federal legislation mandating that all nursing homes receiving Federal funds provide access to dental care, the 1999 National Nursing Home Survey (NNHS) found that only 80 percent of nursing homes offered dental services, and 26 percent of nursing home residents received dental care during the previous 30 days (Vital & Health Statistics, 2002). This later finding can be interpreted in a variety of ways, as it is possible that those reported to have received dental care during the previous 30 days included those that received assistance with daily oral care and/or those who received professional dental services (Dye, Fisher, Yellowitz, Fryar, & Vargas, 2007). Since neither an oral examination was completed nor a definition of dental care was included in the survey, the findings are problematic.

Upon admission to a nursing home, the oral health status of many residents is poor which may be due to the individual having extended periods of time with limited daily oral care and limited professional dental care (Khambu & Levy, 1993; Kiyak et al., 1993; Gift & Atchison, 1995). Many patients are frail or are hospitalized prior to their admission to a nursing home, during which they were likely to modify or neglect their daily routines, including oral care. In addition, some patients become dependent upon others for their daily oral care. Since the role of a hospital is to focus on the treatment of acute medical conditions, little personnel time is expended facilitating daily oral care. And many hospitals provide a disposable toothbrush and/or a toothette (soft foam sponges primarily designed to help moisten a patient's mouth) for the patients' personal use. Anecdotal reports have identified nursing staff and family members erroneously using a toothette to clean natural teeth and/or dentures. Using a toothette in lieu of a toothbrush is likely due to lack of awareness that a toothette provides far less plaque removal than a toothbrush, and without adequate daily oral care, the individuals' oral health status will decline.

To date, two comprehensive oral health surveys of nursing home residents have been completed: one in Australia (Chalmers, Carter, & Spencer, 2004) and the other in Kentucky (Henry, Sallee, & Durham, 2005). In addition, numerous site-specific oral health surveys of nursing home residents have been completed. However, the validity of many of their findings is limited due to sample size, sampling methodology and assessment tool and/or research design. Yet similar to the findings from Australia and Kentucky, these studies have consistently found widespread oral health problems among nursing home residents, including poor oral hygiene, high levels of oral health needs and low rates of dental care utilization (Loesche et al. 1995; Hawkins, Main, & Locker, 1998, Ghezzi & Ship, 2000). Cohen-Mansfield and Lipson (2002) reported that dentists classified 95 percent of the nursing home residents as having some type of dental problem, while Kiyak et al. (1993) found 63.8 percent of nursing home residents to have immediate dental needs, including 9.3 percent with urgent needs. Routine oral hygiene is often the primary need for dentate patients, which is particularly relevant for those who have maintained good oral health throughout their lifetime, as well as what is predicted to be present in future generations of nursing home residents. When compared to independent elders, nursing home residents have a lower self-perception of need for oral health care (Fiske, Gelbier, & Watson, 1990) and a higher need for care as assessed by professionals. Although no data are available, the oral health status of frail and homebound adults is likely to be similar to that of nursing home residents.

Providing Oral Health Care to Nursing Home Residents

As it is the responsibility of every nursing home to arrange for the delivery of dental care for their residents, some facilities contract for care to be delivered to residents, while others have the residents transported to local dental practitioners. Transporting frail and cognitively impaired older adults to a private dental office presents many obstacles for the individual and caregiver, and requires a staff member with skill, confidence and patience to accompany the patient and to ensure their safety. If a personal vehicle is not available or acceptable, an ambulance may be required and can be an added expense. Providing oral health care to nursing home residents unable to be transported to a private dental office can be problematic for both the patient and dentist. Bringing an impaired older adult from a familiar and stable environment to a new setting such as a dental practice can significantly increase the patients' level of confusion both during and following treatment, which increases the difficulty in managing the individual while in the dental practice and upon their return to the nursing home. Sedating impaired patients prior to care can be helpful; however, the resident may require additional supervision following treatment. Whenever possible, it is optimum for nursing home residents to receive their dental care on site.

Health Professionals

Oral Health Professionals

Oral health professionals' attitudes, beliefs and comfort with older adults impact the quantity and type of dental services offered in their practice. Some health care professionals are uncomfortable working with older adults, especially those with cognitive impairments. Wilson et al. (1994) examined dentists' expectations of middle-aged and older patients regarding dental treatment, and found that dentists significantly overestimated older adults' reluctance to receive dental treatment. MacEntee, Weiss, Waxler-Morrison, & Morrison (1987) found that many dentists are reluctant to treat older adults, particularly in long-term care facilities; only 19 percent provided care and 37 percent showed interest in providing care in long-term care facilities (MacEntee et al., 1987). The primary reason dentists reported for their lack of interest in providing dental care in nursing homes was pressure from private practice, concerns about inadequate training, having a small demand and poor conditions in the facilities (MacEntee et al., 1987).)

The shortage of skilled geriatric dental care professionals is part of a larger national shortage of geriatricians. Unlike medical schools and other health professional training programs, dental hygiene and predoctoral dental education programs provide limited didactic training and rarely allow students opportunities to work with medically compromised and cognitively impaired dependent older adults. As such, few dentists are trained to provide care to this population.

Nursing Professionals

The assistance of nursing professionals is fundamental for the daily care of nursing home residents, given their decline in ADLs and IADLs. Nursing home staffs are responsible for the physical, supportive and hygiene procedures necessary for maintaining the health and comfort of residents incapable of completing the tasks themselves. Yet oral health care is not adequately addressed in the personal hygiene and general health protocols in many facilities (Gil-Montoya et al., 2006). The situation is further complicated by nursing professionals describing oral care to be burdensome, unrewarding, problematic and trivial (Coleman, 2005). However, studies have found that nurses and nurse aides do not have the adequate knowledge about oral health (Adams, 1996; Chalmers et al., 2002) and that most nursing assistants provide limited oral care to residents, in particular to those who are dependent and resistant to their efforts (Coleman, 2002; Jablonski, Munro, Grap, & Elswick, 2005).

Providing daily oral care to another person can be difficult, requiring skill, commitment and consistency. Reliance on caregivers who do not have appropriate knowledge, skills or training can have an adverse impact on oral hygiene. Chalmers et al. (2002) found that high carer burden and oral hygiene difficulties have a negative bearing on both oral care and caries prevalence. In many facilities, the seriousness of poor oral health in institutionalized elders is not generally recognized by nursing home staff, and attention to oral hygiene is afforded low priority by nurses (Wardh, Hallberg, Berggren, Andersson, & Sorensen, 2000). In studies where training in oral hygiene has been provided, the ability and willingness of staff to take responsibility for oral care has increased (Frenkel & Needs, 2002), and the oral health of residents showed improvement. However, clear practice and supervisory guidelines have not been established in many facilities. Oral health education and training for all levels of the nursing staff are needed if change is to occur. Due to the high turnover of nursing staff in long-term care facilities, an ongoing oral health education and training program must be maintained.

Interdisciplinary Opportunities: Making a Difference

Oral health care professionals often fail to achieve improvements in the oral health of the community because they do not share their knowledge and expertise with those beyond the dental office, the dental school or the university (DePaola, 1999). As such, limited efforts have been instituted to facilitate the inclusion of oral health into general health, and reduced access to oral health care has been characterized as one of the prices of professional isolation (Haden et al., 2003). This isolation sends the message to other health professionals, policymakers and the public that oral health is not as important as general health (Haden et al., 2003). This isolation is further perpetuated by the limited oral health curricula in most health care professional schools and continuing education programs. Without adequate knowledge and skills, physicians and other primary health care providers do not recognize, or misdiagnose oral conditions (Jones, Siegel, & Schneider, 1998).)

New health care models are needed to decrease the disparities in access to oral health care for older adults. To date, few programs have been successful in addressing older adults' access to oral health care, while some programs have provided comprehensive services to vulnerable elders, and others have provided free oral screening programs. Many access programs work in isolation, and their successes are often limited by the State Practice Acts and the availability of reimbursement. In order to improve the access of oral health care services to older adults, dialogue and collaboration across health disciplines are needed (U.S. DHHS 2000). Integrating oral assessments into the routine services of primary health care providers can improve the quality of care; improve patients' access to and awareness of oral health.

Primary Health Care Providers

Many older adults at high risk for oral disease obtain care from their primary care provider, but not from their oral health care provider. Unlike oral health care for older adults, primary care services are reimbursed by Medicare. Since many older adults often receive frequent care from general health care providers, there may be numerous opportunities for general health care professionals to offer oral health assessments and promote good oral health care. However, most primary care providers have limited knowledge about assessing the oral health status of their patients (Frenckel, 2002) and do not routinely inspect their patients to identify suspicious oral conditions (Amsel, Strawitz, & Engstrom, 1983, Elwood 1985). Health care providers report the following reasons for not assessing the oral cavity of their patients (Morgan, Tsang, Harrington, & Fook, 2001; Maguire, Roberts, Pryce-Howard, & Lloyd-Davies, 1993):

1) Their patients are being seen by dentists.
2) The oral cavity is not their responsibility.
3) Only dentists are responsible for oral health.

During training, most primary health care providers receive little, if any oral health instruction or guidelines for providing an oral assessment. Similar to other assessments, the primary objective of an oral assessment is to distinguish between health and disease. An oral assessment is a systematic oral screening examination that includes both visual assessment and palpation of the head and neck, including the peri-oral and intra-oral hard and soft tissues. Oral assessments are noninvasive, do not require technical equipment and require a short-time period ($\leq$ 2minutes). A comprehensive oral examination completed by a dental professional will include a detailed extra-oral and intra-oral assessment of the hard and soft tissues, radiographs, a medical history review, an assessment of daily oral care designed to provide the patient with a comprehensive treatment plan for care.

Many primary health care providers recognize the connection of general to oral health, but are uncertain how to utilize this information in their practice. Training general health care professionals about oral health care is not a new concept; however, it has not been adopted by many health professional training programs. Oral health care is further distanced from general health care by not being an accepted component of a routine physical assessment protocol. In addition, many health history forms do not include issues related to oral health. Primary health care providers are generally highly trusted and respected by their patients; as such it behooves them to clarify the need for an annual comprehensive examination by a dental professional. And by expanding their oral health knowledge and skill, primary health care providers will be better able to facilitate access to oral health care for older adults.

Training Programs

An oral health training program for primary health providers—physicians, physician assistants, nurse practitioners and all levels of nursing personnel—is critically needed. The goal of this training program is to prepare primary care providers to competently provide oral health assessments, that is, to assess and differentiate common signs and symptoms of oral diseases, to identify disease risk and to know referral source. Identifying the oral health status of older adults often becomes the responsibility of the health care professional. As such, health care providers are well prepared to be trained to provide oral assessments as they are knowledgeable about human anatomy and physiology, physiologic changes associated with aging, signs of inflammation, infection and disease, pharmacology, adverse side effects of medications and the association with general health.

Although an oral assessment can be viewed as a natural extension of a general physical examination, specific didactic and clinical oral health care training is required. Identifying the oral health status of older adults requires substantial familiarity with oral health knowledge and assessment techniques. Oral health training programs are needed in both professional training schools or programs and continuing education programs, and need to include didactic and clinical components.

Embedding oral health into a general health assessment will help both practitioners and their patients recognize that oral health is an integral component of general health, and it will help to remove oral health care from its silo.

In order for oral assessments to be integrated into general health care, professional training programs must adopt the concept and integrate oral health throughout their curricula. In addition, health history and examination forms need to be modified to ensure documentation of recent dental visits and signs and symptoms of disease. Clinical competency examinations can help to provide assurance of training and for practitioners in the field, continuing education programs could meet their needs, with ongoing refresher courses. And collaboration with oral health professionals will be critical to ensure training materials are kept current.

Guidelines for Training

Significant information can be obtained through a systematic evaluation of the hard and soft tissues of the head and neck, and for some, systemic conditions can be identified before symptoms are apparent. By identifying infection, inflammation, disease or trauma in its early stages, the patient has a better chance of having the condition managed before extensive care is needed. With limited oral health training, practitioners can better manage the overall health of their patients.

The following section lists core elements of an oral health care training program, designed for general health care providers. This material is appropriate for all levels of health professional training needs.

Key concepts of an oral health education program for general health care providers should include, but not be limited to the following:

1) Incorporate the oral assessment as a component of a routine physical assessment.
2) A planned, systematic approach ensures thoroughness and improves efficiency.
3) Explain to the patient what is being done and the reason for it.
4) Review signs and symptoms of common oral conditions and diseases with the patient.
5) Instruct patient to report any oral changes they see or feel.
6) Refer unusual and suspicious findings, in particular those present for 2 or more weeks.
7) For the patient, differentiate an oral assessment from a comprehensive examination completed by a dental professional and why the latter is needed.
8) Discuss the need to have an annual or biannual comprehensive oral examination.

A Curriculum Guide to Oral Health for General Health Practitioners

A training program on oral health for primary care providers should include, but not be limited to the following topics:

1. Basic concepts of oral health

   a. Preventive strategies
   b. Daily oral care techniques
   c. Impact of health conditions
   d. Consequences of poor oral health
   e. Age-related changes

2. Clinical presentation of oral anatomy and the variations of normal

   a. Hard and soft tissues

3. Oral disease processes, risk factors and clinical presentation

   a. Caries, coronal and root
   b. Periodontal disease(s)
   c. Oral cancer
   d. Osteonecrosis

4. Clinical presentation of common oral findings

   a. Fixed and removable prostheses
   b. Soft tissue injuries
   c. Reactive and inflammatory processes
   d. Broken teeth, root fragments
   e. Dry mouth and its consequences
   f. Implants

5. Oral manifestations of common systemic diseases
6. Oral assessment techniques

   a. Systematic protocol
   b. Documentation

7. Clinical training

   a. Supervised assessments

8. Equipment/supplies

   a. Lighting

      i. A high-quality focused light is necessary, for example, an otoscope or a small high-quality flashlight. One example (MityLite 1900) is Pelican Products (www.pelican-flashlight.com).

         1. Ambient light and most disposable penlights provide inadequate lighting

      ii. Protective covering for the flashlights allow intra-oral use and reduce bacterial contamination

   b. Gloves

  i. Better the fit, better the tactile ability

 c. Sterile gauze squares (2″ X 2″ or 4″ X 4″)

Pilot Programs

Oral health educational programs for physician assistants and nurse practitioners were recently piloted at the University of Maryland Dental School, supported by the University of Maryland, Maryland Statewide Health Network through the Maryland Cigarette Restitution Funds (Yellowitz, unpulished, 2004). The overall goal of the research programs was to improve the access to oral health care for underserved community-dwelling adults, with an interim goal of assessing knowledge and behavioral changes in the program participants. A similar design was used for the programs; however, the disciplines were trained separately. The programs extended over 9–12 months, and included three 3-hour training sessions. The curriculum presented to each group was designed to provide didactic and clinical training in oral health and oral health assessment, and were based on the previously described curriculum guide.

The program participants were required to provide oral assessments to their patients throughout the length of the study. A secondary goal of the project was to assess the success of these primary health care providers to incorporate oral assessments into their routine practice.

Although designed as pilot programs, a 6-month follow-up survey was completed with one group of participants and found that the majority (65 percent) were still providing oral assessments to their patients.

The program participants' also collected basic demographic data from those examined, maintained a list of 'unusual findings' and referred all patients with 'suspicious lesions' for follow-up care. Individuals identified with a 'suspicious findings present for 2 weeks or more' were referred for follow-up. These individuals were provided a list of local dental clinics and were told that comprehensive oral examinations and biopsies (if needed) were available at free of charge at the dental school, in the Department of Oral Surgery, University of Maryland Dental School. Although thousands of oral assessments were documented, due to the required anonymity of the data collection process, the total number of referred patients who successfully obtained care was not available. Yet in a 9-month project of 13 physicians' assistants, five patients referred for follow-up were diagnosed with oral cancer. Without this program, it is uncertain when these lesions would have been diagnosed.

Although these findings are preliminary, the initial results reveal that this type of training program can be a tremendous asset for those trained and for those they serve. Until oral health is incorporated into training programs of health professionals, the need for this type of program will continue as the population ages and is unable to obtain routine oral assessments. Educational change is needed in dental and health care professionals' training programs to better address oral health disparities in the elderly. However, changing knowledge and changing practice are different and difficult processes that require attention to many logistic and system barriers (Mouradian et al., 2004).

Summary

As a group, the elderly suffer disproportionately from oral disease and access to oral health care. Older adults are faced with numerous barriers to oral health care, ranging from their knowledge and attitudes about oral health to those of general and oral health professionals to financial concerns and health status. These barriers are further complicated for those who are dependent upon others for their daily care and for obtaining professional services. Good oral health requires maintaining good daily oral care, and when not done effectively, oral problems result. Assessing that daily oral care is done thoroughly is difficult for many older adults and their caregivers. Thus, it is recommended that all adults, especially those who are frail and dependent, obtain an annual or biannual comprehensive oral examination. Frequent dental hygiene appointments may also be needed to eliminate factors that predispose older adults to oral disease and to assist them in maintaining their optimal level of oral health. Finally, there is a growing recognition that caregivers of dependent elders, in particular family members, need support to make their situation successful, however information is known about their health status and utilization of health services. Family caregivers, primarily women, are at a greater risk of having poor general and oral health as they often do not take care of themselves in lieu of being a personal caregiver.

In recognition of the Surgeon General's statement that health care professionals should be educated in the importance of oral health to overall health and well-being (U.S. DHHS, 2000), new programs need to be established. There are few successful programs throughout the country focused on improving the oral care for older adults, and most health care professionals and policymakers have not been successful in ensuring that older adults receive an annual oral health examination. To date, there are no national initiatives to address this problem.

Improving access to oral health requires the collaboration of primary health care providers (physicians, physician assistants, nurse practitioners and nurses), that is, general health and oral health professionals. Primarily due to gaps in training, the capacity of general health providers to assess and to promote oral health has largely been untapped (Mouradian et al., 2004). One approach to improve access to oral health care is to optimize the skills, training and practice behaviors of primary health care providers through education and training programs. An integrated education program for primary health care providers can make a difference in the oral health status of older adults. To date, pilot projects have demonstrated that with limited training, primary care professionals will include oral health assessments into their general practice protocols.

The oral health of the elderly becomes potentially more complicated as older adults become frail, homebound or institutionalized or when their access to oral health care is limited. This situation will continue to be a salient public health issue as the population of older and impaired adults increase in size, and the demand for oral health services grows. Oral and general health professionals must educate tomorrow's elderly to recognize that preventive services are a lifelong activity, and dental, dental hygiene and general health programs must institute curricular changes to prepare future practitioners. In addition, continuing education programs are needed to better serve the needs of older adults. Without major changes to professional education programs and public health policies, the barriers to and management of oral health care of frail and institutionalized elderly will remain unchanged in the future.

References

AARP (2006). Ahead of the curve: Emerging trends and practices in family caregiver support, Academic Dental Institutions. *Journal of Dental Education, 67*(5), 563–583.

Administration on Aging, (AOA) U.S. Department of Health and Human Services(2006). A Profile of Older Americans: 2006. This document is only available online at: http://www.aoa.gov/prof/Statistics/profile/2006/2006profile.pdf

Adam, H., & Preston, A. J. (2006). The oral health of individuals with dementia in nursing homes. *Gerodontology, 23*, 99–105.

Adams, R. (1996). Qualified nurses lack adequate knowledge related to oral health, resulting in inadequate oral care of patients on medical wards. *Journal of Advanced Nursing, 24*, 552–560.

Amsel, Z., Strawitz, J. G., & Engstrom, P. F. (1983). The dentist as a referral source of first episode head and neck cancer patients. *Journal the American Dental Association,106*(2), 195–197.

Avlund, K., Holm-Pedersen, P., & Schroll, M. (2001). Functional ability and oral health among older people: A longitudinal study from age 75 to 80. *Journal of American Geriatric Society, 49*(7), 954–962.

Bailit, H., & Beazoglou, T. (2006). The supply of dental services: What are the Issues? *The National AHEC Bulletin, 23*(1), 3–6.

Beck, J. D., & Offenbacher, S. (1998). Oral health and systemic disease: Periodontitis and cardiovascular disease. *Journal* of *Dental Education*, 62(10), 859–870.

Boustani, M., Peterson, B., Hanson, L., Harris, R., & Lohr K. N. (2003). U.S. Preventive Services Task Force. Screening for dementia in primary care: A summary of the evidence for the U.S. Preventive Services Task Force. *Annals of Internal Medicine, 138*(11), 927–933.

Budtz-Jorgensen, E., Chung, J. P., & Rapin, CH. (2001). Nutrition and oral health. *Best Practice & Research in Clinical Gastroenterology, 15*(6), 885–896,

Burt, B. A. (1978). Influences for change in the dental health status of populations: An historical perspective. *Journal of Public Health Dentistry, 38*(4), 272–288

Centers for Disease Control (CDC), National Center Health Statistics (NCHS) 1999. National Nursing Home Survey. Available on line at: http://www.cdc.gov/nchs/data/series/sr_13/sr13_152.pdf

Centers for Medicare & Medicaid Services, US Department of Health and Human Services; www.hhs.gov/MedicareDentalCoverage

Chalmers, J. M., Carter, K. D., & Spencer, J. (2002). Caries incidence and increments in community-living older adults with and without dementia. *Gerodontology, 19*(2), 80–94.

Chalmers, J. M., Carter, K. D., & Spencer, A. J. (2004). Oral health of Adelaide nursing home residents: Longitudinal study. *Australasian Journal on Ageing, 23*(2), 63.

Cohen-Mansfield, J., & Lipson, S. (2002). Pain in cognitively impaired nursing home residents: How well are physicians diagnosing it? *Journal of the American Geriatrics Society, 50*, 1039–1044.

Coleman, P. (2002) Oral health care for the frail elderly. A review of widespread problems and best practices. *Geriatric Nursing, 23*(4);189–199.

Coleman, P. (2005) Opportunities for nursing –dental collaboration: Addressing oral health needs among the elderly. *Nursing Outlook, 53*(1), 33–39.

Coughlin, T. A., McBride, T. D., & Liu, K. (1990). Determinants of transitory and permanent nursing home admissions. *Medical Care, 28*(7), 616–631.

Damiano, P. C., Brown, E. R., Johnson, J. D., & Scheetz, J. P. (1990). Factors affecting dentist participation in a state Medicaid program. *Journal of Dental Education, 11*, 638–643.

Davis, D. M., Fiske, J., Scott, B., & Radford, D. R. (2000). The emotional effects of tooth loss: A preliminary quantitative study. *British Dental Journal, 188*(9), 503–506.

DePaola, D. (1999). Beyond the university: Leadership for the common good. In N. K. Haden, & L. T. Tedesco (Eds.), *Leadership for the future: The dental school in the university* (pp. 92–102). Washington, DC: American Association of Dental Schools (now American Dental Education Association).

Dolan, T. A., & Atchison, K. A. (1993). Implications of access, utilization and need for oral health care by non-institutionalized and institutionalized elderly on the dental delivery system. *Journal of Dental Education, 57*(12), 259–265.

Drury, T. F., Winn, D. M., Snowden, C. B., Kingman, A., Kleinman DV, & Lewis B. (1996). An overview of the oral health component of the 1988–1991 National Health and Nutrition Examination Survey (NHANES III-Phase 1). *Journal of Dental Research, 75* Spec No, 620–630.

Dye, B., Fisher, M. A., Yellowitz, J. A., Fryar, C. D., & Vargas, C. M.(2007). Receipt of dental care, dental status and workforce in US nursing homes: 1997 National Nursing Home Survey. Special Care Dentistry. Accepted for publication.

Elter, J. R., Champagne, C. M., Offenbacher, S., & Beck, J. D. (2004). Relationship of periodontal disease and tooth loss to prevalence of coronary heart disease. *Journal of Periodontology, 75*(6),782–790.

Elwood, J. M. (1985). Factors influencing early diagnosis of cancer of the oral cavity. *Canadian Medical Association, 7*, 651–656.

Ettinger, R. L. (1987). Oral disease and its effect on the quality of life. *Gerodontics, 3*, 103–106.

Fields, J. (2003). *America's families and living arrangements: 2003. Current population reports* (P20–553). Washington, DC: U.S. Census Bureau.

Fiske, J., Gelbier, S., & Watson, R. M. (1990). The benefit of dental care to an elderly population assessed using a socio-dental measure of oral handicap. *British Dental Journal, 168*(4), 153–156.

Fitzpatrick, J. (2000). Oral health care needs of dependent older people: Responsibilities of nurses and care staff. *Journal of Advanced Nursing, 32*(6), 1325–1332r.

Frenkel, H., & Needs, K. (2002).Oral health care and its effect on caregivers' knowledge and attitudes: A randomized controlled trial. *Dentistry and Oral Epidemiology, 30*(2), 91–100.

Geissler, C. A., & Bates, J. F. (1984). The nutritional effects of tooth loss. *American Journal of Clinical Nutrition, 39*, 478–489.

Ghezzi, E. M., & Ship, J. A. (2000). Systemic diseases and their treatments in the elderly: Impact on oral health. *Journal of Public Health Dentistry, 60*(4),289–296.

Gift, H. C., & Atchison, K. A. (1995). Oral health, health, and health-related quality of life. *Medical Care,* Nov; *33*(11 Suppl), NS57–77.

Gil-Montoya, J. A., Ferrerira de Mello, A. L., Cardenas, C. B., & Lopez, I. G. (2006). Oral health protocol for dependent institutionalized elderly. *Geriatric Nursing, 27*(2),95–101.

Haden, N. K., Catalanotto, F. A., Alexander, C. J., Bailit, H., Battrell, A., Broussard, Jr. J., et al. (2003). Improving the oral health status of all Americans: Roles and responsibilities of academic dental institutions: The report of the ADEA president's commission. *Journal of Dental Education, 67*(5), 563–583.

Hawkins, R. J., Main, P. A., & Locker, D. (1998). Oral health status and treatment needs of Canadian adults aged 85 years and over. *Special Care in Dentistry, 18*, 164–169.

Hawkins, R. J. (1999). Functional status and untreated dental caries among nursing home residents aged 65 and over. *Special Care in Dentistry, 19*, 158–163.

Healthy People 2000 at http://odphp.osophs.dhhs.gov/pubs/hp2000.

Helgeson, M. J., Smith, B. J., Johnsen, M., & Ebert, C. (2002). Dental considerations for the frail elderly. *Special Care in Dentistry, 22*(3), 40S–55S.

Henry, R., Sallee, N., & Durham, L. (2005). *Final report: Kentucky elder oral health survey 2005.* Lexington, KY: Division of Dental Public Health, College of Dentistry, University of Kentucky.

Holm-Pedersen, P., Vigild, M., Nitschke, I., & Berkey, D. B. (2005). Dental care for aging populations in Denmark, Sweden, Norway, United Kingdom, and Germany. *Journal Dental Education, 69*(9), 987–997.

Isman, R., & Isman, B. (1997). *Oral health America white paper: Access to oral health services in the US. 1997 and beyond.* Chicago: Oral Health America

Jablonski, R. A., Munro, C. L., Grap, M. J., & Elswick, R. K. (2005). The role of biobehavioral, environmental, and social forces on oral health disparities in frail and functionally dependent nursing home elders. *Biological Research for Nursing, 7*(1), 75–82.

Jones, A. (2002). The national nursing home survey: 1999 summary. *Vital and Health Statistics 13.* 2002 June;(152), 1–116.

Jones, J. A., Lavallee, N., Alman, J., Sinclair, C., & Garcia, R. I.(1993). Caries incidence in patients with dementia. *Gerodontology, 10*(2), 76–82.

Jones, T. V., Siegel, M. J., & Schneider, J. R. (1998). Recognition and management of oral health problems in older adults by physicians: A pilot study. *Journal American Board of Family Practitioners, 11* (6), 474–477.

Joshipura, K. J., Rimm, E. B., Douglass, C. W., Trichopoulos, D., Ascherio, A., & Willett, W. C. (1996). Poor oral health and coronary heart disease. *Journal of Dental Research, 75*, 1631–1636.

Kassab, C., Luloff, A. E., Kelsey, T. W., & Smith, S. M. (1996). The influence of insurance status and income on health care use among the nonmetropolitan elderly. *Journal of Rural Health, 12*(2), 89–99.

Khambu, P., & Levy, S. (1993). Oral hygiene care levels in Iowa intermediate care facilities. *Special Care Dentistry 13*, 209–224.

Kiyak, H., Grayson, M., & Crienan, C. (1993). Oral health problems and needs of nursing home residents. *Community Dentistry Oral Epidemiology, 21*, 49–52.

Kramarow, E., Lentzner, H., Rooks, R., Weeks, J., & Saydah, S. (1999). *Health and aging chartbook. Health United States, 1999.* Hyattsville, MD: National Center for Health Statistics.

Locker, D. (2004). Oral health and quality of life. *Oral Health Preventive Dentistry, 2*(Supplement 1), 247–253.

Locker, D., Clarke, M., & Payne, B. (2000). Self-perceived oral health status, psychological well-being, and life satisfaction in an older adult population. *Journal of Dental Research* Apr; *79*(4),970–975.

Locker, D., & Jokovic, A. (1996). Using subjective oral health status indicators to screen for dental care needs in older. *Community Dental and Oral Epidemiology, 24*(6), 398–402.

Loesche, W. J., Abrams, J., Terpenning, M. S., Bretz, W. A., Dominguez, B. L., Grossman, N. S., et al. (1995). Dental findings in geriatric populations with diverse medical backgrounds. *Oral Surgery Oral Medicine Oral Pathology Oral Radiology and Endodontics*, July; *80*(1), 43–54.

MacEntee, M. E., Weiss, R., Waxler-Morrison, N. E., & Morrison, B. J. (1987). Factors influencing oral health in long term care facilities. *Community Dental and Oral Epidemiology, 15* (6), 314–316.

MacEntee, M. E., (2000). Oral care for successful aging in long-term care. *Journal of Public Health Dentistry, 60*(4), 326–329.

Magaziner, J., German, P., Zimmerman, S. I., Hebel, J. R., Burton, L., Gruber-Baldini, A. L., et al. (2000). The prevalence of dementia in a statewide sample of new nursing home admissions aged 65 and older. The Gerontologist, 40,663–672.

Maguire, B. T., Roberts, E. E., Pryce-Howard, J. N., & Lloyd-Davies, S. R. (1993). *Detecting oral cancer in primary medical and dental care settings. (Abstract)*. San Francisco: Presentation at American Association of Public Health Dentistry scientific session.

Manski, R. J., Goodman, H. S., Reid, B. C., & Macek, M. D. (2004). Dental insurance visits and expenditures among older adults. *American Journal of Public Health, 94*, 759–764.

Marvin, M. (2001). Access to care for seniors – dental concerns. *Journal of the Canadian Dental Association, 67*, 504–507.

Meskin, L. H., Dillenberg, J., Heft, M. W., Katz, R. V., & Martens, L. V. (1990). Economic impact of dental service utilization by older adults. *Journal of the American Dental Association, 120*(6), 665–668.

Mojon, P., Budtz-Jorgensen, E., & Rapin, C. (1999). Relationship between oral health and nutrition in very old people. *Age and Ageing;28*, 463–468.

Mojon, P., & MacEntee, M. I. (1992). Discrepancy between need for prosthodontic treatment and complaints in an elderly edentulous population. *Community Dent Oral Epidemiol, 20*(1), 48–52.

Morgan, R., Tsang, J., Harrington, N., & Fook, L. (2001). Survey of hospital doctors' attitudes and knowledge of oral conditions in older patients. *Journal of Postgraduste Medicine, 77*, 392–394.

Mouradian, W. E., Huebner, C., & DePaola, D. (2004). Addressing health disparities through dental-medical collaborations, part III: Leadership for the public good. *Journal of Dental Education, 68*(5), 505–512.

Murtaugh, C. M., Kemper, P., Spillman, B. C., & Carlson, B. L. (1997). The amount, distribution, and timing of lifetime nursing home use.– *Medical Care, 35*(3), March 1997 204–218.

Lethbridge-Çejku, M., Rose, D., & Vickerie, J. (2004). Summary health statistics for U.S. adults: National Health Interview Survey, National Center for Health Statistics. *Vital Health Stat, 10*(228), 2006.

Norlen, P., Steen, B., Birkhed, D., & Bjorn, A. L. (1993). On the relations between dietary habits, nutrients, and oral health in women at the age of retirement. *Acta Odontol Scand, 51*(5), 277–284.

Oral Health America, A State of Decay, The oral health of older Americans. (2003) www.oralhealthamerica.org/pdf/StateofDecayFinal.pdf

Ritchie, C. S., Joshipura K., Silliman, R. A., Miller, B., & Douglas, C. W. (2000). Oral health problems and significant weight loss among community-dwelling older adults. *The Journals of Gerontology Series A: Biological Sciences and Medical Sciences, 5*5, M366–M371.

Riley, J. L., Gilbert, G. H., Heft, & M. W. (1998). Orofacial pain symptom prevalence: Selective sex differences in the elderly? *Pain* May; *76*(1–2), 97–104.

Sahyoun, N., Pratt, L., Lentzner, H., Dey, A. & Robinson, K. (2001). *The changing profile of nursing home residents : 1985–1997.* Hyattsville, MD: National Center for Health Statistics.

Sahyoun, N. R., Lin, C. L., & Krall, E. (2003). Nutritional status of the older adult is associated with dentition status. *Journal American Dietetic Association 103*(1), 61–66.

Scannapieco, F. A. (1999). Role of oral bacteria in respiratory infection. *Journal of Periodontology, 70*(7), 793–802.

Shay, K. & Ship, J. (1995). The importance or oral health in the older patient. *Journal of the American Geriatric Society, 43*, 1414–1422.

Stanton, M. W. & Rutherford, M. K. (2003). Dental care: Improving access and quality. Rockville (MD): Agency for Healthcare Research and Quality; Research in Action Issue #13. AHRQ Pub No. 03–0040.

Strauss, R. P., & Hunt, R. J. (1993). Understanding the value of teeth to older adults: Influences on the quality of life. *Journal of the American Dent Association, 124*(1), 105–110.

Strayer, M. (1995). Perceived barriers to oral health care among the homebound. *Special Care Dentistry, 15*, 113–118.

Sullivan, D. H., Martin, W., Flaxman, N., & Hagen, J. E. (1993). Oral health problems and involuntary weight loss in a population of frail elderly. *Journal of American Geriatric Society, 41*(7), 725–731.

U.S. Department of Health and Human Services (DHHS). (2000) "Oral Health in America: A Report of the Surgeon General." Rockville, MD: National Institute of Dental and Craniofacial Research, National Institutes of Health, 2000. Online, available at: www. nidr.nih.gov/sgr/execsumm.htm

US Public Health Service for all adults (1994). *Clinicians' handbook of preventive services.* Baltimore, MD: Williams &Wilkins, 1996.

Vargas, C. M., Kramarow, E. A., & Yellowitz, J. A. (2001). The oral health of older Americans. *Aging Trends* (Vol. 3). National Center for Health Statistics.

Vital and health statistics. Public Health Service (2002). The national nursing home survey: 1999 summary. Series 13, No. 152. 125 pp. (PHS) 1723.

Wardh, I., Hallberg, L., Berggren, U., Andersson, L., & Sorensen, S. (2000). Oral health care-low priority in nursing. *Scandinavian Journal of Caring Science, 14*, 127–142.

Weyant, R. J., Newman, A., & Kritchewvsky, S. B. (2004). Periodontal disease and weight loss in older adults. *American Geriatrics Society, 52*, 547–553.

White, B. A. (1994). An overview of oral health status, resources, and care delivery. *Journal Dental Education, 58*, 285–290.

Wolinsky, F. D., Callahan, C. M., Fitzgerald, J. F., & Johnson, R. J. (1992). The risk of nursing home placement and subsequent death among older adults. *Journals of Gerontology, 47:44*, 173–182.

Wilson, M. C., Holloway, P. J. & Sarll, D. W. (1994). Barriers to the provision of complex dental treatment for dentate older people: A comparison of dentists' and patients' views. *British Dental Journal, 177*(4), 130–134.

Yellowitz, J.A. (2004). Unpublished data, University of Maryland Dental School.

Part II
Health and Medical Considerations

Chapter 5
Movement Disorders in Dental Practice

Nina M. Browner and Steven Frucht

Introduction

The purpose of this chapter is to review the classification, clinical phenomenology, diagnosis and treatment of movement disorders. These conditions are characterized by abnormalities in voluntary movements, or by the presence of involuntary movements. Dentists are frequently confronted with movement disorders. Abnormal movements can be located in the orofacial area and thereby complicate dental management, especially in prosthodontics and restorative dentistry. Movement disorders that do not involve oral structures can still affect oral health due to difficulty performing oral hygiene or inability to sustain prolonged and extensive dental procedures.

Movement disorders are collectively attributed to primary degeneration or dysfunction of the basal ganglia, an area of the brain that includes caudate nucleus, putamen, globus pallidus, subthalamic nucleus and substantia nigra, with extensive afferent and efferent connections. Movement disorders are divided into two general groups: hypokinetic and hyperkinetic disorders. The prototype hypokinetic movement disorder is Parkinson's disease (PD), the most common cause of parkinsonism. The main hyperkinetic movement disorders include tremor, dystonia, myoclonus, choreoathetosis and tics. Although these general characterizations are useful, many movement disorders encompass both hyperkinetic and hypokinetic features.

Parkinsonism

Parkinsonism can be classified into three major categories: primary, secondary and parkinson-plus disorders (Table 5.1).

S. Frucht
M.D. 710 West 168th street, NI3 New York, New York 10032, Tel: 212-305-0429, Fax: 212-305-1304
e-mail: sf216@columbia.edu

I.B. Lamster, M.E. Northridge (eds.), *Improving Oral Health for the Elderly*,
© Springer Science+Business Media, LLC 2008

Table 5.1 Classification of Parkinsonism

I. Primary (idiopathic parkinsonism)

    a. Parkinson's disease

II. Atypical parkinsonism (parkinson-plus disorders)

    a. Progressive supranuclear palsy
    b. Multiple system atrophy

        i. Striatonigral degeneration (MSA-P)
        ii. Olivopontocerebellar atrophy (MSA-C)
        iii. Shy-Drager syndrome (MSA-A)

    c. Corticobasal degeneration
    d. Diffuse Lewy body disease

III. Secondary

    a. Drug-induced

        i. Neuroleptics (typical and atypical)
        ii. Metoclopramide
        iii. Lithium
        iv. Calcium channel blockers
        v. Reserpine, tetrabenazine

    b. Toxic

        i. Carbon monoxide
        ii. Manganese
        iii. MPTP

    c. Metabolic

        i. Hypoxia
        ii. Hypocalcemia
        iii. Hepatocerebral degeneration

    d. Infectious

        i. Postencephalitic
        ii. AIDS
        iii. Prion disease

    e. Structural

        i. Tumor
        ii. Hydrocephalus
        iii. Trauma

Parkinson's Disease

Primary parkinsonism or Parkinson's disease (PD) is a progressive neurodegenerative disorder of the central nervous system of unknown etiology, characterized by resting tremor, cogwheel rigidity, bradykinesia (slowness of movements) and postural instability. The incidence of PD increases with age: the median age of onset for idiopathic PD is 62.4 years. Onset before age 30 is rare, but up to 10% of cases of idiopathic PD begin by age 40. In a recent study in the United States, the incidence of PD was 10.9 cases per 100,000 person-years in the general population, and 49.7 per 100,000 person-years for those over age 50 (Bower et al., 1999). For the population over age 40, prevalence is estimated to be approximately 300 per 100,000 in the United States and Canada, with the important caveat that perhaps 40% of cases may be undiagnosed at any given time (Schoenberg et al., 1985). PD appears to be slightly more common in men than in women and may be more common in North American Whites than in Asians or Africans.

The cause of PD is unknown. A current hypothesis suggests that it may be due to a combination of an underlying genetic susceptibility with a superimposed environmental influence, coupled with normal aging. Ten different genetic loci have been associated with PD or variants of classical PD. Several well-confirmed genes are linked to familial PD: alpha-synuclein, parkin, DJ-1, leucine-rich repeat kinase 2 gene (LRRK2), ubiquitin carboxyterminal hydrolase L1 genes (UCH-L1) and pten-induced kinase 1 (PINK1). Three genes have been isolated and cloned, and linked to early-onset PD: alpha-synuclein, parkin and DJ-1. Onset between ages 20 and 40 is called "young-onset" PD, and it is associated with parkin gene mutation on chromosome 6p25.2-27, or DJ-1 gene mutation, both inherited in autosomal recessive pattern (Bonifati et al., 2003; Kitada et al., 1998). A very rare mutation in the alpha-synuclein gene causes autosomal dominant form of PD that presents as young-onset levodopa responsive familial parkinsonism with dementia and rapid symptom progression (Polymeropoulos et al., 1997). Mutations in the LRRK2 gene have recently been identified in families with autosomal dominant late-onset PD (Paisan-Ruiz et al., 2005).

The pathological hallmark of PD is a loss of dopaminergic neurons from substantia nigra pars compacta and accumulation of Lewy bodies (LB)—eosinophlic intracytoplasmic inclusions composed principally of alpha-synuclein, in substantia nigra. As disease progresses, LB can be found in other areas of the brain including the cerebral cortex.

PD manifests with a combination of six cardinal features: tremor at rest, bradykinesia (slow movements or paucity of movements), rigidity, flexed posture, freezing and loss of postural reflexes. At least two of the six cardinal features need to be present before the diagnosis of parkinsonism is made, one of which is bradykinesia or tremor at rest.

Tremor is usually the first symptom recognized by the patient. Tremor is defined as a periodic oscillation of a body part. "Pill-rolling" tremor of the fingers and pronation–supination of the hands is most typical. Tremor also may affect the legs, lips, chin, jaw or tongue. Jaw tremor in PD usually presents with "up-and-down" movement and rarely as "side-to-side" movement. It can cause knocking of the teeth, resulting in a vexing sound and more importantly considerable social embarrassment. Tremor of the tongue and lips may interfere with biting, chewing and swallowing food and saliva, leading to drooling and social embarrassment. Bradykinesia is manifested cranially by masked facies (hypomimia), a decreased frequency of blinking, impaired upward gaze, monotone and soft voice (hypophonia) and drooling of saliva due to decrease spontaneous swallowing. In the limbs, bradykinesia presents with slowing of movements, especially fine motor skills. In the early stages, the symptoms and signs tend to remain on one side of the body but with time, the other side slowly becomes involved as well. In later stages of the disease, progressive cell loss outside of dopaminergic neurons in substantia nigra results in nonmotor symptoms of PD that have a great impact on patient quality of life. These nonmotor symptoms include depression, anxiety, disruption of sleep, postural hypotension, sexual dysfunction, constipation and urinary urgency. Cognitive impairment can be seen early in PD with abnormalities in attention, concentration and visuo-spatial orientation (Dujardin et al., 2001; Uc et al., 2005). Dementia develops in 30% to 70% of patients with PD, becoming an increasing cause of disability over time (Aarsland et al., 2005).

The most common oral manifestations of PD – xerostomia, burning mouth and mucositis – are due to changes in salivatory flow. PD patients have a higher incidence of angular cheilosis and candidiasis due to xerostomia, a side effect of anti-parkinsonian medications rather than PD itself. Nakayama et al. (2004) found that PD patients had more complains of chewing difficulty, denture discomfort and problems with swallowing than controls. They also had fewer of their own teeth, and fewer PD patients cleaned their dentures every day compared to controls. Forty-seven percent of PD patients have difficulty performing oral hygiene due to diminished motor function (Rajput, 1994). Despite xerostomia, patients with PD are not at higher risk for caries (Fukayo et al., 2003).

The diagnosis of idiopathic PD is clinical, based on excluding cases of secondary parkinsonism and atypical parkinsonian syndromes. Currently, no neuroprotective treatment is available for PD. A number of medications are available for symptomatic treatment. The aim of the treatment is to provide reasonable symptom control with a minimum of side effects. In early stages of PD, selegiline, amantadine and anticholinergics have a mild symptomatic benefit. Amantadine is an antiviral drug that improves all PD symptoms. Its exact mechanism of action is unclear but it may augment dopaminergic activity. Side effects of amantadine include xerostomia, urinary hesitancy, leg edema and livedo reticularis. Selegiline blocks monoamine oxidase type B in the brain, one of the two enzymes responsible for metabolizing dopamine in the synaptic cleft, thereby prolonging the effect of dopamine. Its common side effects are insomnia and agitation, thus it is usually taken in the morning. Anticholinergics, such as trihexyphenidil hydrochloride (Artane) and benztropine (Cogentin), may occasionally relieve tremor resistant to other medications. Their common side effects include xerostomia, urinary retention, constipation, confusion and blurred vision. When PD symptoms progress and become more disabling, the mainstay of treatment becomes direct or indirect replacement of dopamine by either giving its precursor, levodopa (since dopamine itself does not cross the blood–brain barrier) or using a direct-acting dopamine agonist (DA) to stimulate postsynaptic dopamine receptors. Four dopamine agonists are available in the United States: two ergot-derived (bromocriptine and pergolide) and two nonergot derived (pramipexole and ropinirole). All four have similar side effects which include orthostatic hypotension, dizziness, leg edema and sleep attacks. The use of pergolide has been reduced due to recent reports of heart valvular disease in its users (Zanettini et al., 2007).

Available since 1961, levodopa remains the most effective medication for PD. When used alone, dopa-decarboxylase converts much of it into dopamine in peripheral tissue, causing skin flushing, nausea and vomiting. Therefore, levodopa is typically given in conjunction with the decarboxylase inhibitor carbidopa, which prevents peripheral conversion of levodopa before it reaches the blood–brain barrier. Levodopa given 3–4 times per day produces stable benefit in PD symptoms. Common side effects of levodopa are orthostatic hypotension, nausea, confusion, hallucinations and motor fluctuations. Within the first 5 years of treatment, at least half of the patients treated with levodopa develop motor fluctuations. These take several forms including end-of-dose wearing off and peak-dose dyskinesias. The pathogenesis of fluctuations is multifactorial and not completely understood. Up to 56% patients may experience dyskinesias, involuntary, random, quick "dance-like" movements at the peak dose of the levodopa effect (Blanchet et al., 1996). Risk factors for developing dyskinesias are younger age of PD onset and higher daily levodopa dose. Any body part can be affected, and neck or mouth involvement is common. Dyskinetic movements of the head consist of jaw closing and opening, lip pursing and smacking and lateral flexion of the neck and can pose challenges for prosthodontits and restorative dentists. As PD progresses, each dose of levodopa typically lasts for shorter period of time and patients note a gradual return of tremor, bradykinesia and sometimes anxiety prior to the next dose, heralding the end-of-dose wearing off phenomena.

Due to advances in imaging and surgical techniques, stereotactic surgery has become an increasingly important part of PD treatment over the past 15 years. Three neuroanatomic targets are considered: thalamus, globus pallidus and subthalamic nucleus. In each location, the surgical procedure can be performed by lesioning or insertion of a deep brain stimulator. Thalamotomy is now rarely used. Pallidal and subthalamic nucleus surgery has been increasingly popular, improving patients "off" times on average by 40% and 70% respectively and decreasing dyskinesias (Volkmann et al., 2001). Postoperative complications include dysarthria, dysphagia, bladder urgency and neuropsychiatric complications such as depression, agitation and permanent cognitive changes (Rodriquez-Oroz et al., 2005). Transplantation of human embryonic dopaminergic neurons into the basal ganglia has recently been tested in clinical trials. No consistent benefit has been seen, and the procedure is currently not recommended for widespread use (Olanow et al., 2003).

Dental treatment of patients with PD requires some special precautions. Patients with PD are not at higher risk for medical emergencies than other age-matched elderly patients, but they require significant modification of treatment plans to accommodate their physical problems (Collins, 1990; Alexander & Gage, 2000). It would be best to see them in the morning and keep appointments as short as possible. Ideally, PD patient should have taken their levodopa dose 60–90 minutes before the appointment so that the treatment can be provided at the peak of the dose. Procedures most likely will take longer than usual to accomplish. Emphasis on preventive measures and early interventions to avoid extensive procedures is wise. Preventive measures and treatment plans should be compatible with the patient's physical, cognitive and behavioral abilities. Clear communication with the patient, caregivers and health care providers is pivotal. Also, emphasis should be placed on dental health education and guidance on maintaining oral hygiene (Clifford & Finnerty, 1995). Dentists can recommend the use of electric toothbrushes and dental products designed for patients with dry mouth. Late in the disease, patients may become homebound or confined to long-term nursing care, requiring dental care to be provided at the patient's location by a mobile dental practice. The dental management of PD patients can be successful when a multidisciplinary approach is followed, including a dietician and speech therapist.

Secondary parkinsonism is usually due to toxins, drugs, vascular disease, trauma, endocrine disorders, normal pressure hydrocephalus or infection. Exposure to dopamine depleting agents such as atypical and typical neuroleptics, calcium channel blockers, valproic acid and lithium is a relatively common cause of drug-induced parkinsonism. A recent study in Minnesota to determine the incidence of parkinsonism found that 20% of cases were drug-induced (Bower, Maraganore, & McDonnell, 1999). Symptoms are reversible soon after the offending medication is stopped. Environmental causes of parkinsonism include very rare cases of manganese poisonings, carbon monoxide and 1-methyl-4-phenyl-1,2,3,6-tetrahydropyridine (MTPT) exposure (Langston et al., 1999; Tanner, 1992). A few cases of postencephalitic parkinsonism were reported in association with West Nile virus and Japanese encephalitis (Sejvar et al., 2003, Pradhan et al., 1999).

Atypical Parkinsonism

The atypical parkinsonian disorders, also known as parkinson-plus syndromes, are characterized by rapidly evolving parkinsonism, poor or transient respond to levodopa, impaired eye movements, early dementia, early dysarthria (slurred speech) and dysphagia (problems with swallowing) and associated dysfunction of other part of nervous system (pyramidal, cerebellar, autonomic nervous system), usually not seen in PD (Table 5.2). Like other neurodegenerative disorders, the pathogenesis of the parkinson-plus syndromes relates to aggregation of

Table 5.2 Diagnosis of Parkinson's Disease

I. Characteristics of Parkinson's disease
a. Rest tremor
b. Bradykinesia
c. Cogwheel rigidity
d. Asymmetry of symptom onset
e. Positive response to levodopa
II. Features suggestive alternative diagnosis
a. Dementia preceding motor symptoms or in the first year
b. Prominent postural instability in the first 3 years after symptoms onset
c. Autonomic nervous system dysfunction
d. Oculomotor abnormalities
e. Documentation of condition known to produce parkinsonism and plausibly connected to the patient's symptoms (such as suitably located focal brain lesion or neuroleptic use within the past 6 months)

intracellular proteins. These include alpha-synuclein and tau protein aggregates. Synucleinopathies include diseases with Lewy body inclusions, such as PD and dementia with Lewy bodies (DLB) and diseases characterized by glial cytoplasmic inclusions, such as multiple system atrophy (MSA). The tauopathies include progressive supranuclear palsy (PSP), corticobasal degeneration (CBD) and frontotemporal dementia with parkinsonism linked to chromosome 17.

Progressive Supranuclear Palsy

PSP was first described by Steele, Richardson and Olszewski in 1964. About 6% of all parkinsonian patients evaluated in specialty clinics fulfilled the clinical criteria for PSP. The average incidence has been estimated to be 5.3 new cases per 100,000 person-year (Bower et al., 1997) and prevalence −1.39 per 100,000 (Golbe et al., 1988). Like PD, PSP occurs more often in men, but its onset in the seventh decade is about 10 years later than the typical onset of PD. PSP can be distinguished from PD by its limited response to levodopa, impaired vertical eye movements, early onset of dysarthria and dysphagia, as well as postural instability. The first presentation of PSP is usually falls, whereas falls occur in later stages of PD. Progressive dysphagia causes most patients to modify their diet, and some eventually need a gastrostomy to maintain adequate nutrition. Dystonia is uncommon, but if present blepharospasm is the most common form of dystonia in PSP. PSP patients also experience "apraxia of eyelid opening", which consists of brief episodes of inability to open the eyes spontaneously on command after the eyes were closed for a few seconds. Its relentlessly progressive course leads to death, usually from aspiration, within 5–8 years. Early onset, presence of falls, slowness and early downward gaze palsy correlates with rapid progression (Santacruz et al., 1998).

Multiple System Atrophy

MSA is a parkinsonian syndrome admixed with varying combination of autonomic nervous system dysfunction, cerebellar, pyramidal and lower motor neuron signs. The average annual incidence is 3.0 cases per 100,000 and prevalence is 4.4 per 100,000 (Bower et al., 1997; Schrag et al., 1999). MSA appears to be more common in men, with first symptoms beginning in the sixth decade; death usually occurs 7–8 years after the initial symptom and approximately 4 years after the onset of neurologic impairment. Features that are helpful in differentiating MSA from other parkinsonian disorders are early-onset falling, orthostatic hypotension, severe dysarthria and dysphonia, excessive snoring and sleep apnea, respiratory stridor, hyperreflexia and extensor plantar responses. Clinicians differentiate three types of MSA, depending on which system dysfunction predominates in the clinical picture: parkinsonism (MSA-P), cerebellar syndrome (MSA-C) or autonomic dysfunction (MSA-A). In one study of 59 patients with MSA, the survival was poorest in MSA-A type, followed by MSA-C and MSA-P types (Saito et al., 1994). About two-thirds of MSA patients respond to levodopa although there is no difference in survival in levodopa responders compared to non-responders.

Corticobasal Degeneration

CBD is an atypical parkinsonian syndrome that usually presents in the seventh decade and never before the age of 45. The most striking features of CBD include marked asymmetry of involvement, unilateral focal rigidity, dystonia (abnormal muscle tone) of the arm and leg and cortical signs, mainly limb apraxia. In some cases, patients develop "alien limb" phenomena, characterized by spontaneous arm levitation (Litvan et al., 1999). As the disease progresses, the arm and leg become functionally impaired and useless, in combination with increased tone leading to contractures. Infrequently, CBD patients have ophthalmoparesis. Cognitive impairment is also present with depression, apathy, irritability and agitation. Patients with CBD rarely benefit from levodopa. The average survival is 7–8 years.

Dementia with Lewy Bodies

DLB is increasingly recognized as a distinct neurodegenerative disorder with variable clinical presentations. Currently, DLB has emerged as the second most common cause of degenerative dementia in the elderly. It clinically overlaps with both PD and AD. Patients with DLB exhibit fluctuating cognitive impairment with pronounced variation in alertness and attention. They may experience recurrent visual hallucination and delusions unrelated to medication's side effects. DLB patients usually have symmetric parkinsonism. Dysarthria, dysphagia and falls develop earlier than in PD (Litvan et al., 1998). The distinction between PD with dementia (20% of all PD patients) and DLB remains unclear and is arbitrarily based on occurrence of dementia and parkinsonism within 1 year of DLB symptoms onset (McKeith et al., 2005).

No curative therapies are available for atypical parkinsonian syndromes. Levodopa may be helpful in MSA and DLB cases, and the dose of medication is usually increased cautiously due to possible worsening of orthostatic hypotension. Botulinum toxin injections may be helpful in dystonia associated with CBD or PSP. Dysphagia is managed by utilizing straws, food thickeners, soft processed food and percutaneous endoscopic gastroscopy. Patients with atypical parkinsonism require multiple social services and may eventually require nursing home placement.

Hyperkinetic Movement Disorders

The clinical presentation and nomenclature of the hyperkinetic movements is extensive, and following the format of this chapter, we will focus on hyperkinetic movement disorders of the orofacial and cervical region which dentists may encounter during their regular office visits. Dentists might be the first medical professionals to recognize the development of involuntary movements in the orofacial region. The hyperkinetic movement disorders discussed in this chapter include tremor, dystonia, choreoathetosis and tics.

Tremor

Tremor is the most common of all movement disorders, defined as involuntary rhythmical oscillation of a body part. Tremor may exist as a manifestation of a single clinical entity (e.g. essential tremor, physiological tremor) or may be a part of a larger spectrum of symptoms constituting a disease state (PD).

Essential tremor (ET) is the most common of all tremor disorders and therefore probably the most common movement disorder. The stated prevalence is quite variable, ranging from 1% to 22% of the older adult population (Findley, 2000). Nearly 2% of individuals over 60 may be affected. Precise numbers are elusive as many people have asymptomatic tremor or do not achieve the age at which the tremor would become prominent enough for them to seek medical attention. ET is a slowly progressive disorder mainly seen in later adulthood, but the first symptoms can be seen as early as the second decade. ET most often affects the hands, and affected individuals often complain of inability to sign checks, eat soup or pour liquid due to hand tremor. Patients may show tongue tremor on protrusion, head tremor of "yes–yes" or "no–no" type, and chin tremor. Legs and trunk may also be involved. Voice disturbance is not uncommon in ET and is thought to be related to vocal cord tremor. Tremor may improve with alcohol in some ET patients. The pathophysiology of ET is poorly understood. It is considered to be a central tremor, arising from central nervous system oscillators, the location of which is unknown (Deuschl & Elble, 2000). Most specialists now use primidone as the first drug of choice for ET, however only 40–50% of patients achieve improvement with primidone. Beta-blockers, short acting propanolol or long acting Inderal were found to be helpful in reducing tremor of ET (Koller et al., 2000a). Benzodiazepines and short acting beta-blockers may reduce tremor prior to public appearances or other stressful situations. In cases of medication resistant ET deep brain stimulation of the vental intermediate nucleus of the thalamus showed marked improvement in 80–90% of patients (Koller et al., 2000b).

Dystonia

Dystonia is defined as a syndrome with sustained muscle contractions frequently causing twisting and repetitive movements or abnormal postures (Fahn et al., 1998). An additional characteristic feature of dystonia is its responsiveness to sensory input. The "geste antagoniste" or sensory trick describes a touch or sensory maneuver that, when applied, reduces or eliminates the dystonia. There are several ways to classify dystonia. Dystonia is classified by the age of onset: (childhood form and adolescence form, both with the age of onset less than 26 years, and adult from) body distribution and etiology. Classification by body area includes focal (involving a single body area), segmental (involving contiguous body areas) and generalized (involving at least one leg, trunk and other body part) forms. Typically, childhood-onset dystonia starts in the lower extremities, with spread to other body parts to become generalized within 5 years. In contrast, in adults focal dystonias predominate and often begin in the upper body (arm, neck or face). Dystonia rarely becomes generalized in adults (Geene et al., 1995). The prevalence of primary generalized dystonia was reported at 3–4 persons per 100,000 in Rochester, Minnesota (Nutt et al., 1988). Focal dystonia is approximately 10 times more frequent with prevalence figures ranging from 6 to 225 cases per 100, 000 persons (Bressman, 2000). With rare exceptions, adult-onset dystonias are idiopathic and sporadic in inheritance. Currently, 13 genetic forms of dystonia have been described (Segawa et al., 1976; Kramer et al., 1999; Waddy et al., 1991). Many of them have additional neurologic findings, including parkinsonism, myoclonus, chorea and spasticity. Of these, only one mutation – DYT 1 – responsible for early-onset autosomal dominant form of generalized dystonia is available for commercial screening. DYT1 is a mutation on gene 9q34 representing a CAG deletion within the coding area for the protein torsin A (Bressman et al., 2000).

The pathophysiology of dystonia is not well understood, and currently, the physiologic inhibitory control of the basal ganglia over the thalamus and cortex is thought to be defective. Dystonia may involve any part of the body, but it has a predilection for head and neck musculature. Blepharospasm is a focal dystonia characterized by involuntary, forceful, bilateral eye closure. Clinical manifestations include increased blinking and spasms under conditions of bright light or stress. This may be infrequent and asymptomatic or sustained causing functional blindness. When blepharospasm coexists with other focal dystonia of the head and neck, it is referred to as Meige syndrome. Oromandibular dystonia (OMD) and facial dystonia are characterized by involuntary movements involving masticatory, lingual and pharyngeal muscles, causing painful spasms, and twisting and jerky movements. Lip retraction, grimacing and tongue protrusion may interfere with food intake as food is pushed out of the mouth. Dystonia may rarely involve pharyngeal muscles leading to dysphagia. Jaw dystonia causes involuntary jaw closure (trismus), jaw opening or lateral deviation. Involuntary jaw closure with trismus causes teeth grinding or clenching and may be so forceful as to cause tooth wear and loss. In one case, rupture of the lingual frenum with hematoma and swelling required urgent evaluation (Blanchet et al., 2005). Patient often use sensory tricks by holding a seed or candy in the mouth, placing a straw or a piece of plastic between the maxillary and mandibular molars on one side, or light touch on a tooth or chin to reduce the intensity of the dystonic spasms.

The most common focal dystonia in adults is torticollis, better termed cervical dystonia. Cervical dystonia presents as a sustained abnormal head posture, sometimes associated with superimposed clonic movements, produced by simultaneous contraction of agonists and antagonists muscle groups. There are several well-recognized head postures including horizontal rotary torticollis with the head turned either left or right, laterocollis, with the ear deviated laterally to the shoulder, anterocollis with the head flexed, or retrocollis with the head extended. Many patients have several patterns of head movement. Dystonia is a dynamic disorder that changes in severity depending on activity or posture. An example of this is writer's cramp, dystonia of the hand and arm, which is present during the action of writing and not at any other activity. Another example of task-specific dystonia is occupational facial dystonia of woodwind and brass musicians, called embouchure dystonia, involving lips, tongue, or jaw that affects musicians only during the act of playing their instruments, and is absent during other activities such as speaking and eating.

No curative therapy is available for dystonia, and treatment is symptomatic. Treatment includes medications, chemodenervation with botulinum toxin and surgery. About 50–85 percent of patients with focal dystonia of the face and neck are successfully treated with botulinum toxin injections (Jost & Kohl, 2001). It is considered the treatment of choice for many focal dystonias, including OMD with bruxism. Several classes of medication are used including high doses of anticholinergic drugs, baclofen, tetrabenazine and clonazepam (Jankovic, 2004). In general, medications are used for generalized dystonia or as an adjunct to botulinum toxin injections in focal dystonias. Clonazepam is a benzodiazepine reported in uncontrolled studies to improve symptoms of dystonia in approximately one-fifth of patients at doses ranging from 1.5 mg to 12 mg per day (Greene et al., 1988). Surgical intervention such as deep brain stimulation of the bilateral globus pallidus is reserved for patients with intractable symptoms and is currently used primarily in patient with generalized dystonia (Lozano & Abosch, 2004). Dentists and prosthodontists are often a key member of the management of oral dystonias. For cases of jaw-closing dystonia clearly responsive to sensory trick, a simple bite-raising soft device fitting between the molars to prevent jaw closure by a few millimeters can improve function (Frucht et al., 1999; Lo et al., 2007). Such devices should be introduced early to prevent tooth wear and temporomandibular joint dysfunction.

Tardive Dyskinesia

Dyskinesia is a general term referring to abnormal involuntary movements. The term tardive dyskinesia (TD) refers to abnormal movements seen as a complication of long-term dopamine receptor antagonist therapy, mainly presenting with rapid stereotypic repetitive movements of oral, buccal and lingual areas. Oro-buccal dyskinesias consist of chewing motions, smacking and licking of the lips, tongue protrusion or constant writhing movements of the tongue when the mouth is held open, which may lead to tongue hypertrophy. Macroglossia is a common clinical sign of TD. The rhythmicity and coordinated pattern of movements is striking. Patients are often unaware of the movements. Dyskinesias may also be accompanied by a feeling of restlessness when patients cannot stay still during the dental procedure, along with constant movements of the fingers, toes and pelvis.

Previous or current exposure to a dopamine receptor blocking (DRB) agent (neuroleptics, metoclopramide, prochlorperazine, etc.) causes TD. The mechanism of TD is not well understood, but currently it is thought that dopamine receptor blockers lead to hypersensitivity of remaining dopamine receptors. Epidemiological studies examining the prevalence of TD have been confounded by factors that affect the detection of the abnormal involuntary movements as well as the variables that affect the prognosis of these movements. Therefore, it is not surprising to find a wide range of prevalence estimations from 0.5% to 65% in the literature (Kane & Smith 1982, Jeste & Wyatt 1982). Kane et al. (1986) showed that the cumulative incidence of TD increases linearly with increasing duration of neuroleptic exposure at least for the first 4–5 years of such exposure. The cumulative incidence of presumptive TD was 6.3% after 1 year of neuroleptic exposure, 11.5% after 2 years, 13.7% after 3 years and 17.5% after 4 years (Chakos et al., 1996). African-Americans are more susceptible to TD than European-Americans. Females are more susceptible, especially in the older population.

It is important to remember that if a patient presents with symptoms of TD and is still on an offending medication, the abrupt discontinuation of the medication may lead to worsening of the symptoms. Rather gradual decrease of the dose to complete discontinuation is a better approach. The movements sometimes persist long after the exposure to neuroleptics. Earlier detection and discontinuation of the offending dopamine receptor blocker increases the chance for clinical remission, thus detection of the stereotypical lip and tongue movements at the dentists' office should be immediately reported to the primary care physician. If neuroleptics cannot be discontinued, or TD persists after offending medication is discontinued, dopamine depletors like tetrabenazine or reserpine can be helpful in minimizing the movements and allowing the brain to heal.

Several case reports describe certain dental conditions, especially edentulousness and poor fitting prostheses as a possible cause for orofacial dyskinesias; however, conclusions regarding the existence of a "dental" subtype of orofacial dystonia are difficult to draw (Koller, 1983; Sutcher et al., 1971; Sankhla et al., 1998; Schrag et al., 1999).

Edentulous Dyskinesia

Edentulousness is thought to be a common cause of oral dyskinesia, although the number of studies on this association is surprisingly low. Koller (1983) compared 75 consecutive edentulous subjects to 75 age-matched controls with natural teeth. Twelve (16%) of the edentulous subjects had oral dyskinesia, whereas none of the control subjects were affected. Stereotyped smacking and pursing of the lips, lateral deviation and protrusion of the tongue, and occasionally lateral deviation and protrusion of the jaw have been documented. Unlike drug-induced dyskinesias, the movements observed were always confined to the oral region and never dystonic, and no tongue movements were recorded when the mouth was open. Sutcher et al. (1971) argued that edentulousness (along with incorrect occlusions produced by inadequate dentures) chronically distort most of the peripheral proprioceptive input from the stomatognatic system necessary for central sensorimotor integration, thereby promoting dyskinesia. Sutcher et al. (1971) reported improvement in four patients after unconventional prosthethic therapy, the benefit of which was repeated anecdotally in a few other cases (Sutcher et al., 1998; Lauciello & Appelbaum, 1977; Kelleher et al., 1998).

Dental Procedure-Related Dystonia

Peripheral trauma precipitating focal dystonia is well recognized and occurs in up to 20% of patients with limb and cervical dystonia, blepharospasm and idiopathic torsion dystonia. Dental intervention represents a peripheral iatrogenic injury to the lower face, and in rare case reports have been implicated as a trigger of oromandibular dystonia (Sankhla et al., 1998; Schrag et al., 1999). The mean latency between the insult and the onset of the movement disorder was less than 3 months, most within hours or days. None of 35 patients reported had ever taken antipsychotic medications, showed brain lesions in basal ganglia or reported a family member with focal dystonia. A coincidence or unmasking effect by the dental procedure of a latent movement disorder cannot be entirely ruled out, nor can a psychogenic disorder.

Chorea

Chorea, derived from the Latin *choreus* meaning "dance", refers to irregular, rapid, nonsustained movements that flow from one body part to another. The movements are unpredictable in timing, direction and distribution. They often involve the lower and upper part of the face and present with brow frowning, winking, lip twitching and pursing. Sometimes patients are unable to maintain sustained contractions, which presents as inability to keep the tongue protruded or dropping objects due to inability to sustain a tight grip. Chorea is a clinical hallmark of Huntington's disease, an autosomal-dominant neurodegenerative disorder associated with CAG trinucleotide repeats in the IT 15 gene on the short arm of chromosome 4. About 10% of HD cases develop before age 20, but the typical peak age at onset occurs in the fourth or fifth decade. The estimated prevalence of HD in the United States is 2–10 per 100,000 population (Kokmen et al., 1994). Chorea rarely requires treatment, and cognitive impairment and psychiatric symptoms are the main causes of patient disability. Dental treatment of patients with HD is hindered by involuntary mouth and jaw movements. Timing and patience may allow a procedure without sedation; however, sedation cannot always be avoided, especially when the extensive procedures are necessary (Bradford et al., 2004; Feeney, 1985).

Tics

Tics can occur as a primary disorder or secondary to an identifiable etiology. Tics occur in children with developmental and chromosomal abnormalities. They also may be associated with infections (encephalitis, Sydneham's chorea, neurosyphilis), drugs (amphetamines, levodopa, antipsychotics), toxins (carbon monoxide), neurodegenerative diseases (Huntington's disease, Wilson's disease, tuberous sclerosis), and head trauma. Although there are many causes of tics, motor and vocal tics are most often associated with Gilles de la Tourette's syndrome (GTS).

GTS is a clinically heterogeneous disorder in which patients manifest a wide spectrum of involuntary movements (motor tics), noises (vocal tics) and behavioral problems. Tics are usually preceded by a sensory urge to move the affected body part. Although the tics can be suppressed voluntarily, the sensory urge builds, resulting in a flurry of tics in rapid succession. Tics are less frequent when the patient is relaxed or concentrating on an enjoyable activity, while stress and anxiety often precipitate and increase the magnitude of tics. Stress and demands of a dental treatment visit may exacerbate tics. Stress can be minimized by dividing dental procedures into small segments and permitting the patient to control the pace of the treatment, allowing the patient to get up, or halt briefly the procedure to dissipate the tension that builds up from the need to suppress the tics.

Motor tics are stereotypic, repetitive movements that may be simple or complex. Examples of simple motor tics include eye blinking, eye rolling, shoulder shrug, lip smacking or lip licking, facial twitching or simultaneous contraction of the lower face and eye blinking, neck jerks, rapid flexion and extension of the arms, hands, trunk or legs. Complex motor tics appear as semi-purposeful movements such as touching oneself or others, hitting the wall, bending to touch the floor, imitating the movements of others (echopraxia) and gesturing obscenely. Vocal tics are analogous to motor tics: simple vocal tics consist of unintelligible sounds such as sniffs, grunts squeaks or shouts, and complex vocal tics consist of words and phrases that are out of context and include phenomena such as repeating one's own words (palilalia), repeating the words of others (echolalia) and using obscene words (coprolalia). Despite popular belief, the presence of coprolalia is rare, affecting less than 10% of patients with GTS (Singer, 1997).

Chronic oral tics may cause severe oral and dental complications. In approximately 20% of patients, tics consist of jaw thrusting, repeat mouth opening, tooth-clicking, bruxism, orofacial pain and dysfunction of the TMJ (Riley & Lang, 1989). Perioral movements may be so severe as to lead to loosening and exfoliation of the permanent teeth due to severe bruxism and the development of chronic non-healing lip and mucosal ulcers. Compulsive touching and manipulation of the oral structures is another common problem. If extreme, it can lead to abraded and friable gingiva and self-extraction of permanent teeth (Woody & Eisenhauer, 1986).

The lifetime prevalence of GTS is unknown, but it is currently estimated at 0.5 per 1000. This rate is probably a gross underestimate because many cases are mild and do not come to medical attention. Boys are affected more commonly than girls (4:1) (Comings et al., 1990). The mean age at onset is 7 years, and 99% of patients have symptoms before the age of 11 years. GTS has been considered a genetic disorder based on the clinical observation that several generations in one family may be affected. However, the lack of complete concordance in monozygotic twins (only 53% compared to dizigotic twin at 8%), suggests that additional factors contribute to the phenotypic expression of GTS. The etiology of the disorder remains unknown. Current models of GTS suggest dysregulation in corticothalamocortical circuitry with abnormal activation and poor suppression of a particular group of striatal neurons leading to the production of stereotyped patterned movements or tics (Mink, 2001).

Obsessive-compulsive disorder (OCD) is a common finding in patient with GTS. More than 25% of pediatrics patients and between 50% and 90% adult GTS patients have obsessive-compulsive symptoms of such magnitude as to also qualify for a diagnosis of OCD. Attention deficit-hyperactivity disorder, characterized by inattention and impulsivity, is observed in 50–60% of children with GTS. Patient with GTS are usually able to function normally with appropriate counseling. Medications are reserved for those whose symptoms impair psychosocial, educational or occupational functioning. The antipsychotics haloperidol and pimozide are frequently prescribed to decrease the number and intensity of motor and vocal tics but are ineffective at controlling behavioral problems of ADHD and OCD. Chemodenervation of particular muscle groups with botulinum toxin injections ameliorates not only the involuntary movements but also the premonitory sensory component (Kwak et al., 2000). ADHD is treated with CNS stimulants such as methylphenidate (Ritalin), control-released methylphenidate (Concerta), dexmethylphenidate (Focalin) and a combination of dextroamphetamine and levoamphetamine (Adderall). Initial concern that stimulants could unmask or exacerbate motor and vocal tics in up to 25% of GTS patients now has been allayed by ample evidence that worsening of the tics is not frequent and usually mild and transient (Kurlan, 2003). Strattera, a norepinephrine reuptake inhibitor, is the only nonstimulant medication used for treatment of the ADHD. Clonidine and guanfacine, the alpha–2 agonists, improve symptoms of ADHD and of impulse control problems. OCD is treated with the selective serotonergic reuptake inhibitors. Surgical treatment of GTS is controversial. The overall experience of stereotactic ablative surgery in the treatment of tics has been rather disappointing. Increasing reports have provided evidence that deep brain stimulation involving thalamus, globus pallidum or other targets could be beneficial to treat severe medically uncontrollable tics (Ackermans et al., 2006; Shahed et al., 2007) A few reports described the contribution of the dentist to the management of the orofacial aspects of GTS (Woody & Eisenhauer, 1986; Friedlander & Cummings, 1992; Leksell & Edvardson, 2005). These cases mainly described the application of dental splints against self-mutilation. A major focus should be on preventive measures, so that extensive treatments can be avoided. If extensive treatments are necessary, one should keep in mind that nitric oxide sedation causes exacerbation of tics and intravenous sedation with midazolam can be used for extensive procedures (Yoshikawa et al., 2002).

Concluding Remarks

From our review, it can be gathered that the described movement disorders can have a profound impact on the provision of oral health care services. Many have facial manifestations as a part of their presentation, and several conditions exclusively affect the oro-facial area. Movements in the oro-facial region can be due to either the disorder itself or secondary to the medications that are being used to alleviate the disorder. By understanding the pathogenesis of the disease, the limitations and problems facing the patients, and the side effects of the drugs used to control the disease, dental offices can effectively manage these patients with less apprehension and stress.

References

Aarsland, D., Zaccai, J., & Brayne, C. (2005). A systematic review of prevalence studies of dementia in Parkinson's disease. *Movement Disorders, 20,* 1255–1263.

Ackermans, L., Temel, Y., Cath, D., van der Linden, C., Bruggerman, R., Kleijer, M., Nederveen, P., Schruers, K., Colle, H., Tijssen, M.A., Visser-Vandewalle, V., & Dutch Flemish Tourette Surgery Study Group. (2006). Deep brain stimulation in Tourette's syndrome: two targets? *Movement Disorders, 21,* 709–713.

Alexander, R.E., & Gage, T.W. (2000). Parkinson's disease: an update for dentists. *General Dentistry, 48,* 572–580.

Blanchet, P.J., Allard, P., Gregoire, L., Tardif, F., & Bernard, P.J. (1996). Risk factors for peak dose dyskinesia in 100 levodopa-treated parkinsonian patients. *Canadian Journal of Neurological Science, 23,* 189–193.

Blanchet, P.J., Rompre, P.H., Lavingne, G.J., & Lamarche, C. (2005). Oral dyskinesia: a clinical overview. *The International Journal of Prosthodontics, 18,* 10–19.

Bonifati, V., Rizzi, P., van Baren, M.J., Schaap, O., Breedveld, G.J., Krieger, E., & Dekker, M.C. (2003). Mutation in DJ-1 gene associated with autosomal recessive early – onset parkinsonism. *Science, 299,* 256–259.

Bower, J.H., Maraganore, D.M., McDonnell, S.K., & Rocca, W.A. (1997). Incidence of progressive supranuclear palsy and multiple system atrophy in Olmsted County, Minnesota 1976–1990. *Neurology, 49,* 1284–1288.

Bower, J.H., Maraganore, D.M., & McDonnell, S.K. (1999). Incidence and distribution of parkinsonism in Olmsted County, Minnesota, 1976–1990. *Neurology, 52,* 1214–1220.

Bradford, H., Britto, L.R., Leal, G., & Katz, J. (2004). Endodontic treatment of a patient with Huntington's disease. *Journal of Endodontics, 30,* 366–369.

Bressman, S.B. (2000). Dystonia update. *Clinical Neuropharmacology, 23,* 239–251.

Bressman, S.B., Sabatti, C., Raymond, D., de Leon D, Klein, C., Kramer, P.L., Brin, M.F., Fahn, S., Breakefield, X., Oselius, L.J., & Risch, N.J. (2000). The DYT1 phenotype and guidelines for diagnostic testing. *Neurology, 54,* 1746–1752.

Chakos, M.H., Alvir, J.M.J., Woerner, M.G., Koreen, A., Geisler, S., Mayerhoff, D., Sobel, S., Kane, J.M., Borenstein. M., & Lieberman, J.A. (1996). Incidence and correlates of tardive dyskinesia in first episode of schizophrenia. *Archives of General Psychiatry, 53,* 313–319.

Clifford, T., & Finnerty, J. (1995). The dental awareness and needs of Parkinson's disease population. *Gerontology, 12,* 99–103.

Collins, R. (1990). Special considerations for the dental patient with Parkinson's disease. *Texas Dentistry Journal, 107,* 31–33.

Comings, D.E., Himes, J.A., & Comings, B.G. (1990). An epidemiologic study of Tourette's syndrome in a single school district. *Journal of Clinical Psychiatry, 51,* 463–469.

Deuschl, G., & Elble, R.J. (2000). The pathophysiology of essential tremor. *Neurology, 54 (suppl. 4),* S14–S20.

Dujardin, K., Defbvre, L., & Grunberg, C. (2001). Memory and executive function in sporadic and familial Parkinson's disease. *Brain, 123,* 115–1160.

Fahn, S., Bressman, S.B., & Marsden, C.D. (1998). Classification of dystonia. *Advances in Neurology, 78,* 1–10.

Feeney, A.W. (1985). Dental treatment considerations for patients with Huntington's chorea: a literature review and case report. *Journal of Connecticut State Dental Association, 59*, 118–123.

Findley, L.J. (2000). Epidemiology and genetics of essential tremor. *Neurology, 54 (suppl 4)*, S8–S13.

Friedlander, A.H., & Cummings, J.L. (1992). Dental treatment of patients with Gilles de la Tourette's syndrome. *Oral Surgery, Oral Medicine and Oral Pathology, 73*, 299–303.

Frucht, S., Fahn, S., Ford, B., & Gelb, M. (1999). A geste antagoniste device to treat jaw – closing dystonia. *Movement Disorders, 14*, 883–886.

Fukayo, S., Nonaka, K., Shimizu, T., & Yano, E. (2003). Oral health of patient with Parkinson's disease: factors related to their better dental status. *Tohoku Journal of Experimental Medicine, 201*, 171–179.

Geene, P., Kahn, U.J., & Fahn, S. (1995). Spread of symptoms in idiopathic torsion dystonia. *Movement Disorders, 10*, 143–152.

Golbe, L.I., Davis, P.H., Schoenberg, B.S., & Duvoisin, R.C. (1988). Prevalence and natural history of progressive supranuclear palsy. *Neurology, 38*, 1031–1034.

Greene, P., Shale, H., & Fahn, S. (1988). Experience with high dosages of anticholinergic and other drugs in the treatment of torsion dystonia. *Advances in Neurology, 50*, 547–556.

Jankovic, J. (2004). Dystonia: medical therapy and botulinum toxin. *Advances of Neurology, 94*, 275–286.

Jeste, D.V., & Wyatt, R.J. (1982). Therapeutic strategies against tardive dyskinesia; two decades of experience. *Archives of Psychiatry, 39*, 803–816.

Jost, W.H., & Kohl, A. (2001). Botulinum toxin: evidence-based medicine criteria in rare indications. *Journal of Neurology, 248 (suppl 1)*, 39–44.

Kane, J.M., & Smith, J.M. (1982). Tardive dyskinesia: prevalence and risk factors, 1959 to 1979. *Archives of General Psychiatry, 39*, 473–481.

Kane, J.M., Woerner, M., Borenstein, M., Wegner, J., & Lieberman, J. (1986). Integrating incidence and prevalence of tardive dyskinesia. *Psychopharmacology Bulletin, 22*, 254–258.

Kelleher, M.G.D., Scott, B.J.J., & Djemal, S. (1998). Case report: Complications of rehabilitation using osseointegrated implants – tardive dyskinesia. *European Journal of Prosthodontics and Restorative Dentistry, 6*, 133–136.

Kitada, T., Asakawa, S., Hattori, N., &Yamamura, Y. (1998). Mutations in the parkin gene cause autosomal recessive juvenile parkinsonism. *Nature, 392*, 605–608.

Kokmen, E., Ozekmekci, F.S, Beard, C.M,, O'Brien, P.C, & Kurland, L.T. (1994). Incidence and prevalence of Huntington's disease in Olmsted County, Minnesota (1950 through 1989). *Archives of Neurology, 51*, 696–698.

Koller, W.C. (1983). Edentulous orodyskinesia. *Annals of Neurology, 13*, 97–99.

Koller, W.C., Hristova, A., & Brin, M. (2000a). Pharmacologic treatment of essential tremor. *Neurology, 54 (suppl 4)*, S30–S38.

Koller, W.C., Pahwa, R., Lyons, K.E., & Wilkinson, S.B. (2000b). Deep brain stimulation of the Vim nucleus of the thalamus for the treatment of tremor. *Neurology, 55 (suppl 6)*, S29–S33.

Kramer, P.L., Mineta, M., Klein, C., Schilling K, de Leon, D., Farlow, M.R., Breakefield, X.O., Bressman, S.B., Dobyns, W.B., Ozelius, L.J, & Brashear. A. (1999). Rapid onset dystonia-parkinsonism: linkage to chromosome 19q13. *Annals of Neurology, 46*, 176–182.

Kurlan, R. (2003). Tourette's syndrome: are stimulants safe? *Current Neurology and Neuroscience Reports, 3*, 285–288.

Kwak, C.H., Hanna, P.A., Jankovic, J. (2000). Botulinum toxin in the treatment of tics. *Archives of Neurology, 57*, 1190–1193.

Langston, J.W., Forno, L.S., Tetrud, J., Reeves, A.G., Kaplan, J.A., & Karluk, D. (1999). Evidence of active nerve cell degeneration in the substantia nigra of human years after 1-methyl-4-phenyl–1,2,3,6–tetrahydropyridine exposure. *Annals of Neurology, 46*, 598–605.

Lauciello, F., & Appelbaum, M. (1977). Prosthodontic implication of tardive dyskinesia. *New York State Dentistry Journal, 43*, 214–217.

Leksell,E., & Edvardson, S. (2005). A case of Tourette syndrome presenting with oral self-injurious behavior. *International Journal of Pediatric Dentistry, 15*, 370–374.

Litvan, I., MacIntyre, A., Goetz, C.G., Wenning, G.K., Jellinger, K., Verny, M., Bartko, J.J., Jankovic, J., McKee, A., Brandel, J.P., Chaudhuri, K.R., Lai, E.C., D'Olhaberriaque, L., Pearce, R.K., & Agid, Y. (1998). Accuracy of the clinical diagnoses of Lewy body disease, Parkinson's disease and dementia with Lewy bodies: a clinicopathologic study. *Archives of Neurology, 55*, 969–978.

Litvan, I., Grimes, D.A., Lang, A.E., Jankovic, J., McKee, A., Verny, M., Jellinger, K., Chaundhuri, K.R., & Pearce, R.K. (1999). Clinical feature differentiating patient with postmortem confirmed progressive supranuclear palsy and corticobasal degeneration. *Journal of Neurology, 246 (suppl 2)*, II1–II5.

Lo, S.E., Gelb, M., & Frucht, S.J. (2007). Geste antagoniste in idiopathic lower cranial dystonia. *Movement Disorders, 22*, 1012–1017.

Lozano, A.M., & Abosch, A. (2004). Pallidal stimulation for dystonia. *Advances in Neurology, 94*, 301–308.

McKeith, I.G., Dickson, D.W., Lowe, J., Emre, M., O'Brien, J.T., Feldman, H., Cummings, J., Duda, J.E., Lippa, C., & Perry, E.K. (2005). Diagnosis and management of dementia with Lewy bodies: third report on the DLB consortium. *Neurology, 65*, 1863–1872.

Mink, J.W. (2001). Basal ganglia dysfunction in Tourette's syndrome: a new hypothesis. *Pediatrics Neurology, 25*, 190–198.

Nakayama, Y., Washio, M., & Mori, M. (2004). Oral health conditions in patients with Parkinson's disease. *Journal of Epidemiology, 14*, 143–150.

Nutt, J.G., Muenter, M.D., Aronson, A., Kurland, L.T., & Melton, L.J. 3rd. (1988). Epidemiology of focal and generalized dystonia in Rochester, Minnesota. *Movement Disorders, 3*, 188–194.

Olanow, C.W., Goetz, C.G., Kordower, J.H., Stoessl, A.J., Sosi, V., Brin, M.F., Shannon, K.M., Nauert, G.M., Perl, D.P., Godbold, J., & Freeman, T.B. (2003). A double-blind controlled trial of bilateral fetal nigral transplantation in Parkinson's disease. *Annals of Neurology, 54*, 403–414.

Paisan-Ruiz, C., Lang, A.E., Kawarai, T., & Sato, C. (2005). LRRK2 gene in Parkinson disease: mutation analysis and case control association study. *Neurology, 65*, 696–700.

Polymeropoulos, M.H., Lavedan, C., & Leroy, E. (1997). Mutation in the alpha-synuclein gene identified in families with Parkinson's disease. *Science, 276*, 2045–2047.

Pradhan, S., Pander, N., Shashank, S., Gupta, R.K., & Mathur, A. (1999). Parkinsonism due to predominant involvement of substantia nigra in Japanese Encephalitis. *Neurology, 53*, 1781–1786.

Rajput, A.H. (1994). Clinical features and natural history of Parkinson's disease (Special consideration of aging). In: D.B. Calne (Eds.), *Neurodegenerative diseases* (pp. 555–571). Philadelphia: WB Saunders.

Riley, D., & Lang, A.E. (1989). Pain in Gilles de la Tourette's syndrome and related tic disorders. *Canadian Journal of Neurological Science, 16*, 439–441.

Rodriquez-Oroz, M.C., Obeso, J.A., Lang, A.E., Houeto, J.L. , Pollak, P., Rehncrona, S., Kulisevsky, J., Albanese, A., Volkmann, J., Hariz, M.I., Quinn, N.P., Speelman, J.D., Guridi, J., Zamarbide, I., Gironell, A., Molet, J., Pascual-Sedno, B., Pidoux, B., Bonnet, A.M., Ajid, Y., Xie, J., Benabid, A.L., Lozano, A.M., Saint-Cyr, J., Romito, L., Contarino, M.F., Scerrati, M., Fraix, V., & Van Blercom, N. (2005). Bilateral deep brain stimulation in Parkinson's disease: a multicentral study with 4 years follow – up. *Brain, 128*, 2240–2249.

Saito, Y., Matsuoka, Y., Takahashi, A., & Ohno, Y. (1994). Survival of patients with multiple system atrophy. *Internal Medicine, 33*, 321–325.

Sankhla, C., Lai, E.C., & Jankovic, J. (1998). Peripherally induced oromandibular dystonia. *Journal of Neurology, Neurosurgery and Psychiatry, 65*, 722–728.

Santacruz, P., Uttl, B., Livan, I., & Grafman, J. (1998). Progressive supranuclear palsy: A survery of the disease course. *Neurology, 50*, 1637–1647.

Schoenberg, B.S., Anderson, D.W., & Haerer, A.F. (1985). Prevalence of Parkinson's disease in the biracial population of Copiah County, Mississippi. *Neurology, 35*, 841–845.

Schrag, A., Ben-Shlomo, Y., & Quinn, N.P. (1999). Prevalence of progressive supranuclear palsy and multiple system atrophy: a cross – sectional study. *Lancet, 354*, 1771–1775.

Schrag, A., Bhatia, K.P, Quinn, N.P, & Marsden, C.D. (1999). Atypical and typical cranial dystonia following dental procedures. *Movement Disorders, 14*, 492–496.

Segawa, M., Hosaka, A., Miyagawa, F., Nomura, Y., & Imai H. (1976). Hereditary progressive dystonia with marked diurnal fluctuation. Advances in *Neurology, 14*, 215–233.

Sejvar, J.J., Haddad, M.B., Tierney, B.C., Campbell, G.L., Marfin, A.A., Van Gerpen, J.A., Fleischauer, A., Leiss, A.A., Stokic, D.S., & Petersen, L.R . (2003). Neurologic manifestations and outcome of West Nile Virus infection. *Journal of American Medical Association, 290*, 511–515.

Shahed, J., Poysky, J., Kenney, C., Simpson, R., & Jankovic, J. (2007). GPi deep brain stimulation for Tourette syndrome improves tics and psychiatric comorbilities. *Neurology, 68*, 159–160.

Singer, C. (1997). Tourette syndrome. Coprolalia and other coprophenomena. *Neurological Clinics, 15*, 299–308.

Sutcher, H., Soderstrom, J., Perry, R., & Das, A. (1998). Tardive dyskinesia: dental prosthetic therapy. *Panminerva medica, 40*, 154–156.

Sutcher, H.D., Underwood, R.B., Beatty, R.A., & Sugar O. (1971). Orofacial dyskinesia – a dental dimension. *Journal of American Medical Association, 216*, 1459–1463.

Tanner, C.M. (1992). Occupational and environmental causes of parkinsonism. *Occupational Medicine, 7*, 503–513.

Uc, E.Y., Rizzo, M., Anderson, S.W., & Qian, S. (2005). Visual dysfunction in Parkinson disease without dementia. *Neurology, 65*, 1907–1913.

Volkmann, J., Allert, N., Vodes, J., Weiss, P.H., Freund, H.J., & Sturm, V. (2001). Safety and efficacy of pallidal or subthalamic nucleus stimulation in advanced PD. *Neurology, 57*, 1354–1358.

Waddy, H.M., Fletcher, N.A,, Harding, A.E., Marsden, C.D. (1991). A genetic study of idiopathic dystonias. *Annals of Neurology, 29*, 320–324.

Woody, R.C., & Eisenhauer, G. (1986). Tooth extraction as a form of self- mutilation in Tourette's disorder. *South Medical Journal, 79*, 1466.

Yoshikawa, F., Takagi, T., Fukayama, H., Miwa, Z., & Umino, M. (2002). Intravenous sedation and general anesthesia for a patient with Gilles de la Tourette's syndrome undergoing dental treatment. *Acta Anasthesiologica Scandinavia, 46*, 1279–1280.

Zanettini, R., Antonini, A., Gatto, G., Gentile, R., Tesei, S., & Pezzoli, G. (2007). Valvular heart disease and the use of dopamine agonists for Parkinson's disease. *New England Journal of Medicine, 356*, 39–46.

Chapter 6
Cognitive Impairment

James M. Noble and Nikolaos Scarmeas

Introduction

Cognitive disorders become more prevalent with age, are medically refractory, reduce life expectancy, and significantly impact effective health interventions in the elderly. As the population ages in the next few decades, the number of patients with cognitive impairment and dementia, most frequently Alzheimer disease (AD), will increase dramatically (Hebert et al. 2003). Oral health problems including periodontal disease, caries, edentulism, and infrequent preventative care also become more prevalent among the elderly. Behaviors associated with cognitive disorders may impact access to appropriate oral health care measures and worsen dental health. Conversely, poor oral health can lead to changes in dietary preference, malnutrition in late life, and may further contribute to dementia. In this chapter, we review barriers to appropriate oral health care and intervention strategies relevant to older patients with cognitive disorders.

Review of Common Diagnoses with Cognitive Impairment

Dementia is the most common cognitive disorder to manifest with advanced age and is defined based on the Diagnostic and Statistical Manual 4th edition (DSM-IV) as cognitive impairment leading to social or occupational dysfunction (Small and Mayeux 2005). Current estimates suggest 24 million people have dementia worldwide. This number will jump to more than 80 million by the year 2040, and areas with rapid development and dense population such as China, India, and Latin America will be most affected (ADI 2006). AD is the most common type of dementia, followed by vascular dementia (VaD), dementia with Lewy bodies (DLB), and dementia with Parkinson disease (PDD), and the group of frontotemporal dementias

J.M. Noble

Department of Neurology Columbia University Medical Center 710 W. 168th St New York, NY, 10032 Tel: 212-305-9194, Fax: 212-305-2526

e-mail: jnoble@neuro.columbia.edu, jn2054@columbia.edu

I.B. Lamster, M.E. Northridge (eds.), *Improving Oral Health for the Elderly*,

© Springer Science+Business Media, LLC 2008

(FTD). In this chapter we briefly review common dementias as well as the neuropsychiatric attributes of other cognitive disorders affecting an aging population, including Huntington disease (HD), the complex picture of normal pressure hydrocephalus (NPH), HIV and other infections, nutritionally related dementias, and the rare prion diseases.

Alzheimer Disease

Alzheimer disease (AD) is the most common form of dementia, representing 60–70% of all patients with dementia. The prevalence increases with age from 5% in the seventh decade to 50% by the tenth decade of life (Gurland et al. 1999; Mayeux 2003b). Recent estimates suggest that in the United States alone, the number of patients affected by AD will jump from 5.1 million in 2010 to 13.2 million by 2050 (Hebert et al. 2003). Current worldwide estimates of Alzheimer disease are 18 million people with an expected doubling to 35 million by 2025; 70% will live in developing nations (Vas et al. 2001). The disease has a slow, insidious onset, initially affecting short-term memory with evidence of other higher cognitive dysfunction including language disturbance, inattention, disorientation, and visuospatial difficulties (Cummings 2004). Mild cognitive impairment (MCI), a related syndrome, represents a transitional stage in cognition different from normal aging. Although it begins with one or more impaired cognitive domains without clear functional impairment, MCI will proceed to dementia, most often AD, at a rate of 10–15% per year—much higher than that of "normal aging" (Hebert et al. 1995; Gurland et al. 1999; Bruscoli and Lovestone 2004; Drachman 2006). Associated psychiatric symptoms with AD can include depression, psychotic delusions (fixed false beliefs which are often suspicious or paranoid in nature), hallucinations (spontaneous perception of visual or auditory phenomena) (Scarmeas et al. 2005b), disruptive behavioral symptoms (ranging from apathy and withdrawal to irritability and anger) (Scarmeas et al. 2007), and sleep–wake cycle abnormalities. AD typically progresses over a range of 3–9 years from the time of diagnosis to death (Aronson et al. 1991; Heyman et al. 1996; Helmer et al. 2001; Wolfson et al. 2001; Waring et al. 2005). Social and physical functions become progressively impaired over this period. Ultimately, neglect of personal hygiene, including dressing, bathing, clothing, and oral health become more prominent as the patient nears an end stage, bedbound state. Death results from malnutrition, secondary infections, and other complications associated with being bedbound, including pneumonia, urinary tract infections, skin ulcers, and pulmonary emboli.

The pathologic hallmarks of brain deposition of neurofibrillary tangles and neuritic plaques are thought to be related to abnormal processing of a neuronal membrane protein, amyloid precursor protein, with excessive accumulation of beta-amyloid. The cause remains unknown. In the sporadic form, which represents 98% of all AD cases, studies suggest a complex interaction of environmental and vascular factors with genetic risk factors, such as the apoE4 allele (Tang et al. 1998;

Mayeux 2003a) and other possible loci (Rogaeva et al. 2007). Three genes are currently known to cause the rare familial AD cases (McKusick 2006).

Current treatment modalities for memory decline are limited to two classes of medications. The most commonly prescribed are the acetylcholinesterase inhibitors (donepezil, galantamine, and rivastigmine). The primary observed side effect of these drugs include gastrointestinal distress including anorexia, nausea, vomiting, and diarrhea. A newer medication, memantine, is an *N*-methyl-D-aspartate (NMDA) receptor antagonist and is indicated for moderate to severe disease; its mechanism is thought to be related to reducing glutamate excitotoxicity in the hippocampus. Depression is most frequently targeted with selective serotonin reuptake inhibitors (SSRIs). For behavioral features, atypical antipsychotics are used with varying tolerability and efficacy (Schneider et al. 2006a) and can have adverse side effects of Parkinson-like or "extrapyramidal" symptoms. Several studies are currently underway investigating disease-modifying therapies which target cellular processing of beta-amyloid.

Vascular Dementia

Vascular dementia is the second most common dementia in the United States and probably the most common in East Asia. Pure VaD is likely infrequent and may be more relevant as a contributing factor in patients with underlying coexisting AD pathology. Cognitive dysfunction in vascular dementia patients is due to cerebrovascular disease, as a constellation of clinically apparent strokes or as "silent" events, affecting areas important to memory or executive function. Risk factors for VaD are common to cardiovascular diseases and include unhealthy lifestyle choices involving diet and infrequent exercise routines. Interestingly, many of the risk factors associated with vascular disease are increasingly recognized as having a strong association with AD without vascular pathology (Luchsinger et al. 2005). Treatment of VaD largely involves medications addressing the underlying risk factors for stroke. Some patients may have a mixed picture of AD plus vascular disease, and these patients may also be prescribed a similar regimen of medications targeting cognitive decline (such as cholinesterase inhibitors) and secondary psychiatric symptoms (SSRIs or antipsychotics). Prognosis in this disease is widely varied and depends largely on the burden of ischemic disease at the time of diagnosis as well as the ability to control various lifelong vascular risk factors (Selnes and Vinters 2006).

Dementia with Lewy Bodies and Parkinson Disease Dementia

Dementia with Lewy bodies (DLB) is the third most common dementia among elderly patients and is defined by poor cognition beginning within a year of the onset of poor motor function, namely parkinsonism (classically a tetrad of rest tremor, rigidity, bradykinesia, and postural and gait disturbance). Patients with DLB often have formed visual hallucinations, fluctuations in alertness and cognition, and other cognitive problems including memory loss. Coexistent sleep disturbances and autonomic signs (manifesting as orthostatic hypotension, arrhythmia, erectile dysfunction, or constipation) further define this illness (McKeith et al. 2005). The related disorder of Parkinson disease with dementia (PDD) is thought to be less common (Miyasaki et al. 2006) and is distinguished from DLB by the appearance of cognitive dysfunction several years after the onset of parkinsonism. PDD and DLB are considered by some to be within a single clinical spectrum of parkinsonism (Langston 2006; Lippa and Emre 2006). Pathologically, each disease is character-ized by the presence of cortical intracytoplasmic inclusions called Lewy bodies. In a substantial proportion of DLB patients, AD pathology insufficient to meet formal criteria for AD may be found concomitant with Lewy bodies.

Treatment options are somewhat limited for DLB and PDD. The movement dis-orders found in either disease can be refractory or less responsive to conventional therapies, including levodopa or dopaminergic agonists, which target the basal gan-glia system. Nonetheless, patients are often continued on these drugs in the hope of some benefit. Memory disturbances are treated with cholinesterase inhibitors used in AD; similarly behavioral disturbances are treated with SSRIs and atypical antipsychotics, and sleep improvement is attempted with benzodiazepines or other sedative-hypnotics (Burn 2006).

The Frontotemporal Dementias

Frontotemporal dementia is overall the fourth most common dementia, but may be as frequent as AD in patients between ages 45 and 64; the mean age of onset is approximately 10 years younger than AD (Scarmeas and Honig 2004). FTD is a clinical spectrum, which can be divided into two broad categories: patients with predominant language disturbance (either comprehension or expression of speech) or frontal-executive dysfunction. The frontal-executive type is notable for behav-ioral or personality changes with impaired insight contributing to abnormal social conduct including impulsivity, joviality, hyper- or hypo-sexuality, and inattention to personal hygiene. Patients may be inattentive and have difficulty planning or executing sequences of a given task. Obsessive-compulsive behavior and depressed mood are also common. "Utilization behavior," or inappropriate unrestrained explo-ration of the immediate environment, can be seen. Motor signs, parkinsonism, and in rare cases motor neuron disease may be present as disease progresses. Relevant to oral health, patients frequently demonstrate hyperorality, overeat, and develop peculiar, sometimes regimented, diets and taste habituations, particularly to sweet foods.

The pathologic characteristics can be thought of in two categories: those with (1) excessive accumulation of intracellular tau (a microtubule binding protein) or (2) the absence of tau, which is further subdivided into either TDP-43 protein-positive or TDP-43 protein-negative pathology (Cairns et al. 2007). Familial cases are common and have been associated with mutations in tau or progranulin processing (Huey et al. 2006). No definitive therapy to slow FTD progression currently exists. Medications targeting psychiatric disturbances, mood, and behavioral control include antipsychotics, SSRIs, and anxiolytics (Neary et al. 2005).

Normal Pressure Hydrocephalus

Dementia associated with hydrocephalus, more commonly known as NPH, is considered to be among the reversible dementias, but remains a rare and controversial diagnosis (Curran and Lang 1994). Patients have a clinical triad of dementia often clinically similar to AD, "magnetic" gait (feet are seemingly stuck to the floor), and urinary incontinence. Formal diagnostic criteria are lacking but a response to one or more of the clinical triad, most often gait (Bugalho and Guimaraes 2006), after large volume cerebrospinal fluid lumbar drainage suggests the diagnosis. Even with strict criteria, only one third have sustained response to treatment with ventriculoperitoneal shunt (Hebb and Cusimano 2001). Medications include those used in other dementias such as cholinesterase inhibitors for memory, SSRIs for depression, and atypical antipsychotics for behavioral disturbance. Anticholinergics for bladder symptoms may be more frequently used in these patients and can further cloud the diagnosis.

Other Cognitive Disorders

HIV-Associated Dementia

Approximately 1 million Americans and 39 million people worldwide are infected with the human immunodeficiency virus (HIV). Dementia in HIV patients may become increasingly more common given improved measures to control HIV disease progression and persistent high disease transmission rates. Years ago HIV supplanted neurosyphilis as the most common primary infectious dementia; today neurosyphilis mostly occurs as an opportunistic infection in HIV patients. Current estimates suggest that as many as 30% of HIV patients have some degree of cognitive impairment and 10% of treated AIDS patients have dementia prior to death (Ghafouri et al. 2006). Cognitive impairment in HIV/AIDS patients can be caused by opportunistic infections affecting areas important to memory. Common examples include involvement of cortical structures such as temporal lobes and hippocampus with other viral infections, white matter changes with either CNS lymphoma or progressive multifocal leukoencephalopathy (PML), and basal ganglia lesions seen with toxoplamosis. Aside from these AIDS-defining illnesses, direct infection of the central nervous system by HIV alone may be the most common cause of cognitive impairment (Sevigny et al. 2005). Additionally, some HIV disease-modifying therapies have been associated with increased risk of cerebrovascular disease (Subsai et al. 2006). The progression of each of these disorders is variable and largely dependent on the course of the underlying opportunistic infection or response of the patient to HIV treatments. As with disorders described above, behavioral problems can be treated with antipsychotics. Treatment strategies for memory deficits are limited but effective response to HIV and opportunistic infectious treatments can lead to some recovery in cognitive function.

Huntington Disease

Although uncommon relative to other cognitive disorders affecting an aging population, Huntington disease affects an estimated 30,000 people in the United States and is distinctive for several reasons: prominent choreiform movements and psychiatric manifestations, every patient has a known autosomal dominant genetic basis for disease, and the widely variable age of onset from early childhood to late adulthood, with potentially decades-long disease duration including a "presymptomatic" stage (Grove et al. 2003; Fahn 2005). Age of onset and disease duration are inversely related to the number of expansion repeats of polyglutamine within the implicated gene for huntingtin protein. As with other diseases affecting cognition, the end stage is phenotypically similar, including profound memory loss, lack of social engagement, and severe rigidity, though distinguished by oculomotor paresis and sometimes increasingly prominent chorea. No effective treatment has been established; behavioral control can be targeted with antidepressants and antipsychotics.

Dementia Related to Vitamin Deficiencies

Diets low in vitamin B12 (cobalamin) and thiamine are seen infrequently in the general population, but persist in the elderly, alcoholics, and patients in developing nations (Buchman 1996). Thiamine deficiency is not uncommon (Harper 2006) and is associated with the Korsakoff amnestic syndrome. Chronic heavy alcohol exposure can be independently neurotoxic, be associated with frequent head trauma, or exacerbate symptomatic vitamin deficiency (Brust 2004). Cobalamin deficiency is screened as a reversible dementia and, in the classic form of subacute combined degeneration, can present with a mixture of cognitive, gait, and sensory dysfunction due to abnormalities in myelin formation affecting signal conduction along CNS white matter tracts (Green and Kinsella 1995). Folate, but not vitamin B6 or B12, deficiency has been shown to be an independent risk factor for the development of AD; the proposed mechanism involves mediation in circulating homocysteine levels (Luchsinger et al. 2007).

Prion Diseases

Although frequently discussed in lay press, prion diseases such as Creutzfeldt–Jakob disease (CJD) are exceedingly rare (Prusiner 2001). The most common human prion disease, sporadic CJD, has an annual incidence of approximately 1 in 1,000,000. Familial variants related to prion protein mutations are even rarer. Fewer than 200 cases of the less frequent new variant CJD (vCJD, associated with ingestion of beef from cows affected by bovine spongiform encephalopathy) have ever been reported, and worldwide surveillance of vCJD and iatrogenic CJD (associated with transmission of prion protein by transplanted tissue) suggests this syndrome is on the decline since the late 1990s (Brown et al. 2006). Both types often have a rapid unremitting dementia with seizures, no known effective treatment, and death typically within a few months to a year from symptom onset.

Epidemiology of Oral Health Problems

Within the WHO policy framework, oral health is included as a major focus, along with tobacco, physical activity, and nutrition, to "protect health throughout the life course." The onus given to the public health world is to: "Promote oral health among older people and encourage women and men to retain their natural teeth for as long as possible. Set culturally appropriate policy goals for oral health and provide appropriate oral health promotion programmes and treatment services during the life course" (Active Ageing: A Policy Framework 2002).

This initiative is no simple matter, and cognitive impairment in elderly patients may make these objectives all the more challenging. The World Health Organization (WHO) gave a recent worldwide population estimate of 600 million people over the age of 60 with an expected doubling of that number by 2025 (UN 2003); three-quarters will live in developing nations. As the population ages, the prevalence of diseases associated with aging such as dementia will also increase. Until recently, the epidemiology of elderly global dental health may have been understudied and its prevalence underappreciated. Estimates of edentulism vary widely worldwide, do not clearly follow socioeconomic patterns (Petersen and Yamamoto 2005), and may be subject to non-uniform methods of ascertainment. Dental health in association with dementia is also understudied; no prospective study has evaluated dental disease in dementia patients. Studies of nursing home patients and small community studies represent our only available data (Chalmers et al. 2002; Nordenram and Ljunggren 2002; Adam and Preston 2006; Rejnefelt et al. 2006).

In focusing on dental disease in the elderly, the first appropriate step is to identify the specific major oral health challenges in the aging population (Petersen and Yamamoto 2005) and how these may restrict social interactions and independence, lead to malnutrition and further dental disease, and ultimately contribute to the development of cognitive dysfunction. Here we review the available literature associating cognitive impairment and oral health and suggest appropriate steps for effective intervention.

Potential Mechanisms of Oral Health Contributing to Cognitive Dysfunction

Edentulism Influencing Cognition via Altered Diet or Other Mechanisms

Tooth loss in the elderly is a global health problem with prevalence as high as 78% in some European countries; persons with low socioeconomic status are disproportionately affected (Petersen 2003). Tooth loss reflects the end stage of a number of oral health diseases, alone or in combination, including caries, periodontal disease, and oral cancers, and can significantly influence diet.

Tooth loss may lead to cognitive impairment through dietary changes. Patients with tooth loss, even with dentures, have inadequate mechanisms for chewing (low masticatory efficiency); a reported maximum load on natural teeth during chewing is 8–15 kilograms (Anderson 1956) while a typical load by sustained dentures is less than 2 kilograms (Yurkstas 1953). As a result, patients with tooth loss and low masticatory efficiency tend to favor a diet low in fiber and essential micronutrients (Sheiham and Steele 2001) and high in saturated fats and cholesterol, possibly due to ease of chewing these foods relative to fiber-rich foods (Walls et al. 2000). These dietary changes, adaptive to low masticatory efficiency, could increase the risk for stroke and dementia. For example, certain dietary patterns, such as adherence to the "Mediterranean diet," characterized by high intake of fiber-rich foods and unsaturated fatty acids, moderately high intake of fish, moderate intake of ethanol, low-to-moderate intake of diary products, and low intake of meat, poultry, and saturated fatty acids, may be protective against the development of AD (Scarmeas et al. 2006a; Scarmeas et al. 2006b). Given differences in dietary profiles of the "Mediterranean diet" and diet associated with edentulism, tooth loss and impaired masticatory efficiency could lead to dietary habits increasing risk for AD; inadequate dentures could further contribute to dietary restrictions. Indeed, this dietary pattern may instead be confounded by a lifelong dietary habituation influenced by taste, economics, social norms, or unhealthy lifestyle decisions associated with tooth loss; tobacco use has been associated with tooth loss (Krall et al. 1999; Services 2000).

Cognitive impairment from tooth loss could arise not only via diet alteration. Tooth loss alone has been associated with a higher risk for stroke (Joshipura et al. 2003). Although the authors proposed that diet resulting from tooth loss could have confounded results, a multivariate model suggested tooth loss had an independent association with stroke. Dementia has been associated with mid-life tooth loss also in a large cohort Swedish twin study (Gatz et al. 2006) and late-life tooth loss in a Japanese case–control study (Kondo et al. 1994). Furthermore, a controlled animal model suggested that in comparison to normal older rats, edentulous older rats were significantly more likely to have poor spatial memory and decreased stimulated acetylcholine release in the parietal cortex (Kato et al. 1997). The mechanism underlying this finding is unclear but the authors suggested that decreased mastication-induced sensory stimulation leads to degeneration of secondary neurons in the spatial pathway of the alveolar and trigeminal nerves (Gobel and Binck 1977;

Gobel 1984) and, through cortical-brainstem circuits, possibly contribute to diminished cortical cholinergic function.

Poor dentition can alter diet, lead to decreased caloric intake, and cause pronounced weight loss. A study of community-dwelling elders in the United States identified edentulism as a risk factor for significant weight loss in a multivariate model (Ritchie et al. 2000). Weight loss in the elderly population is a significant health problem, and patients with dementia may be unrecognized by their caregivers or themselves as being malnourished (Nightingale et al. 1996). Severely demented patients may have prolonged periods of malnutrition until mechanical feedings or calorie-dense dietary supplements are started once weight loss is recognized. Weight loss or decrease in body mass index (BMI) in patients with dementia has been significantly associated with increased mortality (Evans et al. 1991; Nielsen et al. 1991; Wolf-Klein and Silverstone 1994; Cronin-Stubbs et al. 1997; Wang et al. 1997; White 1998; White et al. 1998; Gambassi et al. 1999; Shatenstein et al. 2001; Buchman et al. 2005; Faxen-Irving et al. 2005), higher amount of AD pathology (Buchman et al. 2006), preceding the onset of AD (Johnson et al. 2006). Patients with PD may have pronounced weight loss due to increased energy expenditure related to tremor and muscle rigidity; weight loss can progress despite measures to increase calorie and nutrient content in diet (Lorefat et al. 2006). Dental examinations have not yet been a routine part of studies analyzing weight loss and dementia. Micronutrient deficiencies, such as vitamin B12, thiamine (Hutton et al. 2002), and folate deficiency (Nowjack-Raymer and Sheiham 2003), may also develop as a result of edentulism and contribute to cognitive impairment. Independent of frank dementia, deficiencies in folate, vitamin B6, and vitamin B12 have been associated with cognitive impairment on neuropsychological testing (Elias et al. 2006).

Periodontal Disease, Stroke, and Cognitive Impairment

Periodontal disease is common in America (Machtei et al. 1992; Albandar 2002; Burt 2005) and disproportionately affects men, blacks, and the elderly (Miller et al. 1987; Beck et al. 1990; Machtei et al. 1992). Periodontal disease could impact the overall health of the patient via complex mechanisms mediated by elevated serum cytokines (Roberts et al. 1997; Wu et al. 2000b; Murata et al. 2001; D'Aiuto et al. 2004; Bretz et al. 2005; Bodet et al. 2006), and gene polymorphisms in these cytokines associated with periodontitis (Brett et al. 2005; Agrawal et al. 2006; Babel et al. 2006; Galicia et al. 2006; Kornman 2006). Cytokine elevations have also been associated with cerebrovascular disease (Lalouschek et al. 2006) and AD (Strauss et al. 1992; Wood et al. 1993; Iwamoto et al. 1994; Sheng et al. 1996; Duong et al. 1997; McGeer et al. 2001; Schmidt et al. 2002; Weaver et al. 2002; Frank et al. 2003; Engelhart et al. 2004), as well as risk factors common to both diseases (Jager et al. 2007), and weight loss (Konsman and Dantzer 2001); similarly, AD has also been linked to interleukin gene polymorphisms (Papassotiropoulos et al. 1999;

McGeer and McGeer 2001; Rainero et al. 2004). The association of periodontal disease with systemic illness is reviewed in detail elsewhere in this book (Chapter 12).

Drawing upon this literature, it may be worthwhile to consider the influence of periodontal disease on cognitive function. So far, epidemiologic data of periodontal disease in patients with dementia are limited to a single case–control series which suggested a higher prevalence of periodontitis in patients with dementia but possibly as a late, reactive phenomena due to worse attention to hygiene and higher dental plaque burden (Ship 1992). An attempt to associate periodontal disease and dementia (Stein et al. 2006) suggested several potential mechanisms, and one plausible mechanism is appearing. Elevation of systemic cytokines from chronic periodontitis could influence neurodegenerative change and adversely affect cerebrovascular disease risk. Periodontitis has already been directly linked to cerebrovascular disease (Beck et al. 1996; Wu et al. 2000a; Joshipura et al. 2003; Beck and Offenbacher 2005; Desvarieux et al. 2005) and associated risk factors, including cardiovascular disease (Armitage 2000; Hujoel et al. 2000; Janket et al. 2003; Cueto et al. 2005; Behle and Papapanou 2006) and DM (Shlossman et al. 1990; Lalla et al. 2006; Takeda et al. 2006). Cerebral AD pathology has not been studied or directly linked with periodontal disease.

To date no large cohort has analyzed the prevalence of periodontal disease in dementia patients or long-term risk reduction as a result of presymptomatic oral health interventions. Currently, evidence for treatment of periodontal disease as a therapy to reduce cytokine levels is limited but encouraging. Periodontal care, as a controlled intervention, has been associated with a significant reduction in serum levels of IL-6 (D'Aiuto et al. 2004), serum IL-6 soluble receptor (Offenbacher et al. 2006), and CRP (D'Aiuto et al. 2004; Kadiroglu et al. 2006). Based on the existing literature, further assessment of mid- and late-life prevalence of periodontitis in relation to subsequent development of dementia may be warranted. Until a stronger causal link can be found in rigorous studies, significant doubt may be cast on possible periodontal mechanisms contributing to dementia, given possible confounding unhealthy lifestyle factors associated with the inflammatory cascade, periodontal disease, stroke, and dementia.

Potential Mechanisms of Cognitive Dysfunction Contributing to Worse Oral Health

Cognitive Dysfunction Influences Oral Health Through Diet

Behavioral changes associated with cognitive impairment, including apathy, forgetfulness, and decreased hunger drive, may influence dietary restriction (Morris et al. 1989). The phenomena of sweet cravings, favoring carbohydrate-rich foods over protein-rich foods, and pathologic calorie restriction may be more common in patients with neurodegenerative illness, including AD and FTD (Mungas et al. 1990; Cullen et al. 1997; Ikeda et al. 2002; Greenwood et al. 2005; Seeley et al. 2005).

Table 6.1 Summarizing key potential mechanisms associating oral health and cognitive impairment

Poor oral health contributing to cognitive dysfunction	Cognitive impairments causing barriers to oral health care
Edentulism	*Maintaining appointments*
Poor masticatory efficiency	*Cognitive*
Altered dietary preferences	forgetful of appointments
Malnutrition and weight loss	*Behavioral*
Increased stroke and AD risk from diet	apathy/anxiety/sundowning
Possible increased stroke and AD risk from	*Poor mobility*
tooth loss alone	*Office evaluation*
	Motor
Periodontal Disease	Tremor
Systemic inflammatory response	Bruxism
Increased risk of stroke and vascular factors	Rigidity
Possible increased risk of dementia/AD	Posture
	Somatic reflexes (gag/swallow)
	Aspiration risk
	Communication
	Psychoses, inattention, and forgetfulness
	Reporting pain
	Biting dental staff
	Involving caregivers, especially as care needs advance
	Home care-developing a plan
	Motor
	Tremor
	Apraxia
	Dexterity
	Cognitive
	Inattention to care
	Altered dietary patterns
	Disorders of salivation
	Medications

Although certain taste habituations to sweets could contribute to increased rates of caries and periodontal disease by changes in oral microflora, a case–control study of PD patients craving sweets did not demonstrate such changes (Kennedy et al. 1994).

Neurologic Barriers to Appropriate Oral Health Care in Patients with Cognitive Dysfunction

Several authors have reviewed possible barriers to appropriate health care in the elderly and patients with dementia (Henry and Wekstein 1997; Kaplan 2000; Arai et al. 2003; Chalmers and Pearson 2005; Friedlander et al. 2006). The potential mechanisms are vast and require a comprehensive approach to care. As outlined earlier, abnormalities in cognition and behavior can vary widely according to disease. Dividing the barriers to effective care into specific categories may be worthwhile for systematic approach to the oral care needs of patients with dementia.

Barriers to Scheduling a Plan for Outpatient Care

Before patients with dementia can have an oral health care plan in place, they must first be provided with the advice and tools for effective intervention. Dementia may cause a patient to be more likely to miss an appointment or not seek treatment altogether. In an ambulatory, community-dwelling patient, behavioral problems such as apathy or withdrawal, or mere forgetfulness, may make a patient less likely to visit a health care professional's office. Office visits should be made known to patient as well as caregivers at the time of establishing an appointment. As is done by neurologists caring for patients with dementia, phone contact immediately preceding the appointment may be a simple, cost-effective measure to ensure compliance with attendance. Some patients with dementia are more likely to have behavioral control problems late in the day ("sundowning"), so late afternoon appointments should be avoided. Earlier appointments in the morning or afternoon office session will also decrease the chances of prolonged wait times and agitation (Ocasio et al. 2000), though a patient should not be awakened for the purposes of attending an earlier morning appointment. In patients with more advanced disease and still living at home, transportation to a dentist's office may be more difficult due to poor cooperation with caregivers or because of complete physical dependence for transfer from a bed to wheelchair or stretcher. In these patients, arranging for ambulette/ambulance service may obviate a physical barrier to transport. Should a patient with dementia miss an appointment, a concerted effort by the office staff should be made to identify the reason an appointment was not kept. Discussions with a patient's neurologist or caregivers may be warranted to make an as needed (prn) antipsychotic or anxiolytic available immediately before transport or office visit. The plan outlined above for initial visits, including transportation arrangements and reminders, should be used with each return to the office, with re-consultation with home caregivers and physicians as dementia progresses.

Barriers to Office Dental Examination

Motoric Barriers

As degenerative neurologic diseases progress, physical barriers may emerge as significant hurdles to office examination. Several associated neurologic phenomena include tremor, rigidity, abnormal posture, and defective swallowing increasing aspiration risk. Tremor can generally be divided into two categories: tremor at rest and tremor with action. Tremor at rest is most commonly associated with parkinsonism, less commonly AD (Scarmeas et al. 2004; Scarmeas et al. 2005a), and typically abolishes with action. A rest tremor, however, can re-emerge when the affected limb retains a relatively fixed position. Tremor with action is typically seen with essential tremor and abolishes at rest. Either types of tremor can affect the hands, arms, legs, neck, and jaw. Jaw tremor, which is mostly associated with PD, may pose a significant physical barrier for examination and office cleaning. Parkinsonian jaw tremor may fluctuate, sometimes wildly, with dopaminergic treatments or independently of them as disease progresses. A head/neck "no" tremor is mostly associated with essential tremor and may only become problematic in advanced cases. Cradling the head in the arm at the elbow may be a useful, simple technique to reduce head movements (Jolly et al. 1989).

Bruxism (teeth-grinding) and orobuccal dyskinesias (irregular, non-rhythmic, non-stereotyped involuntary movements) are movement disorders of the face seen in patients with neurodegenerative diseases. Most commonly, they are associated with an adverse response, either idiosyncratic or dose-related, to various antipsychotic class medications. These movements can also occur as a hyperkinetic, or "overshoot," effect of levodopa or dopamine agonist treatments for PD or DLB. These movements are reportedly more frequent with the older "typical" class antipsychotics but are associated with the newer "atypical" antipsychotics also (Schneider et al. 2006b). Bruxism is most commonly seen after exposure to these drugs though it can be due to a personal affectation or stereotypy. Edentulous dyskinesias are seen without known antipsychotic exposure and are thought to be self-stimulatory, partially involuntary phenomena seen after tooth loss; they often remit with dentures in place.

Rigidity, or increased muscle tone, is seen in many neurodegenerative diseases (Scarmeas et al. 2004; Scarmeas et al. 2005a) and may preclude jaw opening sufficient for effective examination. Muscle relaxants may aide to increase mouth aperture. Body rigidity, manifesting as stooped posture, can be a feature in many neurodegenerative illnesses, in particular PD or DLB, but can be overcome briefly volitionally. Some patients with advanced PD or AD may have significant kyphosis, or remain in a near fetal position, requiring near complete supination of the patient in the dental chair and could contribute to aspiration risk. As rigidity and postural changes become more pronounced with disease progression, often so will impairment in somatic reflexes, both voluntary and involuntary, such as a weak gag reflex or poor swallowing (Pfeiffer 2003). Aspiration risk may be compounded by these slowed reflexes while a patient is supinated during office examination. Therefore, the use of sprayed water should be minimized, and wound closure should assure minimal risk for blood aspiration (Friedlander et al. 2006).

Cognitive and Communication Barriers

Behavioral disturbances associated with dementia may emerge or regress and adversely impact oral care. With advanced disease, psychotic or unsafe behaviors

(Scarmeas et al. 2005b; Scarmeas et al. 2007) or intellectual rigidity (Franks and Hedegard 1973) may impair patients from undertaking new preventative health strategies. With each step of the treatment plan, caregivers should be involved and participate in surrogate informed consent for procedures.

Effective communication of the dental plan with a patient with dementia may be difficult. A specifically outlined, goal-directed course of each step of care during office visits should be presented to the patient and caregiver to improve communication. Once a patient is situated within the office environment, eliminating background distraction, frequently re-orientating the patient to the situation and context as needed, using simple directed questions (as opposed to open-ended discussion) with repeated rephrasing to assure clarity, and encouraging the presence of home care providers in the treatment room may also be effective tools to improving a potentially difficult patient interaction (Friedlander et al. 2006). Allowing additional time with the patient may be necessary, although the appointment itself may be unpredictably shorter or require several breaks during care (Ostuni and Mohl 1995).

Patients with cognitive impairment may have fewer complaints of dental pain or other dental problems clearly evident on examination, despite substrate for experiencing pain; lack of dental and pain complaints may be due to memory dysfunction, language impairment, or unawareness of self. Instead of taking a typical history of dental complaints, in a mildly affected patient, directed questioning during examination at individual sites may provide more insight into the current state of disease. As dementia progresses patients may become less communicative, and the dentist may have to rely upon behaviors noticed by the caregivers such as abnormal facial or mouth movements and guarding or avoidant behaviors (Friedlander et al. 2006). As disease progresses, dental professionals must become more reliant on astute examination, as pain expression can be inconsistent or absent (Lapeer 1998).

An often cited problem within the literature involving dental care of patients with dementia is the threat of a patient biting a practitioner during periods of uncontrolled aggression. In advanced dementia, aggression can become a problematic form of psychotic behavior (Scarmeas et al. 2007). Biting can also be a manifestation of an involuntary frontal-release phenomena or "primitive reflex" with or without seemingly voluntary behavior. The "bulldog" sign is an oral grasp reflex, akin to a hand or foot grasp reflex (involuntary grasping at an object placed in the patient's hand). The reflex is considered present (pathologic) when a tongue blade is placed between the front teeth and the patient automatically bites (without prompting) and is unable to quickly release the grip on the blade; use of this test could more predictably suggest the risk of biting. Biting injury could be reduced using rubber bite blocks or similar devices but this should be weighed against possibly exacerbating agitation and patient stress. Appropriate pharmacologic intervention, coordinated with the patient's neurologist (i.e., either with a planned dose of an antipsychotic, anxiolytic, or perhaps muscle relaxant), may also be indicated. Risks associated with each of these medications should be tempered with the potential benefit to successful dental intervention.

Meaningful verbal interaction with patients with advanced cognitive disease may not be possible, and out of necessity, complete direction will increasingly become directed to personal caregivers; involvement of caregivers at each step of oral care is of utmost importance (Kocaelli et al. 2002). Invasive procedures involving general anesthesia may become necessary as patient non-compliance with office intervention escalates or becomes impossible due to other motoric reasons as outlined above. If possible, the need for restorative or invasive procedures should be addressed as early as possible in disease to avoid unnecessary operative risk later in the course of cognitive dysfunction (Niessen and Jones 1987).

Even with the most astute attention to preventative care, patients with advanced dementia may need to have interventions requiring chemical or physical restraint or generalized anesthesia. The context of these aggressive interventions should be considered on an individualized basis with explicit involvement of home caregivers (Shuman and Bebeau 1996). Analgesia and sedation must be carefully considered in the elderly and patients with dementia. The pharmacokinetics of many agents used in anesthesia is significantly prolonged due to age-related changes in renal and hepatic function. Patients with dementia may be more vulnerable to developing postoperative delirium (a waxing and waning acute confusion state) after seemingly low or normal doses of commonly prescribed analgesics and opioids (Moore and O'Keeffe 1999). Although the mechanism is unclear, patients with neurodegenerative illness, particularly PD and AD patients, frequently cite prolonged or incomplete recovery periods after procedures involving general anesthesia. Postoperative aggressive physical rehabilitation should be considered for the patient, even if periprocedural inpatient hospitalization is not anticipated.

Barriers to Dental Care at Home

Motoric Barriers

"Major components of oral hygiene and home care programs...require muscle-eye-coordination, digital dexterity and tongue–cheek–lip control. Tremor and the associated loss and/or lessening of the above faculties mitigate against effective oral hygiene procedures" (Kaplan 2000). Although the author was describing Parkinson patients, his summary of neurologic barriers is applicable to most dementing illnesses. The physical neurologic phenomena associated with impaired oral health care at home include arm/hand tremor, apraxia, rigidity, and decreased fine motor movements.

Tremor affecting the arms may be present either as a rest tremor of PD, re-emerging when a limb is held in a fixed position, or as a manifestation of severe essential tremor. When severe in amplitude and pervasiveness, either type could potentially disturb fine motor movements required of effective home dental care such as brushing, successfully guiding floss between the teeth, and denture care. Spontaneous self-report of this problem may be underemphasized in the literature.

Although tremor can be relatively refractory to medications, aggressively addressing tremor with the patient's neurologist may be worthwhile.

Apraxia, or an inability or difficulty to complete a single task or series of tasks despite normal gross motor and primary sensory functions (Brazis et al. 2001), is frequently seen in patients with dementia. The basic dysfunction is an inability to organize, sequence, or recall the steps required to complete a task. Apraxic patients lose programmed information, and recovery with instructions or routines would be unexpected. Simple tasks such as steps in preparing to brush the teeth or the movements of toothbrushing could be impaired. Caregivers likely need to be involved with each cleaning once a significant degree of apraxia is identified.

Prominent motor symptoms other than tremor, such as difficulty with dexterous and repetitive motions, along with jaw and arm muscle rigidity (Kieser et al. 1999; Chiappelli et al. 2002; Scarmeas et al. 2004), may pose greater barriers to dental care. Rigidity is a constant resistance to motion and is not specific to movement disorders. Rigidity usually accompanies loss of fine motor movement (dexterity) by reduction in amplitude and precision fine motor movements. Patients with stroke, tumor, or demyelinating disease may have the neck, a single limb, or side affected, whereas patients with diffuse brain disease such as AD or VaD may have increased tone throughout. Rigidity in PD usually affects one limb or side with subsequent progression to the opposite side; the severity on the initially affected side may be worse for the duration of the illness. Medications, such as dopaminergic class agents and muscle relaxants, may help in treating rigidity.

Cognitive and Communication Barriers

As cognitive impairment worsens in patients with dementia, self-care declines and patients have an increasing dependency on others for assistance with basic skills such as feeding and routine hygiene. Infrequent toothbrushing and inappropriate denture care may be the earliest signs to indicate impairment with self dental care. Inability to rinse the mouth or sit at a table for meals may be subtle yet strong indicators of cognitive impairment warranting increased vigilance toward appropriate dental care (Arai et al. 2003).

Disorders of Salivation in Patients with Cognitive Impairment

"Absent the antibacterial, lubricating, remineralizing, and buffering action of saliva, the patient is at increased risk of developing caries, periodontal disease and dysfunctions of speech, chewing, swallowing, and taste" (Kaplan 2000). Xerostomia affects the health of present teeth and can adversely affect the use of dentures through dry mouth leading to irritation and denture-related sores. Xerostomia commonly develops in older patients who often take one or more medications associated with xerostomia (Thomson et al. 2000), but may also be present independent of medication use, in older patients with neurodegenerative diseases. In patients with cognitive impairment, xerostomia occurs as a consequence of (1) dysautonomia associated with some neurodegenerative diseases, (2) atypical antipsychotics used for aggressive behavior, delusions, and hallucinations, or (3) anticholinergics used for urinary incontinence, or less commonly as a part of regimen for parkinsonism.

Independent of medication use, patients with AD have been shown to have submandibular gland hyposalivation, while parotid gland function appears unaffected (Ship et al. 1990; Ship and Puckett 1994). The reason for selected salivatory gland dysfunction is unclear but could be related to differential hypothalamic innervation of the submandibular and facial salivatory nuclei. Interestingly, salivatory acetylcholinesterase activity may mirror decline in cortical cholinergic activity. One small study suggested differences in the catalytic activity of the acetylcholinesterase enzyme in the saliva of elderly patients. Patients with either poor response to cholinesterase inhibitor therapy or more rapidly progressing AD had lower enzymatic activity than age-matched controls (Sayer et al. 2004). Some have recommended saliva substitutes or simply increasing the frequency of small mouthfuls of water or juice throughout the day to combat idiopathic and medication-associated xerostomia (Jolly et al. 1989). Sialorrhea may also be seen in patients with advanced PD, although this may reflect a hypoactive swallowing reflex in patients with normal salivation or hyposalivation, rather than true hypersalivation.

Interventions for Decreasing Oral Health Barriers at Home

Introducing an effective plan of preventative dental care can have a significant impact on morbidity and mortality associated with cognitive impairment. A randomized controlled multicenter nursing home study from Japan, comparing caregiver versus self dental care after each meal, had significantly lower mortality, less frequent pneumonia, and slower decline in MMSE scores (Yoneyama et al. 2002). However, incorporation of simple home dental care can prove quite difficult without a directed plan.

Once a plan of care is established in the office, physical barriers and cognitive problems associated with dementing illnesses may pose significant barriers to effective care at home. One center has attempted to create a screening tool in order to individualize treatment based on recognized impairments in home dental care tasks and simple cognitive tests (Nordenram et al. 1997). Other clinical screening tools with the same target include dental hygiene and cognitive indices useful for both the dentist and home caregivers (Niessen et al. 1985; Doherty et al. 1994; Chiappelli et al. 2002).

Ultimately, an effective homecare program should target a patient's remaining abilities and involve the patient's caregivers early. One such strategy includes teaching one-handed preventative strategies to patients whose limbs are affected by tremor, rigidity, or weakness. For instance, denture care can be accomplished by affixing a nailbrush to a surface by suction cup and moving the denture alone

(Jolly et al. 1989). Other simple interventions such as use of electric toothbrushes may obviate the need for fine or repetitive motions. Topical stannous fluoride gel preparations have been advocated for preventive theraphy both as a daily treatment (Jolly et al. 1989) and as part of 3-month routine dental office visits (Friedlander and Jarvik 1987). Mouthwashes are generally discouraged given the risk of aspiration, but if the patient is still capable, non-alcohol-based preparations using chlorhexidine or an admixture of baking soda and water have been suggested. Chlorhexidine laden brushes may be a worthwhile alternative (Ransier et al. 1995).

Physical trauma as a consequence of orobuccal dyskinesias may occur within dental practice and can be prevented by an appropriate device (Hussein 1989). Involvement of speech pathologists to aid prosthodontic design in individuals can be worthwhile, as the dentist's goals of reducing interocclusal distance to favor ridge preservation and lessen masticatory pressure may conflict with goals of speech production (Kaplan 2000).

Medications Used in Dementia and Their Impact on Oral Health

As discussed throughout the chapter, a number of different classes of drugs may be used to treat cognitive, behavioral, and motor dysfunction in patients with neurodegenerative illness. Many of these medications have implications for dental care.

Currently, the only two classes of medications for the treatment of memory loss include the acetylcholinesterase inhibitors (AchI, including rivastigmine, donepezil, and galantamine) and the NMDA antagonist memantine. AchI class medications act centrally and increased salivation (due to peripheral acetylcholinesterase inhibition) is a possible adverse event. Memantine has not been associated with salivatory dysfunction. Toothache has been rarely associated with donepezil (Product-Information).

Atypical antipsychotics commonly used in dementia patients with behavioral disturbance include risperidone, quetiapine, olanzapine, and zisprasidone. This class of medications has been associated with dyskinesia, akathisia (an inner restlessness), and parkinsonism, most often manifesting with rigidity (Schneider et al. 2006b). Hypersalivation has been reported with risperidone and olanzapine (Product-Information); risperidone has also been associated with hyposalivation (Product-Information). Weight gain and the metabolic syndrome may be an adverse side effect of the atypical antipsychotics; dietary implications are unclear. This finding has the potential to adversely affect cerebrovascular risk factors including diabetes, hypertension, and stroke, as well as periodontitis. Benzodiazepines are also prescribed for behavioral control and anxiety and may be useful in the setting of dental phobia; they have no associated oral health side effects.

Mood disorders and sleep disturbance frequently accompany neurodegenerative disorders and need to be treated. Selective serotonin reuptake inhibitors (SSRIs) are the predominant class of medication prescribed for depression in patients with dementia. Tricyclic antidepressants (TCAs) and atypical antidepressants (including buproprion, trazodone, venlafaxine, nefazadone, and mirtazipine) are also tried either for depressive symptoms or more frequently for sleep disturbance. All antidepressants, but particularly the TCAs and mirtazipine, have been associated with significant xerostomia (Keene et al. 2003). Dysgeusia and hypogeusia have been associated with TCAs (Schiffman et al. 1998) and the sedative-hypnotic eszopiclone (Product-Information). Another sedative-hypnotic zolpidem has been associated with xerostomia (Product-Information). Ramelteon, the first agent in the class of melatonin receptor agonists, has been associated with dysgeusia (Product-Information).

Patients with parkinsonism arguably have the widest array of pharmacologic interventions of the neurodegenerative illnesses. Among the many medications used to treat complex movement and behavioral problems with PDD and DLB, levodopa and dopaminergic agents, which may lead to dyskinesias, psychoses, and salivatory changes, are most often associated with xerostomia. Again, reports of sialorrhea with these agents may instead reflect hypoactive swallowing reflexes rather than true hypersalivation.

Conclusions

Poor oral health, including edentulism and periodontal disease, may be an unrecognized risk factor contributing to the development of cognitive impairment through dietary changes, malnutrition, and a systemic inflammatory response associated with increased risk of stroke and AD. The many neurodegenerative illnesses pose unique, complex barriers to effective oral health care based on cognitive, motoric, and behavioral abnormalities in each disease. We have tried to identify key diseases of epidemiologic importance, barriers for effective treatment in patients with dementia, and consolidate potential interventions unique to these patients (Summarized in Table 6.1). Improving preventative strategies focusing on periodontal disease and caries, tailoring late-disease interventions based on the stage and characteristics of dementing illness, and involving caregivers in both daily preventative care and during office consultation could significantly improve the oral health of patients with cognitive impairment and potentially impact the development or progression of some dementing illnesses.

Acknowledgments Dr James M. Noble is supported by Public Health Service Grant #5-T32-NS07153-23 and a grant from Charles L. and Ann Lee Saunders Brown. Dr Nikolaos Scarmeas is supported by Alzheimer's Association grant IIRG-04-1353, NIH grant AG028506 and the Taub Institute for Research in Alzheimer's Disease and the Aging Brain. The authors would like to thank Karen S. Marder, M.D., M.P.H, and David A. Noble, D.D.S., for their assistance with preparation of this manuscript.

References

Active Ageing: A Policy Framework (2002). World Health Organization: 1–60.

Adam, H. and Preston, A. J. (2006). "The oral health of individuals with dementia in nursing homes." *Gerodontology* **23**(2): 99–105.

ADI. (January 25, 2006). "Common Questions." http://www.alz.co.uk/alzheimers/faq.html Retrieved December 11, 2006.

Agrawal, A. A., Kapley, A., Yeltiwar, R. K. and Purohit, H. J. (2006). "Assessment of single nucleotide polymorphism at IL-1A + 4845 and IL-1B+3954 as genetic susceptibility test for chronic periodontitis in Maharashtrian ethnicity." *J Periodontol* **77**(9): 1515–21.

Albandar, J. M. (2002). "Periodontal diseases in North America." *Periodontol 2000* **29**: 31–69.

Anderson, D. J. (1956). "Measurement of stress in mastication. I." *J Dent Res* **35**(5): 664–70.

Arai, K., Sumi, Y., Uematsu, H. and Miura, H. (2003). "Association between dental health behaviours, mental/physical function and self-feeding ability among the elderly: a cross-sectional survey." *Gerodontology* **20**(2): 78–83.

Armitage, G. C. (2000). "Periodontal infections and cardiovascular disease–how strong is the association?" *Oral Dis* **6**(6): 335–50.

Aronson, M. K., Ooi, W. L., Geva, D. L., Masur, D., Blau, A. and Frishman, W. (1991). "Dementia. Age-dependent incidence, prevalence, and mortality in the old old." *Arch Intern Med* **151**(5): 989–92.

Babel, N., Cherepnev, G., Babel, D., Tropmann, A., Hammer, M., Volk, H.-D. and Reinke, P. (2006). "Analysis of Tumor Necrosis Factor-α, Transforming Growth Factor-β, Interleukin-10, IL-6, and Interferon-γ Gene Polymorphisms in Patients With Chronic Periodontitis." *J Periodontol* **77**(12): 1978–83.

Beck, J., Garcia, R., Heiss, G., Vokonas, P. S. and Offenbacher, S. (1996). "Periodontal disease and cardiovascular disease." *J Periodontol* **67**(10 Suppl): 1123–37.

Beck, J. D., Koch, G. G., Rozier, R. G. and Tudor, G. E. (1990). "Prevalence and risk indicators for periodontal attachment loss in a population of older community-dwelling blacks and whites." *J Periodontol* **61**(8): 521–28.

Beck, J. D. and Offenbacher, S. (2005). "Systemic effects of periodontitis: epidemiology of periodontal disease and cardiovascular disease." *J Periodontol* **76**(11 Suppl): 2089–100.

Behle, J. H. and Papapanou, P. N. (2006). "Periodontal infections and atherosclerotic vascular disease: an update." *Int Dent J* **56**(4 Suppl 1): 256–62.

Bodet, C., Chandad, F. and Grenier, D. (2006). "*Porphyromonas gingivalis*-induced inflammatory mediator profile in an ex vivo human whole blood model." *Clin Exp Immunol* **143**(1): 50–57.

Brazis, P. W., Masdeu, J. C. and Biller, J. (2001). Cerebral Hemispheres. *Localization in Clinical Neurology*. Philadelphia, Lippincott Williams & Wilkins: 453–522.

Brett, P. M., Zygogianni, P., Griffiths, G. S., Tomaz, M., Parkar, M., D'Aiuto, F. and Tonetti, M. (2005). "Functional gene polymorphisms in aggressive and chronic periodontitis." *J Dent Res* **84**(12): 1149–53.

Bretz, W. A., Weyant, R. J., Corby, P. M., Ren, D., Weissfeld, L., Kritchevsky, S. B., Harris, T., et al. (2005). "Systemic inflammatory markers, periodontal diseases, and periodontal infections in an elderly population." *J Am Geriatr Soc* **53**(9): 1532–37.

Brown, P., Brandel, J. P., Preece, M. and Sato, T. (2006). "Iatrogenic Creutzfeldt-Jakob disease: the waning of an era." *Neurology* **67**(3): 389–93.

Bruscoli, M. and Lovestone, S. (2004). "Is MCI really just early dementia? A systematic review of conversion studies." *Int Psychogeriatr* **16**(2): 129–40.

Brust, J. C. M. (2004). Ethanol. *Neurological Aspects of Substance Abuse*. J. C. M. Brust. Philadelphia, Elsevier Inc.: 317–425.

Buchman, A. L. (1996). "Vitamin supplementation in the elderly: a critical evaluation." *Gastroenterologist* **4**(4): 262–75.

Buchman, A. S., Schneider, J. A., Wilson, R. S., Bienias, J. L. and Bennett, D. A. (2006). "Body mass index in older persons is associated with Alzheimer disease pathology." *Neurology* **67**(11): 1949–54.

Buchman, A. S., Wilson, R. S., Bienias, J. L., Shah, R. C., Evans, D. A. and Bennett, D. A. (2005). "Change in body mass index and risk of incident Alzheimer disease." *Neurology* **65**(6): 892–97.

Bugalho, P. and Guimaraes, J. (2006). "Gait disturbance in normal pressure hydrocephalus: A clinical study." *Parkinsonism Relat Disord* **13**(7): 434–7.

Burn, D. J. (2006). "Cortical Lewy body disease and Parkinson's disease dementia." *Curr Opin Neurol* **19**(6): 572–79.

Burt, B. (2005). "Position paper: epidemiology of periodontal diseases." *J Periodontol* **76**(8): 1406–19.

Cairns, N. J., Bigio, E. H., Mackenzie, I. R., Neumann, M., Lee, V. M., Hatanpaa, K. J., White, C. L. 3rd, Schneider, J. A., Grinberg, L. T., Halliday, G., Duyckaerts, C., Lowe, J. S., Holm, I. E., Tolnay, M., Okamoto, K., Yokoo, H., Murayama, S., Woulfe, J., Munoz, D. G., Dickson, D. W., Ince, P. G., Trojanowski J. Q., Mann, D. M.(2007) Consortium for Frontotemporal Lobar Degeneration. Neuropathologic diagnostic and nosologic criteria for frontotemporal lobar degeneration: consensus of the Consortium for Frontotemporal Lobar Degeneration. *Acta Neuropathol (Bed)*. **114**(1): 5–22.

Chalmers, J. and Pearson, A. (2005). "Oral hygiene care for residents with dementia: a literature review." *J Adv Nurs* **52**(4): 410–19.

Chalmers, J. M., Carter, K. D. and Spencer, A. J. (2002). "Caries incidence and increments in community-living older adults with and without dementia." *Gerodontology* **19**(2): 80–94.

Chiappelli, F., Bauer, J., Spackman, S., Prolo, P., Edgerton, M., Armenian, C., Dickmeyer, J. and Harper, S. (2002). "Dental needs of the elderly in the 21st century." *Gen Dent* **50**(4): 358–63.

Cronin-Stubbs, D., Beckett, L. A., Scherr, P. A., Field, T. S., Chown, M. J., Pilgrim, D. M., Bennett, D. A. and Evans, D. A. (1997). "Weight loss in people with Alzheimer's disease: a prospective population based analysis." *Bmj* **314**(7075): 178–79.

Cueto, A., Mesa, F., Bravo, M. and Ocana-Riola, R. (2005). "Periodontitis as risk factor for acute myocardial infarction. A case control study of Spanish adults." *J Periodontal Res* **40**(1): 36–42.

Cullen, P., Abid, F., Patel, A., Coope, B. and Ballard, C. G. (1997). "Eating disorders in dementia." *Int J Geriatr Psychiatry* **12**(5): 559–62.

Cummings, J. L. (2004). "Alzheimer's disease." *N Engl J Med* **351**(1): 56–67.

Curran, T. and Lang, A. E. (1994). "Parkinsonian syndromes associated with hydrocephalus: case reports, a review of the literature, and pathophysiological hypotheses." *Mov Disord* **9**(5): 508–20.

D'Aiuto, F., Parkar, M., Andreou, G., Suvan, J., Brett, P. M., Ready, D. and Tonetti, M. S. (2004). "Periodontitis and systemic inflammation: control of the local infection is associated with a reduction in serum inflammatory markers." *J Dent Res* **83**(2): 156–60.

Desvarieux, M., Demmer, R. T., Rundek, T., Boden-Albala, B., Jacobs, D. R., Jr., Sacco, R. L. and Papapanou, P. N. (2005). "Periodontal microbiota and carotid intima-media thickness: the Oral Infections and Vascular Disease Epidemiology Study (INVEST)." *Circulation* **111**(5): 576–82.

Doherty, S. A., Ross, A. and Bennett, C. R. (1994). "The oral hygiene performance test: development and validation of dental dexterity scale for the elderly." *Spec Care Dentist* **14**(4): 144–52.

Drachman, D. A. (2006). "Aging of the brain, entropy, and Alzheimer disease." *Neurology* **67**(8): 1340–52.

Duong, T., Nikolaeva, M. and Acton, P. J. (1997). "C-reactive protein-like immunoreactivity in the neurofibrillary tangles of Alzheimer's disease." *Brain Res* **749**(1): 152–56.

Elias, M. F., Robbins, M. A., Budge, M. M., Elias, P. K., Brennan, S. L., Johnston, C., Nagy, Z. and Bates, C. J. (2006). "Homocysteine, folate, and vitamins B6 and B12 blood levels in relation to cognitive performance: the Maine-Syracuse study." *Psychosom Med* **68**(4): 547–54.

Engelhart, M. J., Geerlings, M. I., Meijer, J., Kiliaan, A., Ruitenberg, A., van Swieten, J. C., Stijnen, T., Hofman, A., Witteman, J. C. and Breteler, M. M. (2004). "Inflammatory proteins in plasma and the risk of dementia: the Rotterdam study." *Arch Neurol* **61**(5): 668–72.

Evans, D. A., Smith, L. A., Scherr, P. A., Albert, M. S., Funkenstein, H. H. and Hebert, L. E. (1991). "Risk of death from Alzheimer's disease in a community population of older persons." *Am J Epidemiol* **134**(4): 403–12.

Fahn, S. (2005). Huntington Disease. *Merritt's neurology*. L. P. Rowland. Philadelphia, Lippincott Williams & Wilkins: 803–807.

Faxen-Irving, G., Basun, H. and Cederholm, T. (2005). "Nutritional and cognitive relationships and long-term mortality in patients with various dementia disorders." *Age Ageing* **34**(2): 136–41.

Frank, R. A., Galasko, D., Hampel, H., Hardy, J., de Leon, M. J., Mehta, P. D., Rogers, J., Siemers, E. and Trojanowski, J. Q. (2003). "Biological markers for therapeutic trials in Alzheimer's disease. Proceedings of the biological markers working group; NIA initiative on neuroimaging in Alzheimer's disease." *Neurobiol Aging* **24**(4): 521–36.

Franks, A. S. T. and Hedegard, B. (1973). *Aging and Oral Health*. Oxford, Blackwell Scientific.

Friedlander, A. H. and Jarvik, L. F. (1987). "The dental management of the patient with dementia." *Oral Surg Oral Med Oral Pathol* **64**(5): 549–53.

Friedlander, A. H., Norman, D. C., Mahler, M. E., Norman, K. M. and Yagiela, J. A. (2006). "Alzheimer's disease: psychopathology, medical management and dental implications." *J Am Dent Assoc* **137**(9): 1240–51.

Galicia, J. C., Tai, H., Komatsu, Y., Shimada, Y., Ikezawa, I. and Yoshie, H. (2006). "Interleukin-6 receptor gene polymorphisms and periodontitis in a non-smoking Japanese population." *J Clin Periodontol* **33**(10): 704–709.

Gambassi, G., Landi, F., Lapane, K. L., Sgadari, A., Mor, V. and Bernabei, R. (1999). "Predictors of mortality in patients with Alzheimer's disease living in nursing homes." *J Neurol Neurosurg Psychiatry* **67**(1): 59–65.

Gatz, M., Mortimer, J. A., Fratiglioni, L., Johansson, B., Berg, S., Reynolds, C. A. and Pedersen, N. L. (2006). "Potentially modifiable risk factors for dementia in identical twins." *Alzheimer's and Dementia: J Alzheimer's Assoc* **2**(2): 110–117.

Ghafouri, M., Amini, S., Khalili, K. and Sawaya, B. E. (2006). "HIV-1 associated dementia: symptoms and causes." *Retrovirology* **3**: 28.

Gobel, S. (1984). "An electron microscopic analysis of the trans-synaptic effects of peripheral nerve injury subsequent to tooth pulp extirpations on neurons in laminae I and II of the medullary dorsal horn." *J Neurosci* **4**(9): 2281–90.

Gobel, S. and Binck, J. M. (1977). "Degenerative changes in primary trigeminal axons and in neurons in nucleus caudalis following tooth pulp extirpations in the cat." *Brain Res* **132**(2): 347–54.

Green, R. and Kinsella, L. J. (1995). "Current concepts in the diagnosis of cobalamin deficiency." *Neurology* **45**(8): 1435–40.

Greenwood, C. E., Tam, C., Chan, M., Young, K. W., Binns, M. A. and van Reekum, R. (2005). "Behavioral disturbances, not cognitive deterioration, are associated with altered food selection in seniors with Alzheimer's disease." *J Gerontol A Biol Sci Med Sci* **60**(4): 499–505.

Grove, M., Vonsattel, J. P., Mazzoni, P. and Marder, K. (2003). "Huntington's disease." *Sci Aging Knowledge Environ* **2003**(43): dn3.

Gurland, B. J., Wilder, D. E., Lantigua, R., Stern, Y., Chen, J., Killeffer, E. H. and Mayeux, R. (1999). "Rates of dementia in three ethnoracial groups." *Int J Geriatr Psychiatry* **14**(6): 481–93.

Harper, C. (2006). "Thiamine (vitamin B1) deficiency and associated brain damage is still common throughout the world and prevention is simple and safe!" *Eur J Neurol* **13**(10): 1078–82.

Hebb, A. O. and Cusimano, M. D. (2001). "Idiopathic normal pressure hydrocephalus: a systematic review of diagnosis and outcome." *Neurosurgery* **49**(5): 1166–84; discussion 1184–86.

Hebert, L. E., Scherr, P. A., Beckett, L. A., Albert, M. S., Pilgrim, D. M., Chown, M. J., Funkenstein, H. H. and Evans, D. A. (1995). "Age-specific incidence of Alzheimer's disease in a community population." *Jama* **273**(17): 1354–59.

Hebert, L. E., Scherr, P. A., Bienias, J. L., Bennett, D. A. and Evans, D. A. (2003). "Alzheimer disease in the US population: prevalence estimates using the 2000 census." *Arch Neurol* **60**(8): 1119–22.

Helmer, C., Joly, P., Letenneur, L., Commenges, D. and Dartigues, J. F. (2001). "Mortality with dementia: results from a French prospective community-based cohort." *Am J Epidemiol* **154**(7): 642–48.

Henry, R. G. and Wekstein, D. R. (1997). "Providing dental care for patients diagnosed with Alzheimer's disease." *Dent Clin North Am* **41**(4): 915–43.

Heyman, A., Peterson, B., Fillenbaum, G. and Pieper, C. (1996). "The consortium to establish a registry for Alzheimer's disease (CERAD). Part XIV: Demographic and clinical predictors of survival in patients with Alzheimer's disease." *Neurology* **46**(3): 656–60.

Huey, E. D., Grafman, J., Wassermann, E. M., Pietrini, P., Tierney, M. C., Ghetti, B., Spina, S., et al. (2006). "Characteristics of frontotemporal dementia patients with a Progranulin mutation." *Ann Neurol* **60**(3): 374–80.

Hujoel, P. P., Drangsholt, M., Spiekerman, C. and DeRouen, T. A. (2000). "Periodontal disease and coronary heart disease risk." *Jama* **284**(11): 1406–10.

Hussein, S. B. (1989). "Use of a gum shield for Parkinson's disease patients." *Br Dent J* **166**(9): 320.

Hutton, B., Feine, J. and Morais, J. (2002). "Is there an association between edentulism and nutritional state?" *J Can Dent Assoc* **68**(3): 182–87.

Ikeda, M., Brown, J., Holland, A. J., Fukuhara, R. and Hodges, J. R. (2002). "Changes in appetite, food preference, and eating habits in frontotemporal dementia and Alzheimer's disease." *J Neurol Neurosurg Psychiatry* **73**(4): 371–76.

Iwamoto, N., Nishiyama, E., Ohwada, J. and Arai, H. (1994). "Demonstration of CRP immunoreactivity in brains of Alzheimer's disease: immunohistochemical study using formic acid pretreatment of tissue sections." *Neurosci Lett* **177**(1–2): 23–26.

Jager, J., Gremeaux, T., Cormont, M., Le Marchand-Brustel, Y. and Tanti, J. F. (2007). "Interleukin-1{beta}-induced insulin resistance in adipocytes through down-regulation of insulin receptor substrate-1 expression." *Endocrinology* **148**(1): 241–51.

Janket, S. J., Baird, A. E., Chuang, S. K. and Jones, J. A. (2003). "Meta-analysis of periodontal disease and risk of coronary heart disease and stroke." *Oral Surg Oral Med Oral Pathol Oral Radiol Endod* **95**(5): 559–69.

Johnson, D. K., Wilkins, C. H. and Morris, J. C. (2006). "Accelerated weight loss may precede diagnosis in Alzheimer disease." *Arch Neurol* **63**(9): 1312–17.

Jolly, D. E., Paulson, R. B., Paulson, G. W. and Pike, J. A. (1989). "Parkinson's disease: a review and recommendations for dental management." *Spec Care Dentist* **9**(3): 74–78.

Joshipura, K. J., Hung, H. C., Rimm, E. B., Willett, W. C. and Ascherio, A. (2003). "Periodontal disease, tooth loss, and incidence of ischemic stroke." *Stroke* **34**(1): 47–52.

Kadiroglu, A. K., Kadiroglu, E. T., Sit, D., Dag, A. and Yilmaz, M. E. (2006). "Periodontitis is an important and occult source of inflammation in hemodialysis patients." *Blood Purif* **24**(4): 400–404.

Kaplan, D. (2000). Oral Health, Dental Care and Quality of Life Issues in Parkinson's Disease. *Parkinson's Disease and Quality of Life.* L. Cote, L. L. Sprinzeles, R. Elliott and A. H. Kutscher. Binghamton, NY, The Haworth Press: 87–92.

Kato, T., Usami, T., Noda, Y., Hasegawa, M., Ueda, M. and Nabeshima, T. (1997). "The effect of the loss of molar teeth on spatial memory and acetylcholine release from the parietal cortex in aged rats." *Behav Brain Res* **83**(1–2): 239–42.

Keene, J. J., Jr., Galasko, G. T. and Land, M. F. (2003). "Antidepressant use in psychiatry and medicine: importance for dental practice." *J Am Dent Assoc* **134**(1): 71–79.

Kennedy, M. A., Rosen, S., Paulson, G. W., Jolly, D. E. and Beck, F. M. (1994). "Relationship of oral microflora with oral health status in Parkinson's disease." *Spec Care Dentist* **14**(4): 164–68.

Kieser, J., Jones, G., Borlase, G. and MacFadyen, E. (1999). "Dental treatment of patients with neurodegenerative disease." *N Z Dent J* **95**(422): 130–34.

Kocaelli, H., Yaltirik, M., Yargic, L. I. and Ozbas, H. (2002). "Alzheimer's disease and dental management." *Oral Surg Oral Med Oral Pathol Oral Radiol Endod* **93**(5): 521–24.

Kondo, K., Niino, M. and Shido, K. (1994). "A case-control study of Alzheimer's disease in Japan–significance of life-styles." *Dementia* **5**(6): 314–26.

Konsman, J. P. and Dantzer, R. (2001). "How the immune and nervous systems interact during disease-associated anorexia." *Nutrition* **17**(7–8): 664–68.

Kornman, K. S. (2006). "Interleukin 1 genetics, inflammatory mechanisms, and nutrigenetic opportunities to modulate diseases of aging." *Am J Clin Nutr* **83**(2): 475S–483S.

Krall, E. A., Garvey, A. J. and Garcia, R. I. (1999). "Alveolar bone loss and tooth loss in male cigar and pipe smokers." *J Am Dent Assoc* **130**(1): 57–64.

Lalla, E., Kaplan, S., Chang, S. M., Roth, G. A., Celenti, R., Hinckley, K., Greenberg, E. and Papapanou, P. N. (2006). "Periodontal infection profiles in type 1 diabetes." *J Clin Periodontol* **33**(12): 855–62.

Lalouschek, W., Schillinger, M., Hsieh, K., Endler, G., Greisenegger, S., Marculescu, R., Lang, W., Wagner, O., Cheng, S. and Mannhalter, C. (2006). "Polymorphisms of the inflammatory system and risk of ischemic cerebrovascular events." *Clin Chem Lab Med* **44**(8): 918–23.

Langston, J. W. (2006). "The Parkinson's complex: parkinsonism is just the tip of the iceberg." *Ann Neurol* **59**(4): 591–96.

Lapeer, G. L. (1998). "Dementia's impact on pain sensation: a serious clinical dilemma for dental geriatric care givers." *J Can Dent Assoc* **64**(3): 182–84, 187–92.

Lippa, C. F. and Emre, M. (2006). "Characterizing clinical phenotypes: the Lewys in their life or the life of their Lewys?" *Neurology* **67**(11): 1910–11.

Lorefat, B., Ganowiak, W., Wissing, U., Granerus, A. K. and Unosson, M. (2006). "Food habits and intake of nutrients in elderly patients with Parkinson's disease." *Gerontology* **52**(3): 160–68.

Luchsinger, J. A., Reitz, C., Honig, L. S., Tang, M. X., Shea, S. and Mayeux, R. (2005). "Aggregation of vascular risk factors and risk of incident Alzheimer disease." *Neurology* **65**(4): 545–51.

Luchsinger, J. A., Tang, M. X., Miller, J., Green, R. and Mayeux, R. (2007). "Relation of higher folate intake to lower risk of Alzheimer disease in the elderly." *Arch Neurol* **64**(1): 86–92.

Machtei, E. E., Christersson, L. A., Grossi, S. G., Dunford, R., Zambon, J. J. and Genco, R. J. (1992). "Clinical criteria for the definition of "established periodontitis"." *J Periodontol* **63**(3): 206–14.

Mayeux, R. (2003a). "Apolipoprotein E, Alzheimer disease, and African Americans." *Arch Neurol* **60**(2): 161–63.

Mayeux, R. (2003b). "Epidemiology of neurodegeneration." *Annu Rev Neurosci* **26**: 81–104.

McGeer, E. G., Yasojima, K., Schwab, C. and McGeer, P. L. (2001). "The pentraxins: possible role in Alzheimer's disease and other innate inflammatory diseases." *Neurobiol Aging* **22**(6): 843–48.

McGeer, P. L. and McGeer, E. G. (2001). "Polymorphisms in inflammatory genes and the risk of Alzheimer disease." *Arch Neurol* **58**(11): 1790–92.

McKeith, I. G., Dickson, D. W., Lowe, J., Emre, M., O'Brien, J. T., Feldman, H., Cummings, J., et al. (2005). "Diagnosis and management of dementia with Lewy bodies: third report of the DLB Consortium." *Neurology* **65**(12): 1863–72.

McKusick, V. A. (December 18, 2006). "Alzheimer Disease." *Online Mendelian Inheritance in Man*, from http://www.ncbi.nlm.nih.gov/entrez/dispomim.cgi?cmd=entry&id=104300.

Miller, A. J., Brunelle, J. A., Carlos, J. P., Brown, L. J. and Löe, H. (1987). *Oral Health of United States Adults*. Bethesda, MD, U.S. Department of Health & Human Services, Public Health Service, National Institutes of Health.

Miyasaki, J. M., Shannon, K., Voon, V., Ravina, B., Kleiner-Fisman, G., Anderson, K., Shulman, L. M., Gronseth, G. and Weiner, W. J. (2006). "Practice Parameter: Evaluation and treatment of depression, psychosis, and dementia in Parkinson disease (an evidence-based review). Report of the Quality Standards Subcommittee of the American Academy of Neurology." *Neurology*.

Moore, A. R. and O'Keeffe, S. T. (1999). "Drug-induced cognitive impairment in the elderly." *Drugs Aging* **15**(1): 15–28.

Morris, C. H., Hope, R. A. and Fairburn, C. G. (1989). "Eating habits in dementia. A descriptive study." *Br J Psychiatry* **154**: 801–806.

Mungas, D., Cooper, J. K., Weiler, P. G., Gietzen, D., Franzi, C. and Bernick, C. (1990). "Dietary preference for sweet foods in patients with dementia." *J Am Geriatr Soc* **38**(9): 999–1007.

Murata, T., Miyazaki, H., Senpuku, H. and Hanada, N. (2001). "Periodontitis and serum interleukin-6 levels in the elderly." *Jpn J Infect Dis* **54**(2): 69–71.

Neary, D., Snowden, J. and Mann, D. (2005). "Frontotemporal dementia." *Lancet Neurol* **4**(11): 771–80.

Nielsen, H., Lolk, A., Pedersen, I., Autzen, M., Sennef, C. and Kragh-Sorensen, P. (1991). "The accuracy of early diagnosis and predictors of death in Alzheimer's disease and vascular dementia–a follow-up study." *Acta Psychiatr Scand* **84**(3): 277–82.

Niessen, L. C. and Jones, J. A. (1987). "Professional dental care for patients with dementia." *Gerodontology* **6**(2): 67–71.

Niessen, L. C., Jones, J. A., Zocchi, M. and Gurian, B. (1985). "Dental care for the patient with Alzheimer's disease." *J Am Dent Assoc* **110**(2): 207–209.

Nightingale, J. M., Walsh, N., Bullock, M. E. and Wicks, A. C. (1996). "Three simple methods of detecting malnutrition on medical wards." *J R Soc Med* **89**(3): 144–48.

Nordenram, G. and Ljunggren, G. (2002). "Oral status, cognitive and functional capacity versus oral treatment need in nursing home residents: a comparison between assessments by dental and ward staff." *Oral Dis* **8**(6): 296–302.

Nordenram, G., Ryd-Kjellen, E., Ericsson, K. and Winblad, B. (1997). "Dental management of Alzheimer patients. A predictive test of dental cooperation in individualized treatment planning." *Acta Odontol Scand* **55**(3): 148–54.

Nowjack-Raymer, R. E. and Sheiham, A. (2003). "Association of edentulism and diet and nutrition in US adults." *J Dent Res* **82**(2): 123–26.

Ocasio, N. A., Solomowitz, B. H. and Sher, M. R. (2000). "Dental management of the patient with Alzheimer's disease." *N Y State Dent J* **66**(3): 32–35.

Offenbacher, S., Lin, D., Strauss, R., McKaig, R., Irving, J., Barros, S. P., Moss, K., Barrow, D. A., Hefti, A. and Beck, J. D. (2006). "Effects of Periodontal Therapy During Pregnancy on Periodontal Status, Biologic Parameters, and Pregnancy Outcomes: A Pilot Study." *J Periodontol* **77**(12): 2011–2024.

Ostuni, E. and Mohl, G. (1995). "Communicating more effectively with the confused or demented patient." *Gen Dent* **43**(3): 264–66.

Papassotiropoulos, A., Bagli, M., Jessen, F., Bayer, T. A., Maier, W., Rao, M. L. and Heun, R. (1999). "A genetic variation of the inflammatory cytokine interleukin-6 delays the initial onset and reduces the risk for sporadic Alzheimer's disease." *Ann Neurol* **45**(5): 666–68.

Petersen, P. E. (2003). "The World Oral Health Report 2003: continuous improvement of oral health in the 21st century–the approach of the WHO Global Oral Health Programme." *Community Dent Oral Epidemiol* **31 Suppl 1**: 3–23.

Petersen, P. E. and Yamamoto, T. (2005). "Improving the oral health of older people: the approach of the WHO Global Oral Health Programme." *Community Dent Oral Epidemiol* **33**: 81–92.

Pfeiffer, R. F. (2003). "Gastrointestinal dysfunction in Parkinson's disease." *Lancet Neurol* **2**(2): 107–16.

Product-Information AMBIEN(R) Oral Tablet, zolpidem tartrate oral tablet. Sanofi-Synthelabo Inc, New York, NY, 2004.

Product-Information Aricept package insert (Eisai—US). Rev Rec 4/1/99., 4/98.

Product-Information Lunesta (TM), eszopiclone. Sepracor, Inc, Marlborough, MA, 2004.

Product-Information Risperdal(R) risperidone. Janssen Pharmaceutica Products, L.P., Titusville, NJ, 2004.

Product-Information ROZEREM(TM) oral tablets, ramelteon oral tablets. Takeda Pharmaceutical Company, Lincolnshire, IL, 2005.

Product-Information Zyprexa(R), olanzapine. Eli Lilly & Company, Indianapolis, IN, 2003.

Prusiner, S. B. (2001). "Shattuck lecture–neurodegenerative diseases and prions." *N Engl J Med* **344**(20): 1516–526.

Rainero, I., Bo, M., Ferrero, M., Valfre, W., Vaula, G. and Pinessi, L. (2004). "Association between the interleukin-1alpha gene and Alzheimer's disease: a meta-analysis." *Neurobiol Aging* **25**(10): 1293–298.

Ransier, A., Epstein, J. B., Lunn, R. and Spinelli, J. (1995). "A combined analysis of a toothbrush, foam brush, and a chlorhexidine-soaked foam brush in maintaining oral hygiene." *Cancer Nurs* **18**(5): 393–96.

Rejnefelt, I., Andersson, P. and Renvert, S. (2006). "Oral health status in individuals with dementia living in special facilities." *Int J Dent Hyg* **4**(2): 67–71.

Ritchie, C. S., Joshipura, K., Silliman, R. A., Miller, B. and Douglas, C. W. (2000). "Oral health problems and significant weight loss among community-dwelling older adults." *J Gerontol A Biol Sci Med Sci* **55**(7): M366–M371.

Roberts, F. A., McCaffery, K. A. and Michalek, S. M. (1997). "Profile of cytokine mRNA expression in chronic adult periodontitis." *J Dent Res* **76**(12): 1833–839.

Rogaeva, E., Meng, Y., Lee, J. H., Gu, Y., Kawarai, T., Zou, F., Katayama, T., et al.(2007). "The neuronal sortilin-related receptor SORL1 is genetically associated with Alzheimer disease." *Nat Genet.* Feb;**39**(2): 168–77.

Sayer, R., Law, E., Connelly, P. J. and Breen, K. C. (2004). "Association of a salivary acetylcholinesterase with Alzheimer's disease and response to cholinesterase inhibitors." *Clin Biochem* **37**(2): 98–104.

Scarmeas, N., Albert, M., Brandt, J., Blacker, D., Hadjigeorgiou, G., Papadimitriou, A., Dubois, B., et al. (2005a). "Motor signs predict poor outcomes in Alzheimer disease." *Neurology* **64**(10): 1696–703.

Scarmeas, N., Brandt, J., Albert, M., Hadjigeorgiou, G., Papadimitriou, A., Dubois, B., Sarazin, M., et al. (2005b). "Delusions and hallucinations are associated with worse outcome in Alzheimer disease." *Arch Neurol* **62**(10): 1601–608.

Scarmeas, N., Brandt, J., Blacker, D., Albert, M., Hadjigeorgiou, G., Dubois, B., Devanand, D., Honig, L. and Stern, Y. (2007). "Disruptive behavior as predictor in Alzheimer's disease." *Archives of Neurology* [in press].

Scarmeas, N., Hadjigeorgiou, G. M., Papadimitriou, A., Dubois, B., Sarazin, M., Brandt, J., Albert, M., et al. (2004). "Motor signs during the course of Alzheimer disease." *Neurology* **63**(6): 975–82.

Scarmeas, N. and Honig, L. (2004). "Frontotemporal degenerative dementias." *Clin Neurosci Res* **3**(6): 449–60.

Scarmeas, N., Stern, Y., Mayeux, R. and Luchsinger, J. A. (2006a). "Mediterranean Diet, Alzheimer Disease, and Vascular Mediation." *Arch Neurol* **63**(12): 1709–17.

Scarmeas, N., Stern, Y., Tang, M. X., Mayeux, R. and Luchsinger, J. A. (2006b). "Mediterranean diet and risk for Alzheimer's disease." *Ann Neurol* **59**(6): 912–21.

Schiffman, S. S., Graham, B. G., Suggs, M. S. and Sattely-Miller, E. A. (1998). "Effect of psychotropic drugs on taste responses in young and elderly persons." *Ann N Y Acad Sci* **855**: 732–37.

Schmidt, R., Schmidt, H., Curb, J. D., Masaki, K., White, L. R. and Launer, L. J. (2002). "Early inflammation and dementia: a 25-year follow-up of the Honolulu-Asia Aging Study." *Ann Neurol* **52**(2): 168–74.

Schneider, L. S., Dagerman, K. and Insel, P. S. (2006a). "Efficacy and adverse effects of atypical antipsychotics for dementia: meta-analysis of randomized, placebo-controlled trials." *Am J Geriatr Psychiatry* **14**(3): 191–210.

Schneider, L. S., Tariot, P. N., Dagerman, K. S., Davis, S. M., Hsiao, J. K., Ismail, M. S., Lebowitz, B. D., et al. (2006b). "Effectiveness of atypical antipsychotic drugs in patients with Alzheimer's disease." *N Engl J Med* **355**(15): 1525–38.

Seeley, W. W., Bauer, A. M., Miller, B. L., Gorno-Tempini, M. L., Kramer, J. H., Weiner, M. and Rosen, H. J. (2005). "The natural history of temporal variant frontotemporal dementia." *Neurology* **64**(8): 1384–90.

Selnes, O. A. and Vinters, H. V. (2006). "Vascular cognitive impairment." *Nat Clin Pract Neurol* **2**(10): 538–47.

Services, U. S. D. o. H. a. H. (2000). Oral Health in America: A Report of the Surgeon General. D. o. H. a. H. Services. Rockville, MD, National Institutes of Health, National Institute of Dental and Craniofacial Research.

Sevigny, J. J., Chin, S. S., Milewski, Y., Albers, M. W., Gordon, M. L. and Marder, K. (2005). "HIV encephalitis simulating Huntington's disease." *Mov Disord* **20**(5): 610–13.

Shatenstein, B., Kergoat, M. J. and Nadon, S. (2001). "Anthropometric changes over 5 years in elderly Canadians by age, gender, and cognitive status." *J Gerontol A Biol Sci Med Sci* **56**(8): M483–M488.

Sheiham, A. and Steele, J. (2001). "Does the condition of the mouth and teeth affect the ability to eat certain foods, nutrient and dietary intake and nutritional status amongst older people?" *Public Health Nutr* **4**(3): 797–803.

Sheng, J. G., Ito, K., Skinner, R. D., Mrak, R. E., Rovnaghi, C. R., Van Eldik, L. J. and Griffin, W. S. (1996). "In vivo and in vitro evidence supporting a role for the inflammatory cytokine interleukin-1 as a driving force in Alzheimer pathogenesis." *Neurobiol Aging* **17**(5): 761–66.

Ship, J. A. (1992). "Oral health of patients with Alzheimer's disease." *J Am Dent Assoc* **123**(1): 53–58.

Ship, J. A., DeCarli, C., Friedland, R. P. and Baum, B. J. (1990). "Diminished submandibular salivary flow in dementia of the Alzheimer type." *J Gerontol* **45**(2): M61–M66.

Ship, J. A. and Puckett, S. A. (1994). "Longitudinal study on oral health in subjects with Alzheimer's disease." *J Am Geriatr Soc* **42**(1): 57–63.

Shlossman, M., Knowler, W. C., Pettitt, D. J. and Genco, R. J. (1990). "Type 2 diabetes mellitus and periodontal disease." *J Am Dent Assoc* **121**(4): 532–36.

Shuman, S. K. and Bebeau, M. J. (1996). "Ethical issues in nursing home care: practice guidelines for difficult situations." *Spec Care Dentist* **16**(4): 170–76.

Small, S. A. and Mayeux, R. (2005). Delirium and Dementia. *Merritt's neurology*. L. P. Rowland. Philadelphia, Lippincott Williams & Wilkins: 3–8.

Stein, P. S., Scheff, S. and Dawson, D. R. (2006). "Alzheimer Disease and Periodontal Disease: Mechanisms Underlying a Potential Bi-directional Relationship." *Grand Rounds Oral-Sys Med* **1**(3): 14–24.

Strauss, S., Bauer, J., Ganter, U., Jonas, U., Berger, M. and Volk, B. (1992). "Detection of interleukin-6 and alpha 2-macroglobulin immunoreactivity in cortex and hippocampus of Alzheimer's disease patients." *Lab Invest* **66**(2): 223–30.

Subsai, K., Kanoksri, S., Siwaporn, C., Helen, L., Kanokporn, O. and Wantana, P. (2006). "Neurological complications in AIDS patients receiving HAART: a 2-year retrospective study." *Eur J Neurol* **13**(3): 233–39.

Takeda, M., Ojima, M., Yoshioka, H., Inaba, H., Kogo, M., Shizukuishi, S., Nomura, M. and Amano, A. (2006). "Relationship of serum advanced glycation end products with deterioration of periodontitis in type 2 diabetes patients." *J Periodontol* **77**(1): 15–20.

Tang, M. X., Stern, Y., Marder, K., Bell, K., Gurland, B., Lantigua, R., Andrews, H., Feng, L., Tycko, B. and Mayeux, R. (1998). "The APOE-epsilon4 allele and the risk of Alzheimer disease among African Americans, whites, and Hispanics." *Jama* **279**(10): 751–55.

Thomson, W. M., Chalmers, J. M., Spencer, A. J. and Slade, G. D. (2000). "Medication and dry mouth: findings from a cohort study of older people." *J Public Health Dent* **60**(1): 12–20.

UN (2003). The United Nations Population Division. World Population Prospects: The 2002 Revision. New York, United Nations.

Vas, C. J., Rajkumar, S., Tanyakitpisl, P. and Chandra, V. (2001). *When Old Age Becomes a Disease*, World Health Organization.

Walls, A. W., Steele, J. G., Sheiham, A., Marcenes, W. and Moynihan, P. J. (2000). "Oral health and nutrition in older people." *J Public Health Dent* **60**(4): 304–307.

Wang, S. Y., Fukagawa, N., Hossain, M. and Ooi, W. L. (1997). "Longitudinal weight changes, length of survival, and energy requirements of long-term care residents with dementia." *J Am Geriatr Soc* **45**(10): 1189–195.

Waring, S. C., Doody, R. S., Pavlik, V. N., Massman, P. J. and Chan, W. (2005). "Survival among patients with dementia from a large multi-ethnic population." *Alzheimer Dis Assoc Disord* **19**(4): 178–83.

Weaver, J. D., Huang, M. H., Albert, M., Harris, T., Rowe, J. W. and Seeman, T. E. (2002). "Interleukin-6 and risk of cognitive decline: MacArthur studies of successful aging." *Neurology* **59**(3): 371–78.

White, H. (1998). "Weight change in Alzheimer's disease." *J Nutr Health Aging* **2**(2): 110–112.

White, H., Pieper, C. and Schmader, K. (1998). "The association of weight change in Alzheimer's disease with severity of disease and mortality: a longitudinal analysis." *J Am Geriatr Soc* **46**(10): 1223–227.

Wolf-Klein, G. P. and Silverstone, F. A. (1994). "Weight loss in Alzheimer's disease: an international review of the literature." *Int Psychogeriatr* **6**(2): 135–42.

Wolfson, C., Wolfson, D. B., Asgharian, M., M'Lan, C. E., Ostbye, T., Rockwood, K. and Hogan, D. B. (2001). "A reevaluation of the duration of survival after the onset of dementia." *N Engl J Med* **344**(15): 1111–116.

Wood, J. A., Wood, P. L., Ryan, R., Graff-Radford, N. R., Pilapil, C., Robitaille, Y. and Quirion, R. (1993). "Cytokine indices in Alzheimer's temporal cortex: no changes in mature IL-1 beta or IL-1RA but increases in the associated acute phase proteins IL-6, alpha 2-macroglobulin and C-reactive protein." *Brain Res* **629**(2): 245–52.

Wu, T., Trevisan, M., Genco, R. J., Dorn, J. P., Falkner, K. L. and Sempos, C. T. (2000a). "Periodontal disease and risk of cerebrovascular disease: the first national health and nutrition examination survey and its follow-up study." *Arch Intern Med* **160**(18): 2749–755.

Wu, T., Trevisan, M., Genco, R. J., Falkner, K. L., Dorn, J. P. and Sempos, C. T. (2000b). "Examination of the relation between periodontal health status and cardiovascular risk factors: serum total and high density lipoprotein cholesterol, C-reactive protein, and plasma fibrinogen." *Am J Epidemiol* **151**(3): 273–82.

Yoneyama, T., Yoshida, M., Ohrui, T., Mukaiyama, H., Okamoto, H., Hoshiba, K., Ihara, S., et al. (2002). "Oral care reduces pneumonia in older patients in nursing homes." *J Am Geriatr Soc* **50**(3): 430–33.

Yurkstas, A. (1953). "The effect of masticatory exercise on the maximum force tolerance of individual teeth." *J Dent Res* **32**(3): 322–27.

Chapter 7
Musculoskeletal Conditions

Jennifer L. Kelsey

Musculoskeletal disorders are common and have a large impact on the quality of life of older adults. Data from the U.S. National Health Interview Survey indicate that musculoskeletal impairments (defined as chronic or permanent defects representing a decrease or loss of ability to perform various functions) are the most frequent type of impairment in the United States and are second only to hearing impairments in persons of age 65 years and older. Table 7.1 shows that among those of age 65 years and older, more than 20% have a musculoskeletal impairment, including about 10% attributed primarily to the back or spine, 8% to the lower extremity or hip, and 3% to the upper extremity or shoulder (Praemer, Furner, & Rice, 1999).

Musculoskeletal conditions are the leading cause of disability among persons of age 65 years and older (Lawrence et al., 1998). In the National Health Interview Survey, older persons reported an average of 20 days of restricted activity and 7 days in bed per year for each of their musculoskeletal impairments. Impairments of the lower extremity and hip had the greatest impact, resulting in 31 days of restricted activity and 9 bed days per year per impairment on average. About a third of nursing home residents report musculoskeletal impairments, with arthritis and osteoporosis being most frequent (Praemer et al., 1999).

Musculoskeletal injuries are also a major problem for older individuals. Among non-institutionalized persons of age 65 years and older, each year 2% report experiencing a fracture and 2% a dislocation or sprain. Fractures are even more frequent among nursing home residents. Among female nursing home residents of age 65 years and older, each year 5% experience a hip fracture and 4% suffer a fracture of another skeletal site (Praemer et al., 1999).

J.L. Kelsey

University of Massachusetts Medical School, Department of Medicine (Division of Preventive and Behavioral Medicine) and Department of Family Medicine and Community Health Worcester MA 01655

e-mail: jennykelsey@comcast.net

I.B. Lamster, M.E. Northridge (eds.), *Improving Oral Health for the Elderly*,
© Springer Science+Business Media, LLC 2008

Table 7.1 Percent prevalence of self-reported musculoskeletal impairments in persons of age 65 years and older, United States, 1995

Site of impairment	Prevalence
Back or spine	9.6%
Hip or lower extremity	7.7%
Shoulder or upper extremity	3.1%
All musculoskeletal impairments	20.4%

Adapted from Praemer et al. (1999).

People with musculoskeletal conditions use a large amount of medical care. In the United States, musculoskeletal conditions account for 17% of all visits to physicians in office-based practice, 15% of hospital outpatient visits, and 26% of emergency department visits. Among older individuals, the rate of hospitalizations for musculoskeletal conditions ranges from 3% per year in persons 65–74 years to 5% in the age range 75–84 years to 8% in those of age 85 years and older. Among those of age 65 years and older, fractures account for 36% of musculoskeletal-related hospitalizations. Older women are especially likely to be hospitalized for musculoskeletal conditions, and over a 10-year period have a greater than 50% chance of being hospitalized with a musculoskeletal condition (Praemer et al., 1999).

A survey in the United Kingdom found that 17% of adults report a long-standing musculoskeletal disorder (Bowling, 1996). The most important areas of daily life affected by long-standing musculoskeletal disorders are ability to get around, stand, walk, and go shopping (24%) and to participate in social and leisure-time activities (24%). Another study in England (Thompson, Anderson, & Wood, 1974) found that many of the elderly with musculoskeletal disorders live alone. Half of them have difficulty with stairs, one-third say they would not be able to attract attention even in the event of an emergency, and 20% say they are dependent on others for such everyday tasks as taking a bath, doing housework, and getting out of the house. Thus, being able to obtain medical or dental care can be a problem for older people with musculoskeletal disorders.

Musculoskeletal disorders may affect oral health in several ways. First, the disease process itself may involve some component of the oral cavity. Second, the treatment for a musculoskeletal disorder may affect the oral cavity. Finally, the disability associated with many musculoskeletal conditions can limit a person's ability to practice good oral hygiene and to obtain proper dental and medical care. This chapter will discuss the occurrence, risk factors, clinical course, and impact on oral health of the most common musculoskeletal disorders in older adults, including those primarily of bone (osteoporosis, osteoporotic fractures, and Paget's disease), those primarily of joints (osteoarthritis and rheumatoid arthritis), and low back and neck pain, which can involve various structures in and around the spine. Less common conditions that involve the musculoskeletal system and that can affect oral health will be discussed briefly at the end.

Diseases Primarily of Bone

Osteoporosis and Associated Fractures

Public Health and Clinical Aspects

Osteoporosis is a skeletal disorder characterized by compromised bone strength, predisposing to an increased risk of fracture (Osteoporosis Prevention, Diagnosis, and Therapy, 2000). Bone mineral content (grams) and bone mineral density (grams per square-centimeter) are usually measured by dual-energy X-ray absorptiometry (DXA) of the spine, hip, distal forearm, and whole body. On the basis of DXA measurements people are classified in relation to means and standard deviations for young adults of the same sex. Those with *T*-scores above the threshold of 1.0 standard deviations below the mean for young adults of the same sex are considered normal, those with *T*-scores between 1.0 and 2.5 standard deviations below the mean for young adults are considered to have osteopenia, and those with *T*-scores of 2.5 or more standard deviations below the mean for young adults of the same sex are considered to have osteoporosis (World Health Organization, 1994). Ultrasound of the heel and CT scan are also sometimes used to measure bone status.

It is important to recognize that bone mineral density and bone mineral content are not the only indicators of bone quality. Other aspects of bone quality include structural properties such as bone geometry (e.g., size and shape), microarchitecture (e.g., trabecular thickness and connectivity, cortical thickness, and porosity), and material properties such as mineralization (e.g., mineral-to-matrix ratio and crystal size), collagen composition (e.g., type and cross-links), and damage accumulation (e.g., microfractures) (Seeman & Delmas, 2006). These properties are not routinely measured.

Using the World Health Organization definition, about 20% of postmenopausal white women in the United States have osteoporosis in their femoral neck (Looker et al., 1997). Table 7.2 shows the estimated lifetime risks of fractures of the hip, vertebrae, and distal forearm for an average 50-year-old white woman and white man in the United States. About 40% of white women and 13% of white men experience a fracture at one of these three sites during their lifetime (Melton, Chrischilles, Cooper, Lane, & Riggs, 1992).

Table 7.2 Estimated lifetime risk, in percent, of fracture in 50-year-old white women and men

Fracture site	Women	Men
Hip fracture	17.5%	6.0%
Clinically diagnosed vertebral fracture	15.6%	5.0%
Distal forearm fracture	16.0%	2.5%
Any of the above	39.7%	13.1%

Adapted from Melton et al. (1992).

Bone mass in later adulthood, when osteoporotic fractures most often occur, depends on bone mass in young adulthood, when bone mass is at its peak, and on the extent of bone loss after the peak is reached. A particularly rapid rate of bone loss occurs in the years immediately following menopause, especially in the spine (Recker, Lappe, Davies, & Heaney, 2000). Heredity is an important determinant of bone mass in childhood, adolescence, and early adulthood, but the role of genetics in loss of bone mass with age and in association with menopause is less certain. Probably multiple genes are involved, each with a small effect (Peacock, Turner, Econs, & Foroud et al., 2002). Evidence suggests that weight, physical activity, calcium intake, and possibly other nutrients also affect bone mass in childhood, adolescence, and early adulthood, but to a lesser extent than heredity (Bonjour & Rizzoli, 2001; Specker, Namgung, & Tsang, 2001).

Osteoporosis-associated hip fractures are particularly common and disabling in older people. These fractures are strongly associated with increasing age, the female gender, and the white race (Cummings et al., 1995; Villa, Nelson, & Nelson 2001). Because they are more common in women than men, most studies of risk factors to date have been undertaken in women, so the discussion below refers to women.

The risk for hip fracture increases as bone mineral density decreases (Cummings et al., 1995). Other risk factors include prolonged corticosteroid use, oophorectomy, very low concentrations of endogenous estradiol, prolonged immobility, a history of a previous fracture, a maternal history of hip fracture, a history of falls, a fall from a standing height or greater, a fall that is sideways or straight down, a fall in which the person lands on the hip, poor neuromuscular function, poor self-rated health, poor vision, long hip axis length, use of psychotropic drugs, and cigarette smoking (Cummings et al., 1995; Cummings et al., 1998b; Faulkner et al., 1993; Grisso et al., 1991; Grisso et al., 1994; Hayes et al., 1993; Nevitt & Cummings, 1993; Seeman, 2001). Probable risk factors include tallness, a recent increase in the frequency of falls, high alcohol consumption, and high caffeine consumption (Cummings et al., 1995; Nevitt & Cummings, 1993; Schwartz, Nevitt, Brown, & Kelsey, 2005; Seeman, 2001). Relatively strong established protective factors include use of menopausal hormone therapy and obesity, and to a lesser extent calcium supplements, adequate dietary calcium consumption, adequate vitamin D intake, adequate vitamin D metabolism, physical activity, and use of thiazide diuretics (Beck, Shaw, & Snow, 2001; Cauley & Salamone, 2001; Cumming, 1990; Cummings et al., 1995; Gregg, Cauley, Seeley, Ensrud, & Bauer, 1998; Jackson, et al., 2006; Writing Group for the Women's Health Initiative Investigators, 2002). Most of the risk factors and protective factors can be related to one or more of the following attributes: bone strength, the occurrence of a fall, the protective response during the fall, the orientation of the fall, and the presence of local shock absorbers (Cummings & Nevitt, 1989).

Risk factors for fractures of other common sites have some similarities to and some differences from the risk factors for hip fracture. Proximal humerus fractures also tend to occur in elderly women with low bone mass who are prone to fall, but frailty does not appear to be a strong risk factor (Chu et al., 2004). Distal forearm fractures most often occur in relatively healthy, active women with low bone mass who are prone to fall and who can break a fall with their outstretched hand (Kelsey et al., 2005). The incidence does not increase much with age in middle-aged and older adults. Foot fractures often occur in women with foot problems and visual impairments. Low bone mass is associated with only a slightly increased risk for foot fracture, and the incidence does not increase much with age (Luetters et al., 2004). Vertebral fractures are strongly associated with low bone mass. Only about one-third of clinically diagnosed vertebral fractures occur as the result of a fall. Rather, the majority are attributed to compression loading from such activities as lifting and changing positions (Cooper, Atkinson, O'Fallon, & Melton, 1992). Incidence rates increase steeply with age (Cooper et al., 1992; European Prospective Osteoporosis Study (EPOS) Group, 2002; van der Klift, de Laet, McCloskey, Hofman, 2002). Whether frailty is a risk factor is uncertain.

Because only a small amount of protection against loss of bone mass is provided by increased dietary calcium consumption, calcium supplements, and physical activity, much attention has focused on the use of pharmaceutical agents to retard loss of bone mass and to reduce the risk of fractures in older people. Until a few years ago, menopausal hormone therapy had been widely used for this purpose, as it had been found to maintain bone mass and reduce fracture risk. However, in 2002 the results of the Women's Health Initiative randomized trial showed that although estrogen/progestin indeed afforded substantial protection against fractures in postmenopausal women, estrogen/progestin was associated with an increased risk for other diseases such as breast cancer, coronary heart disease, and pulmonary embolism (Writing Group for the Women's Health Initiative Investigators, 2002). Because the risks outweigh the benefits for most women, estrogen/progestin compounds are no longer recommended for the prevention of osteoporosis and associated fractures. Other agents currently used for retarding loss of bone mass and possibly reducing the risk for fractures are bisphosphonates, the selective estrogen receptor modulator raloxifene, calcitonin, and, for severe osteoporosis, parathyroid hormone. Of these agents, bisphosphonates are of greatest interest to those concerned with oral health.

Bisphosphonates are currently relatively widely used for the treatment and prevention of osteoporosis. Bisphosphonates slow bone resorption, which in turn retards bone formation and thereby slows bone remodeling. By slowing bone remodeling, loss of bone mass is prevented or at least retarded. Alendronate is incorporated into the skeleton without being degraded, where its half-life is up to 12 years (Lin, Russell, & Gertz, 1999). Alendronate, risedronate, pamidronate, zoledronic acid, and ibandronate are called aminobisphosphonates because they contain a nitrogen side chain.

In 1997, oral alendronate was the first bisphosphonate to be approved by the U.S. Food and Drug Administration for the prevention of loss of bone mass in recently postmenopausal women. Alendronate has been shown in randomized controlled trials to preserve bone mineral density in the hip and vertebrae. It reduces the risk for vertebral, hip, and other fractures in women who have already experienced at least one vertebral fracture (Black et al., 1996) and in women whose hip bone mineral density is more than 2.5 standard deviations below the mean for healthy young women (Cummings et al., 1998a). However, it does not reduce the risk for hip and other non-vertebral fractures in women without a previous vertebral fracture and whose bone density is above 2.5 standard deviations below the mean for healthy young women. Thus, slowing bone remodeling may indeed be beneficial for women with very low bone mass, but bisphosphonates do not appear to reduce the risk for fracture among those whose bone mass is not very low, possibly because adverse effects on bone are occurring as well. For instance, one report indicated that severe suppression of bone turnover may develop during long-term bisphosphonate therapy, resulting in delayed healing of non-spine fractures (Odvina et al., 2005). Richer et al. (2005) have reported depressed modulus of elasticity, an indicator of bone strength, following bisphosphonate therapy, especially long-term therapy. The possibility of long-term unanticipated effects of bisphosphonate on other health outcomes needs to be monitored. In addition, data from an extension of an earlier randomized trial of alendronate suggest that little benefit on bone mineral density and fracture risk is gained by using alendronate for an additional 5 years after the first 5 years of treatment, except for those at very high risk of clinical vertebral fracture (Black et al., 2006).

Bisphosphonates, mostly in oral form, are also used in the treatment of Paget's disease and certain other bone diseases. Intravenously administered bisphosphonates are used to treat patients with multiple myeloma and metastatic cancer to the bones, such as breast, prostate, lung, and renal cell carcinomas. Their use in these cancer patients has resulted in a reduction in skeletal complications such as pathologic fractures, spinal cord compression, and hypercalcemia, and in less need for subsequent radiotherapy or surgery to bone (Woo, Hellstein, & Kalmar, 2006).

Bisphosphonates and Oral Health

A side effect of bisphosphonates of particular concern to dental professionals is osteonecrosis of the jaw. No universally accepted definition of osteonecrosis of the jaw has been established, but it consists of areas of bone death that do not heal. Osteonecrosis generally appears as an area of exposed alveolar bone in the mandible or maxilla. Usually the area of exposed bone has developed after a tooth extraction or oral injury. Osteonecrosis of the jaw was first reported in association with bisphosphonate therapy in 2003 (Marx, 2003), mainly among patients with multiple myeloma or breast cancer who were receiving high doses of the intravenous bisphosphonates pamidronate or zoledronic acid, especially after recent dental pathology, trauma, or oral surgery. One of the 36 cases in this series was using a bisphosphonate for osteoporosis. Another series of 63 patients with osteonecrosis of the jaw was reported soon thereafter (Ruggiero, Mehrotra, Rosenberg, & Engroff, 2004). Again, most of the cases were cancer patients who had received intravenous bisphosphonates, but a few had taken oral alendronate or risedronate for osteoporosis.

In a review of 368 cases reported in the literature through January 2006, Woo et al. (2006) found that 65% occurred in the mandible only, 26% in the maxilla only, and 9% in both. Most lesions were on the posterior lingual mandible near the mylohyoid ridge. Sixty percent of the cases occurred after a tooth extraction or other dentoalveolar surgery, and the other 40% occurred spontaneously. The spontaneous cases tended to occur in patients wearing dentures, a potential source of local trauma. Ninety-four percent of the cases had been treated with intravenous bisphosphonates (primarily pamidronate and zoledronic acid), and 85% of patients had multiple myeloma or metastatic breast cancer. The other 15% of patients were taking oral bisphosphonates for osteoporosis or Paget's disease.

Most information on risk factors comes from follow-up of cancer patients. The most important risk factors are type (pamidronate or zoledronic acid) and total dose of bisphosphonate and a history of trauma, dental surgery, or dental infection (Badros et al., 2006; Woo et al., 2006). Clodronate, a non-aminobisphosphonate, has not been implicated (Woo et al., 2006). Risk increases with longer length of follow-up after initiation of bisphosphonate treatment (Badros et al., 2006; Bamias et al., 2005; Woo et al., 2006). One study (Badros et al., 2006) reported a greater risk in older people. Because of the association with length of use, there is concern that more cases of osteonecrosis of the jaw will be seen among users of oral bisphosphonates as their length of use becomes greater.

The jaw may be affected for two main reasons (Woo et al., 2006). First, the jaw bones are separated from the oral environment by only a thin mucosa and periosteum. Minor trauma can cause local damage to the mucosa and underlying periosteum. Trauma to the periosteum may also lead to osteonecrosis in patients wearing dentures or dental prostheses and in patients with prominent exostoses. Second, teeth are infected by bacteria that cause caries and periodontal disease. Because the teeth are separated from bone by only a thin layer of connective tissue, infections can readily be transmitted to underlying bone. Woo et al. (2006) postulate that bisphosphonate-associated osteonecrosis of the jaws is the result of marked suppression of bone metabolism that results in accumulation of microdamage in the jawbones, which are thereby biomechanically weakened. Repair of bone following trauma and infection is slowed because of the bisphosphonate, resulting in localized bone necrosis. Other medications and diseases may enhance the likelihood of persistence and progression of the condition.

Table 7.3 presents the recommendations of Woo et al. (2006) for managing this problem in dental patients according to their current status regarding bisphosphonate therapy. Before initiation of bisphosphonate therapy, it is important to eliminate active infections and to decrease the likelihood of future infections and the need for future dentoalveolar surgery, such as tooth extractions. Those who are already receiving intravenous bisphosphonate therapy should be evaluated on a case-by-case basis. No effective treatment is available for patients who have developed osteonecrosis of the jaw. Treatment focuses on control of pain and infection and careful local removal of dead bone, but not wide excision of lesions. Reduction of pain and regression and occasionally resolution of the osteonecrosis have been seen when patients are treated with antibiotics and the mouthrinse chlorhexidine, when use of bisphosphonates is stopped, and when loose pieces of necrotic bone are removed (Woo et al., 2006). It is not known whether bisphosphonate therapy should be halted; the half-life is so long, at least for alendronate (Lin et al., 1999), that its withdrawal may not have an effect for years.

Table 7.3 Recommendations to dental professionals for managing patients on bisphosphonate therapy

Type of patient	Recommended treatment
(1) On oral bisphosphonate therapy or about to begin intravenous bisphosphonate therapy or having received intravenous bisphosphonate therapy for less than 3 months and with no osteonecrosis of the jaw	(a) Treat active oral infections, eliminate sites at high risk for infection, non-restorable teeth, and teeth with substantial periodontal bone loss; (b) encourage routine dental care, including biannual oral examinations and dental cleaning, minimization of periodontal inflammation, provision of routine restorative care of teeth with caries, and provision of endodontic therapy where indicated
(2) Having received intravenous bisphosphonate therapy for 3 months or more and with no osteonecrosis of the jaw	(a) Seek alternatives to surgical procedures with appropriate local and systemic antibiotics; (b) undertake extractions and other surgery using as little bone manipulation as possible, using appropriate local and systemic antibiotics, and with follow-up to ensure healing
(3) With osteonecrosis of the jaw	(a) Follow recommendations for group (2) above; (b) consider additional imaging studies; (c) remove dead bone as necessary with minimal trauma to adjacent tissue; (d) prescribe oral rinses; (e) prescribe systemic antibiotics; (f) prescribe systemic analgesics as needed; (g) prescribe a soft acrylic stent; (h) suggest cessation of bisphosphonate therapy until osteonecrosis heals or the underlying disease progresses

Adapted from Woo et al. (2006).

A task force of the American Society of Bone and Mineral Research (Shane et al., 2006) has made the following recommendations in dealing with the problem of osteonecrosis of the jaw among persons with osteoporosis and Paget's disease:

(1) If possible, patients about to begin oral bisphosphonate therapy for osteoporosis or Paget's disease should have a dental examination before or soon after starting therapy. If oral surgery or other invasive dental procedures are planned, it would be best if they could be done before or soon after beginning bisphosphonates.
(2) Patients taking oral bisphosphonates for the treatment of osteoporosis and Paget's disease should be informed about the low risk of developing osteonecrosis of the jaw in association with oral surgery and other dental procedures.
(3) Patients taking oral bisphosphonates for the treatment of osteoporosis and Paget's disease should follow the same dental hygiene and dental care recommendations as the general population.
(4) Patients receiving oral bisphosphonates for the treatment of osteoporosis and Paget's disease should inform their dentist that they are taking these medications. They should also inform their physician if they are planning to have oral surgery or invasive dental procedures.

(5) Dental surgery should be limited to what is required for good dental health and undertaken only when more conservative non-surgical therapies are not appropriate.
(6) Patients with suspected osteonecrosis of the jaw should be referred to a dentist or an oral surgeon for evaluation and treatment.
(7) Some health care professionals recommend stopping bisphosphonates for several weeks before and after dentoalveolar surgery, although it is not known whether this practice would actually reduce the risk of developing osteonecrosis of the jaw. Because of the very long half-life of bisphosphonates in bone, this practice would probably not have an adverse effect on the treatment of osteoporosis or Paget's disease.

In addition, case reports have described severe oral ulcerations in patients who have sucked alendronate tablets or kept the tablet on the tongue for a short time (Demerjian, Bolla, & Spreux, 1999; Gonzales-Moles & Bagan-Sebastian, 2000). Taking the tablets in the manner recommended should eliminate this problem.

Osteoporosis and Periodontal Disease

Although most studies are small and cross-sectional, findings are for the most part quite consistent that mandibular and maxillary bone mineral densities, as well as specifically alveolar bone mineral density or reduced alveolar bone height, are modestly correlated with bone mineral density of other skeletal sites (Geurs, Lewis, & Jeffcoat, 2003; Jacobs, Ghyselen, Koninckx, & van Steenberghe, 1996; Jeffcoat, Lewis, Reddy, Wang, & Redford, 2000; Jonasson, 2005; Jonasson, Bankvall, & Kiliaridis, 2001; Kribbs, 1990; Kribbs, Chesnut, Ott, & Kilcoyne, 1989; Kribbs, Chesnut, Ott, & Kilcoyne, 1990; Southard, Southard, Schlechte, & Meis, 2000; Streckfus, Johnson, Nick, Tsao, & Tucci, 1997; Tezal et al., 2000; von Wowern, Klausen, & Kollerup, 1994; Wactawski-Wende et al., 1996). In addition, dense mandibular alveolar trabecular patterns have been found to be strongly correlated with higher skeletal bone mineral density (Jonasson et al., 2001; White & Rudolph, 1999), and in one study (Jonasson et al., 2001) more strongly associated with skeletal bone mineral density than is alveolar bone mineral density. Also, hormone replacement therapy is associated with higher bone mineral density in mandibular alveolar bone, as with other skeletal sites (Jacobs et al., 1996), and low endogenous estrogen concentration is associated with lower alveolar bone density (Payne, Zachs, Reinhardt, Nummikoski, & Patil, 1997).

Only a few longitudinal studies have been undertaken of the association of mandibular and maxillary bone mineral densities with bone mineral density in other skeletal sites, but the results tend to be consistent with those of the cross-sectional studies. Jonasson, Jonasson, & Kiliaridis (2006) reported a correlation between loss of forearm bone mineral density and loss of mandibular alveolar bone mass over a 5-year period. In this study the change in the bucco-lingual thickness of the alveolar process was correlated with change in bone mineral density of the forearm, but not with change in alveolar bone mass, possibly because more time is needed for the latter change to occur. A small longitudinal study ancillary to the Women's Health Initiative found a correlation between hip osteoporosis at baseline and subsequent loss of alveolar bone, particularly in women with periodontitis at baseline (Geurs et al., 2003). A small 2-year longitudinal study found that osteoporotic and osteopenic women exhibited a higher frequency of loss of alveolar bone height and of crestal and subcrestal density relative to women with normal lumbar spine bone mineral density (Geurs et al., 2003).

Results are mixed as to whether or not bone mineral density in various skeletal sites is correlated with tooth loss (Elders, Habets, Netelenbos, van der Linden, & van der Stelt, 1992; Krall, Dawson-Hughes, Papas, & Garcia, 1994; Mohammad, Bauer, & Yeh, 1997; Streckfus et al., 1997; Taguchi et al., 1999). However, tooth loss can occur for several reasons, and thus is not a good marker for periodontal disease. Unfortunately, studies of other markers of periodontal disease in relation to bone mineral density have also been inconclusive. For instance, von Wowern et al. (1994) found more frequent loss of attachment in women with osteoporotic fractures, but no difference in plaque or gingival bleeding. Tezal et al. (2000) reported a trend toward an association between bone mineral density at several skeletal sites and clinical attachment. In another study, attachment loss was correlated with tooth loss, but not with bone mineral density in the vertebrae or proximal femur (Hildebolt et al., 1997). Lundstrom, Jendle, Stenstrom, Toss, & Ravald (2001), in a study of a small number of 70-year-old women, found no significant correlations between low hip bone mineral density and gingival bleeding, probing pocket depths, gingival recession, or marginal bone level, and Weyant et al. (1999) reported at most weak associations between low bone mineral density at various skeletal sites and indicators of periodontal disease.

Three large prospective cohort studies have found that use of hormone replacement therapy is associated with less tooth loss (Grodstein, Colditz, & Stampfer, 1996; Krall, Dawson-Hughes, Hannan, Wilson, & Kiel, 1997; Paganini-Hill, 1995). Whether this apparent protective effect is mediated by lower bone loss among users of replacement estrogen or some other effect of estrogen, such as on inflammation, pathogen growth, or salivary function, is uncertain. Also, it is possible that the women using hormone replacement therapy had other attributes that put them at lower risk for tooth loss. A small 2-year longitudinal study found that women characterized as deficient in endogenous estrogen had a trend toward a higher frequency of sites with attachment loss than the non-estrogen-deficient group (Geurs et al., 2003).

Finally, an ancillary study of the Study of Osteoporotic Fractures (Famili, Cauley, Suzuki, & Weyant, 2005) reported no difference in subsequent change in bone mineral density of the hip in women who were dentate versus edentulous or between women with versus without periodontal disease.

In summary, mandibular and maxillary bone mineral densities are moderately correlated with bone mineral density elsewhere in the skeleton. This modest correlation suggests that decreases in jaw bone mineral density are partly the result of systemic factors and partly the result of local factors. However, whether low bone mineral density in the jaw results in other adverse changes, such as more missing teeth, gingival bleeding, greater probing pocket depth, and gingival recession, is unclear at present. Large, long-term longitudinal studies are needed to clarify these issues. Also, among various indicators of poor bone quality, it is possible that low bone mineral density is not the best predictor of periodontal disease, but that some other indicator, such as trabecular thickness, will be a preferred measure.

Paget's Disease

Public Health and Clinical Aspects

Paget's disease, the second most frequent disease of bones, is a thickening and weakening of bone that occurs when the normal balance of bone formation and bone loss is disrupted. Large, highly active bone resorbing cells (osteoclasts) produce abnormal bone resorption. The bone forming cells (osteoblasts) try to repair this damage, but the new bone that is formed is structurally disorganized, weaker, and prone to fracture and deformities (U.S. Department of Health and Human Services, 2004). Paget's disease can affect any part of the skeleton, but most frequently involves the spine, skull, pelvis, and legs. Osteoarthritis in adjacent joints is common, and neurological, cardiovascular, and metabolic complications may occur. Diagnosis should be based on X-rays of affected bones and at least one measurement of bone metabolic activity (Lyles, Siris, Singer, & Meunier, 2001). The most common neurological complication is hearing loss in patients with Paget's disease of the temporal bone. Osteosarcoma and other sarcomas occur in about 1% of Paget's disease patients, a percentage that is much higher than in the general population (Lyles et al., 2001).

The incidence of Paget's disease increases with age and occurs in 1.5–3.0% of people of age 60 years and older in the United States (Lyles et al., 2001). Males and females are affected with approximately equal frequency. Only about 10% of affected people have symptoms, usually consisting of aching pain caused by small fractures or from nerve compression. Sometimes visible deformities develop, such as an enlarged skull or curvature of the femur of lower leg.

The causes are unknown, although the disease appears to run in families (Morales-Piga, Rey-Rey, Corres-Gonzales, Garcia-Sagredo, & Lopez-Abente, 1995; Siris, Ottman, Flaster, & Kelsey, 1991). A slow viral infection of osteoclasts with paramyxoviruses has been suggested in the etiology of Paget's disease (Friedrichs et al., 2002), but there is no firm evidence for this view.

A survey of mostly long-term patients with Paget's disease has documented the strong adverse effect of the disease on the quality of life (Gold, Boisture, Shipp, Pieper, & Lyles, 1996). Hearing loss and bowed limbs were the most frequently reported complications. Forty-seven percent of the surveyed patients reported feelings of depression, and 42% said their health was only fair or poor.

Non-pharmacologic treatment may include use of walking aids, shoe lifts, and orthotics. Physical therapy may also be of help. In addition, bisphosphonates are often used to decrease bone resorption and slow bone turnover. The doses used are usually higher than those used in the treatment of osteoporosis (Lyles et al., 2001).

Paget's Disease and Oral Health

The jaw is affected in about 17% of cases (Woo & Schwartz, 1995). In early stages of the disease, loss of bone around the base of the teeth can result in loosening of the teeth and eventual tooth loss. More often, overgrowth of bone with spreading of the teeth and malocclusion occurs. Edentulous patients often have trouble with the proper fit of dentures. Other complications include root resorption, hyperplasia of the cementum, excessive bleeding on extraction, and osteomyelitis. Tooth extractions may be difficult because of hyperplasia of the cementum. Infections are a frequent complication following dental procedures (Kaplan, Horowitz, & Quinn, 1993). Because of the many potential oral complications, some dentists tend to avoid patients with Paget's disease (Kaplan, Haddad, & Singer, 1994). In addition, patients who are using bisphosphonates for Paget's disease have an elevated risk for osteonecrosis of the jaw, as described above.

Diseases Primarily of Joints

Osteoarthritis

Public Health and Clinical Aspects

Osteoarthritis, sometimes called degenerative joint disease, is a gradual deterioration of the joint cartilage with proliferation and remodeling of subchondral bone. Although often thought of as primarily a disease of cartilage, any of the joint tissues may be involved, including subchondral bone, synovium, joint capsule, periarticular muscles, sensory nerve endings, ligaments, and the meniscus where present (Brandt, Radin, Dieppe, & van de Putte, 2006). The usual symptoms are pain and stiffness, accompanied by loss of function. The course of the disease is variable and may differ from one joint to another. Radiographic criteria for population studies (Council for International Organizations of Medical Sciences, 1963), as well as clinical criteria (Altman et al., 1986; Altman et al., 1990; Altman et al., 1991), have been established.

Radiologic grade and symptomatology are correlated, but only moderately so. For instance, the First National Health and Nutrition Examination Survey (National Center for Health Statistics, 1979) found that among those with severe osteoarthritis of the hip as measured by radiograph, only 57% reported pain in or around the hips on most days for at least 1 month; among those with moderate radiologic osteoarthritis, 28% were thus affected, while 7% of those with questionable or no evidence of osteoarthritis in the hips had pain with this degree of frequency.

Several pathologic features of osteoarthritis, including the proliferative bone changes, may represent attempted repair responses in an injured joint. Osteophytes, for example, may result from a reactive response of cartilage and bone to abnormal mechanical loading, conferring protection to a damaged joint by reducing instability (Arden & Nevitt, 2006; Dieppe, 1999).

Single joints may be affected, with the knees, hands, feet, hips, and spine most commonly involved (Kellgren & Lawrence, 1958). Generalized osteoarthritis is defined as having three or more joint groups affected, and the term secondary osteoarthritis is used to categorize osteoarthritis resulting from trauma or congenital, developmental, or systemic disorders involving the joints.

In Western countries osteoarthritis is a leading cause of pain and physical disability in older people. As the populations of developing countries age, osteoarthritis will become an increasing burden in these populations as well. The World Health Organization predicts that osteoarthritis will become the fourth leading cause of disability worldwide by the year 2020 (Woolf & Pfleger, 2003).

The strongest risk factor for osteoarthritis is age (Table 7.4), and on autopsy, some cartilage damage is almost universal in older people. After about age 45–50 years, females are affected more frequently than males. Several factors contribute to the increase in incidence and prevalence with age, including accumulated wear and tear, stress from superincumbent weight, increased joint instability from ligamentous laxity, increased vulnerability of the joints to mechanical insults, and decreased resilience and reparative capacity of cartilage (Arden & Nevitt, 2006).

Wear and tear and repetitive loading of joints, particularly in certain occupations and sports, are strong risk factors. For instance, it has long been noted that miners often develop osteoarthritis of the elbows and knees (Lawrence, 1955), cotton pickers of the fingers, farmers of the hips (Lawrence, 1961), and dockers of the fingers, elbows, and knees (Partridge & Duthrie, 1968). Specific activities on the job that predisposed to knee and hip osteoarthritis are knee bending, squatting, kneeling, stair climbing, heavy lifting, and carrying heavy loads (Coggon et al., 2000; Cooper, McAlindon, Coggon, Egger, & Dieppe, 1994; Felson et al., 1991).

Congenital and developmental disorders and injuries involving joints, particularly if not treated early, greatly increase the likelihood of developing osteoarthritis in the affected joint (Felson, 1988). Prior inflammatory joint disease is also a risk factor. Increased grip strength appears to increase the risk for osteoarthritis of the hands (Chaisson, Zhang, Sharma, & Felson, 2000), whereas muscle weakness may be a risk factor for other sites such as the knees and hips (Slemenda et al., 1998). Heavy body weight is associated with an increased risk for osteoarthritis of

Table 7.4 Percent prevalence of X-ray evidence of osteoarthritis of the hands and/or feet by age and sex, United States, 1960–1962

Age (years)	Females	Males
18–24	1.6%	7.2%
25–34	6.2%	13.6%
35–44	19.6%	30.2%
45–54	46.3%	47.0%
55–64	75.2%	63.2%
65–74	84.7%	75.8%
75–79	89.8%	80.9%
Total	37.3%	37.4%

Source: National Center for Health Statistics (1966).

several sites, especially the knees and hands (Carman, Sowers, Hawthorne, & Weissfeld, 1994; Davis, Ettinger, & Neuhaus, 1988; Hochberg et al., 1995). Nutritional factors, high bone mineral density, and low concentrations of serum estradiol have been linked to osteoarthritis in some studies (Arden & Nevitt, 2006), but the evidence is not conclusive.

Genetic susceptibility is thought to play a role in the etiology of osteoarthritis (Loughlin, 2001; Arden & Nevitt, 2006). Multiple genes are likely to be involved. Polymorphisms of the type II collagen gene (Col2A1) are of particular interest, since type II collagen is a major constituent of the articular cartilage. The vitamin D and estrogen receptor genes are probably contributory as well. Genes encoding other structural proteins of the cartilage matrix and bone and cartilage growth factors are under study.

Preventive measures include weight loss, reduction in the workplace of repetitive mechanical stress on joints, and prevention and early treatment of congenital and developmental diseases involving joints. To decrease pain and stiffness and to reduce functional limitations, several steps may be taken, depending on the severity of the disease (Jüni, Reichenbach, & Dieppe, 2006). The first steps to control symptoms are usually patient education about weight, exercise, and lifestyle. Early in the disease process, simple analgesics, rubefacients, and nutriceuticals may also be beneficial. If these are not helpful, the patient may start to use non-steroidal anti-inflammatory agents and may be referred for physical or occupational therapy. Other steps may involve steroid injections into joints or minor surgery. Finally, joint replacement surgery of the hips and knees has been highly successful for those with severe osteoarthritis in these joints.

Osteoarthritis and Oral Health

Osteoarthritis of the temporomandibular joint, the joint between the temporal bone of the skull and the mandible of the jaw, is one cause of temporomandibular joint dysfunction. The temporomandibular joint contains a piece of cartilage called a disk that keeps the skull and the lower jawbone apart. When this cartilage disk degenerates, a grating sensation is felt as the mandible and temporal bones rub against each other when the mouth is opened and closed. With severe osteoarthritis of this joint, the person is not able to open the mouth wide. Temporomandibular joint dysfunction is covered in Chapter 17.

The activity and mobility limitation associated with osteoarthritis of various joints can affect both dental hygiene and the frequency of visits to dentists. Because of their disabilities, people with osteoarthritis may be unable to maintain proper oral hygiene, resulting in accumulation of plaque and calculus, thus increasing the likelihood of dental caries and periodontal disease (Pokrajac-Zirojevic, Slack-Smith, & Booth, 2002). Certain medications such as corticosteroids may suppress the immune system, thereby increasing the risk for periodontal infections, delayed wound healing, and prolonged bleeding time.

In addition, a large national survey in Australia (Pokrajac-Zirojevic et al., 2002) found that persons who reported that they had osteoarthritis were less likely to have

Table 7.5 Percentage of persons reporting having visited a dental professional within the past 2 years by self-reported Arthritis Status, Australia, 1995

Arthritis status	Percentage having visited a dental professional
Osteoarthritis ($N = 3091$)	57%
Rheumatoid arthritis ($N = 1193$)	55%
No arthritis ($N = 49544$)	72%

Source: Pokrajac-Zirojevic et al. (2002).

visited a dental professional within the past 2 years than persons from the general population without arthritis (57% versus 72%) (Table 7.5). When they did visit a dentist, those who reported osteoarthritis were more likely to require extractions and fillings than those without arthritis. They were also more likely to visit the dentist for restorative and prosthodontic treatment involving construction and insertion of dentures, as well as denture repairs, and denture and teeth cleaning. They were less likely to see dentists for routine check-ups and preventive treatment. Thus, persons with osteoarthritis need further education on the importance to their health of routine dental visits, despite the possible inconvenience of the visit.

Rheumatoid Arthritis

Public Health and Clinical Aspects

Rheumatoid arthritis is an inflammatory disease that damages the synovial tissue connecting bones and joints. The synovitis results in destruction of articular cartilage and bony erosion. The symptoms typically are stiffness, pain, and swelling of multiple joints, most commonly of the hands and wrists. Systemic manifestations of rheumatoid arthritis, including vascular, renal, and eye complications, may also be present. The diagnostic classification system generally used is the 1987 American College of Rheumatology revised criteria (Arnett et al., 1988).

The clinical course is variable, but as the disease progresses, most people with rheumatoid arthritis develop functional limitations, physical disabilities, and sometimes early mortality. Rheumatoid arthritis frequently results in work disability. Physical demands of the job, older age, low functional capacity, and lower educational attainment are associated with work disability (de Croon et al., 2004).

The prevalence in the United States and Western Europe is around 0.5–1.0% (Lawrence et al., 1998; Uhlig & Kvien, 2005). Females are affected more frequently than males, although this differential decreases with age. Over the age of 60 years, women are affected about 1.5 times more often than men (Rasch, Hirsch, Paulose-Ram, & Hochberg, 2003). In this older population, prevalence increases with age: 1.6–1.9% of older adults are affected in the age group 60–69 years, while 2.5–2.8% are affected among those of age 70 years and older. The incidence of rheumatoid arthritis appears to be decreasing in many parts of the world (Kvien, Uhlig, Ødegård, & Heiberg, 2006; Uhlig & Kvien, 2005).

Rheumatoid arthritis is considered to be of autoimmune etiology, and genetic factors are important. Familial aggregation and a higher concordance in monozygotic than dizygotic twins is seen. The genetic system that has been the subject of most study is the major histocompatibility complex (MHC). The human leukocyte antigen (HLA)–DR4 was the first allele to be associated with rheumatoid arthritis (Stastny, 1978). It is now known that the incidence and severity of rheumatoid arthritis are associated with a specific amino acid sequence on several HLA-DRB1 alleles, called the rheumatoid arthritis shared epitope (Gregersen, Silver, & Winchester, 1987; Kvien, Uhlig, Ødegård, & Heiberg, 2006; Ollier, Harrison, & Symmons, 2001). Other possible susceptibility genes are under study, but they are unlikely to be as important as the MHC genes. The role of infectious agents has been explored, but no agent has been definitively linked with rheumatoid arthritis (Albani & Carson, 1997). Oral contraceptives may retard the progression from mild to severe disease (Spector & Hochberg, 1990). Previous blood transfusion, obesity, and cigarette smoking may be associated with increased risks (Costenbader, Feskanich, Mandl, & Karlson, 2006; Ollier et al., 2001; Symmons et al., 1997).

Conventional treatment of rheumatoid arthritis has mainly relied on drugs to alleviate symptoms, such as non-steroidal anti-inflammatory agents and corticosteroids. These drugs improve symptoms and signs, but they do little to alter the structural progression and long-term disability associated with the disease. Disease-modifying drugs, including gold, penicillamine, and sulfasalazine, are thought to act by inhibition of cytokines, but these drugs produce a slow response and a high level of toxicity. They have generally not been taken for long periods of time. Methotrexate has somewhat better properties, but is still not used for long periods of time. Nevertheless, use of these drugs early in the course of the disease and escalation of therapy on the basis of objective evidence of continued disease activity have greatly improved the course of the disease (Emery, 2006). In addition, the discovery that the proinflammatory cytokine tumor necrosis factor α (TNF-α) plays a major role in the pathogenesis of the disease has led to the use of TNF-α antagonists in the treatment of rheumatoid arthritis. These agents have been shown to be highly effective in reducing symptoms and signs and in inhibiting structural damage in patients who have not responded to disease modifying antirheumatic drugs, including methotrexate. Use of both methotrexate and anti-TNF-α has brought about the best results (Breedveld et al., 2006).

Rheumatoid Arthritis and Oral Health

As with osteoarthritis, rheumatoid arthritis can affect oral health in several ways (Pokrajac-Zirojevic et al., 2002). Because of the usual involvement of the hands, personal oral hygiene may be difficult. This poor dental hygiene, along with the inflammatory reactions in the disease process, results in an increased risk for periodontal infections and dental caries. Mercado, Marshall, Klestov, & Bartold, (2000) in fact found a high prevalence (62.5%) of advanced periodontal disease in patients with rheumatoid arthritis. Immunosuppressive agents used in the treatment of rheumatoid arthritis also increase the risk for infections, delayed wound healing, and prolonged bleeding time. In addition, dry mouth frequently occurs in rheumatoid arthritis patients (Arneberg, Bjertness, Storhaug, Glennas, & Bjerkhoel, 1992). Rheumatoid arthritis can also contribute to the occurrence of temporomandibular joint dysfunction (Wolfe, Katz, & Michaud, 2005), as discussed in Chapter 17. Finally, people with rheumatoid arthritis are less likely to visit a dental professional than persons without arthritis. In the Australian study by Pokrajac-Zirojevic et al. (2002), only 55% of those with rheumatoid arthritis had visited a dental professional within the past 2 years, compared to 72% of persons without arthritis (Table 7.5). When they did visit a dentist, those with rheumatoid arthritis were considerably more likely than those without arthritis to have extractions, prosthodontic treatment, denture maintenance and repairs, and denture and teeth cleaning and polishing.

Low Back and Neck Pain

Public Health and Clinical Aspects

About 75–85% of people in Western countries experience some form of low back pain during their lifetime. In the United States, 15–20% of adults are affected during the course of a year, about 1% are chronically disabled because of back pain, and another 1% are temporarily disabled. Back pain is the most frequently reported reason for a physician visit in the United States (Andersson, 1998).

Most low back problems resolve within 2–4 weeks, and close to 90% resolve within 12 weeks (Andersson, 1998). However, recurrences are common, and low back pain often becomes a chronic problem with intermittent, usually mild exacerbations (Cassidy, Côté, Carroll, & Kristman 2005; Deyo & Weinstein, 2001). In a study of English patients seen by general practitioners for low back pain, after 1 year only 25% had no disability even though the majority was no longer seeking care for their problem from their practitioner (Croft, Macfarlane, Papageorgiou, Thomas, & Silman, 1998). In a small proportion of cases, the pain becomes constant and severe. In one study, 25% of cases accounted for 90% of the costs (Snook, 1982). Thus, low back pain that starts during the working years may persist into older age.

The specific condition responsible for low back pain is often not known. However, given that different low back disorders have different etiologies and clinical courses, combining all causes of low back pain can be misleading. Conditions commonly causing low back pain include sprains and strains, arthritic disorders, disc herniations, spinal stenosis, spondylolysis and spondylolisthesis, and facet abnormalities, but because most studies combine all types of low back pain, for the most part low back pain as a whole will be considered here.

The strongest predictor of low back pain is a history of low back pain (Lagerström, Hansson, & Hagberg, 1998; Papageorgiou et al., 1996; Van Poppel, Koes, Deville, Smid, & Bouter, 1998). First episodes of low back pain most frequently occur among persons in the age range 20–39 years, but the proportion of the population reporting low back pain (either old or new) is relatively constant across the working years (Biering-Sorenson, 1982; Guo, Tanaka, Halperin, &

Cameron, 1999). Over the age of 60 years, the prevalence of low back pain increases among women, probably in association with spinal osteoporosis and osteoarthritis. Low back pain occurs more frequently in persons of lower than higher socioeconomic status, mainly because of their greater likelihood of working in jobs requiring heavy manual labor.

People in jobs with a high degree of heavy manual labor are at high risk for low back pain (Punnett et al., 2005). The elevated risk appears to occur mainly in jobs requiring heavy lifting (e.g., 25 pounds or more), especially if bending and twisting are required while lifting, if objects are held away from the body, and if the knees are not bent while lifting (Andersson, 1981; Hales & Bernard, 1996; Hoogendoorn et al., 2000; Kelsey et al., 1984c; Liira, Shannon, Chambers, & Haines, 1996). Jobs involving motor vehicle driving and exposure to other forms of whole-body vibration also entail an increased risk (Bovenzi & Hulshof, 1999; Pope, Magnusson, & Wilder, 1998). Psychological factors such as low social support in the workplace and low job satisfaction may be associated with an increased risk (Hoogendoorn et al., 2000).

Non-occupational driving also confers an increased risk (Kelsey et al., 1984a; Lings and Leboeuf-Yde, 2000; Pope et al., 1998), as does cigarette smoking (Leboeuf-Yde, 1999). Associations have been reported between tallness and low back pain with sciatica or herniated lumbar intervertebral disc (Heliövaara, Mäkelä, Knekt, Ollimpivaara, & Aromaa, 1991) and between narrow spinal canals and herniated lumbar intervertebral disc (Heliövaara, Vanharanta, Korpi, & Troup, 1986). A recent review (Lis, Black, Korn, & Nordin, 2006) suggests that prolonged sitting by itself does not increase the risk for low back pain, but that sitting in combination with other exposures such as whole-body vibration and awkward posture does increase the risk.

Preventing the occurrence of low back pain is difficult. One approach is to modify exposures in the workplace, such as reducing the amount of weight to be lifted and minimizing bending and twisting motions while lifting. Using strength testing to select workers for heavy manual jobs and using exercises to strengthen back and abdominal muscles and improve overall fitness can be beneficial (Keyserling, Herrin, Chaffin, Armstrong, & Foss, 1980; Lahad, Malter, Berg, & Deyo, 1994). Although not yet the subject of formal evaluation, other helpful measures are likely to be smoking cessation, moving around from time to time in situations requiring prolonged exposure to one position, and vibration dampening. Also potentially beneficial would be motor vehicles with adjustable seat positioning and good lumbar support, reduction of the driving time of professional drivers, and better ergonomic properties of motor vehicles (Krause, Rugulies, Ragland, & Syme, 2004; Pope et al., 1998; Porter & Gyi, 2002). Approaches that do not seem to work are screening workers on the basis of low back X-rays and medical examinations, training workers to bend their knees while lifting (because of poor compliance), and wearing lumbar supports in high-risk occupations (Jellema, van Tulder, van Poppel, Nachemson, & Bouter, 2001; Snook, 1982).

Of particular importance in prevention of long-term disability for many people with acute low back pain is continuation of normal activities to the extent tolerated and a prompt return to work (Malmivaara et al., 1995; Nachemson, 1983). For instance, in a 12-week trial that compared various outcomes following random-ization to bed rest for 2 days, back mobilizing exercises, or resumption of normal activities as tolerated, those randomly assigned to resume their normal activities had the fewest number of sick days, the lowest intensity of pain, the lowest score on a back-disability index, the greatest ability to work, and the highest degree of lumbar flexion (Malmivaara et al., 1995).

Neck pain affects 60–70% of people during their lifetime (Côté, Cassidy, & Carroll, 1998), and the number of people affected appears to have been increas-ing in the United States. As with low back pain, a variety of conditions can cause neck pain, and recurrences are common. Risk factors have not been well studied, but to some extent appear to be similar to those associated with low back pain: previous low back or neck pain, prolonged exposure to awkward positions, and possibly heavy lifting, cigarette smoking, frequent diving from a board, motor vehicle driving, and exposure to other sources of whole-body vibration (Croft et al., 2001; Kelsey et al., 1984b; Krause et al., 1997; Magnusson, Pope, Wilder, & Areskoug, 1996; Smedley et al., 2003). Little research has been done on prevention, but probably of benefit would be reductions in heaving lifting, cigarette smoking, prolonged time spent in awkward positions such as at video display terminals, motor vehicle driving, and exposure to other forms of whole-body vibration.

Low Back and Neck Pain and Oral Health

No known direct link exists between low back pain and oral health, except that some of those with back pain have decreased mobility. Thus, like individuals with arthritis, they are probably less likely to visit a dental professional for routine care.

Regarding the neck, physiological links exist between the cervical spine and the masticatory system such that functional integration between the mandibular and the head–neck motor systems occurs during jaw motion (Häggman-Henrikson, Zafar, & Eriksson, 2002). Natural jaw function depends on simultaneous movement in the temporomandibular, atlanto-occipital, and cervical spine joints (Eriksson, Häggman-Henrikson, Nordh, & Zafar, 2000; Zafar, 2000). Activation of jaw and neck muscles brings about these coordinated movements. Because of this interde-pendence, injury to any of these joints can affect jaw function (Häggman-Henrikson et al., 2002). Patients with temporomandibular disorders may seek care for pain and dysfunction in the neck region, and patients with cervical spine disorders may present with pain and dysfunction in the jaw–face region. Injury to the head–neck area, as in whiplash injury, can affect this integrated jaw–neck function and thus compromise jaw function. Trauma to the neck can also contribute to temporo-mandibular dysfunction, thereby affecting mandibular mobility and mouth opening capacity (Klobas, Tegelberg, & Axelsson, 2004). Dentists should look for cervical dysfunction in patients with temporomandibular dysfunction. In addition, occlusal disorders, often related to masticatory dysfunction, are common and may cause neck pain that responds to dental treatment, especially in persons with abnormal craniocervical posture, signs linking the neck pain to mastication, and symptoms of masticatory dysfunction (Catanzariti, Debuse, & Duquesnoy, 2005). Physicians dealing with neck pain should thus keep in mind masticatory and occlusal disorders as possible causes.

Less Common Conditions that May Affect Oral Health

Osteomyelitis

Osteomyelitis is a rare condition in which bacteria or fungi infect bone and bone marrow. Acute osteomyelitis usually develops when pathogenic bacteria, most commonly *Staphylococcus aureus*, reach the metaphyseal blood vessels of bone through the blood stream (Cunha, 2002). Pathogenic bacteria in the smaller arterioles of the metaphyses of bone multiply, leading to microabscess formation. The abscesses usually occur in the medullary cavity of bone, the metaphyseal space, or subperiosteal space. Eventually fragments of infected dead bone form without a blood supply. Acute osteomyelitis can generally be cured with antibiotic therapy alone. However, if this process becomes chronic, extensive bone destruction occurs. *Staphylococcus aureus* may be involved, but gram-negative organisms are also frequently seen. Surgery is often required in addition to antibiotics. Older adults are at high risk because of the frequent occurrence of other predisposing diseases, such as peripheral vascular disease, diabetes mellitus, and poor dentition, and because of surgical procedures that are frequently performed in elderly persons, such as dental extractions, open-heart surgery, and joint replacement (Cunha, 2002).

Osteomyelitis of the mandible is usually seen in elderly patients with poor dentition or periodontal disease. Abscesses around the periodontal membrane and adjacent bone are common, and the abscess may extend deeper into the bone. The organisms usually responsible are those of the oropharyngeal anaerobic flora, such as *Actinomyces, Eikenella*, and *Peptostreptococcus*. Abscesses may occur locally or spread to the brain through the blood stream. Treatment, in addition to appropriate antibiotics, entails removal of the diseased tooth and root along with excision of the dead bone tissue (Cunha, 2002). Osteomyelitis may also occur in association with alendronate-induced osteonecrosis of the jaw, as described above.

Fracture of the Mandible

Across all ages, fracture of the mandible most commonly occurs as a result of violent crimes such as assault and gunshot wounds and, less commonly, motor vehicle accidents. In older individuals, however, falls and motor vehicle accidents are the most common causes of mandibular fractures and other maxillofacial injuries (King, Scianna, & Petruzzelli, 2004; Rehman & Edmondson, 2002; Sidal & Curtis, 2006). Thus, preventive efforts focusing on falls and motor vehicle accidents should reduce the frequency of these injuries in older populations.

Multiple Myeloma

Multiple myeloma is a cancer characterized by uncontrolled multiplication of abnormal plasma cells in the bone marrow. The annual incidence rate is about 6 per 100,000 in the United States and survival is poor (Ries & Devesa, 2006). Incidence and mortality rates increase steeply with age, and it usually occurs in persons older than 50–60 years of age. Although multiple myeloma is not technically a musculoskeletal condition, plasma cells produce cytokines that cause weakening of bone, leading to pain and fractures. Bone pain, especially during movement, is in fact often the main symptom of multiple myeloma. The weakening of the bone can lead to fracture. Bisphosphonates are often used in the treatment of multiple myeloma to strengthen bone and reduce hypercalcemia. The doses of bisphosphonates are high, thus leading to an increased risk of osteonecrosis of the jaw (see above).

Conclusion

It is important for dental and medical health professionals to keep in mind that several diseases of the musculoskeletal system can involve the oral cavity as part of the disease process. In addition, drugs used to treat several musculoskeletal disorders, including bisphosphonates for osteoporosis and Paget's disease and corticosteroids for the arthritic disorders, can increase the risk for oral disease. Finally, many musculoskeletal conditions, whether or not they directly affect oral health, make it more difficult for people to perform effective personal oral hygiene and also to get around, thus reducing the likelihood that they will receive office-based professional dental care. Those concerned with the health of older people need to be aware of these special problems caused by musculoskeletal conditions.

References

Albani, S., & Carson, D. A. (1997). Etiology and pathogenesis of rheumatoid arthritis. In W. J. Koopman (Ed.), *Arthritis and allied conditions. A textbook of rheumatology* (pp. 979–992). Baltimore: Williams & Wilkins.

Altman, R., Asch, E., Bloch, D., Bole, G., Borenstein, D., Brandt, K., et al. (1986). Development of criteria for the classification and reporting of osteoarthritis. Classification of osteoarthritis of the knee. Diagnostic and therapeutic criteria committee of the American rheumatism association. *Arthritis and Rheumatism, 29*, 1039–1049.

Altman, R., Alarcón, G., Appelrouth, D., Bloch, D., Borenstein, D., Brandt, K., et al. (1990). The American College of Rheumatology criteria for the classification and reporting of osteoarthritis of the hand. *Arthritis and Rheumatism, 33*, 1601–1610.

Altman, R., Alarcón, G., Appelrouth, D., Bloch, D., Borenstein, D., Brandt, K., et al. (1991). The American College of Rheumatology criteria for the classification and reporting of osteoarthritis of the hip. *Arthritis and Rheumatism, 34*, 505–514.

Andersson, G. B. J. (1981). Epidemiologic aspects of low-back pain in industry. *Spine, 6*, 53–60.

Andersson, G. B. J. (1998). Epidemiology of low back pain. *Acta Orthopaedica Scandinavica Supplement, 281*, 28–31.

Arden, N., & Nevitt, M. C. (2006) Osteoarthritis: Epidemiology. *Best Practice & Research Clinical Rheumatology, 20*, 3–25.

Arneberg P., Bjertness E., Storhaug, K., Glennas, A., & Bjerkhoel, F. (1992). Remaining teeth, oral dryness and dental health habits in middle-aged Norwegian rheumatoid arthritis patients. *Community Dentistry and Oral Epidemiology, 20*, 292–296.

Arnett, F. C., Edworthy, S. M., Bloch, D. A., McShane, D. J., Fries, J. F., Cooper, N. S., et al. (1988). The American Rheumatism Association 1987 revised criteria for the classification of rheumatoid arthritis. *Arthritis and Rheumatism, 31*, 315–324.

Badros, A., Weikel, D., Salama, A., Goloubeva, O., Schneider, A., Rapoport, A., et al. (2006). Osteonecrosis of the jaw in multiple myeloma patients: clinical features and risk factors. *Journal of Clinical Oncology, 24*, 945–952.

Bamias, A., Kastritis, E., Bamia, C., Moulopoulos, L. A., Melakopoulos, I., Bozas, G., et al. (2005). Osteonecrosis of the jaw in cancer after treatment with bisphosphonates: Incidence and risk factors. *Journal of Clinical Oncology, 23*, 8580–8587.

Beck, B. R., Shaw, J., & Snow, C. M. (2001). Physical activity and osteoporosis. In R. Marcus, D. Feldman, & J. Kelsey (Eds.), *Osteoporosis* (pp 701–720). San Diego: Academic Press.

Biering-Sorenson, F. (1982). Low back trouble in a general population of 30-, 40-, 50-, and 60-year old men and women. Study design, representativeness, and basic results. *Danish Medical Bulletin, 29*, 289–299.

Black, D. M., Cummings, S. R., Karpf, D. B., Cauley, J. A., Thompson, D. E., Nevitt, M. C., et al. (1996). Randomised trial of alendronate on risk of fracture in women with existing vertebral fractures. Fracture Intervention Trial Research Group. *Lancet, 348*, 1535–1541.

Black, D. M., Schwartz, A. V., Ensrud, K. E., Cauley, J. A., Levis, S., Quandt, S. A., et al. (2006). Effects of continuing or stopping alendronate after 5 years of treatment. The fracture intervention trial long-term extension (FLEX): A randomized trial. *Journal of the American Medical Association, 296*, 2927–2938.

Bonjour, J.-P., & Rizzoli, R. (2001). Bone acquisition in adolescence. In R. Marcus, D. Feldman, & J. Kelsey (Eds.), *Osteoporosis* (pp. 621–638). San Diego: Academic Press.

Bovenzi, M., & Hulshof, C. T. J. (1999). An updated review of epidemiologic studies on the relationship between exposure to whole-body vibration and low back pain (1986–1997). *International Archives of Occupational and Environmental Health, 72*, 351–365.

Bowling, A. (1996). The effects of illness on quality of life: Findings from a survey of households in Great Britain. *Journal of Epidemiology and Community Health, 50*, 149–155.

Brandt, K. D., Radin, E. L., Dieppe, P. A., & van de Putte, L. (2006). Yet more evidence that osteoarthritis is not a cartilage disease (Editorial). *Annals of the Rheumatic Diseases, 65*, 1261–1264.

Breedveld, F. C., Weisman, M. H., Kavanaugh, A. F., Cohen, S. B., Pavelka, K., van Vollenhoven, R., et al. (2006). The PREMIER study: A multicenter randomized, double-blind clinical trial of combination therapy with adalimumab plus methotrexate versus methotrexate alone or adalimumab alone in patients with early, aggressive rheumatoid arthritis and who had not had previous methotrexate therapy. *Arthritis and Rheumatism. 54*, 26–37.

Carman, W. J., Sowers, M., Hawthorne, V. M., & Weissfeld, L. A. (1994). Obesity as a risk factor for osteoarthritis of the hand and wrist: A prospective study. *American Journal of Epidemiology, 139*, 119–129.

Cassidy, J. D., Côté, P., Carroll, L. J., & Kristman, V. (2005). Incidence and course of low back pain episodes in the general population. *Spine, 30*, 2817–2823.

Catanzariti, J. F., Debuse, T., & Duquesnoy, B. (2005). Chronic neck pain and masticatory dysfunction. *Joint, Bone, Spine: Revue du Rhumatisme, 72*, 515–519.

Cauley, J. A., & Salamone, L. M. (2001). Postmenopausal endogenous and exogenous hormones, degree of obesity, thiazide diuretics, and risk of osteoporosis. In R. Marcus, D. Feldman, & J. Kelsey (Eds.), *Osteoporosis* (pp 741–769). San Diego: Academic Press.

Chaisson, C. E., Zhang, Y., Sharma, L., & Felson, D. T. (2000). Higher grip strength increases the risk of incident radiographic osteoarthritis in proximal hand joints. *Osteoarthritis and Cartilage, 8, Supplement A*, S29–32.

Chu, S. P., Kelsey, J. L., Keegan, T. H. M., Sternfeld, B., Prill, M., Quesenberry, C. P. Jr., et al. (2004). Risk factors for proximal humerus fracture. *American of Epidemiology, 160*, 360–367.

Coggon, D., Croft, P., Kellingray, S., Barrett, D., McLaren, M., & Cooper, C. (2000). Occupational physical activities and osteoarthritis of the knee. *Arthritis and Rheumatism, 43*, 1443–1449.

Cooper, C., Atkinson, E. J., O'Fallon, W. M., & Melton, L. J. III. (1992). Incidence of clinically diagnosed vertebral fractures: a population-based study in Rochester, Minnesota, 1985–1989. *Journal of Bone and Mineral Research, 7*, 221–227.

Cooper, C., McAlindon, T., Coggon, D., Egger, P., & Dieppe, P. (1994). Occupational activity and osteoarthritis of the knee. *Annals of the Rheumatic Diseases, 53*, 90–93.

Costenbader, K. H., Feskanich, D., Mandl, L. A., & Karlson, E. W. (2006). Smoking intensity, duration, and cessation, and the risk of rheumatoid arthritis in women. *American Journal of Medicine, 119*, 503–511.

Côté, P. Cassidy, J. D., & Carroll, L. (1998). The Saskatchewan Health and Back Pain Survey. The prevalence of neck pain and related disability in Saskatchewan adults. *Spine, 23*, 1689–1698.

Council for International Organizations of Medical Sciences (1963). *The epidemiology of chronic rheumatism. Atlas of standard radiographs of arthritis* (Vol. 2). Oxford: Blackwell.

Croft, P. R., Macfarlane, G. J., Papageorgiou, A. C., Thomas, E., & Silman A J. (1998). Outcome of low back pain in general practice: A prospective study. *British Medical Journal, 316*, 1356–1359.

Croft, P. R., Lewis, M., Papageorgiou, A. C., Thomas, E., Jayson, M. I., Macfarlane, G. J., et al. (2001). Risk factors for neck pain: A longitudinal study in the general population. *Pain, 93*, 317–325.

Cumming, R. G. (1990). Calcium intake and bone mass: A quantitative review of the evidence. *Calcified Tissue International, 47*, 194–201.

Cummings, S. R., & Nevitt, M. C. (1989). A hypothesis: the causes of hip fracture. *Journal of Gerontology Medical Sciences, 44*, M107–111.

Cummings, S. R., Nevitt, M. C., Browner, W. S., Stone, K., Fox, K. M., Ensrud, K. E., et al. (1995). Risk factors for hip fracture in white women. *New England Journal of Medicine, 332*, 767–773.

Cummings, S. R., Black, D. M., Thompson, D. E., Applegate, W. B., Barrett-Connor, E., Musliner, T. A., et al. (1998a). Effect of alendronate on risk of fracture in women with low bone density but without vertebral fractures: Results from the fracture intervention trial. *Journal of the American Medical Association, 24*, 2077–2082.

Cummings, S. R., Browner, W. S., Bauer, D., Stone, K., Ensrud, K., Jamal, S., et al. (1998b). Endogenous hormones and the risk of hip and vertebral fractures among older women. Study of Osteoporotic Fractures Research Group. *New England Journal of Medicine, 339*, 733–738.

Cunha, B. A. (2002). Osteomyelitis in elderly patients. *Aging and Infections Diseases, 35*, 287–293.

Davis, M. A., Ettinger, W. H., & Neuhaus, J. M. (1988). The role of metabolic factors and blood pressure in the association of obesity with osteoarthritis of the knee. *Journal of Rheumatology, 15*, 1827–1832.

de Croon, E. M., Sluiter, J. K., Nijssen, T. F., Dijkmans, B. A. C., Lankhorst, G. J., Frings-Dresen, M. H. W. (2004). Predictive factors of work disability in rheumatoid arthritis: A systematic literature review. *Annals of the Rheumatic Diseases, 63*, 1362–1367.

Demerjian, N., Bolla, G., & Spreux, A. (1999). Severe oral ulcerations induced by alendronate. *Clinical Rheumatology, 18*, 349–350.

Deyo, R. A., & Weinstein, J. N. (2001). Low back pain. *New England Journal of Medicine, 344*, 363–370.

Dieppe, P. (1999). Subchondral bone should be the main target for the treatment of pain and disease progression in osteoarthritis. *Osteoarthritis and Cartilage, 7*, 325–326.

Elders, P. J., Habets, L. L., Netelenbos, J. C., van der Linden, L. W., & van der Stelt, P. F. (1992). The relation between periodontitis and systemic bone mass in women between 46 and 55 years of age. *Journal of Clinical Periodontology, 19*, 492–496.

Emery, P. (2006). Treatment of rheumatoid arthritis. *British Medical Journal, 332*, 152–155.

Eriksson, P. O., Häggman-Henrikson, B., Nordh, E., & Zafar, H. (2000). Coordinated mandibular and head-neck movements during rhythmic jaw activities in man. *Journal of Dental Research, 79*, 1378–1384.

European Prospective Osteoporosis Study (EPOS) Group. (2002). Incidence of vertebral fracture in Europe: Results from the European Prospective Osteoporosis Study (EPOS). *Journal of Bone and Mineral Research, 17*, 716–724.

Famili, P., Cauley, J., Suzuki, J. B., & Weyant, R. (2005). Longitudinal study of periodontal disease and edentulism with rates of bone loss in older women. *Journal of Periodontology, 76*, 11–15.

Faulkner, K. G., Cummings, S. R., Black, D., Palermo, L., Glüer, C-C., & Genant, H. K. (1993). Simple measurement of femoral geometry predicts hip fracture: The study of osteoporotic fractures. *Journal of Bone and Mineral Research, 8*, 1211–1217.

Felson, D. T. (1988). Epidemiology of hip and knee osteoarthritis. *Epidemiologic Reviews, 10*, 1–28.

Felson, D. T., Hannan, M. T., Naimark, A. Berkeley, J., Gordon, G., Wilson, P. W., et al. (1991). Occupational physical demands, knee bending, and knee osteoarthritis: Results from the Framingham study. *Journal of Rheumatology, 18*, 1587–1592.

Friedrichs, W. E., Reddy, S. V., Bruder, J. M., Cundy, T., Cornish, I. J., Singer, F. R., et al. (2002). Sequence analysis of measles virus nucleocapsid transcripts in patients with Paget's disease. *Journal of Bone and Mineral Research, 17*, 145–151.

Geurs, N. C., Lewis, C. A., & Jeffcoat, M. K. (2003). Osteoporosis and periodontal disease progression. *Periodontology, 2000, 32*, 105–110.

Gold, D. T., Boisture, J., Shipp, K. M., Pieper, C. F., & Lyles, K. W. (1996). Paget's disease of bone and quality of life. *Journal of Bone and Mineral Research, 11*, 1897–1904.

Gonzales-Moles, M. A., & Bagan-Sebastian, J. V. (2000). Alendronate-related oral mucosa ulcerations. *Journal of Oral Pathology & Medicine, 29*, 514–518.

Gregersen, P. K., Silver, J., & Winchester, R. J. (1987). The shared epitope hypothesis. An approach to understanding the molecular genetics of susceptibility to rheumatoid arthritis. *Arthritis and Rheumatism, 30*, 1205–1213.

Gregg, E. W., Cauley, J. A, Seeley, D. G., Ensrud, K. E., & Bauer, D. C. (1998). Physical activity and osteoporotic fracture risk in older women. *Annals of Internal Medicine, 129*, 81–88.

Grisso, J. A., Kelsey, J. L., Strom, B. L., Chiu, G. Y., Maislin, G., O'Brien, L. A., et al. (1991). Risk factors for falls as a cause of hip fracture in women. The Northeast Hip Fracture Study Group. *New England Journal of Medicine, 324*, 1326–1331.

Grisso, J. A., Kelsey. J. L., Strom, B. L., O'Brien, L. A., Maislin, G., LaPenn, K., et al. (1994). Risk factors for hip fracture in black women. The Northeast Hip Fracture Study Group. *New England Journal of Medicine, 330*, 1555–1559.

Grodstein, F., Colditz, G. A., & Stampfer, M. J. (1996). Post-menopausal hormone use and tooth loss: A prospective study. *Journal of the American Dental Association, 127*, 370–377.

Guo, H-R., Tanaka, S., Halperin, W. E., & Cameron, L. L. (1999). Back pain prevalence in US industry and estimates of lost workdays. *American Journal of Public Health, 89*, 1029–1035.

Häggman-Henrikson, B., Zafar, H., & Eriksson, P-O. (2002). Disturbed jaw behavior in whiplash-associated disorders during rhythmic jaw movements. *Journal of Dental Research, 81*, 747–751.

Hales, T. R., & Bernard, B. P. (1996). Epidemiology of work-related musculoskeletal disorders. *Orthopedic Clinics of North American, 27*, 679–709.

Hayes, W. C., Myers, E. R., Morris, J. N., Gerhart, T. N., Yett, H. S., & Lipsitz, L. A. (1993). Impact near the hip dominates fracture risk in elderly nursing home residents who fall. *Calcified Tissue International, 52*, 192–198.

Heliövaara, M., Vanharanta, J., Korpi, J., & Troup, J. D. G. (1986). Herniated lumbar disc syndrome and vertebral canals. *Spine, 11*, 433–435.

Heliövaara, M., Mäkelä, M., Knekt, P., Ollimpivaara, & Aromaa, A. (1991). Determinants of sciatica and low-back pain. *Spine, 16*, 608–614.

Hildebolt, C. F., Pilgram, T. K., Dotson, M., Yokoyama-Crothers, N., Muckerman, J., Hauser, J., et al. (1997). Attachment loss with postmenopausal age and smoking. *Journal of Periodontal Research, 32*, 619–625.

Hochberg, M. C., Lethbridge-Cejku, M., Scott, W. W. Jr., Reichie, R., Plato, C. C., & Tobin, J. D. (1995). The association of body weight, body fatness and body fat distribution with osteoarthritis of the knee: Data from the Baltimore longitudinal study of aging. *Journal of Rheumatology, 22*, 488–493.

Hoogendoorn, W. E., Bongers, P. M., de Vet, H. C., Douwes, M., Koes, B. W., Miedema, M. C., et al. (2000). Flexion and rotation of the trunk and lifting at work are risk factors for back pain: Results of a prospective cohort study. *Spine, 25*, 3087–3092.

Jackson, R. D., LaCroix, A. Z., Gass, M., Wallace, R. B., Robbins, J., Lewis, C. E., et al. (2006). Calcium plus vitamin D supplementation and the risk of fractures. *New England Journal of Medicine, 354*, 669–683.

Jacobs, R., Ghyselen, J., Koninckx, P., & van Steenberghe, D. (1996). Long-term bone mass evaluation of mandible and lumbar spine in a group of women receiving hormone replacement therapy. *European Journal of Oral Sciences, 104*, 10–16.

Jeffcoat, M. K., Lewis, C. E., Reddy, M. S., Wang, C-Y., & Redford, M. (2000). Post-menopausal bone loss and its relationship to oral bone loss. *Periodontology, 23*, 94–102.

Jellema, P., van Tulder, M. W., van Poppel, M. N., Nachemson, A. L., & Bouter, L M. (2001). Lumbar supports for prevention and treatment of low back pain: A systematic review within the framework of the Cochrane Back Review Group. *Spine, 26*, 377–386.

Jonasson, G. (2005). Mandibular alveolar bone mass, structure and thickness in relation to skeletal bone density in dentate women. (2005). *Swedish Dental Journal Supplement, 177*, 1–63.

Jonasson, G., Bankvall, G., & Kiliaridis, S. (2001). Estimation of skeletal bone mineral density by means of the trabecular pattern of the alveolar bone, its interdental thickness, and the bone mass of the mandible. *Oral Surgery, Oral Medicine, Oral Pathology, Oral Radiology & Endodontics, 92*, 346–352.

Jonasson, G., Jonasson, L., & Kiliaridis, S. (2006). Changes in the radiographic characteristics of the mandibular alveolar process in dentate women with varying bone mineral density: A 5-year prospective study. *Bone, 38*, 714–721.

Jüni, P., Reichenbach, S., & Dieppe, P. (2006). Osteoarthritis: rational approach to treating the individual. *Best Practice & Research Clinical Rheumatology. 20*, 721–740.

Kaplan, F. S., Horowitz, S. M., & Quinn, P. D. (1993). Dental complication of Paget's disease: The need for hard facts about hard tissues (Editorial). *Calcified Tissue International, 53*, 223–224.

Kaplan, F. S., Haddad, J. G., & Singer, F. R. (1994). Paget's disease: Complications and controversies (Editorial). *Calcified Tissue International, 55*, 75–78.

Kellgren, J. H., & Lawrence, J. S. (1958). Osteo-arthrosis and disk degeneration in an urban population. *Annals of the Rheumatic Diseases, 17*, 388–397.

Kelsey, J. L., Githens, P. B., O'Connor, T., Weil, U., Calogero, J. A., Holford, T. R., et al. (1984a). Acute prolapsed lumbar intervertebral disc: An epidemiologic study with special reference to driving automobiles and cigarette smoking. *Spine, 9*, 608–613.

Kelsey, J. L., Githens, P. B., Walter, S. D., Southwick, W. O., Weil, U. Holford, T. R., et al. (1984b). An epidemiologic study of acute prolapsed cervical intervertebral disc. *Journal of Bone and Joint Surgery, 66A*, 907–914.

Kelsey, J. L., Githens, P. B., White A. A, III, Holford, T .R., Walter, S. D., O'Connor, T., et al. (1984c). An epidemiological study of lifting and twisting on the job and risk for acute prolapsed lumbar intervertebral disc. *Journal of Orthopaedic Research, 2*, 61–66.

Kelsey, J. L., Prill, M. M., Keegan, T. H. M., Tanner, H. E., Bernstein, A. L., Quesenberry, C. P., Jr., et al. (2005). Reducing the risk for distal forearm fracture: Preserve bone mass, slow down, and don't fall! *Osteoporosis International, 16*, 681–690.

Keyserling, W. M., Herrin, G. D., Chaffin, D. B., Armstrong, T. J., & Foss, M. L. (1980). Establishing an industrial strength testing program. *American Industrial Hygiene Association Journal, 41*, 730–736.

King, R. E., Scianna, J. M., & Petruzzelli, G. J. (2004). Mandible fracture patterns: A suburban trauma center experience. *American Journal of Otolaryngology, 25*, 301–307.

Klobas, L., Tegelberg, A., & Axelsson, S. (2004). Symptoms and signs of temporomandibular disorders in individuals with chronic whiplash-associated disorders. *Swedish Dental Journal, 28*, 29–36.

Krall, E. A., Dawson-Hughes, B., Papas, A. & Garcia, R. I. (1994). Tooth loss and skeletal bone density in healthy postmenopausal women. *Osteoporosis International, 4*, 104–109.

Krall, E. A., Dawson-Hughes, B., Hannan, M. T., Wilson, P. W. F., & Kiel, D .P. (1997). Postmenopausal estrogen replacement and tooth retention. *American Journal of Medicine, 102*, 536–542.

Krause, N., Ragland, D. R., Greiner, B. A., Fisher, J. M., Holman, B. L., & Selvin, S. (1997). Physical workload and ergonomic factors associated with prevalence of back and neck pain in urban transit operators. *Spine, 22*, 2117–2126.

Krause, N., Rugulies, R., Ragland, D. R., & Syme, L. S. (2004). Physical workload, ergonomic problems, and incidence of low back injury: A 7.5-year prospective study of San Francisco transit operators. *American Journal of Industrial Medicine, 46*, 570–585.

Kribbs, P J. (1990). Comparison of mandibular bone in normal and osteoporotic women. *Journal of Prosthetic Dentistry, 63*, 218–222.

Kribbs, P. J., Chesnut, C. H. III, Ott, S. M., & Kilcoyne, R. F. (1989). Relationships between mandibular and skeletal bone in an osteoporotic population. *Journal of Prosthetic Dentistry, 62*, 703–707.

Kribbs, P. J., Chesnut, C. H. III, Ott, S. M., & Kilcoyne, R. F. (1990). Relationships between mandibular and skeletal bone in a population of normal women. *Journal of Prosthetic Dentistry, 63*, 86–89.

Kvien, T. K., Uhlig,T., Ødegård, S.,& Heiberg, M. S. (2006). Epidemiological aspects of rheumatoid arthritis. The sex ratio. *Annals of the New York Academy of Sciences, 1069*, 212–222.

Lagerström, M., Hansson, T., & Hagberg, M. (1998). Work-related low-back problems in nursing. *Scandinavian Journal of Work, Environment, and Health, 24*, 449–464.

Lahad, A., Malter, A. D., Berg, A. O., & Deyo, R. A. (1994). The effectiveness of four interventions for the prevention of low back pain. *Journal of the American Medical Association, 272*, 1286–1291.

Lawrence, J. S. (1955). Rheumatism in coal minters. Part III. Occupational factors. *British Journal of Industrial Medicine, 12*, 249–261.

Lawrence, J. S. (1961). Rheumatism in cotton operatives. *British Journal of Industrial Medicine, 18*, 270–276.

Lawrence, R. C., Hemlick, C. G., Arnett, F. C., Deyo, R. A., Felson, D. T., Giannini, E. H., et al. (1998). Estimates of the prevalence of arthritis and selected musculoskeletal disorders in the United States. *Arthritis and Rheumatism, 41*, 778–799.

Leboeuf-Yde, C. (1999). Smoking and low back pain. A systematic literature review of 41 journal articles reporting 47 epidemiologic studies. *Spine, 15*, 1463–1470.

Liira, J. P., Shannon, H. S., Chambers, L. W., & Haines, T. A. (1996). Long-term back problems and physical work exposures in the 1990 Ontario Health Survey. *American Journal of Public Health, 86*, 382–387.

Lin, J.H., Russell, G., & Gertz, B. (1999). Pharmacokinetics of alendronate: An overview. *International Journal of Clinical Practice Supplement, 101*, 18–26.

Lings, S., & Leboeuf-Yde, C. (2000). Whole-body vibration and low back pain: A systematic, critical review of the epidemiological literature 1992–1999. *International Archives of Occupational and Environmental Health, 73*, 290–297.

Lis, A. M., Black, K. M., Korn, H., & Nordin, M. (2006). Association between sitting and occupational LBP. *European Spine Journal, 16*:283–298, 2007.

Looker, A. C., Orwoll, E. D., Johnston, C. C., Jr., Lindsay, R. L., Wahner, H. W., Dunn, W. L., et al. (1997). Prevalence of low femoral bone density in older U.S. adults from NHANES III. *Journal of Bone and Mineral Research, 12*, 1761–1768.

Loughlin, J. (2001). Genetic epidemiology of primary osteoarthritis. *Current Opinion in Rheumatology, 13,* 111–116.

Luetters, C. M., Keegan, T. H. M., Sidney, S., Quesenberry, C. P. Jr., Prill, M., Sternfeld, B., et al. (2004). Risk factors for foot fracture among individuals aged 45 years and older. *Osteoporosis International, 15,* 957–963.

Lundstrom, A., Jendle, J., Stenstrom, B., Toss, G., & Ravald, N. (2001). Periodontal conditions in 70-year old women with osteoporosis. *Swedish Dental Journal, 25,* 89–96.

Lyles, K. W., Siris, E. S., Singer, F. R., & Meunier, P. J. (2001). A clinical approach to diagnosis and management of Paget's disease of bone. *Journal of Bone and Mineral Research, 16,* 1379–1387.

Magnusson, M. L., Pope, M. H., Wilder, D. G., & Areskoug, B (1996). Are occupational drivers at an increased risk for developing musculoskeletal disorders? *Spine, 12,* 710–717.

Malmivaara, A., Häkkinen, U., Aro T., Heinrichs, M. L., Koskenniemi, L., Kuosma, E., et al. (1995). The treatment of acute low back pain – bed rest, exercises, or ordinary activity? *New England Journal of Medicine, 332,* 351–355.

Marx, R. E. (2003). Pamidronate (Aredia) and zoledronate (Zometa) induced alveolar necrosis of the jaws: a growing epidemic. *Journal of Oral and Maxillofacial Surgery, 61,* 1115–1117.

Melton, L. J. III, Chrischilles, E. A., Cooper, C., Lane, A. W., & Riggs, B. L. (1992) How many women have osteoporosis? *Journal of Bone and Mineral Research, 7,* 1005–1010.

Mercado F., Marshall, R. I., Klestov, A. C., & Bartold, P. M. (2000). Is there a relationship between rheumatoid arthritis and periodontal disease? *Journal of Clinical Periodontology, 27,* 267–272.

Mohammad, A. R., Bauer, R. L., & Yeh, C. K. (1997). Spinal bone density and tooth loss in a cohort of postmenopausal women. *International Journal of Prosthodontics, 10,* 381–385.

Morales-Piga, A. A., Rey-Rey, J. S., Corres-Gonzales, J., Garcia-Sagredo, J. M., & Lopez-Abente, G. (1995). Frequency and characteristics of familial aggregation of Paget's disease of bone. *Journal of Bone and Mineral Research, 10,* 663–670.

Nachemson, A. (1983). Work for all: those with low back pain as well. *Clinical Orthopaedics and Related Research, 179,* 77–85.

National Center for Health Statistics. (1966). Osteoarthritis in adults by selected demographic characteristics, United States, 1960–1962.*Vital & Health Statistics Series 11,* Number 20.

National Center for Health Statistics. (1979). Basic data on arthritis: knee, hip and sacroiliac joints, in adults ages 25–74 years: United States, 1971–1975.*Vital & Health Statistics Series 11,* Number 213.

Nevitt, M. C., & Cummings, S. R. (1993). Type of fall and risk of hip and wrist fractures: The study of osteoporotic fractures. *Journal of the American Geriatric Society, 41,* 1226–1234.

Odvina, C. V., Zerwekh, J. E., Rao, D. S., Maalouf, N., Gottschalk, F. A., & Pak, C. Y. (2005). Severely suppressed bone turnover: A potential complication of alendronate therapy. *Journal of Clinical Endocrinology and Metabolism, 90,* 1294–1301.

Ollier, W. E. R., Harrison, B., & Symmons, D. (2001). What is the natural history of rheumatoid arthritis? *Best Practice & Research Clinical Rheumatology, 15,* 27–48.

Osteoporosis Prevention, Diagnosis, and Therapy. (2000). *NIH Consensus Statement, 17,* 1–36.

Paganini-Hill, A. (1995). The benefits of estrogen replacement therapy on oral health. The Leisure World Cohort. *Archives of Internal Medicine, 155,* 2325–2329.

Papageorgiou A. C., Croft, P. R., Thomas, E., Ferry, S., Jayson, M. I. V., & Silman, A. J. (1996). Influence of previous pain experience on the episode incidence of low back pain: Results from the South Manchester back pain study. *Pain, 66,* 181–185.

Partridge, R. E. H., & Duthrie, J. J. R. (1968). Rheumatism in dockers and civil servants: A comparison of heavy manual workers and sedentary workers. *Annals of the Rheumatic Diseases, 27,* 559–568.

Payne, J. B., Zachs, N. R., Reinhardt, R. A., Nummikoski, P. V., & Patil, K. (1997). The association between estrogen status and alveolar bone density changes in postmenopausal women with a history of periodontitis. *Journal of Periodontology, 68,* 24–31.

Peacock, M., Turner, C. H., Econs, M. J., & Foroud T. (2002). Genetics of osteoporosis. *Endocrine Reviews, 23*, 303–326.

Pokrajac-Zirojevic, V., Slack-Smith, L. M., & Booth, D. (2002). Arthritis and use of dental services: A population based study. *Australian Dental Journal, 47*, 208–213.

Pope, M. H., Magnusson, M., & Wilder, D. B. (1998). Kappa delta award. Low back pain and whole body vibration. *Clinical Orthopaedics and Related Research, 354*, 241–248.

Porter, J. M., & Gyi, D. E. (2002). The prevalence of musculoskeletal troubles among car drivers. *Occupational Medicine, 52*, 4–12.

Praemer, A., Furner, S., & Rice, D. P. (1999). *Musculoskeletal conditions in the United States.* Rosemont IL: American Academy of Orthopaedic Surgeons.

Punnett, L., Prüss-Üstün, A., Nelson, D. I., Fingerhut, M. A., Leigh, J., Tak, S. et al. (2005). Estimating the global burden of low back pain attributable to combined occupational exposures. *American Journal of Industrial Medicine, 48*, 459–469.

Rasch, E. K., Hirsch, R., Paulose-Ram, R., & Hochberg, M. C. (2003). Prevalence of rheumatoid arthritis in persons 60 years of age and older in the United States: Effect of different methods of case classification. *Arthritis and Rheumatism, 48*, 917–926.

Recker, R., Lappe, J., Davies, K., & Heaney, R. (2000). Characterization of perimenopausal bone loss: A prospective study. *Journal of Bone and Mineral Research, 15*, 1965–1973.

Rehman, K., & Edmondson, H. (2002). The causes and consequences of maxillofacial injuries in elderly people. *Gerodontology, 19*, 60–64.

Richer, E., Lewis, M. A., Odvina, C. V., Vazquez, M. A., Smith, B. J., Peterson, R. D., et al. (2005). Reduction in normalized bone elasticity following long-term bisphosphonate treatment as measured by ultrasound critical angle reflectometry. *Osteoporosis International, 16*, 1384–1392.

Ries, L. A. G., & Devesa, S. S. (2006). Cancer incidence, mortality, and patient survival in the United States. In D. Schottenfeld & J. F. Fraumeni (Eds.). *Cancer epidemiology and prevention* (pp. 139–173). New York: Oxford University Press.

Ruggiero, S. L., Mehrotra, B., Rosenberg, T. J., & Engroff, S. L. (2004). Osteonecrosis of the jaws associated with use of bisphosphonates: A review of 63 cases. *Journal of Oral and Maxillofacial Surgery, 62*, 527–534.

Schwartz, A. V., Nevitt, M. C., Brown, B. W., Jr., & Kelsey, J. L. (2005). Increased falling as a risk factor for fracture among older women: The study of osteoporotic fractures. *American Journal of Epidemiology, 161*, 180–185.

Seeman, E. (2001). Effects of tobacco and alcohol use on bone. In R. Marcus, D. Feldman, & J. Kelsey (Eds.), *Osteoporosis* (pp 771–794). San Diego: Academic Press.

Seeman, E., & Delmas, P. D. (2006). Bone quality – the material and structural basis of bone strength and fragility. *New England Journal of Medicine, 354*, 2250–2261.

Shane, E., Goldring, S., Christakos, S., Drezner, M., Eisman, J., Silverman, S., et al. (2006). Osteonecrosis of the jaw: More research needed (Editorial). *Journal of Bone and Mineral Research, 21*, 1503–1505.

Sidal, T., & Curtis, D. A. (2006). Fractures of the mandible in the aging population. *Special Care in Dentistry, 26*, 145–149.

Siris, E. S., Ottman, R., Flaster, E., & Kelsey, J. L. (1991). Familial aggregation of Paget's disease of bone. *Journal of Bone and Mineral Research, 6*, 495–500.

Slemenda, C., Hoffman, D. K., Brandt, K. D., Katz, B. P., Mazzuca, S. A., Braunstein, E. M., et al. (1998). Reduced quadriceps strength relative to body weight: A risk factor of knee osteoarthritis in women? *Arthritis and Rheumatism, 41*, 1951–1959.

Smedley, J., Inskip, H., Trevelyan, F., Buckle, P., Cooper, C., & Coggon, D. (2003). Risk factors for incident neck and shoulder pain in hospital nurses. *Occupational and Environmental Medicine, 60*, 864–869.

Snook, S. H. (1982). Low back pain in industry. In A. A. White III & S. L. Gordon (Eds.), *American academy of orthopaedic surgeons symposium on idiopathic low back pain* (pp. 23–38). St. Louis: C.V. Mosby.

Southard, K. A., Southard, T. E., Schlechte, J A., & Meis, P. A. (2000). The relationship between the density of the alveolar processes and that of post-cranial bone. *Journal of Dental Research, 79*, 964–969.

Specker, B. L., Namgung, R., & Tsang, R. C. (2001). Bone mineral acquisition *in utero*, during infancy, and throughout childhood. In R. Marcus, D. Feldman, & J. Kelsey (Eds.), *Osteoporosis* (pp 599–620). San Diego: Academic Press.

Spector, T. D., & Hochberg, M. C. (1990). The protective effect of the oral contraceptive pill on rheumatoid arthritis: an overview of the analytic epidemiological studies using meta-analysis. *Journal of Clinical Epidemiology, 43*, 1221–1230.

Stastny, P. (1978). Association of the B-cell alloantigen DRw4 with rheumatoid arthritis. *New England Journal of Medicine, 298*, 869–871.

Streckfus, C. F., Johnson, R. B., Nick, T., Tsao, A., & Tucci, M. (1997). Comparison of alveolar bone loss, alveolar bone density and second metacarpal bone density, salivary and gingival crevicular fluid interleukin-6 concentrations in healthy premenopausal and postmenopausal women on estrogen therapy. *Journal of Gerontology. Series A, Biological Sciences and Medical Sciences, 52*, M343–351.

Symmons, D. P., Bankhead, C. R., Harrison, B. J., Brennan, P., Barrett, E. M., Scott, D. G., et al. (1997). Blood transfusion, smoking and obesity as risk factors for the development of rheumatoid arthritis: Results from a primary care-based incident case-control study in Norfolk, England. *Arthritis and Rheumatism, 40*, 1955–1961.

Taguchi, A., Suei, Y., Ohtsuka, M., Otani, K., Tanimoto, K., & Hollender, L. G. (1999). Relationship between bone mineral density and tooth loss in elderly Japanese women. *Dento Maxillo Facial Radiology, 28*, 219–223.

Tezal, M, Wactawski-Wende, J., Grossi, S. G., Ho, A. W., Dunford, R., & Genco R. J. (2000). The relationship between bone mineral density and periodontitis in postmenopausal women. *Journal of Periodontology, 71*, 1492–1498.

Thompson, M., Anderson, M., & Wood, P. H. N. (1974). Locomotor disability – a study of need in an urban community (Abstract). *British Journal of Preventive and Social Medicine, 28*, 70–71.

Uhlig, T, & Kvien, T. K. (2005). Is rheumatoid arthritis disappearing? *Annals of the Rheumatic Diseases, 64*, 7–10.

U.S. Department of Health and Human Services. (2004). *Bone health and osteoporosis: A report of the Surgeon General*. Rockville, MD: U.S. Department of Health and Human Services, Office of the Surgeon General.

Van der Klift, M., de Laet, C. E. D. H., McCloskey, E. V., Hofman, A., & Pols, H. A. P. (2002). The incidence of vertebral fractures in men and women: The Rotterdam study. *Journal of Bone and Mineral Research, 17*, 1051–1056.

Van Poppel, M. N., Koes, B. W., Deville, W., Smid, T., & Bouter, L. M. (1998). Risk factors for back pain incidence in industry: A prospective study. *Pain, 77*, 81–86.

Villa, M. L., Nelson, L., & Nelson, D. (2001). Race, ethnicity, and osteoporosis. In R. Marcus, D. Feldman, & J. Kelsey (Eds.), *Osteoporosis* (pp 569–584). San Diego: Academic Press.

Von Wowern, N., Klausen, B., & Kollerup, G. (1994). Osteoporosis: A risk factor in periodontal disease. *Journal of Periodontology, 65*, 1134–1138.

Wactawski-Wende, J., Grossi, S. G., Trevisan, M., Genco, R. J., Tezal, M., Dunford, R. G., et al. (1996). The role of osteopenia in oral bone loss and periodontal disease. *Journal of Periodontology, 67*, 1076–1084.

Weyant, R. J., Pearlstein, M. E., Churak, A. P., Forrest, K., Famili, P. & Cauley, J. A. (1999). The association between osteopenia and periodontal attachment loss in older women. *Journal of Periodontology, 70*, 982–991.

White, S. C., & Rudolph, D. J. (1999). Alterations of the trabecular pattern of the jaws in patients with osteoporosis. *Oral Surgery, Oral Medicine, Oral Pathology, Oral Radiology & Endodontics, 88*, 628–635.

Wolfe F., Katz, R. S., & Michaud, K. (2005). Jaw pain: Its prevalence and meaning in patients with rheumatoid arthritis, osteoarthritis, and fibromyalgia. *Journal of Rheumatology, 32*, 2421–2428.

Woo, S-B., Hellstein, J. W., & Kalmar, J. R. (2006). Systemic review: Bisphosphonates and osteonecrosis of the jaws. *Annals of Internal Medicine, 144*, 753–761.

Woo, T. S., & Schwartz, H. C. (1995). Unusual presentation of Paget's disease of maxilla. *British Journal of Oral & Maxillofacial Surgery, 33*, 98–100.

Woolf, A. D., & Pfleger, B. (2003). Burden of major musculoskeletal conditions. *Bulletin of the World Health Organization, 81*, 646–656.

World Health Organization. (1994). Assessment of fracture risk and its application to screening for postmenopausal osteoporosis. Geneva, Switzerland, World Health Organization. *WHO Technical Report Series, 843*, 1–129.

Writing Group for the Women's Health Initiative Investigators. (2002). Risks and benefits of estrogen plus progestin in healthy postmenopausal women: Principal results from the Women's Health Initiative randomized controlled trial. *Journal of the American Medical Association, 288*, 321–333.

Zafar, H. (2000). Integrated jaw and neck function in man. Studies of mandibular and head-neck movements during jaw opening-closing tasks. *Swedish Dental Journal Supplement, 143*, 1–41.

Chapter 8
Cardiovascular, Cerebrovascular Diseases and Diabetes Mellitus: Co-morbidities that Affect Dental Care for the Older Patient

Neerja Bhardwaj, Shelly Dubin, Huai Cheng, Mathew S. Maurer, and Evelyn Granieri

The prevalence of chronic disease increases with age. Consistent with the high prevalence is often substantial morbidity and mortality. Among the most common chronic diseases in older adults are those associated with micro- and macrovascular disorders. This chapter emphasizes those syndromes, and focuses on diabetes, major cardiovascular diseases and risk factors, and on cerebrovascular disease. Each of these disorders has significant implications in the management of older adults undergoing dental care. Because these co-morbidities are frequently coexistant and complex, familiarity with their management will continue to be increasingly important to dentists caring for older adults.

Diabetes Mellitus

Diabetes is the sixth leading cause of death in the United States and affects both the micro- and macrovasculature. The overall risk of death from diabetes is twice that of people without diabetes from the same age cohort. Persons with diabetes have a two to four times higher death rate from heart disease than adults without diabetes. Diabetes is a disorder of carbohydrate metabolism secondary to defects in insulin secretion or resistance to the action of insulin or both, resulting in elevated plasma glucose levels (American Diabetes Association, 2004). The incidence and prevalence of diabetes mellitus increase with age. According to the Center for Disease Control, the prevalence of diabetes, in 2005, in adults over the age of 60 in the United States, is 10.3 million or 20.9% (American Diabetes Association, 2004; National Center for Health Statistics, 2006). Alarmingly, there are a large number

N. Bhardwaj

Division of Geriatric Medicine and Aging, Department of Medicine, Columbia University Medical Center, New York, USA

I.B. Lamster, M.E. Northridge (eds.), *Improving Oral Health for the Elderly*,
© Springer Science+Business Media, LLC 2008

of older adults between the ages of 60 and 74, almost 11%, who have the disease but are undiagnosed (American Diabetes Association, 2004).

The two most common types of diabetes mellitus (DM) are type I and type II. Older adults are usually diagnosed with type II diabetes. Type II diabetes mellitus accounts for 90%–95% of adult diabetes and is caused by inadequate secretion of insulin as well as poor tissue response to insulin. An elderly person with type II diabetes mellitus usually does not require insulin but may often be required to diet and exercise. Type I diabetes accounts for 5%–10% of all diabetes and is a result of autoimmune destruction of the β-cells of the pancreas, resulting in little or no production of insulin. This typically occurs in a younger cohort of patients.

The diagnosis of diabetes is made when a patient exhibits classic symptoms: polyuria, polydipsia, weight loss, blurred vision and serum glucose of 200 mg/dl at any time of the day, or an 8-hour fasting plasma glucose (FPG) of 126 mg/dl, or a 2-hour oral glucose tolerance test (OGTT) resulting in a plasma glucose 200 mg/dl. The OGTT requires the ingestion of 75 g of glucose in 300 ml of water administered after an overnight fast (American Diabetes Association, 2004). The American Diabetes Association recommends the FPG as it is inexpensive and less complex for the patient. The World Health Organization recommends the OGTT as it provides additional information for differentiation of impaired glucose metabolism, and the unmasking of impaired glucose tolerance. OGTT is specifically recommended in high risk groups (Metcalf & Scragg, 2000). Impaired glucose tolerance is considered pre-diabetes and has an association with cardiovascular disease. Table 8.1 summarizes the diagnostic criteria for diabetes.

The first line of treatment for the newly diagnosed patient with type II diabetes is lifestyle modification such as control of blood pressure, lipids, weight loss and smoking cessation. When management cannot be achieved with lifestyle changes, there are multiple oral agents available to achieve glycemic control (Table 8.2).

Insulin is the oldest hypoglycemic agent available and is used in the management of the Type I patient or in concert with oral agents when oral agents alone cannot achieve glycemic control. Banting and Best first discovered insulin in the 1920s which was commercially produced using purified bovine (cow) and porcine (pig) insulin. In the 1980s technology advanced such that human insulin could be commercially produced. Human insulin is not recognized by the body as a foreign agent and therefore has decreased the risk of adverse reaction.

Table 8.1 Diagnosis criteria for diabetes

Normal FPG	Impaired FPG	Diabetes
FPG < 100 mg/dl	FPG ≥ 100 and < 126 mg/dl (IFG)	FPG ≥ 126 mg/dl
2-hPG < 140	2-hPG ≥ 140 and < 200 mg/dl (IGT)	2-h PG ≥ 200 mg/dl
		Casual plasma glucose ≥ 200 mg/dl

Table 8.2 Oral medications for treatment of Diabetes Mellitus

Generic Name	Trade Name	Dosage	Mechanism
Sulfonylureas			Enhance insulin secretion
First generation			
Acetohexamide	Dymelor	500–750 mg	
Chlorpropamide	Diabinese	250–275 mg	
Tolazimide	Tolinase	250–500 mg	
Tolbutamide	Orinase	1000–2000 mg	
Second Generation			
Glemeperide	Amaryl	4 mg	
Glipizide	Glucotrol	10–20 mg	
Glipizide SR	Glucotrol XL	5–10 mg	
Glyburide	Diabeta, micronase	5–20 mg	
Glyburide, micronized	Glynase	3–12 mg	
Alpha-glucosidse inhibitor			Decrease glucose absorption
Acarbose	Precose	50–100 mg tid	
Biguanide			Decrease hepatic glucose production
Metformin	Glucophage	1500–2550 mg divided	
Thiazolidinedione			Enhance insulin sensitivity
Troglitazone	Rezulin	400–600 mg	
Pioglitizone	Actos	15–45 mg	
Rosiglitazone	Avandia	4 mg qd-bid	
Combinations			
Glipizide and Metformin	Metaglip	2.5/250–5/500	
Glyburide and metformin	Glucovance	1.25/250–5/500	
Rosiglitazone and metformin	Avandamet	1/500–4/1000	

Health Maintenance and Diabetes

There are additional complications associated with DM besides those that are related to the cardiovascular system. Diabetic retinopathy is responsible for 12,000–24,000 cases of blindness each year. In the United States and Puerto Rico, diabetes is also the leading cause of renal failure, with 153,730 people who have end-stage kidney disease due to diabetes and are on chronic dialysis or have a kidney transplant. In 2002 82,000 amputations were performed on people with diabetes. There is also an increased association of periodontal disease in diabetics (Genco, 1996; Fontana et al., 1999). These complications dictate the health measures necessary for the maintenance of the health and well being of the patient with diabetes. The maintenance regimen needs to include a dilated eye exam by an ophthalmologist once a year. Podiatric care to evaluate foot care and prevention of diabetic foot ulcers is also recommended. Patients need to be taught how to cut their nails and to examine the skin between the toes for any lesions or signs of infection.

There is a strong connection between diabetes and periodontal disease, and it therefore important for persons with diabetes to have regular dental maintenance. It is beneficial for the dentist to determine the severity of the disease and the degree of control achieved. When dental procedures are required the patient should be advised to eat in the morning and take his or her insulin and/or oral agent. When treating a patient with a history of poor glycemic control it is important to consult with the managing clinician. Patients on oral agents do not require special care prior to procedures unless they have multiple co-morbidities and complications from the disease. Patients undergoing procedures that would require them not to eat prior to the procedure should not take their oral hypoglycemics on the day of the procedure and these agents should be reinitiated at the time that the diet is resumed.

The measurement of glycemic control is the hemoglobin A_1C (A_1C). The recommendation by the American Geriatrics Society for an elderly individual is maintenance of A_1C at 7% or lower. For the frail elderly patient with life expectancy of less than 5 years and others with multiple co-morbidities, tight control of glycemic levels may outweigh the benefits of the recommended A_1Cs (American Diabetes Association, 2004). In these cases one would want to avoid the potential of hypoglycemic events with a rigid medical regimen for glycemic control, which can be more detrimental to a patient's health, then allowing the blood sugars run at a higher level.

Acute Complications of Diabetic Mellitus

Diabetic ketoacidosis (DKA) can occur in patients with established diabetes or present as the initial manifestation of newly diagnosed diabetes. DKA results from insulin deficiency and excess of glucagon, catecholamines, cortisol and growth hormone. The diagnosis of DKA is made with the presentation of symptoms and/or physical findings that include

Symptoms
Nausea/vomiting
Thirst/polyuria
Abdominal pain
Shortness of breath
Lethargy/cerebral edema/coma

Physical Findings
Tachycardia
Dry mucous membranes
Dehydration/hypotension
Kussmaul respirations
Abdominal tenderness

DKA occurs because of inadequate insulin administration, infection, drugs (e.g. cocaine) or infarction (cerebral, coronary, mesenteric or peripheral) (Durso, 2006). The elderly diabetic patient with suspected DKA is a medical emergency and requires transfer to an emergency medical center.

Elderly persons with type II diabetes can develop nonketotic diabetic acidosis or a hyperglycemic hyperosmolar state (HHS). HHS is caused by a hyperglycemic state in the setting of deficient fluid intake. The elevated serum glucose levels cause an osmotic diuresis that in turn elevates the plasma glucose levels. A slow repletion of the body fluid volume in an acute care setting is the specified treatment.

Hypertension

Hypertension is an extremely common condition among older adults. The prevalence of hypertension in noninstitutionalized older women aged 55–64, 65–74 and 75 years and older was 53.9%, 72.7% and 83.1%, respectively. Older men have a slightly lower prevalence of hypertension (National Center for Health Statistics, 2006). It has been observed that systolic blood pressure (SBP) and diastolic blood pressure (DBP) increases as people get older (Fagard, 2002). However, elevation of DBP reaches the plateau when a person is around 60 years old. This contributes to a wide pulse pressure and isolated systolic hypertension (i.e. SBP $\geq$ 140 mmHg and DBP $\leq$ 90 mmHg), which are mainly seen in older adults (Fagard, 2002).

The diagnostic criteria of hypertension in adults including older adults are usually based on the Joint National Committee on Prevention, Detection, Evaluation and Treatment of High Blood Pressure (JNC). According to the classification of hypertension of JNC 7 report in 2003 (Table 8.3), hypertension is defined as either SBP $\geq$ 140 mmHg or DBP $\geq$ 90 mmHg (Chobanian et al., 2003). One of the major changes during the last decades is the definition of hypertension from $\geq$ 160/95 mmHg to $\geq$ 140/90 mmHg (Table 8.3). The JNC 7 and previous JNC reports were well accepted in the oral healthcare community (Muzyka & Glick, 1997; Glick, 1998; Aubertin, 2004; Herman, Konzelman, & Prisant, 2004).

Hypertension is a significant cardiovascular risk factor. In older adults, hypertension is associated with increased cardiovascular morbidity and mortality (Fagard, 2002). This increased morbidity and mortality could be reduced by lowering blood pressure (BP) as has been demonstrated in several randomized controlled trials (Leonetti & Zanchetti, 2002). The trend of uncontrolled hypertension in adults, mainly in older adults, has not been improved in the past decades despite there being hundreds of antihypertensive drugs on the market (Hajjar & Kotchen, 2003). Older adults with hypertension often visit their dentists. This provides dentists an opportunity to diagnose hypertension in older adults.

BP is determined by flow (cardiac output) and by peripheral vascular resistance. The mechanism of hypertension, including hypertension in older adults, is still unclear. Hypertension with an unknown or multifactorial etiology is called essential hypertension. Increased salt sensitivity, reduced aortic elasticity, baroreceptor

Table 8.3 Classification and Management of Hypertension for Adults

BP Classification	Systolic BP (mmHg)		Diastolic BP (mmHg)	Lifestyle Modification†	Management* With Compelling Indication	Initial Drug Therapy With Compelling Indication
Normal	<120	and	<80	Encourage		
Prehypertension	120–139	or	80–89	Yes	No antihypertensive drug indicated	Drug(s) for the compelling indications‡
Stage 1 hypertension	140–159	or	90–99	Yes	Thiazide-type diuretics for most; may consider ACE inhibitor, ARB, β-blocker, CCB or combination	Drug(s) for the compelling indications. Other antihypertensive drugs (thiazide-type diuretics and ACE inhibitor, ARB, β-blocker, CCB) as needed
Stage 2 hypertension	≥160	or	≥100	Yes	2-Drug combination for most (usually Thiazide-type diuretics and ACE inhibitor, ARB, β-blocker, CCB)	Drug(s) for the compelling indications. Other antihypertensive drugs (thiazide-type diuretics and ACE inhibitor, ARB, β-blocker, CCB) as needed

Abbreviations: ACE=angiotensin-converting enzyme; ARB=angiotensin-receptor blocker; BP=blood pressure; CCB=calcium channel blocker.

*Treatment determined by highest BP category; treat patients with chronic kidney disease or diabetes mellitus to BP goal of less than 130/80 mmHg; Initiate drug therapy for patients with orthostatic hypotension should be cautious.

†Lifestyle modification includes weight reduction, diet, physical activity and moderate of alcohol consumption.

‡ Thiazide-type diuretics and ACE inhibitor, ARB, β-blocker and aldosterone antagonist are indicated for hear failure; ACE inhibitor, ARB, β-blocker and aldosterone antagonist are indicated for post-myocardial infarction; Thiazide-type diuretics and ACE inhibitor, ARB, β-blocker are indicated for high coronary disease risk or diabetes mellitus; Thiazide-type diuretics and ACE inhibitor are indicated for recurrent stroke prevention (Chobanian V et al. 2003)

sensitivity and several other physiologic changes are potential mechanisms for hypertension in older adults (Burris, 1991). However, it is clear that the aging-related elevation of SBP and DBP is not physiologic and should not be considered as benign.

The concept of SBP and DBP introduced by Korotkoff is still used today. The first phase of Korotkoff sounds, heard as clear and tapping sounds, is defined as SBP. DBP is defined as the Korotkoff sounds begin to disappear or to muffle. The indirect BP measurement, i.e. the auscultatory method, is often used to diagnose hypertension (Chobanian et al., 2003). Accurately and properly measuring BP requires multiple steps and cautions (Williams et al., 2004; World Hypertension League, 2007). A mercury sphygmomanometer or semiautomatic device is often used to measure BP. According to Williams, the cuff sizes, including small adults, standard adults, large adults and adult thigh cuff, are used based on the arm circumference. The BP measuring device should be properly maintained, calibrated and validated. Both the patient and the provider should avoid talking during the measurement procedure. One should lower the mercury column at 2 mm/s and read the BP to the nearest 2 mmHg. Both sitting and standing BP should be recorded. A BP reading should be measured at least twice (Williams et al., 2004). Some patients may have elevated BP in the practitioner's office, however the patients' BP returns to normal in their homes. This is called white-coat hypertension (Chobanian et al., 2003; Williams et al., 2004). BP in older adults often varies and is termed labile hypertension (Williams et al., 2004). This can be detected by 24-hour ambulatory BP monitoring (ABPM) (Williams et al., 2004). However, ABPM is not routinely recommended for every person with hypertension (Williams et al., 2004).

The diagnosis of hypertension often requires three separate blood pressure readings (Bolli, 2005). Depending on BP level, which may identify a patient with hypertensive urgency or emergency, and/or the presence of target organ damage, such as diabetes, chronic kidney disease or macrovascular damage, some patients can be diagnosed with hypertension on the initial visit while others will require continued followed up or need an ambulatory BP monitor or home blood pressure monitoring. As Bolli suggested, diagnosing hypertension needs multiple visits depending on the initial BP level and co-existence of diabetes mellitus. Patients may need three to five clinic visits to diagnose hypertension based on JNC VII criteria (Bolli, 2005).

A systematic evaluation of hypertension is generally approached by history, physical examination, laboratory tests and imaging studies. The initial evaluation of a patient with hypertension includes identifying the causes of hypertension (drugs, renal diseases, pheochromocytoma and other secondary causes of hypertension), contributory factors (overwight, excess salt intake, physical inactivity and stress), complications of hypertension (renal insufficiency, heart failure and others) and other cardiovascular risk factors (smoking, diabetes mellitus, cholesterol level and etc) (Williams et al., 2004). The evaluation starts by asking about the history of hypertension and medications, especially cardiovascular and pain medications such as nonsteroidal anti-inflammatory drugs (NSAIDS). Persons with hypertension are often asymptomatic (Chobanian et al., 2003; Williams et al., 2004). Cardiovascular risk factors and common identifiable causes should be the focus of the initial evaluation (Williams et al., 2004). A key aspect of the physical examination is correct blood pressure measurement. Routine tests include urine analysis, basic metabolic panels, lipid profile and electrocardiogram. Imaging studies are used for certain patients (Chobanian et al., 2003; Williams et al., 2004) to evaluate for secondary causes.

Improving health outcomes is the major goal in treating hypertension in older adults. Randomized controlled trials (RCTs) have shown that lowering BP reduces cardiovascular morbidity and mortality (Leonetti & Zanchetti, 2002). An algorithm for the treatment of hypertensive adults is shown in Figure 8.1 (Chobanian et al., 2003). In general nonpharmacologic interventions are initiated first and then drug therapy is employed if nonpharmacologic interventions fail. The goal is to lower BP to the target level.

Nonpharmacologic interventions for blood pressure management includes weight reduction, DASH (Dietary Approaches to Stop Hypertension) diet, dietary sodium reduction, physical activity and moderation of alcohol consumption (Chobanian et al., 2003). It is important to reduce the cardiovascular risk factors such as smoking mentioned above. Lifestyle modifications such as physical activity and weight reduction are also beneficial to other cardiovascular diseases.

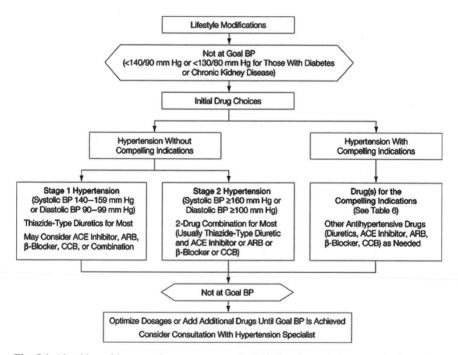

Fig. 8.1 Algorithm of hypertension management in JNC 7 and permission was obtained from JAMA (Aram V. Chobanian et al., 2003)

Initial antihypertensive drug therapy is chosen depending upon blood pressure level and compelling indications which is simplified in Figure 8.1 (Chobanian et al., 2003). The common compelling indications are heart failure, post-myocardial infarction, high coronary disease risk factor, diabetes mellitus, chronic kidney disease and recurrent stroke prevention (Chobanian et al., 2003). The classifications of antihypertensive drugs include thiazide diuretics, loop diuretics, β-blockers, α-blockers, combined α- and β-blockers, ACE inhibitors, angiotensin receptor blockers (ARBs), calcium channel blockers (CCBs), central acting agents, and direct vasodilators (Chobanian et al., 2003). The commonly used drugs are easily found in most drug books. For older adults, thiazide diuretics or calcium channel blockers are often the initial drug choice (Chobanian et al., 2003; Williams et al., 2004). Adding any medication, including antihypertensive drugs, could easily cause drug–drug and drug–disease interactions because many older adults consume multiple medications to treat their multiple co-morbidities. A "start low and go slow" approach for any drug, including antihypertensive drugs is warranted. In general, quickly lowing BP in an asymptomatic older adult with hypertension, to a target level, i.e. ≤ 140/90 mmHg in a short time such as hours or days may be harmful.

Hypertensive Emergency (or Crisis) and Urgency

Hypertensive emergency or crisis is defined as a sudden increase in SBP and DBP associated with acute target organ damage that requires immediate management (Varon & Marik, 2003; Flanigan & Vitberg, 2006). Target organ damage includes hypertensive encephalopathy, acute left ventricular failure with pulmonary edema, dissecting aortic aneurysm, acute myocardial ischemia, and acute renal failure. Such patients need to be admitted to a critical care unit to lower the blood pressure (Varon & Marik, 2003; Flanigan & Vitberg, 2006). Hypertensive urgency is defined as a significantly elevated BP without acute target organ damage. SBP is usually > 180 mmHg or DBP > 110 mmHg. In this situation, any elective dental procedure should be postponed. A medical consultation is recommended.

Dentists and Special Concerns in Hypertension

Hypertension is one of the most common reasons for a medical consultation prior to a dental procedure (Jainkittivong, Yeh, Guest, & Cottone, 1995). It is important that a hypertension history be ascertained for every dental patient. Pain, anxiety, stress and epinephrine-containing local anesthetics might be associated with elevated heart rate and BP. As shown in one study, a simple dental check-up increased SBP and DBP by 7–9 and 3–4 mmHg, respectively. Dental extractions have been shown to increase SBP and DBP by 7–9 and 3–4 mmHg, respectively (Brand, 1999). Control of pain, anxiety, and stress, and appropriate sedation results in less BP elevation during procedures. A low concentration of epinephrine

(1:80,000–1:100,000) is considered safe (Muzyka & Glick, 1997; Glick, 1998; Bader, Bonito, & Shugars, 2002; Brown, 2002; Aubertin, 2004; Herman, Konzelman, & Prisant, 2004). BP monitoring during a long dental procedure is recommended if patients have long-standing hypertension. If a patient complains of dental pain and BP reaches a severe level, i.e. SBP $\geq$ 180 mmHg or DBP $\geq$ 110 mmHg and has no symptoms such as headache, or chest pain, better pain control should be initiated. If dental pain is under good control, but the BP is still high, 100–200 mg of labetalol, or 0.1–0.2 mg of clonidine can be given orally. However, elective dental procedures should be postponed if patients have severe hypertension or uncontrolled hypertension, i.e. SBP $\geq$ 180 mmHg or DBP $\geq$ 110 mmHg measured before the dental procedure. However, there are no recognized or published criteria, based on absolute BP levels, to indicate when the urgent dental care should proceed (Muzyka & Glick, 1997; Glick, 1998; Aubertin, 2004; Herman, Konzelman, & Prisant, 2004).

Many cardiovascular drugs can cause adverse oral effects. They include dry mouth (associated with β-blockers or diuretics), loss of taste (associated with ACE inhibitors), bluish lips (associated with antianginal agents), angioedemma of face, tongue or glottis (associated with ARB), gingival enlargement or bleeding (associated with CCBs), stomatitis or gingivitis (associated with lipid lowering agents) (Aubertin, 2004). Lichenoid reactions, similar in appearance to oral lichen planus, have been associated with thiazide diuretics, ACE inhibitors, propranolol, furosemide, spironolactone and labetalol. A dentist should first review the patient's antihypertensive drugs and identify possible associations with oral adverse effects prior to considering primary oral or dental disease.

Coronary Artery Disease and Heart Failure

The incidence and prevalence of heart failure and coronary artery disease are increasing, both of which are strikingly age-dependent, with prevalence rates for heart failure in adults over 80 years of age approaching 10% (Senni et al., 1998; Forman & Rich, 2003). The mortality rates are increasing exponentially with advance in age in all major demographic subgroups of the U.S. population. It has been projected that these rates will continue well into the twenty-first century. Although several factors have contributed to the rise in these disorders, principal among them is the progressive aging of the population.

A good history remains of substantial value in establishing the diagnosis of these conditions despite the recent advances in laboratory measurements. The provider's initial examination, despite the subjective nature of much of the information gathered, can be used to identify patients likely to benefit from further evaluation and treatment.

Ischemic Heart Disease

While it is typical for patients with ischemic heart disease to note a characteristic chest pain, compatible with angina, only 70%–80% of patients with acute

Table 8.4 Categories of Angina

Angina Categories	Description
Definite angina	Substernal discomfort that precipitated by exertion, with a typical radiation to the shoulder, jaw or inner aspect of the arm, often associated with diaphoreisis or shortness of breath and relieved by rest or nitroglycerin in less than 10 minutes.
Probable angina	Patients have most of the features of definite angina, but are atypical in some aspects [i.e. atypical radiation of pain, nitroglycerin not always effective, not associated with other symptoms, nor is the pain was relieved only after 15–20 minutes of rest.]
Probably not angina	An atypical overall pattern of chest pain that does not fit the description of definite angina.
Definitely not angina	Chest pain that is unrelated to activity appeared to be clearly of non-cardiac origin and was not relieved by nitroglycerin. Features suggesting a diagnosis of not angina include: pleuritic pain, pain localized with one finger, pain reproduced by movement or palpation of chest wall or arms, constant pain lasting for days, very brief episodes of pain lasting a few seconds or less, and pain radiating into the lower extremities.

myocardial infarction (AMI) present with ischemic type chest discomfort (Lusiani, Perrone, Pesavento, & Conte, 1994; Ahto et al., 1998). Accordingly, providers should be aware of clinical characteristics that are an independent predictor of significant coronary artery disease including advanced age, male gender, type of chest pain (definite or probably angina, Table 8.4), diabetes mellitus, smoking, hyperlipidemia and a previous history of myocardial infarction. Additionally, particularly in the elderly, an acute myocardial infarction or unstable coronary syndrome can manifest clinically not with chest pain but rather by symptoms of acute left ventricular failure and chest tightness or by marked weakness or frank syncope (Lusiani, Perrone, Pesavento, & Conte, 1994; Nowak, 1997). Persons with diabetes (women in particular) have been noted in many studies to have atypical presentation of acute ischemic syndromes (Yoshino et al., 1983) and in some instances, the pain of acute ischemic events may begin in the epigastrium and simulate a variety of abdominal disorders. This fact often causes a myocardial infarction to be misdiagnosed as "indigestion". Thus, acute myocardial infarction or an unstable coronary syndrome should be suspected in any older patient who presents with ischemic type chest pain (definite or probable angina) that is prolonged (i.e. >10–20 minutes), occurs at rest or with less activity than usual and in those patients with significant risk factors despite atypical presentations.

In patients with a high likelihood of an acute ischemic syndrome based on historical information, dental procedures should be delayed until more definitive evaluations, typically including a 12 lead electrocardiogram and serial cardiac enzymes, are performed. These additional evaluations should be obtained as rapidly as possible to help confirm the diagnosis, stratify patients with regard to risk, and identify the presenting cardiac rhythm and site of potential myocardial ischemia or infarction (Antman et al., 2004).

The treatment of patients with ischemic heart disease is relatively simple if the proper steps are taken. In general, a preventive approach to the treatment of these patients will serve to prevent untoward outcomes and provide safe and simple delivery of dental care for older cardiovascular patients. First, obtain blood pressure measurements to screen for undiagnosed hypertension and to identify patients in whom further medical therapy is warranted prior to dental procedures. Second, establish what medications the patient is taking along with the dose and timing and note any potential drug interactions and side effects (Table 8.5). Third, the use of short (less than 1 hour) and morning appointments along with pre-medication to alleviate anxiety should be considered. Additionally, the use of intra-operative nitrous oxide and oxygen is also a reasonable strategy for patients with ischemic heart disease. Finally, effective local anesthesia is vital, in order to avoid undue stress that can promote ischemic events, while following guidelines for the administration of epinephrine (Leviner et al., 1992; Perusse, Goulet, & Turcotte, 1992; Mask, 2000). For patients with ischemic coronary syndromes, a fresh supply of nitroglycerin should be available. In the event of the development of cardiovascular symptoms during dental treatment, all work should be stopped and emergency measures should be instituted if necessary.

Among patients with unstable angina or a recent (within 1 month) myocardial infarction or recent coronary artery bypass operation, elective dental procedures should in general be avoided (Eagle et al., 2002), and necessary dental treatment should be conservative in its approach, aimed at treating pain or underlying infection. In such patients, prior to proceeding with definitive dental interventions, consultation with the physician is strongly advisable and during such procedures, attention to the comfort of the patient in order to reduce anxiety and pain could include any and all of the following: short appointments, comfortable dental chair and positioning, monitoring of vital signs pretreatment, good communication, oral sedation and adequate intra-operative and postoperative pain control (Leviner et al., 1992).

Patients with an acute coronary syndrome include those whose clinical presentations span the range of diagnoses from unstable angina to MI without ST elevation (NSTEMI) and finally, MI with ST elevation (STEMI). The distinguishing underlying pathophysiologic process in this spectrum of disorders is the presence of underlying occluding thrombosis. Patients with STEMI have a high likelihood of a coronary thrombus occluding the infarct artery, with a coronary thrombus possible present in more than 90% of patients with STEMI, while only 1% of patients with stable angina and about 35%–75% of patients with unstable angina or NSTEMI have a coronary thrombosis (Antman et al., 2004).

Oxygen is very effective initial therapy for patients with potential acute ischemic syndrome and can be administered at nasal flow rates of 4–6 Liters/minute but for patients with evidence of chronic pulmonary disease, lower flow rates may be prudent. For patients with suspected acute ischemic syndromes nd patients with evidence of chronic pulmonary disease, lower flow rates may be prudent. Aspirin has been shown to have a significant reduction in mortality and reinfarction rates

Table 8.5 Drugs Employed Commonly for Cardiovascular Conditions

Drug	Mechanism of Action	Dental/Oral Consideration	Non-Dental Issues
Anti-platelet Agents			
Aspirin	Inhibits prostaglandin synthesis via cyclooxygenase inactivation	• Rare cases of stomatitis with excessive use orally	• Common Side Effects, are gastrointestinal: dyspepsia, nausea/vomiting and ulcer • Other adverse effects include bleeding, tinnitus
Ticlopidine (Ticlid)	ADP-Induced Aggregation Inhibitor	• No significant effects	• Rarely used because of potential for life-threatening hematological adverse reactions, including neutropenia, agranulocytosis, thrombotic thrombocytopenic purpura (TTP) and aplastic anemia
Clopidigril (Plaxix)	ADP-Induced Aggregation Inhibitor	• No significant effects	• Gastrointestinal hemorrhage (2%, 2.7% with aspirin), ulcer, agranulocytosis (less than 1%), Thrombotic thrombocytopenic purpura (rare)
Dyrpidimole (Persantine)	Not fully elucidated, may involve its ability to increase endogenous concentrations of adenosine, which is a coronary vasodilator and a platelet aggregation inhibitor and of cyclic adenosine monophosphate (cAMP), which decreases platelet activation.	• No significant effects	• ECG abnormal (15.9%), abdominal discomfort, dizziness

Table 8.5 (continued)

Drug	Mechanism of Action	Dental/Oral Consideration	Non-Dental Issues
ACE Inhibitors			
Benazepril (Lotensin) Captopril (Capoten) Enalapril (Vasotec) Fosinopril (Monopril) Lisinopril (Prinivil, Zestril) Moexipril (Univasc) Perindopril (Aceon) Qunapril (Accupril) Ramipril (Altace) Trandolapril (Mavik)	Competitive inhibition of angiotensin I-converting enzyme (ACE) activity, resulting in a decreased rate of conversion of angiotensin I to angiotensin II, which is a potent vasoconstrictor.	• Head and neck angioedema has been reported in patients treated with angiotensin-converting enzyme inhibitors, and these effects may occur at any time during the course of therapy. • More frequent in Black patients • Oral ulceration • Burning pain of oral mucosa	• Hypotension, hyperkalemia, Nausea and vomiting, Dizziness, cough (typically dry, nonproductive, tickling and persistent, and worse at night), fatigue. • Reduced effectiveness in setting of chronic NSAID use.
ARBs			
Candesartan (Atacand) Eprosartan (Tevetan) Irbesartan (Avapro) Telmisartan (Mycardis) Valsartan (Diovan) Losartan (Cozaar)	Inhibition of angiotensin II AT1 receptors	• No significant effects	• Hypotension, in heart failure patients (common), dizziness, headache

Table 8.5 (continued)

Drug	Mechanism of Action	Dental/Oral Consideration	Non-Dental Issues
Beta Blockers			
Acebutolol (Sectral)	Competive inhibition of catecholamines for beta adrenergic receptors ($\beta 1$ and/or $\beta 2$). Some have alpha blocking properties and antioxidant mechanisms.	• No significant effects	• Asthma with status asthmaticus (rare), atrioventricular block, bradyarrhythmia, edema, hypotension, syncope, hyperglycemia, weight gain, dizziness, headache, insomnia, somnolence, and fatigue.
Atenolol (Tenormin)			
Betaxolol (Kerlone)			
Bisoprolol (Zebeta)			
Bucindolol*			
Carvedilol (Coreg)*			
Labetalol (Normodyne)			
Metoprolol (Toprol)*			
Nadolol (Corgard)			
Penbutolol (Levatol)			
Pindolol (Visken)			
Propranolol (Inderal)			
Timolol			

Table 8.5 (continued)

Drug	Mechanism of Action	Dental/Oral Consideration	Non-Dental Issues
Calcium Channel Blockers Amlodipine (Norvasc) Bepridil (Vascor) Diltiazem (Cardizem, Cartia, Tiazac) Felodipine (Plendil) Isradipine (Dynacirc) Nicardipine (Cardene) Nifedipine (Procardia) Nimodipine Verapamil	Decrease and/or block calcium entry either in heart muscle or vascular smooth muscle resulting in variable degrees of decreasing heart rate, decreased contractility and vasodilation depending on whether drug has predominately cardiac versus peripheral effects	• Gingival hyperplasia • Dry mouth	• Peripheral edema, hypotension, bradyarrhythmia, palpitations, dizziness, Headache, fatigue
Digoxin (Digoxin, Lanoxin)	Inhibits sodium-potassium ATPase and results in increase contractility and slow conduction through AV node.	• No significant effects	• Blurred or yellow vision, confusion (suspect toxicity; rare) • Dizziness, mental depression, feeling of not caring, headache, loss of appetite, seeing or hearing things that are not there, and/or weakness; irregular or slow heartbeat, palpitations

Table 8.5 (continued)

Drug	Mechanism of Action	Dental/Oral Consideration	Non-Dental Issues
Thiazide Diuretics HCTZ Chlorthalidone (Diuril) Metolazone (Zaroxalyn)	Diuresis by blocking the reabsorption of sodium and chloride in the distal tubule resulting in an altered sodium balance and a reduction in extracellular water and plasma volume.	• Dry mouth • Loss of appetite	• Hypotension, electrolytes abnormal, hyperglycemia, Hyperuricemia
Loop Diuretics Furosemide (Lasix) Bumetanide (Bumex) Torsemide (Demadex)	Reversibly bind to the sodium, potassium, chloride co-transport mechanism thereby inhibiting the to reabsorb salt resulting in a higher osmolality and also decreases the kidney's ability to reabsorb water.	• Dry mouth • Loss of appetite	• Photosensitivity, Pruritus, Rash, Urticaria, Metabolic: Electrolyte imbalance (14–60%), Hyperglycemia, hyperuricemia (40%), muscle cramp and hypotension.
Aldosterone Antagonists Spironolactone (Aldactone) Eplerenone (Inspira)	Competitive inhibition of aldosterone for intracellular mineralocorticoid receptors, which results in natriuresis and potassium retaining action.	• Dry mouth	• Gynecomastia (not for Eplerenone), hyperkalemia, diarrhea, nausea and vomiting.
Nitrates Isosorbide dinitrates (Isordil) Isosorbide mononitrate (Imdur)	Venous and arterial vasodilators with primary mechanism being reduction in preload.	• Dry mouth	• Orthostatic hypotension, dizziness, syncope and headadache

Table 8.5 (continued)

Drug	Mechanism of Action	Dental/Oral Consideration	Non-Dental Issues
Intravenous Inotropes/Vasodilators			
Dobutamine	Stimulation of beta adrenergic receptors (β1 and β2).	• No significant effects	• Hypotension, arrhythmias
Milrinone (Primacor)	Cyclic AMP specific phosphodiesterase (PDE) inhibitor.	• No significant effects	• Hypotension, arrhythmias, thrombocytopenia
Natrecor	Natrecor is a synthetic analogue of human BNP which results in vasodilatation.	• No significant effects	• Hypotension
Statins			
Atorvastatin (Lipitor)	Competitive inhibitor of the enzyme 3-hydroxy-3-methylglutaryl coenzyme A reductatase (HMG-CoA reductase)	• No significant effects	• Hepatotoxicity (not common) and drug-induced myopathy, Rhabdomyolysis (rare)
Fluvastatin (Lescol)			
Lovastatin (Mevacor)			
Pravastatin (Pravachol)			
Rosuvastatin (Crestor)			
Simvastatin (Zocor)			

* Approved for use in Heart Failure

(15% and 31%, respectively) in eight trials for patients with acute myocardial infarction (Antman et al., 2004), and thus should be prescribed to all patients with acute ischemic syndromes in a dental office, assuming no contraindications, while awaiting for more definitive evaluation.

The treatment for acute ischemic heart disease has become increasingly focused on invasive cardiovascular procedures both in the acute setting for immediate reperfusion in the setting of an ST segment elevation myocardial infarction, and in the chronic setting for treatment of chronic coronary artery stenosis. Coronary stents have had a significant impact on reducing rates of restenosis, which was the Achilles heel of percutaneous coronary angioplasty. After stent placement, with either bare metal or drug eluding stents, patients are maintained with combined antiplatelet regimens, typically including aspirin and Plavix (Berger et al., 1999). While the risk of in-stent thrombosis with bare metal stents was defined to be highest in the first few weeks after placement (Berger et al., 2002), which resulted in combined antiplatelet therapy for this period, the risk of thrombosis for drug eluding stents appear to remain elevated for months and potentially even years after placement (Berger, Bell, Grill, Melby, & Holmes, 1998; Roberts & Redding, 2000). While the exact mechanism is not known, it may be related to the use of polymers which are employed in the manufacturing of these stents to affix the active drug compound and may contribute to inflammation and thrombosis (Aggarwal et al., 1996; Colombo et al., 2003). Accordingly, the duration of antiplatlet recommended has been extended for at least 9 months and potentially longer for patients undergoing placement of a drug eluding stent (2006).

As a result of the wider use of more aggressive antiplatelet therapy and the wider application of anticoagulants (warfarin and low molecular weigh heparins), the issue of discontinuing these therapies prior to dental surgeries has become more common. In general, the scientific data does not support routine discontinuation of oral anticoagulation therapy for dental patients (Kamien, 2006). Rather it has been shown that when appropriate care is provided for potential excess bleeding, in the absence of an International Normalized Ratio (INR) > 4.0, routine discontinuation of these drugs before dental care can place these patients at unnecessary medical risk. However, the literature on the risk/benefit ratio of discontinuing antiplatetlet therapy in patients undergoing dental procedures with drug eluding stents is lacking. Given the increasing concerns about in-stent thrombosis in this population and the attending associated risks, discontinuation of antiplatelet therapy prior to the currently recommended period should be done in consultation with the cardiovascular consultant.

Heart Failure

Heart failure is a complex clinical syndrome that can result from any structural or functional cardiac disorder that impairs the ability of the heart to meet the demands of the body. The cardinal manifestations of heart failure (HF) are dyspnea and fatigue, which typically result in a reduced exercise tolerance and fluid retention.

This may lead to pulmonary congestion and peripheral edema. Since not all patients have volume overload at the time of evaluation, the term "heart failure" is preferred over the older term "congestive heart failure" and reminds practitioners to not ignore symptoms compatible with the diagnosis simply because of the absence of edema.

The New York Heart Association (NYHA) Function Class is the most commonly employed method to quantify the degree of functional limitation and has important prognostic implications. The NYHA system assigns patients to one of four functional classes, depending on the degree of effort needed to elicit symptoms: patients may have symptoms of HF at rest (class IV), on less-than-ordinary exertion (class III), on ordinary exertion (class II), or only at levels of exertion that would limit normal individuals (class I). Individuals with decompensated heart failure (e.g. class IV) should not undergo elective dental procedures. Patients with class III heart failure, undergoing dental procedures can usually receive office based dental treatment after consultation with the medical consultant with or without modifications including short, stress-free appointments with supplemental oxygen.

Therapy for heart failure has evolved over the past three decades and typically consists of diuretics for volume control, angiotensin converting enzyme inhibitors or angiotensin receptor antagonists as well as β-blockers which both have significant neurohormonal benefits (see Table 8.6). An increasing number of patients with heart failure are receiving biventricular pacemakers with an implantable cardiac defib-

Table 8.6 Cardiac Conditions Associated With Endocarditis

High-risk category	Moderate-risk category	Negligible-risk category (no greater risk than the general population)
Prosthetic cardiac valves, including bioprosthetic and homograft valves	Most other congenital cardiac malformations (other than above)	Isolated secundum atrial septal defect
Previous bacterial endocarditis	Acquired valvar dysfunction (e.g., rheumatic heart disease)	Surgical repair of atrial septal defect, ventricular septal defect, or patent ductus arteriosus (without residua beyond 6 mo)
Complex cyanotic congenital heart disease (e.g., single ventricle states, transposition of the great arteries, tetralogy of Fallot)	Hypertrophic cardiomyopathy	Previous coronary artery bypass graft surgery
Surgically constructed systemic pulmonary shunts or conduits	Mitral valve prolapse with valvar regurgitation and/or thickened leaflets	Mitral valve prolapse without valvar regurgitation
		Physiologic, functional, or innocent heart murmurs
		Previous rheumatic fever without valvar dysfunction
		Cardiac pacemakers (intravascular and epicardial) and implanted defibrillators

rillator (ICD) for management of life threatening arrhythmias. These devices are equipped with a left ventricular lead, which stimulates the left ventricle in case of delayed electrical conduction (e.g. a left bundle branch block). This so called cardiac resynchronization therapy decreases morbidity and mortality in selected patients (Bradley et al., 2003). While biventricular pacers and implantable cardiac defibrillators (BiV/ICDs) are safe in the dental office even in case of discharge, certain precautions should be noted. The modern dental office comprises a variety of electromagnetic devices that can interfere with pacemaker function. One study (Miller, Leonelli, & Latham, 1998) evaluated the effect of dental equipment on dual-chamber pacemaker function with bipolar leads programmed to DDD mode (pacing of both the atria and ventricles) and a single-chamber pacemaker with a unipolar lead programmed to VVI mode (set to pace the ventricle only), all set at maximum sensitivity. Pacemaker inhibition was noted while the pacemaker was near an electrosurgical unit, the ultrasonic bath cleaner, and the ultrasonic scaler (Trenter & Walmsley, 2003; Balfry, 2005). Electromagnetic interference (EMI) was absent with standard operation of the amalgamator, the electric pulp tester, a composite curing light, dental hand pieces and/or drills, the electric toothbrush, the dental chair and light, ultrasonic instruments, a radiography unit, and an ultrasonic scaler. Accordingly, dental providers should recognize the possibility for EMI in patients with pacemakers and defibrillators. For the nonpacemaker-dependent patient, dental procedures are safe, but for the pacemaker-dependent patient who cannot avoid interaction with interference-causing dental equipment, the patient's pacemaker should be programmed to asynchronous pacing mode before the dental procedure is initiated. Data on the patient with an ICD is lacking and dentists are encouraged to discuss the clinical strategy in such patients with the consulting cardiologist.

Atrial Fibrillation

Atrial Fibrillation is a common atrial tachycardia. It is characterized by an extremely rapid atrial rate without any discrete P waves on the electrocardiographic (EKG) tracing. It occurs when there are multiple small foci in the atria continuously discharging and contracting. It is commonly associated with patients who have hypertension, ischemic heart disease, thyrotoxicosis or rheumatic heart disease. The incidence of atrial fibrillation increases with age. The prevalence of atrial fibrillation has been shown to occur in more than 10% people over the age of 80 years. (Wolf, Abbott, & Kannel, 1987; Krahn, Manfreda, Tate, Mathewson, & Cuddy, 1995).

In controlling atrial fibrillation either rate or rhythm control is acceptable. Studies have not demonstrated that one method is more superior to the other with regard to decreasing incidence of embolic complication. This has been demonstrated by the AFFIRM and RACE trials (Van et al., 2002; Wyse et al., 2002). One must keep in mind that antiarrhythmic control may be associated with more adverse drug reactions and concomitant hospitalizations in older persons. If a patient cannot tolerate the side effects of the antiarrhythmics and is not very symptomatic with the atrial fibrillation, it is reasonable to just maintain rate control.

Rate control can be achieved with intravenous β-blockers and/or calcium channel blockers. These drugs both slow conduction in the AV node by prolonging the refractory period in the node. Digoxin is not as effective when used as monotherapy and is associated with more toxicity. However, digoxin when used in combination with either a β-blocker or calcium channel blocker may enhance the effect of both drugs. If atrial fibrillation is known to be occurring for less than 48 hours, conversion to sinus rhythm may be attempted without significant concern regarding thromboembolic risk. This is often difficult to predict since most patients are not sure of the exact timing of when their symptoms occurred. Often it is best to assume the arrhythmia has been present for longer then 48 hours. In this event it is important to ensure there is not a thrombus in the heart before attempting cardioversion. This may be done by a transesophageal echo (TEE) or by simply treating as if a thrombus is present by anticoagulating the patient for about 3 weeks and then attempting cardioversion. If a patient is seen not to have a thrombus by TEE, cardioversion may be attempted in a controlled manner immediately, however anticoagulation should be maintained for 4 weeks after the cardioversion, assuming the patient remains in normal sinus rhythm.

Antiarrhythmic medications may be used to restore sinus rhythm but they are modestly effective. These medications may have complications such as inducing arrhythmias such as torsades de pointes, and other toxicities in the liver and lung, neurologic abnormalities, thyroid disorders and gastrointestinal upset. The longer a patient has been in atrial fibrillation the more difficult it will be to try to convert her or him to a sinus rhythm. A patient may be considered for radioablation of the atrial fibrillation when the rhythm is not controllable with conventional methods and symptoms are persistent and severe. This is a newer form of therapy and may provide a "cure" for a patient in atrial fibrillation. One study demonstrated success rates of 88% in 6 months in patients with paroxysmal atrial fibrillation, however the follow-up was limited in this study and the patients were considerable younger than those in everyday practice (Oral et al., 2003).

Patients with atrial fibrillation are at increased risk of developing thrombi, possibly leading to thromboembolism. This puts patients at risk of developing an ischemic stroke by an embolic event. Stroke risk is increased 5-fold in the absence of rheumatic heart disease and 20-fold in the presence of rheumatic heart disease (Trumble & Taffet, 2007). Atrial fibrillation is accountable for one-sixth of all ischemic strokes in people over the age of 60 years (Wolf, Abbott, & Kannel, 1991). Patients with this dysrhythmia should be anticoagulated to prevent the event of an embolic stroke. Anticoagulation in older individuals carries greater risk because of potential to develop adverse drug effects, and hemorrhagic events especially in the event of falling.

Warfarin is the drug of choice for anticoagulation in patients with chronic atrial fibrillation. Numerous studies have shown that warfarin, when at a therapeutic range, will reduce the likelihood of developing a stroke. The requirement of consistently having to check coagulation levels to monitor warfarin therapy may make this a difficult drug for some patients to take. Aspirin can be used as an alternative though it is not as efficacious as warfarin therapy in reducing the incidence of strokes.

The laboratory test used to monitor the anticoagulant effect of warfarin is International Normalized Ratio or INR (Hirsh & Poller, 1994). The INR is the prothrombin time ratio obtained by testing a given sample using the World Health Organization reference thromboplastin. Prothrombin measures the activity of coagulation factors II, VII and X. A target INR of 2.5 with an acceptable range of 2.0–3.0 has been recommended by the American Geriatrics Association (American Geriatrics Society, 2007). There is an increase in complications with INR greater than 4.0 and the drug is not as efficacious when the INR is less than 2.0. In elderly patients it is especially important to monitor their INR levels due to concerns of polypharmacy. Many elderly patients are on a multitude of medications, which may have drug–drug interactions with warfarin. Some of the medications that affect cytochrome P-450 system in the liver that may interfere with warfarin metabolism are phenytoin, steroids, ranitidine and propylthioruracil (Dharmarajan, Varma, Akkaladevi, Lebelt, & Norkus, 2006). The goal for therapy is to reduce thromboembolic events with a safe blood level without jeopardizing the patient's health to bleeding complications.

Many older dental patients who present for a dental procedure will be on warfarin. It is important for a dentist to know how to be able to manage a patient on anticoagulation and to be able to safely proceed with a dental procedure. There is concern that warfarin may increase bleeding risks during a procedure. Overall outcomes for a patient will vary with age, other comorbidities, and the invasiveness of the procedure. Ultimately the risk of cessation or decreasing the dose of warfarin needs to be considered since this may increase the chances of a patient developing a thromboembolic event.

Literature has shown that if the INR is within therapeutic range (INR 2–3) that it is safe for a patient to undergo a dental procedure (McIntyre, 1966; Wahl, 1998; Cannon & Dharmar, 2003). Carter et al. described in their extensive review of studies concerning dental extraction of anticoagulated patients that the majority of the cases had PT values that were either on the low side of the therapeutic range or were virtually normal. Their concern was that larger patient groups should be studied before the technique of not stopping anticoagulation during a procedure can be fully advocated (Carter, Goss, Lloyd, & Tocchetti, 2003). Ultimately it was proposed in their study that most ambulatory patients could safely proceed for their dental procedure on anticoagulation.

Valvular Heart Disease

The prevalence of valvular heart disease increases with age. In the general population, moderate or severe valve disease was identified in 615 of 11,915 adults (5.1%). While there was no difference in the frequency of valve diseases between men and women, the prevalence increased with age, from 0.7% (95% CI 0.5–1.0) in 18–44 year olds to 13.3% (11.7–15.0) in the 75 years and older group ($p < 0.0001$). The national prevalence of valve disease, corrected for age and sex distribution from the U.S. 2000 population was estimated to be 2.5% (2.2–2.7) (Nkomo et al., 2006). Fibrocalcific changes of the heart, including mitral annular calcification (MAC), aortic annular calcification (AAC) and aortic valve sclerosis (AVS) among 3929 community dwelling elderly individuals 3929 participants in the Cardiovascular Health Study (CHS) with a mean age 76 ± 5 years of whom 60% were women was found in 1640 (42%) subjects, 1710 (44%), AVS in 2114 (54%) of subjects, respectively (Barasch et al., 2006). Thus, for dental care providers who encounter a growing population of older individuals, knowledge regarding the diagnosis, evaluation and management, particularly as it relates to anticoagulation and endocarditis prophylaxis is imperative.

For a complete review of major valve disorders in the geriatric population, the dental care provider is referred to several recent reviews (Segal, 2003a,b). Many therapies including administration of prophylactic antibiotics to a dental patient with a history of heart murmur, rheumatic fever or mitral valve prolapse rely on a reliable diagnosis of heart valve disease. However, reliance on historical information has been shown to be questionable in as many as 65% of patients who report a history of valvular heart disease actually had no evidence of a pathological heart murmur during previous physical examinations (Guggenheimer, Orchard, Moore, Myers, & Rossie, 1998). Another study indicated that only 14% of patients who had cardiac murmur and usually received antibiotic prophylaxis required prophylaxis (Ching, Straznicky, & Goss, 2005). Additionally, in older individuals, who have a high prevalence of cognitive impairment, historical information regarding valvular disease requiring prophylaxis may not be reliable (Randall et al., 2001). Accordingly, self-reported history of heart valve disease should not be the sole criterion for antibiotic pre-medication. Rather, clinical examination of the older individual, coupled with review of medical histories with medical providers and echocardiographic imaging is required for appropriate therapeutic interventions (Kilmartin, 1994). In general, any diastolic murmur or a systolic murmur that is associated with either symptoms or signs of cardiovascular disease (heart failure, syncope, angina) or a systolic murmur, which on exam is holosytolic, occurs in early or late systole regardless of intensity, or occurs in mid-systole and is louder than grade II out of VI, should be considered pathologic and evaluated with echocardiography (Bonow et al., 2006).

Endocarditis Prophylaxis

Established guidelines for the prevention of bacterial endocarditis have been published and are available through numerous internet sites (Dajani et al., 1997; Bonow et al., 2006). Notably, the frequency of bacteremia has been shown to be highest with dental and oral procedures in comparison with procedures that involve the genitourinary tract and the gastrointestinal tract, thereby emphasizing the importance of prophylactic measures for individuals at risk.

Recent guidelines recommend the following patients to receive antibiotic prophylaxis: patients with prosthetic cardiac valve, previous infective endocarditis, some forms of congenital heart disease (CHD), and cardiac transplant recipients who develop cardiac valvulopathy. The forms of congenital heart disease that are included are unrepaired cyanotic CHD (such as palliative shunts and conduits), completely repaired congenital heart defect with prosthetic material or device during the first 6 months after the procedure, and repaired CHD with residual defects at the site or adjacent to the site of a prosthetic patch or prosthetic device (which inhibit endothelialization). Antibiotic prophylaxis are no longer required for any other form of CHD except for the conditions mentioned above (Wilson et al., 2007). Among older adults, high-risk patients typically are those with prosthetic cardiac valves, including bioprosthetic and homograft valves, and those with previous bacterial endocarditis. The presence of a pacemaker or automatic implantable defibrillator (AICDs), previous coronary artery bypass surgery or the placement of a coronary stent, while very common in older individuals, are not indications for endocarditis prophylaxis. However, it should be noted that discussion as to the possible need for antibiotic prophylaxis of patients with pacemakers, AICDs and stents largely is missing from the literature and there is some evidence that if required, antibiotic prophylaxis may only be needed during the first few weeks after placement. For older individuals who may have concomitant cognitive difficulties and who require prophylaxis, the American Heart Association has developed a bacterial endocarditis wallet card that can be provided to patients to facilitate care (http://www.americanheart.org/ presenter. html?identifier=3003000).

Anticoagulation

Guidelines for anticoagulation of patients with prosthetic valves both in the presence of normal sinus rhythm and of atrial fibrillation have been established (Salem et al., 2004). Unfortunately, there is wide variation in the management of patients with mechanical prosthetic valves who are taking anticoagulants and who require noncardiac surgery including dental procedures. Practically, any approach to the adjustment or discontinuation of anticoagulation should take into account both the degree of surgical trauma during oral and maxillofacial surgery and the risk of thromboembolism associated with the prosthetic valve and the alteration in anticoagulation.

Temporary discontinuation of high-intensity oral anticoagulant treatment is not recommended in patients undergoing dental surgery. This policy is not based on solid data from randomized clinical trials but on expert consensus. One prospective cohort study that evaluated bleeding and thromboembolic complications in patients with prosthetic heart valves and INR values between 2.0 and 4.5, who underwent dental procedures after a 2-day suspension of warfarin treatment, found no major bleeding complications occurred in the week after the procedure; no thromboembolic events and no cases of bacterial endocarditis in the 3 months after the procedure but minor bleeding requiring local measures occurred in two patients. The INR during the 2-day period in which warfarin was held decreased by approximately 1.0 U (from 2.95 ± 0.59 to 1.87 ± 0.46). INR values returned to the therapeutic range in 90% of cases within 7 days of re-initiation of warfarin therapy with an average time spent at INR less than 2.0 being 28 hours (Bussey & Lyons, 1998; Russo, Corso, Biasiolo, Berengo, & Pengo, 2000; Kamien, 2006). Accordingly, 2 days of suspending warfarin prior to a dental procedure in subjects with a prosthetic valve appears to be a simple and safe policy.

In summary, for minor surgery, no adjustment of anticoagulation is needed if the International Normalized Ratio (INR) is less than 4.0, especially if local haemostatic methods and tranexamic acid mouthwashes are used (Bussey & Lyons, 1998; Johnson, Granberry, Thomas, & Smith, 2000; Russo, Corso, Biasiolo, Berengo, & Pengo, 2000; Webster & Wilde, 2000a ; Kamien, 2006). In fact, topical antifibrinolytic agents can negate the need to alter systemic anticoagulation during dental surgery (Bussey & Lyons, 1998). An alternative is to hold warfarin for 2 days prior to the procedure and reinstitute immediately after the procedure is completed. For major surgery, warfarin is usually discontinued in the perioperative period and depending on the risks of thrombosis, low-molecular-weight heparin can be utilized. For emergency surgery, partial reversal of anticoagulation with low-dose parenteral vitamin K is an additional option.

Stroke

Stroke is a generic term to describe a cerebrovascular accident (CVA). Stroke is defined as a sudden focal neurologic deficit caused by an interruption of oxygenated blood to the brain. This may be caused by ischemia (80%–85% of all strokes) or hemorrhage (15%–20% of all strokes). In ischemic strokes there is often a blood vessel occlusion leading to neuronal cell death or damage. Hemorrhagic strokes are caused by rupture of a blood vessel. This leads to hemorrhage, elevated intracranial pressure, and possible mass effect. In addition, patients may suffer stroke-like symptoms but without permanent neurologic deficits. This is called a transient ischemic attack (TIA) and the symptoms resolve within 24 hours. Patient with TIAs are at increased risk for developing strokes, with a risk of up to 5%–6% a year.

Five percent of the population over the age of 65 years has suffered from a CVA. It is the third leading cause of death in the United States (Hoyert, Kochanek, & Murphy, 1999). Stroke is a leading cause of disability for survivors, and these disabilities are common medical conditions a dentist will encounter in older adult patients. Stroke affects 700,000 Americans annually and costs $30 billion a year in medical costs and lost wages (Hall, 2007). Although the overall incidence of stroke has been decreasing nationally, the risk of stroke continues to increase with age, approximately doubling with each decade of life. The incidence of CVA for men is 2.1 per 1000 at ages 55–64 years, 4.5 per 1000 at ages 65–74 years, and 9.3 per 1000 at ages 75–84 years (Louis, 2007).

It is important to quickly assess a patient for a stroke so that immediate treatment can be started. Most patients present with sudden loss of focal brain function. A patient may present with symptoms of weakness, numbness, visual changes, dysarthria, aphasia, apraxia, slow response, cranial nerve palsies, nausea, vomiting, severe hypertension, and decreased level of consciousness. It is important to immediately call emergency services and have the patient transported to the nearest emergency department if a patient presents with such symptoms.

In the dental office one can place the patient flat, give oxygen if the patient is hypoxic, and try to ascertain how long the symptoms have been present. The exact timing of when the stroke-like symptoms started will be helpful in determining whether the patient is a candidate for thrombolytic therapy if they have had an ischemic event. Studies have demonstrated that laying a patient flat may help flow through stenosed blood vessels (Toole, 1968; Caplan & Sergay, 1976; Adams et al., 2003).

There are a number of therapies that can be initiated post stroke to help decrease the chances of a repeat CVA. A patient can benefit from lipid lowering agents, cessation of smoking, blood pressure reduction, and management of diabetes, obesity and the metabolic syndrome. Studies have shown that hypertension is the most common and important stroke risk factor (Collins et al., 1990; MacMahon et al., 1990). An increase of blood pressure over 110/75 mmHg will increase the incidence of both coronary disease and CVA (MacMahon et al., 1990; Lewington, Clarke, Qizilbash, Peto, & Collins, 2002). Lowering diastolic blood pressure by just 5–6 mmHg has been shown to decrease strokes by 35%–40% over the course of 5 years of therapy (Collins et al., 1990). Smoking has been shown to double the risk of strokes (Kawachi et al., 1993).

Antiplatelet therapy is used for both primary and secondary prevention of stroke and during the initial management of acute ischemic stroke. There are several agents on the market that have been shown to lower the risk of stroke such as aspirin, dipyridamole and clopidogrel. Aspirin is the most commonly used medication for the treatment and prevention of stroke. Aspirin is a cyclooxygenase enzyme inhibitor that reduces the production of thromboxane A2. Thromboxane A2 stimulates platelet aggregation which helps in the formation of thrombus and contributes to the increase of atherosclerotic disease. Aspirin has been shown to be effective in the prevention of ischemic stroke in numerous trials, up to a 25% reduction, in comparison to placebo (Antithrombotic Trialists' Collaboration, 2002). Some patients may be at an increased risk of stroke by simply stopping aspirin therapy for a few days. One study showed that 13 of 289 patients hospitalized for ischemic CVA had recently (within 6–10 days) stopped their antiplatelet therapy; most were on aspirin (Hirsh et al., 1995).

The ideal dose of aspirin that should be prescribed is controversial. Low dose aspirin has been shown to be as effective as higher doses. Many studies recommend a dose between 50 and 325 mg/day for most patients to maximize the benefit of treatment with little bleeding risk. A meta-analysis of 195 trials demonstrated that doses of aspirin between 75 and 150 mg/day were as effective in risk reduction for stroke as daily doses of 150–325 mg/day (Antithrombotic Trialists' Collaboration, 2002).

There are other antiplatelet agents that can be used in addition to aspirin to prevent future strokes. However, these agents are more expensive and have their own side effects. Clopidogrel is a drug that inhibits platelet aggregation, which is ADP-dependent. Clopidogrel has been shown to decrease risk of stroke, MI, or vascular disease by 5.3% annually in the CAPRIE trial (1996). The results were similar to what was found in aspirin therapy. The side effects of clopidogrel are similar to that of aspirin as well. Clopidogrel was shown to have a lower frequency of gastric upset or bleeding in comparison to aspirin, but a higher percentage of rash and diarrhea (McQuaid & Laine, 2006). Aspirin and clopidogrel taken together for patients with a TIA or stroke did not offer any benefits in comparison to taking clopidogrel alone. However it was shown that combination therapy increased bleeding complications with a three-fold increase in life-threatening hemorrhaging and two-fold increase in other major hemorrhages (Diener et al., 2004).

Dipyridamole impairs platelet function by inhibiting platelet phophodiesterase activity and increases the availability of adenosine. The second European Stroke Prevention Study (ESPS-2) showed that Dipyridamole in combination with aspirin is more effective than aspirin alone in the prevention of stroke. There was a relative risk reduction of 23%, 95% CI 9.2–37 with the combination therapy (Diener et al., 1996). There was no difference in risk of death or bleeding complications with the combination group in comparison to the aspirin monotherapy group. The major side effect of dipyridamole is headache.

In general younger patients have a better prognosis and recovery than older patients following a stroke. Recovery of function is greatest within the first 3 months post stroke. A concern many dentists may have with an elderly patient who has had a stroke is the timing of proceeding with an elective procedure. Some sources recommend at least 2 weeks should elapse before an elective procedure is done (Sundt, Sandok, & Whisnant , 1975). It has been recommended to wait up to 6 months post stroke before considering a dental procedure since the risk of recurrent stroke is high during this period (Little, Falace, Miller, & Rhodus, 2007). If a dentist is in doubt with what to do for their patient and whether it is safe to proceed with a procedure, a medical consultation is advised.

Post-stroke patients should have their blood pressure monitored along with their oxygenation during a procedure and having pain control maintained (Little et al., 2007). Post-stroke patients may suffer from continued neurologic deficits. Some oral manifestations include aphasia, weak palate, difficulty swallowing, and orofacial musculature paralysis. Patients may have difficulty maintaining good oral hygiene if they have suffered damage in their coordination or in the strength in their upper extremities.

Summary

As the population of the U.S. ages, dentists will provide care to an increasing number of older adults with diabetes, cardiovascular and cerebrovascular diseases. All of these conditions have implications for oral health care. Dentists must be aware of the diagnosis and management, both of the acute and chronic manifestations of these diseases. Each time an older adult presents for dental care, dentists must ascertain a history and review of appropriate systems and insure that blood pressure, coagulation status and blood glucose levels are at acceptable levels. Co-management of these older adults with a medical provider will assist the dentist and help assure that optimal dental care of older adults is provided.

References

Adams, H. P., Jr., Adams, R. J., Brott, T., del Zoppo, G. J., Furlan, A., Goldstein, L. B., et al. (2003). Guidelines for the early management of patients with ischemic stroke: A scientific statement from the Stroke Council of the American Stroke Association. *Stroke, 34*, 1056–1083.

Aggarwal, R. K., Ireland, D. C., Azrin, M. A., Ezekowitz, M. D., de Bono, D. P., & Gershlick, A. H. (1996). Antithrombotic potential of polymer-coated stents eluting platelet glycoprotein IIb/IIIa receptor antibody. *Circulation, 94*, 3311–3317.

Ahto, M., Isoaho, R., Puolijoki, H., Laippala, P., Romo, M., & Kivela, S. L. (1998). Prevalence of coronary heart disease, associated manifestations and electrocardiographic findings in elderly Finns. *Age Ageing, 27*, 729–737.

American Diabetes Association, (2004) Diagnosis and classification of diabetes mellitus. *Diabetes Care, 27 Suppl 1*, S5-S10.

American Geriatrics Society. (2007). Clinical practice guidelines. The use of oral anticoagulants (warfarin) in older people. *J. Am. Geriatr. Soc., 50*, 1439–1445.

Antman, E. M., Anbe, D. T., Armstrong, P. W., Bates, E. R., Green, L. A., Hand, M., et al. (2004). ACC/AHA guidelines for the management of patients with ST-elevation myocardial infarction–executive summary: A report of the American College of Cardiology/American Heart Association Task Force on Practice Guidelines (Writing Committee to Revise the 1999 Guidelines for the Management of Patients with Acute Myocardial Infarction). *Circulation, 110*, 588–636.

Aubertin, M.A. (2004). The hypertensive patient in dental practice: Updated recommendations for classification, prevention, mornitoring, and dental mangement. Gen. Dent. [November–December], 544–552.

Bader, J. D., Bonito, A. J., & Shugars, D. A. (2002). A systematic rview of cardiovascular efects of epinephrine on hypertensive dental patients. *Oral Surg. Oral Med. Oral Pathol. Oral Radiol. Endod., 93*, 647–653.

Balfry, G. (2005). Pacemakers and ultrasonic scalers. *Br. Dent. J., 199*, 625.

Barasch, E., Gottdiener, J. S., Larsen, E. K., Chaves, P. H., Newman, A. B., & Manolio, T. A. (2006). Clinical significance of calcification of the fibrous skeleton of the heart and aortosclerosis in community dwelling elderly. The Cardiovascular Health Study (CHS). *Am. Heart J., 151*, 39–47.

Berger, P. B., Bell, M. R., Grill, D. E., Melby, S., & Holmes, D. R., Jr. (1998). Frequency of adverse clinical events in the 12 months following successful intracoronary stent placement in patients treated with aspirin and ticlopidine (without warfarin). *Am. J. Cardiol., 81*, 713–718.

Berger, P. B., Bell, M. R., Rihal, C. S., Ting, H., Barsness, G., Garratt, K., et al. (1999). Clopidogrel versus ticlopidine after intracoronary stent placement. *J. Am. Coll. Cardiol., 34*, 1891–1894.

Berger, P. B., Mahaffey, K. W., Meier, S. J., Buller, C. E., Batchelor, W., Fry, E. T., et al. (2002). Safety and efficacy of only 2 weeks of ticlopidine therapy in patients at increased risk of coronary stent thrombosis: Results from the Antiplatelet Therapy alone versus Lovenox plus Antiplatelet therapy in patients at increased risk of Stent Thrombosis (ATLAST) trial. *Am. Heart. J., 143*, 841–846.

Blood clots a late hazard for drug-coated stents. The benefits of drug-coated stents come with a price–long term use of clot-preventing drugs (2006). *Harv. Heart Lett., 16*, 1–3.

Bolli, P. (2005). Applying the 2005 Canadian Hypertension Education Program recommendations: 1. Diagnosis of hypertension. Martin Myers and Donals McKay for the Canadian Hypertension Education Program. *CMAJ, 173(5)*, 480–482.

Bonow, R. O., Carabello, B. A., Kanu, C., de, L. A., Jr., Faxon, D. P., Freed, M. D., et al. (2006). ACC/AHA 2006 guidelines for the management of patients with valvular heart disease: A report of the American College of Cardiology/American Heart Association Task Force on Practice Guidelines (writing committee to revise the 1998 guidelines for the management of patients with valvular heart disease): developed in collaboration with the Society Of Cardiovascular Anesthesiologists: Endorsed by the Society for Cardiovascular Angiography and Interventions and the Society of Thoracic Surgeons. *Circulation, 114*, e84–e231.

Bradley, D. J., Bradley, E. A., Baughman, K. L., Berger, R. D., Calkins, H., Goodman, S. N., et al. (2003). Cardiac resynchronization and death from progressive heart failure: A meta-analysis of randomized controlled trials. *JAMA, 289*, 730–740.

Brand, H. S. (1999). Cardiovascular responses in patients and dentists during dental treatment. Int. Dent. J, 49, 60–66.

Brown, R. S. (2002). Epinephrine and local anesthesia revisited. *Oral Surg Oral Med Oral Pathol Oral Radiol Endod, 100(4)*, 401–408.

Burris, J. F. (1991). Caring for older patients with high blood pressure. *Am. Fam. Physian., 44(1)*, 137–144.

Bussey, H. I., & Lyons, R. M. (1998). Controversies in antithrombotic therapy for patients with mechanical heart valves. *Pharmacotherapy, 18*, 451–455.

Cannon, P. D., & Dharmar, V. T. (2003). Minor oral surgical procedures in patients on oral anticoagulants–a controlled study. *Aust. Dent. J., 48*, 115–118.

Caplan, L. R., & Sergay, S. (1976). Positional cerebral ischaemia. *J. Neurol. Neurosurg. Psychiatry., 39*, 385–391.

CAPRIE Steering Committee, (1996) A randomised, blinded, trial of clopidogrel versus aspirin in patients at risk of ischaemic events (CAPRIE).*Lancet, 348*, 1329–1339.

Carter, G., Goss, A. N., Lloyd, J., & Tocchetti, R. (2003). Current concepts of the management of dental extractions for patients taking warfarin. *Aust. Dent. J., 48*, 89–96.

Ching, M., Straznicky, I., & Goss, A. N. (2005). Cardiac murmurs: Echocardiography in the assessment of patients requiring antibiotic prophylaxis for dental treatment. *Aust. Dent. J., 50*, S69–S73.

Chobanian, A. V., Bakris, G. L., Black, H. R., Cushman, W. C., Green, L. A., & Izzo, J. L., Jr. (2003). The seventh report of the Joint National Committee on Prevention, Detection, Evaluation, and Treatment of high blood pressure. *JAMA, 289*, 2560–2572.

Collaborative meta-analysis of randomised trials of antiplatelet therapy for prevention of death, myocardial infarction, and stroke in high risk patients (2002). *BMJ, 324*, 71–86.

Collins, R., Peto, R., MacMahon, S., Hebert, P., Fiebach, N. H., Eberlein, K. A., et al. (1990). Blood pressure, stroke, and coronary heart disease. Part 2, short-term reductions in blood pressure: Overview of randomised drug trials in their epidemiological context. *Lancet, 335*, 827–838.

Colombo, A., Drzewiecki, J., Banning, A., Grube, E., Hauptmann, K., Silber, S., et al. (2003). Randomized study to assess the effectiveness of slow- and moderate-release polymer-based paclitaxel-eluting stents for coronary artery lesions. *Circulation, 108*, 788–794.

Dajani, A. S., Taubert, K. A., Wilson, W., Bolger, A. F., Bayer, A., Ferrieri, P., et al. (1997). Prevention of bacterial endocarditis: Recommendations by the American Heart Association. *J. Am. Dent. Assoc., 128*, 1142–1151.

Dharmarajan, T. S., Varma, S., Akkaladevi, S., Lebelt, A. S., & Norkus, E. P. (2006). To anti-coagulate or not to anticoagulate? A common dilemma for the provider: Physicians' opinion poll based on a case study of an older long-term care facility resident with dementia and atrial fibrillation. *J. Am. Med. Dir. Assoc., 7*, 23–28.

Diener, H. C., Bogousslavsky, J., Brass, L. M., Cimminiello, C., Csiba, L., Kaste, M., et al. (2004). Aspirin and clopidogrel compared with clopidogrel alone after recent ischaemic stroke or transient ischaemic attack in high-risk patients (MATCH): Randomised, double-blind, placebo-controlled trial. *Lancet, 364*, 331–337.

Diener, H. C., Cunha, L., Forbes, C., Sivenius, J., Smets, P., & Lowenthal, A. (1996). European Stroke Prevention Study. 2. Dipyridamole and acetylsalicylic acid in the secondary prevention of stroke. *J. Neurol. Sci., 143*, 1–13.

Durso, S. C. (2006). Using clinical guidelines designed for older adults with diabetes mellitus and complex health status. *JAMA, 295*, 1935–1940.

Eagle, K. A., Berger, P. B., Calkins, H., Chaitman, B. R., Ewy, G. A., Fleischmann, K. E., et al. (2002). ACC/AHA Guideline Update for Perioperative Cardiovascular Evaluation for Noncardiac Surgery–Executive Summary. A report of the American College of Cardiology/American Heart Association Task Force on Practice Guidelines (Committee to Update the 1996 Guidelines on Perioperative Cardiovascular Evaluation for Noncardiac Surgery). *Anesth. Analg., 94*, 1052–1064.

Fagard, R. H. (2002) Epidemiology of hypertension in the elderly. *Am J Geriatr Cardiol, 11*, 23–28.

Flanigan, J. S., & Vitberg. D. (2006). Hypertensive emargency and severe hypertension: What to treat, who to treat, and how to treat. *Med. Clin. North Am., 90*, 439–451.

Fontana, G., Lapolla, A., Sanzari, M., Piva, E., Mussap, M., De, T. S., et al. (1999). An immunological evaluation of type II diabetic patients with periodontal disease. *J. Diabetes Complicat., 13*, 23–30.

Forman, D. E., & Rich, M. W. (2003). Heart failure in the elderly. *Congest. Heart Fail., 9*, 311–321.

Genco, R. J. (1996). Current view of risk factors for periodontal diseases. *J. Periodontol., 67*, 1041–1049.

Glick, M. (1998). New guidelines for prevention, detection, evalustion and treatment of high blood pressure. *J. Am. Dent. Assoc., 129(November)*, 1588–1594.

Guggenheimer, J., Orchard, T. J., Moore, P. A., Myers, D. E., & Rossie, K. M. (1998). Reliability of self-reported heart murmur history: Possible impact on antibiotic use in dentistry. *J. Am. Dent. Assoc., 129*, 861–866.

Hajjar, I., & Kotchen, T. A. (2003). Trends in prevalence, awareness, treatment, and control of hypertension in the United states, 1988–2000. *JAMA, 290(2)*, 199–206.

Hall, K. N. (2007). Stroke syndromes. In D. Cline, O. J. Ma, J. E. Tintinalli, G. D. Kelen, & J. S. Stapczynski (Eds.), *Emergency medicine: A comprehensive study guide, companion handbook* (5th ed., pp. 718–724). New York: McGraw-Hill.

Herman, W. W., Konzelman, J. L., Jr., & Prisant, L. M. (2004). New national guidelines on hypertension. A summary for dentistry. *J. Am. Dent. Assoc., 135(May)*, 576–584.

Hirsh, J., & Poller, L. (1994). The international normalized ratio. A guide to understanding and correcting its problems. *Arch. Intern. Med., 154*, 282–288.

Hirsh, J., Dalen, J. E., Fuster, V., Harker, L. B., Patrono, C., & Roth, G. (1995). Aspirin and other platelet-active drugs. The relationship among dose, effectiveness, and side effects. *Chest, 108*, 247S–257S.

Hoyert, D. L., Kochanek, K. D., & Murphy, S. L. (1999). Deaths: Final data for 1997. *Natl. Vital Stat. Rep., 47*, 1–104.

Jainkittivong, A., Yeh, C.-K., Guest, G. F., & Cottone, J. A. (1995). Evaluation of medical consultation in a predoctoral dental clinic. *Oral Surg. Oral Med. Oral Pathol. Oral Radiol. Endod 80(4)*, 409–413.

Johnson, J. T., Granberry, M. C., Thomas, A. R., & Smith, E. S. (2000). Anticoagulation management in mechanical heart valve patients who undergo dental procedures. *J. Ark. Med. Soc., 97*, 128–131.

Kamien, M. (2006). Remove the tooth, but don't stop the warfarin. *Aust. Fam. Physician, 35*, 233–235.

Kawachi, I., Colditz, G. A., Stampfer, M. J., Willett, W. C., Manson, J. E., Rosner, B., et al. (1993). Smoking cessation and decreased risk of stroke in women. *JAMA, 269*, 232–236.

Kilmartin, C. M. (1994). Managing the medically compromised geriatric patient. *J. Prosthet. Dent., 72*, 492–499.

Krahn, A. D., Manfreda, J., Tate, R. B., Mathewson, F. A., & Cuddy, T. E. (1995). The natural history of atrial fibrillation: Incidence, risk factors, and prognosis in the Manitoba Follow-Up Study. *Am. J. Med., 98*, 476–484.

Leonetti, G., & Zanchetti, A. (2002). Results of antihypertensive treatment trials in the elderly. *Am. J. Geriatr. Cardiol., 11(57)*, 41–47.

Leviner, E., Tzukert, A. A., Mosseri, M., Fisher, D., Yossipovitch, O., Pisanty, S., et al. (1992). Perioperative hemodynamic changes in ischemic heart disease patients undergoing dental treatment. *Spec. Care Dentist., 12*, 84–88.

Lewington, S., Clarke, R., Qizilbash, N., Peto, R., & Collins, R. (2002). Age-specific relevance of usual blood pressure to vascular mortality: A meta-analysis of individual data for one million adults in 61 prospective studies. *Lancet, 360*, 1903–1913.

Little, J., Falace, D. A., Miller, C. S., & Rhodus, N. L. (2007). Neurological diseases. In *Dental management of the medically compromised patient* (6th ed., pp. 417–438). St. Louis, Missouri: Mosby.

Louis, E. (2007). Neurological diseases and disorders. In *Geriatric review syllabus* (5th ed., pp. 294–305). New York: American Geriatrics Society.

Lusiani, L., Perrone, A., Pesavento, R., & Conte, G. (1994). Prevalence, clinical features, and acute course of atypical myocardial infarction. *Angiology, 45*, 49–55.

MacMahon, S., Peto, R., Cutler, J., Collins, R., Sorlie, P., Neaton, J., et al. (1990). Blood pressure, stroke, and coronary heart disease. Part 1, Prolonged differences in blood pressure: Prospective observational studies corrected for the regression dilution bias. *Lancet, 335*, 765–774.

McIntyre, H. (1966). Management, during dental surgery, of patients on anticoagulants. *Lancet, 2*, 99–100.

McQuaid, K. R., & Laine, L. (2006). Systematic review and meta-analysis of adverse events of low-dose aspirin and clopidogrel in randomized controlled trials. *Am. J. Med., 119*, 624–638.

Mask, A. G., Jr. (2000). Medical management of the patient with cardiovascular disease. *Periodontology 2000, 23*, 136–141.

Metcalf, P. A., & Scragg, R. K. (2000). Comparison of WHO and ADA criteria for diagnosis of glucose status in adults. *Diabetes Res. Clin. Pract., 49*, 169–180.

Miller, C. S., Leonelli, F. M., & Latham, E. (1998). Selective interference with pacemaker activity by electrical dental devices. *Oral Surg. Oral Med. Oral Pathol. Oral Radiol. Endod., 85*, 33–36.

Muzyka, B. C., & Glick, M. (1997). The hypertensive dental patient. *J. Am. Dent. Assoc., 128(August)*, 1109–1120.

National Center for Health Statistics (12-18-2006a). US Health 2005. CDC. 12-18-2006.

Nkomo, V. T., Gardin, J. M., Skelton, T. N., Gottdiener, J. S., Scott, C. G., & Enriquez-Sarano, M. (2006). Burden of valvular heart diseases: A population-based study. *Lancet, 368*, 1005–1011.

Nowak, K. A. (1997). Atypical chest pain in the elderly. *Nurse Pract., 22*, 11, 14.

Oral, H., Scharf, C., Chugh, A., Hall, B., Cheung, P., Good, E., et al. (2003). Catheter ablation for paroxysmal atrial fibrillation: Segmental pulmonary vein ostial ablation versus left atrial ablation. *Circulation, 108*, 2355–2360.

Perusse, R., Goulet, J. P., & Turcotte, J. Y. (1992). Contraindications to vasoconstrictors in dentistry: Part I. Cardiovascular diseases. *Oral Surg. Oral Med. Oral Pathol., 74*, 679–686.

Randall, C. W., Kressin, N. R., Garcia, R. I., Sims, H., Kazis, L., & Jones, J. A. (2001). Heart murmurs: Are older male dental patients aware of their existence? *J. Am. Dent. Assoc., 132*, 171–176.

Roberts, H. W., & Redding, S. W. (2000). Coronary artery stents: Review and patient-management recommendations. *J. Am. Dent. Assoc., 131*, 797–801.

Russo, G., Corso, L. D., Biasiolo, A., Berengo, M., & Pengo, V. (2000). Simple and safe method to prepare patients with prosthetic heart valves for surgical dental procedures. *Clin. Appl. Thromb. Hemost., 6*, 90–93.

Salem, D. N., Stein, P. D., Al-Ahmad, A., Bussey, H. I., Horstkotte, D., Miller, N., et al. (2004). Antithrombotic therapy in valvular heart disease–native and prosthetic: The Seventh ACCP Conference on Antithrombotic and Thrombolytic Therapy. *Chest, 126*, 457S–482S.

Segal, B. L. (2003a). Valvular heart disease, part 1. Diagnosis and surgical management of aortic valve disease in older adults. *Geriatrics, 58*, 31–35.

Segal, B. L. (2003b). Valvular heart disease, part 2. Mitral valve disease in older adults. *Geriatrics, 58*, 26–31.

Senni, M., Tribouilloy, C. M., Rodeheffer, R. J., Jacobsen, S. J., Evans, J. M., Bailey, K. R., et al. (1998). Congestive heart failure in the community: A study of all incident cases in Olmsted County, Minnesota, in 1991. *Circulation, 98*, 2282–2289.

Sundt, T. M., Sandok, B. A., & Whisnant, J. P. (1975). Carotid endarterectomy. Complications and preoperative assessment of risk. *Mayo Clin. Proc., 50*, 301–306.

Toole, J. F. (1968). Effects of change of head, limb and body position on cephalic circulation. *N. Engl. J. Med., 279*, 307–311.

Trenter, S. C., & Walmsley, A. D. (2003). Ultrasonic dental scaler: Associated hazards. *J. Clin. Periodontol., 30*, 95–101.

Trumble, T., & Taffet, G. (2007). Cardiac problems. In T. Yoshikawa, E. Cobbs, & K. Brumel-Smith (Eds.) *Practical ambulatory geriatrics* (St. Louis: Mosby).

Van Gelder, I., Hagens, V. E., Bosker, H. A., Kingma, J. H., Kamp, O., Kingma, T., et al. (2002). A comparison of rate control and rhythm control in patients with recurrent persistent atrial fibrillation. *N. Engl. J. Med., 347*, 1834–1840.

Varon, J., & Marik. P. E. (2003). Clinical review: The management of hypertensive crises. *Crit. Care, 7(5)*, 374–384.

Wahl, M. J. (1998). Dental surgery in anticoagulated patients. *Arch. Intern. Med., 158*, 1610–1616.

Webster, K., & Wilde, J. (2000). Management of anticoagulation in patients with prosthetic heart valves undergoing oral and maxillofacial operations. *Br. J. Oral Maxillofac. Surg., 38*, 124–126.

Williams, B., Poulter, N. R., Brown, M. J., Davis, M., Potter, J. F., Sever, P. S., et al. (2004). British Hypertension Society guielines-guidelinee for management of hypertension: Report of the fourth working party of the British Hypertension Society, 2004-BHS-IV.. *J. Human. Hyperten., 18*, 139–185.

Wilson, W., Taubert, K. A., Gewitz, M., Lockhart, P. B., Baddour, L. M., Levison, M., et al. (2007). Prevention of infective endocarditis: Guidelines from the American Heart Association: A guideline from the American Heart Association Rheumatic Fever, Endocarditis and Kawasaki Disease Committee, Council on Cardiovascular Disease in the Young, and the Council on Clinical Cardiology, Council on Cardiovascular Surgery and Anesthesia, and the Quality of Care and Outcomes Research Interdisciplinary Working Group. *J. Am. Dent. Assoc., 138*, 739–760.

Wolf, P. A., Abbott, R. D., & Kannel, W. B. (1987). Atrial fibrillation: A major contributor to stroke in the elderly. The Framingham Study. *Arch. Intern. Med., 147*, 1561–1564.

Wolf, P. A., Abbott, R. D., & Kannel, W. B. (1991). Atrial fibrillation as an independent risk factor for stroke: The Framingham Study. *Stroke, 22*, 983–988.

World Hypertension League. (2007). Measuring your blood pressure.

Wyse, D. G., Waldo, A. L., DiMarco, J. P., Domanski, M. J., Rosenberg, Y., Schron, E. B., et al. (2002). A comparison of rate control and rhythm control in patients with atrial fibrillation. *N. Engl. J. Med., 347*, 1825–1833.

Yoshino, H., Matsuoka, K., Nishimura, F., Kimura, M., Okada, M., Ogino, T., et al. (1983). Painless myocardial infarction in diabetics. *Tohoku J. Exp. Med., 141 Suppl*, 547–554.

Chapter 9
Geriatric Pharmacology: Principles and Implications for Oral Health

Brian C. Scanlan

Development of more effective pharmacologic therapies and preventive measures has played a substantial role in the observed increased longevity of the U.S. population. Advances in the medical treatment of cardiovascular disease are major contributors to the current trend. The signs of adverse effects of an array of agents useful in preventing life-altering conditions present first in the dental office. Xerostomia, dysguesia, periodontitis and root caries are unintended consequence of established therapy for cardiovascular disease, cancer, infection and behavior illness. Judicious application of drug therapies by medical and dental providers as well as heightened awareness of potential adverse oral effects is necessary to providing quality care to elderly patients.

Demographics of Aging

In 2006, the U.S. population exceeded 300 million. For the previous half century, the annual growth rate averaged 1.2%. The number of persons 65 years of age and older increased at nearly twice that rate, and the cohort of those aged 75 and older grew the fastest, increasing by an average of 2.8% annually (National Center for Health Statistics, 2006). Current projections are that in the first third of this century, the aging of the baby boomers will swell the ranks of those 65–74 to 10% of the total population. By mid-century, the U.S. population over the age of 75 is expected to reach 12% and will exceed the number of those aged 65–74. As they reach 65, men and women can expect to live up to an additional of 17–20 years, respectively.

While accounting for less than 20% of the total population, the elderly received one-third of all prescriptions, and their treatment consumed over 40% of the annual national prescription drug expenditure in the late 1990s (Stagnitti et al., 2003).

B.C. Scanlan
Associate Professor of Clinical Medicine New York Medical College St. Vincent's Hospital Manhattan 153 West 11th Street, NR1218 New York, NY 10011
Tel: 212-604-7147, Fax: 212-604-2128
e-mail: bscanlan@svcmcny.org

I.B. Lamster, M.E. Northridge (eds.), *Improving Oral Health for the Elderly*,
© Springer Science+Business Media, LLC 2008

Ninety percent of all persons aged 65 or more use at least one prescription drug and the average older patient uses four pharmaceutical agents.

With a rise in life expectancy, the elderly can expect to contend with multiple chronic conditions. Large-scale studies designed to define the parameters of successful aging have demonstrated that chronic disease and the coexistence of multiple chronic conditions, or comorbidity, is the rule beyond the seventh decade of life. The MacArthur Successful Aging Study found comorbidity in over 60% of women and nearly 50% of men studied (Berkman et al., 1993). The interaction of chronic disease, pharmacologic therapy and aging makes it difficult for the clinician to determine the source of many common clinical problems.

Chronic illness and comorbidity come with advanced age. Almost all of the over 500 elderly (age 70–100) subjects of a cross-sectional study in Berlin suffered from at least one chronic illness (Baltes & Mayer, 1999). Half of the study population suffered from painful arthritis, highlighting the chronic need for analgesic agents in this population. Both the Berlin Aging Study and the MacArthur Study of Successful Aging document the persistence of self-perceived health in a majority of elderly persons despite having to contend with inevitable challenges to their health. Therapeutic decisions, those of either commission or of omission, all too often add to the care burden of the elderly patients.

Adverse Drug Events and Polypharmacy

The combined influence of comorbidity and simultaneous chronic use of multiple agents increases the likelihood of clinically significant adverse drug events (ADEs), drug–drug and drug-disease interaction. A crucial component of geriatric assessment is a careful review of all pharmacologic agents the patient may be using, including over-the-counter preparations, supplements, herbal and homeopathic agents. Patients are much less likely to consider nonprescription agents "medications" and report their use. Nonetheless, these agents can have significant clinical adverse effects, such as unanticipated normalization of the coagulation profile (INR) in a patient with atrial fibrillation and using St. John's wort for depression along with warfarin. The opposite effect on the action of warfarin may result from simultaneous use of an OTC form of ranitidine for gastroesophageal reflux symptoms.

The elderly are at four times greater risk of ADEs than the general population, and nearly 90% of their ADEs leading to hospitalization are preventable (Beijer & de Blaey, 2002). In one review, an estimate of nearly 20% of medications prescribed before admission and implicated in hospitalization for ADEs lacked clear indication (Dormann et al., 2003). Age, female gender, low body weight, polypharmacy, liver and kidney dysfunction are all risk factors for ADEs. Surveillance of nationwide emergency department visits precipitated by outpatient ADEs revealed a rate of 2.4 ADEs per 1000 population (Budnitz et al., 2006). Patients aged 65 and older were more than twice as likely to present with adverse drug events (4.9/1000) and nearly seven times more likely to require hospitalization for the event. Over half of the events requiring hospitalization of the elderly patients resulted from toxicity to drugs normally monitored regularly in the outpatient setting, chiefly warfarin, insulin and digoxin. Other commonly prescribed "older drugs, used poorly" included nonsteroidal antiinflammatory agents, aspirin, clopidogrel, several antibiotics, narcotic analgesics and acetaminophen.

Times of transition in care, such as hospital discharge or transfer, are associated with heightened risk for various adverse events, two-thirds those involving prescribed drugs (Forster et al., 2003). In their study of 400 consecutive discharges to home from a general medical service, Forster and colleagues identified discrete system deficiencies associated with significant, preventable ADEs (Forster et al., 2003). The majority of the events documented were preventable or remediable; however, 3% of post-discharge events resulted in permanent disability. Reviewers identified poor communication between patient and physician, between the hospital and community providers and several other errors of monitoring and implementation dependent on the providers' communication skills. The paradox of a nation awash in cell phones, voice mail, handheld computers and plain old pen and paper unable to convey vital information regarding drug safety is staggering.

Significant risk of ADEs persists in the long-term care setting. Nearly one-half of the ADEs were preventable in a nested case-control study of residents of large skilled nursing facilities in New England and Canada (Gurwitz et al., 2005). The majority of the events occurred at the stages of ordering or monitoring. Drugs associated with the highest risk were antipsychotic agents, anticoagulants, diuretics and antiepileptics.

The Beers criteria provide a useful tool for avoiding the use of agents that are either ineffective or present substantially higher risk to elderly patients than existing alternatives (Fick et al., 2003). First developed from study of prescribing patterns for institutionalized elderly patient, the current revision of the criteria provides additional guidance by identifying agents with heightened risk of ADEs for patients with specific medical conditions. Table 9.1 lists the most common classes of drugs and examples in each class associated with high risk of ADEs in the elderly. Analgesics, psychotropic agents, anticholinergic agents and drugs that provide symptomatic relief generally pose significant risk to elderly patients, and therefore the clinician must carefully assess the potential benefit against this risk before prescribing these agents.

In a comprehensive review of issues in geriatric pharmacology, Vestal (1997) identifies a diverse set of risk factors for polypharmacy in this population. Among them are the propensity for providers to prescribe and the tendency to continue agents that lack clear indication or efficacy, especially if another provider has prescribed the drug. Both are understandable consequences of the increasing availability of an armamentarium of effective drugs for conditions with significant morbidity and the shift toward specialist-based care. Both influences in the absence of the primary care model or a multidisciplinary team approach to care could further fragment care delivery and promote the incidence of ADEs (Murray & Callahan, 2003).

In Japan, where the use of a regular physician is relatively less common than in the United States, a study of ambulatory geriatric patients determined the risk

Table 9.1 Potentially Inappropriate Medications for Elderly Patients

Class	Drug
Analgesics	
Nonsteroidal antiinflammatory drugs (NSAIDs)	
	ketrolac
	indomethacin
Narcotic analgesics	
	meperidine
	pentazocin
Agents for symptom relief	
Antiemetics	
	trimethobenzamide
Muscle relaxants and antispamodics	
	carisoprodol
	chorzoxazone
	orphenadrine
	metaxalone
	cyclobenzaprine
	methocarbamol
Antispasmodics (gastrointestinal)	
	hycyamine
	propantheline
	belladonna
	dicyclomine
Psychotropic agents	
Benzodiazepines (long-acting)	
	chlordiazepoxide
	diazepam
	flurazepam
Benzodiazepines (shorter-acting)	
	oxazepam
	alprazolam
	temazepam
	triazolam
	lorazepam
Antidepressants	
	doxepin
	amitriptyline
Antidepressants (SSRI)	
	fluoxetine
Anticholinergics/antihistamines	
	diphenhydramine
	hydroxyzine
	cyproheptadine
	promethazine
	chlorpheniramine

of polypharmacy (i.e., use of ≥ 5drugs). Subjects without a primary care provider were 2.5 times more likely to meet the criterion for polypharmacy than those with this form of continuity of care, despite comparable comorbidity, impairment of functional status and frequency of office visits (Tsuji-Hayashi et al., 1999).

Polypharmacy is virtually unavoidable in the course of following the advice of existing prevention and treatment guidelines for elderly persons, that is, if polypharmacy is defined solely by the number of medications in use. Strict adherence to existing clinical practice guidelines may in itself produce added stress and undesirable effects (Boyd et al., 2005), as most are not designed with older patients with comorbidities in mind. ADEs, complicated treatment regimens and cost are among the potential adverse outcomes of this approach. Foremost, in the minds of clinicians, as they prescribe for this vulnerable population should be the risks posed by polypharmacy and comorbidity.

Polypharmacy may also result from omitting or failing to prescribe highly effective agents. For example, overestimation of the risks of prescribing aspirin to a diabetic patient and subsequently withholding it may needlessly heighten the risk of developing new chronic conditions (e.g., stroke, myocardial infarction) requiring their own pharmacotherapy. An array of symptoms related to the new condition (e.g., limb spasticity associated with a stroke) then may lead to symptomatic treatment, itself a risk factor for adverse drug events.

Pharmacology of Aging – Pharmacokinetics and Pharmacodynamics

Understanding of age-related structural and functional changes affords providers with a means of differentiating the impact of disease states on individuals and the consequences of therapeutic decisions. The pharmacokinetic and pharmacodynamic changes attributable to aging itself can assist clinicians in effective and safe clinical decision-making.

Defined age-related changes in drug absorption, distribution, metabolism and elimination are of varying clinical significance. Aging affects absorption through the gastrointestinal tract, and the skin changes through several influences (Bressler & Bahl, 2003) affecting the amount of various drugs reaching the circulation (bioavailability) or how rapidly the drug reaches peak concentration after oral administration. Digoxin provides an example of the latter. When initiating treatment of elderly patients, the clinician can expect a slower rise to an effective level of this and other beneficial agents in an elderly patient.

Reduced gastric acidity in elderly patients may decrease absorption of ionized drugs that require exposure to an acidic milieu (e.g., fluconazole, itraconazole, iron sulfate). While the aging small bowel displays marked decrease in its absorptive surface and blood flow, the clinical significance of the changes may be negligible. Aging skin not only wrinkles but also may provide a less efficient conduit for transdermal delivery systems and delay the achievement of effective plasma concentration. The importance of this observation has implications for providing prompt pain control when employing fentanyl in this form for an elderly individual. The relatively low frequency of clinically significant events related to the changes in absorption suggests the presence of significant reserve capacity in various organ systems.

Changes in body composition associated with aging can affect the distribution of drugs. The ratio of body fat to lean body mass increases in both men and women with aging. The change results in increased volume distribution and half-life of lipid soluble agents, accounting in part for the heightened effects of benzodiazepines and their high potential for ADEs in elderly subjects. Concomitant reduction in lean body mass and total body water can lead to higher peak serum concentrations for a given dose of water-soluble agents (e.g., alcohol) in the elderly. Hypoalbuminemia associated with advanced age can effect the distribution of drugs highly bound to plasma proteins. Particularly in the setting of malnutrition and chronic illness, the deficiency of plasma albumin can lead to unanticipated toxicity due to an augmented free fraction. This factor commonly complicates phenytoin and warfarin dose adjustment.

Hepatic metabolism declines with aging due primarily to a 20–50% decline in liver mass. The increase in sensitivity to warfarin in the elderly correlates more closely with the decline in liver mass than with chronological age. Drugs extracted at high rates on the first pass through the liver, a category including several β-blockers, calcium channel blockers and morphine, may have unanticipated augmented effects as a consequence of a 10–15% decline in liver perfusion that is part of normal aging. With this phase of liver metabolism diminished, a given dose of these agents achieve greater circulating levels and resulting end organ effects.

Aging contributes less to differences in hepatic oxidative (phase I) metabolism than the influence of genetic variation. ADEs associated with this aspect of liver function are far more frequently due to polypharmacy and resulting drug interactions than to age-related changes in the liver. In one review of a large pharmacy management database encompassing five million patients, nearly 10% of the patients reviewed filled prescriptions for multiple medications linked to QT-prolongation or for agents that inhibited hepatic clearance of the medications, thus increasing their risk of a fatal dysrhythmia (Curtis et al., 2003). More than 20% of the subjects in the study were elderly. Consideration of potential adverse interactions at this level between commonly prescribed agents is warranted, if a patient experiences an unanticipated delay or exuberance of effects to a seemingly judicious dose of an agent.

Advanced age is associated with impaired renal clearance of drugs. Renal plasma flow decreases by about 1% annually after age 50. The number of functioning glomeruli declines by nearly one-third on average with advanced age. The Cockcroft–Gault equation and other formulae for estimating the influence of age on creatinine clearance (Cockcroft & Gault, 1976) (Levey et al., 1999) provide clinical tools for adjusting dosing of agents dependent on the kidneys for elimination. Dosage or dosing interval adjustment is critical for nephrotoxic drugs, such as aminoglycosides and vancomycin, as well as drugs with narrow therapeutic indices, such as digoxin and lithium.

In addition to changes in how elderly patients influence the drugs they take (pharmacokinetics), there are less well-defined and less frequently studied age-related changes in how drugs affect older patients at the site of action (pharmacodynamics). Enhanced sensitivity to anxiolytic agents, hypnotics and narcotic analgesics frequently results in unintended prolonged effects and ADE when an elderly patient receives a seemingly prudent dose of an appropriate agent. Benzodiazepines present an instructive illustration. Body composition changes lead to prolonged half-life of these agents and permit prolonged exposure to the sensitized receptors and can result in delirium, somnolence, and falls with injury. Blunted sensitivity to both β-adrenergic agonists (e.g., albuterol) and β-blockers (e.g., metoprolol) associated with aging can delay the anticipated response to treatment for bronchospasm and hypertension respectively.

Aging and Oral Health

The oral health of the elderly is a joint responsibility of primary care providers and dental professionals (Shenkin & Baum, 2001). While it is not typically a chief focus of medical providers, there is increasing awareness among geriatricians of the importance of oral health on the functional condition, general health and well-being of their patients. The persistent trend of decreased rates of edentulousness brings with it a rise in the prevalence of periodontitis, which affects over one-third of the community-dwelling adult population and disproportionately higher rates among the poor and disadvantaged. Common geriatric conditions, such as cerebrovascular disease, stroke, dementia and chronic pain may impede the ability of the elderly patient to maintain adequate dental hygiene. Treatments for many geriatric syndromes may further threaten oral health by impeding the performance of essential activities of daily living or by promoting the accumulation of plaque. Persistent oral health problems were the focus of an investigation among participants of the Geisinger Rural Aging Study (Bailey et al., 2004). Subjects with persistent problems with chewing, swallowing and mouth pain were far more likely to have lower Healthy Eating Index scores than counterparts without these problems. In addition, medication use was significantly greater (4.2 vs 2.6 medications on average) and comorbidity (7.0 vs 4.2 chronic conditions) was more prevalent in the subjects with substantial oral health problems than those without.

Improvements in oral hygiene and public health measures have reduced the risk of edentulousness in old age (Ship, 1999; Beltrán-Aguilar et al., 2005), while prevalence of tooth loss remains high. The gain in this area is due largely to reduction in dental caries, but the risk for caries and periodontal disease remains high after age 65. Edentulousness and tooth loss can have widespread medical, functional, nutritional and social implications for individuals.

Problems with mastication in elderly patients are more likely the consequence of dentition than age. Worn cusps or ill-fitting dentures can result in fatigue while chewing, nutritional deficiencies and increased risk of aspiration pneumonia from swallowing larger food boluses. Angular chelitis, oral candidiasis and frank oral mucosal injury are associated with denture use. The latter augments the reduced protective function of the mucosa resulting from age-associated thinning, vascular compromise and decreased general immune competency.

Salivary Gland Function with Aging

In healthy, nonmedicated individuals, the number of acinar cells of the major salivary glands (i.e., parotid, submandibular and sublingual) declines with age while gland function, measured by volume produced, remains normal (Ship et al., 1995) (Ghezzi et al., 2000). Each glands unique distribution of mucous and serous cells contributes elements to the whole saliva that lubricates the oral mucosa, promotes remineralization of the teeth and provides protection from microbial infection. Preservation of normal salivary function is fundamental to the health of the oral mucosa, the teeth and the periodontium. Preparation of the food bolus for deglutition and facilitation of taste are relatively minor functions of the saliva that can have a major impact on general health and well-being.

Medical conditions associated with salivary gland dysfunction include Sjörgren's syndrome, an autoimmune disorder of exocrine tissue; Alzheimer's disease, with associated submandibular gland dysfunction; sequelae of radiation therapy for head and neck cancer and dehydration.

The elderly are at increased risk for dehydration through a variety of age-related and disease-specific influences (Ayus & Arieff, 1996). Age affects the experience of thirst and response to it and age-related changes in renal tubular function diminish the ability to concentrate the urine and thus converse water. With the decline in total body water that occurs with aging, smaller volumes of water deprivation may result in a more profound response in an older patient. The steady decline in renal blood flow and glomerular filtration rate after age 50 also influence the ability of older individuals to adapt to changes in hydration. The direct influence of medication, particularly diuretics for treatment of hypertension and congestive heart failure, may promote dehydration. Cognitive impairment and functional impairment may influence access to water.

A study of the effects of dehydration on salivary gland function compared the stimulated and unstimulated responses of parotid salivary flow in healthy young (ages 20–40) and older (ages 60–80) (Ship & Fischer, 1997). Parameters measured at baseline, after a 24-hour fast and 1 hour after intravenous rehydration included stimulated and unstimulated parotid salivary flow rates. Both groups experienced decreased flow rates during the dehydration phase and neither groups unstimulated flow rate returned to baseline levels with rehydration thus suggesting an age-independent influence of dehydration on the salivary function of healthy adults.

Caloric intake correlates strongly with parotid flow rates in otherwise health adults. In a large ($N = 1006$) community-based study of an age-stratified population, investigators sought to define the effect of age on salivary function

(Yeh et al., 1998). They studied six cohorts divided by age from 35 to over 75 and measured stimulated and unstimulated flow rates along with additional parameters including height, caloric intake and saliva protein content. Age and caloric intake were both significant influences on stimulated and unstimulated submandibular and sublingual flow rates and that protein content of unstimulated saliva increased with age.

The Baltimore Longitudinal Study of Aging sought to differentiate the influences of age, menopause, hormone replacement therapy (HRT) and medication on parotid salivary function (Ghezzi et al., 2000). Age was a statistically significant predictor of decrease stimulated parotid flow rates, however the influence of just one xerostomic medication was much more profound, the equivalent of "14 years of aging." Neither menopause nor HRT displayed any consistent correlation with flow rates. The findings underline the relatively powerful influence of medication effects versus disease states or aging on the prevalence of dry mouth. Xerostomia is a consequence of systemic disease or therapy for conditions, rather than a phenomenon of aging.

Xerostomia

In a randomized controlled cross-over study of 18 healthy young subjects and 18 healthy older persons with a mean age over 70, investigators found no significant age or gender differences in glycopyrrolate stimulated flow rates or xerostomic symptoms (Ghezzi & Ship, 2003). The older subjects, however, experienced prolonged recovery and longer duration of suppression of parotid flow rates, providing support to "the secretory reserve hypothesis of salivary function." The authors concluded that xerostomic agents have a relatively greater importance in generating xerostomia than age-related decline in function.

Prolonged recovery and longer duration of suppression may reflect impaired ability to adapt to environmental demands typical of a variety of physiologic systems as we age. Chronic exposure to the extremes of the environment over time impairs the ability to respond to external challenges through internal regulation (Seeman et al. 2001). The accumulation of an "allostatic load" may influence an elderly patient's ability to adapt to pharmacological challenges, despite the presence of "reserve" function in organ systems.

The autonomic nervous system controls the flow of saliva through the action of acetylcholine, the chief neurotransmitter of the parasympathetic nervous system. Through its action on a number of specific receptors (i.e., muscarinic), acetylcholine influences innervated smooth muscle, cardiac muscle and exocrine glands, such as the major salivary glands. Anticholinergic agents that block specific receptors may produce a syndrome including xerostomia, excessive sedation, weakness, urinary retention, constipation, hypotension, increased fall risk and delirium. The syndrome may further compromise performance of activities of daily living, dental hygiene practices, undermine nutrition and adequate hydration.

Diphenhydramine is a sedating antihistamine with pronounced sedative and anticholinergic effects included in many OTC preparations for symptomatic relief of

colds and sleep disturbance. A cohort study of over 400 inpatients in a university hospital setting revealed that the 27% of patients receiving the drug during their stay were at significantly heightened risk for delirium, for placement of an in-dwelling urinary catheter and for prolonged length of stay (Agostini et al., 2001). It is indicated solely for allergy symptoms, particularly pruritis in elderly patients, and when prescribed, it is vital to document the appropriate indication and to use the lowest effective dose while monitoring the patient for ADEs.

A cohort study of cognitively intact outpatients at an Iowa Veterans Affairs Medical Center with a mean age greater than 74 and prescribed five or more medications found that the use of anticholinergic agents was common (27.1%). Dry mouth and constipation were significantly more prevalent in those taking these agents. While the rate of frank ADE was low (0.8%), the use of antihistamines, tricyclic antidepressants and muscle relaxants often lacked clear indication (Ness et al., 2006).

Antihistamines and other anticholinergic agents are among the most prominent examples of literally hundreds of prescription and OTC pharmaceuticals that may promote xerostomia (Butt, 1991). The use of multiple medications increases the risk of the compounded influence of several agents with modest xerostomic characteristics producing pronounced symptoms.

Significant overlap exists between medications with high potential for adverse effects in the elderly and those commonly associated with xerostomia (Table 9.2 and Table 9.3). Meperidine, a narcotic analgesic without indication in the elderly population, provides an example of a xerostomic agent with great potential for other ADEs.

Chronic pain and acute pain are common phenomena for elderly persons. The Berlin Aging Study found chronic painful arthritis in 50% of its study population after age 70. Analgesics from acetaminophen to an array of narcotic analgesics are among the most frequently prescribed agents in this population. The potential for adverse effects from meperidine far exceed its utility as an analgesic. Since the chief site of metabolism is the liver, its half-life may double in elderly patients simply by virtue of advanced age, and additional liver impairment through established or transient conditions extends its duration of action even further. Normeperidine is a metabolite of meperidine that relies on the kidneys for elimination. Its levels increase with acute or chronic impairment of renal function and this in turn may induce confusion, frank delirium or seizures. Effective alternatives for pain relief are abundant and consequently the use of meperidine in the elderly is contraindicated.

A study of the influence of the number of xerostomic medications on oral health suggests the cardinal role of saliva in preserving dental health. A cross-sectional study of subjects from Veterans Affairs facilities using at least one xerostomic agent found they were nearly three times likely to demonstrate more mucosal inflammation and higher rates of coronal and root caries (Janket et al., 2003).

Excluding agents that have direct and pronounced anticholinergic effects, particularly those employed in symptomatic treatment, is a relatively straightforward approach when confronted with patients with xerostomia. As the array of drugs in Table 9.2 demonstrates, discontinuing medications with established efficacy and benefit to patients with glaucoma, hypertension, congestive heart failure, depression

Table 9.2 Frequently Prescribed Agents Associated with Xerostomia

Generic name	Common proprietary name	Class	Chief indication
		Alpha adrenergic agents	
brimonidine	Alphagan	alpha2 agonist	glaucoma
clonidine	Catapres	alpha agonist – central	hypertension
midodrine		alpha agonist – peripheral	orthostatic hypotension
phenylephrine		adrenergic agonist	nasal congestion
prazosin	Minipres	alpha blocker	hypertension
terazosin	Hytrin	alpha antagonist	hypertension, prostatic hypertrophy
tizanidine	Zanaflex	alpha agonist – central	spasticity
		Beta adrenergic agents	
albuterol		brochodilator, beta-agonist	asthma
atenolol	Tenormin	beta blocker	hypertension
levalbuterol	Xopenex	beta2 agonist, bronchodilator	asthma
nadolol	Corgard	beta blocker	hypertension
		Analgesic agents	
butorphanol	Stadol	narcotic agonist-antagonist	pain
celecoxib	Celebrex	NSAID* – COX 2	inflammation, pain
diphenoxylate	Lomotil	narcotic analgesic	diarrhea
fentanyl	Duragesic	narcotic analgesic	pain
hydrocodone		narcotic analgesic, antitussive	pain, cough
hydromorphone	Dilaudid	narcotic analgesic	pain
meperidine	Demerol	narcotic analgesic	pain
methadone		narcotic analgesic	pain, narcotic dependency
morphine		narcotic analgesic	pain
nabumtone	Relafen	NSAID	inflammation, pain
oxaprozin	Daypro	NSAID	inflammation, pain
piroxicam	Feldene	NSAID	inflammation, pain
sulindac	Clinoril	NSAID	inflammation, pain
tramadol	Ultram	analgesic	pain
		Antibiotics	
isoniazid			tuberculosis
metronidazole	Flagyl		infection, pseudomembranous colitis
moxifloxacin	Avelox		infection
ofloxacin	Floxin		infection
		Anticholinergic agents	
atropine	Lomotil		diarrhea
clidinium			irritable bowel syndrome
hyocyamine	Levsin	antispasmodic	irritable bowel syndrome

Table 9.2 (continued)

Generic name	Common proprietary name	Class	Chief indication
ipratropium	Atrovent		asthma, COPD**
oxybutinin	Ditropan		urinary incontinence
tolterodine	Detrol		urinary incontinence
		Anticonvulsants	
carbamazepine	Tegretol		seizures, trigeminal neuralgia
gabapentin	Neurontin		neuropathic pain
pregabalin	Lyrica		neuropathic pain, seizures
		Antidepressants	
amitriptyline	Elavil	tricyclic antidepressant	depression, neuropathic pain
bupropion	Wellbutrin	antidepressant	depression, smoking cessation
citalopram	Celexa	antidepressant	
desipramine		tricyclic antidepressant	
doxepine	Sinequan	tricyclic antidepressant	
duloxetine	Cymbalta	antidepressant	
escitalopram	Lexapro	antidepressant	
fluoxetine	Prozac	antidepressant, SSRI***	
fluvoxamine	Luvox	antidepressant	
imipramine	Tofranil	tricyclic antidepressant	
maprotiline	Ludiomil	tetracyclic antidepressant	
mirtazapine	Remeron	antidepressant	
nortriptyline	Aventyl	tricyclic antidepressant	
paroxetine	Paxil	antidepressant, SSRI	
phenelzine	Nardil	antidepressant	
sertraline	Zoloft	antidepressant, SSRI	
St. John's Wort		antidepressant (over the counter)	
trazadone		antidepressant	
venlafaxine	Effexor	antidepressant	
		Antihistamines	
cetirizine	Zyrtec		rhinitis, pruritis
chlorpheniramine			pruritis, rhinitis
cyproheptadine	Periactin		allergy
desloratadine	Clarinex		rhinitis
diphenhydramine	Benadryl		pruritis
hydroxyzine	Atarax		pruritis
loratadine	Claritin		rhinitis
meclizine	Antivert		motion sickness, nausea
nizatidine	Axid	histamine-H2 antagonist	dyspepsia, PUD****
		Anti-Parkinson's agents	
amantadine	Symmetrel	anti-Parkinson's, antiviral	Parkinsonism, influenza A infection

Table 9.2 (continued)

Generic name	Common proprietary name	Class	Chief indication
pergolide	Permax	ergot alkaloid	Parkinson's disease
ropinirole	Requip	dopamine agonist	Parkinson's disease
selegiline	Eldepryl	anti-Parkinson's	Parkinson's disease
trihexyphenidyl		anticholinergic, anti-Parkinson's	Parkinsonism, dystonia, EPS****
Antipsychotic agents			
aripiprazole	Abilify	atypical antipsychotic	schizophrenia, mania
chlorpromazine			
clozapine	Clozaril		
fluphenazine	Prolixin		
haloperidol	Haldol		
mesoridazine	Serentil		
olanzapine	Zyprexa	atypical antipsychotic	
perphenazine	Trilafon		
quetiapine	Seroquel	atypical antipsychotic	
risperidone	Risperdol	atypical antipsychotic	
trifluoperazine	Stelazine		
ziprasidone	Geodon	atypical antipsychotic	
Benzodiazepines			
alprazolam	Ativan		anxiety
clorazepate	Tranxene		anxiety
Diuretics			
amiloride			hypertension, heart failure
chlorthalidone			hypertension, heart failure
hydrochlorothiazide			hypertension
indapamide			hypertension
metolazone	Zaroxolyn		hypertension, heart failure, edema
triamterene			hypertension
Hypnotics			
eszopiclone	Lunesta		sleep disturbance
zaleplon	Sonata		sleep disturbance
zolpidem	Ambien		sleep disturbance
Muscle relaxants			
baclofen			spasticity
botulinum toxin	Botox		blepharospasm, hyperhidrosis
cyclobenzaprine	Flexeril		spasticity
orphenadrine	Norflex		spasticity
Miscellaneous agents			
bicalutamide	Casodex	antiandrogen	advanced prostate cancer
isosorbide dinitrate	Isordil	nitrate	angina
nitroglycerin		nitrate	angina
beclomethasone		anti-inflammatory, corticosteroid	asthma, rhinitis
budesonide		anti-inflammatory, corticosteroid	asthma, rhinitis

Table 9.2 (continued)

Generic name	Common proprietary name	Class	Chief indication
methylphenidate	Ritalin	CNS stimulant	attention deficit disorder, narcolepsy
memantine	Namenda	NMDA****** antagonist	dementia
loperamide	Imodium	antidiarrheal	diarrhea
loperamide	Imodium	antidiarrheal	diarrhea
esomeprazole	Nexium	proton pump inhibitor	dyspepsia, PUD
disopyramide	Norpace	antiarrhythmic	dysrhythmia
vardenafil	Levitra	phosphodiesterase inhibitor	erectile dysfunction
calcitriol		1,25 OH Vitamin D	hypocalcemia in renal failure
ergocalciferol		Vitamin D2	supplement
dicyclomine	Bentyl	antispasmodic	irritable bowel syndrome
lithium		antimania agent	mania
zolmitriptan	Zomig	anti-migraine agent	migraine
scopolamine		belladonna alkaloid	motion sickness, nausea
prochlorperazine	Compazine	antiemetic, antipsychotic	nausea
promethazine	Phenergan	antiemetic, anticholinergic	nausea, allergy
sucralfate	Carafate	sucrose sulfate complex	PUD

*Nonsteroidal antiinflamatory drug
**Chronic obstructive pulmonary disease
***Selective serotonin reuptake inhibitor
****Peptic ulcer disease
*****Extrapyramidal syndrome
******N-methyl-D-aspartate

and other life-altering conditions becomes a more complex task. A team effort that fosters interaction, communication and cooperation between all professionals engaged in the care of the patient is essential to providing optimal management of all the patient's conditions.

The quality of the initial assessment of the geriatric patient predicts the risk of iatrogenic complication of medical therapy, whether initiated in the physician's office, hospital or dental office. In addition to a careful review of all prescription and OTC drugs taken by the patient, the initial assessment should also include evaluation of the patient's functional status, cognitive function and nutritional status. Each of these aspects of the patient's condition can have a profound effect on the adherence to a regimen as well as the effect of the chosen therapy. Impaired performance of activities of daily living and compromised cognitive function place individuals at particularly high risk for drug-related delirium and other adverse effects. Female gender, low body weight, advanced age, liver dysfunction and renal impairment present risk for adverse drug effects. Without recognizing these characteristics in their patients, providers are at risk of inappropriate prescribing.

Table 9.3 Potentially Inappropriate Medications for Elderly Patients Associated with Xerostomia

Antidepressants
Fluoxetine
Amitriptyline
Imipramine
Doxepin

Antispasmodics
Orphenadrine
Cyclobenzaprine
Oxybutinin (short-acting form)
Tolteridine

Antispasmodics (gastrointestinal)
Hyocyamine
Dicyclomine
Clindinium

Analgesics
Meperidine
Pentazocin
Naproxen
Piroxicam

Antihistamines
Chlorpheniramine
Diphenhydramine
Cyproheptadine
Trimethobenzamide

Antihypertensives
Methyldopa
Clonidine

Benzodiazepines
Alprazolam
Diazepam
Flurazepam
Triazolam

Miscellaneous
Thioridazine
Disopyramide
Atropine

Drugs Commonly Used in the Dental Office

Effective management of acute pain is the best method of avoiding the development of chronic pain, which affects up to 40% of community-dwelling elderly persons (Chodosh et al., 2001). NSAIDs are among the most frequently prescribed drugs for pain. Their use may be appropriate and sufficient for pain management for dental conditions when hemostasis is less of a concern. Since elderly patients have substantially elevated risk for peptic ulcer disease, dental providers should be aware of their patient's history of peptic ulcer disease. NSAIDs relieve pain at lower doses than are required for an antiinflammatory effect. Prescribers should avoid long-acting agents and those with pronounced central nervous system effects, such as piroxicam and indomethacin respectively. Untoward renal effects of NSAIDs are also a concern and are most likely to occur in patients with preexisting chronic kidney disease, congestive heart failure, liver disease or diuretic use.

Narcotic analgesics are effective for the management of significant pain, and elderly patients tolerate them reasonably well when they are prescribed appropriately. Finding an effective pain-relieving dose while avoiding constipation, delirium, falls and other adverse effects can nonetheless be daunting. The concept of "start low and go slow" applies to the use of narcotics in the elderly due to the enhanced pharmacodynamic effects in this population. Meperidine and codeine are agents best avoided in the elderly. Meperidine has prominent adverse central nervous system effects and codeine, a relatively weak analgesic with a propensity for a range of adverse effects that often exceeds the pain relief it provides.

The principles of antibiotic usage are the same for elderly patients regardless of the clinical setting. Allergy is common with antibiotic use and a careful history is essential to the effort to avoid major and minor allergic complications. When possible, clinicians should use specific identification of infectious agents to guide the choice of antibiotics. The current epidemics of methacillin resistant *Staphylococcus aureus* (MRSA) and *Clostridium difficile* infection, once limited to inpatient populations, are now concerns in long-term care settings and the community at large. Precise and succinct use of antimicrobials is a major safeguard against these complications of therapy for infection. When culture and susceptibility data are not available, providers must exercise the appropriate index of suspicion for specific causative agents and prescribe accordingly. Dosage adjustment for impaired renal function is essential for aminoglycocides, vancomycin, ciprofloxacin and other antibiotics dependent on this route of elimination. Interaction between antibiotics and warfarin mediated by alteration of intestinal flora or by cytochrome P450 effects may lead to unanticipated inhibition or augmentation of warfarin's effects.

Conclusion

Primary providers of medical and dental care have a shared responsibility to their elderly patients in the pursuit of safe and high quality care. Their collaboration offers the patient the best opportunity for meeting oral health objectives and aging successfully. Challenges come with the successes of the past, such as the decline in edentulousness, the reduction of cardiovascular morbidity and increased life span. The growing numbers of effective pharmacological agents and the complexity of chronic disease management can only reinforce the need for more effective multidisciplinary systems of care for our aging population. It is imperative that dental practitioners be familiar with current drug usage, including drug interactions and adverse side effects. These are particularly important considerations for older adult patients.

References

Agostini, J.V., Leo-Summers, L.S. & Inouye, S.K. (2001). Cognitive and other adverse effects of diphenhydramine use in hospitalized older patients. *Archives of Internal Medicine*, 161(17), 2091–2097.

Ayus, J.C. & Arieff, A.I. (1996). Abnormalities of water metabolism in the elderly. *Seminars in Nephrology*, 16(4), 277–288.

Bailey, R.L., Ledikwe, J.H., Smiciklas-Wright, H., Mitchell, D.C. & Jensen, G.L. (2004). Persistent oral health problems associated with comorbidity and impaired diet quality in older adults. *Journal of the American Dietary Association*, 104(8), 173–176.

Baltes, P.B. & Mayer, K.V. (1999) *The Berlin Aging Study*. Cambridge: Cambridge University Press.

Beijer, H.J. & de Blaey, C.J. (2002). Hospitalisations caused by adverse drug reactions (ADR): a meta-analysis of observational studies. *Pharmacy World and Science*, 24(2), 46–54.

Beltrán-Aguilar, E.D., Barker, L.K., Canto, M.T., Dye, B.A., Gooch, B.F., Griffin, S.O. et al. (2005). Surveillance for dental caries, dental sealants, tooth retention, edentulism, and enamel fluorosis – United States, 1988–1994 and 1999–2002. *Mortality and Morbidity Weekly Reports*, 54(03), 1–44.

Berkman, L.F., Seeman, T.E., Albert, M., Blazer, D., Kahn, R., Mohs, R. et al. (1993). High, usual and impaired functioning in community-dwelling older men and women: findings from the MacArthur Foundation Research Network on Successful Aging. *Journal of Clinical Epidemiology*, 46(10), 1129–1140.

Boyd, C.M., Darer, J., Boult, C., Fried, L.P., Boult, L. & Wu, A.W. (2005). Clinical practice guidelines and quality of care for older patients with multiple comorbid diseases. *Journal of the American Medical Association*, 294, 716–724.

Bressler, R. & Bahl, J.J. (2003). Principles of drug therapy for the elderly patient. *Mayo Clinic Proceedings*, 78, 1564–1577.

Budnitz, D.S., Pollock, D.A., Weidenbach, K.N., Mendelsohn, A.B., Schroeder, T.J. & Annest, J.L. (2006). National surveillance of emergency department visits for outpatient adverse drug events. *Journal of the American Medical Association*, 296(15), 1858–1866.

Butt G.M. (1991). Drug-induced xerostomia. *Journal of the Canadian Dental Association*, 57(5), 391–393.

Chodosh, J., Ferrell, B.A., Shekelle, P.G. & Wenger, N.S (2001). Quality indicators for pain management in vulnerable elders. *Annals of Internal Medicine*, 135(8 pt 2), 731–735.

Cockcroft, D.W. & Gault, M.H. (1976). Prediction of creatinine clearance from serum creatinine. *Nephron*, 16(1), 31–41.

Curtis, L.H., Ostbye, T., Sendersky, V., Hutchinson, S., Allen LaPointe, N.M., Al-Khatib, S.M. et al. (2003). Prescription of QT-prolonging drugs in a cohort of about 5 million outpatients. *American Journal of Medicine*, 114(2), 135–141.

Dormann, H., Criegee-Rieck, M., Neubert, A., Egger, T., Geise, A. Krebs, S. et al. (2003). Lack of awareness of community-acquired adverse drug reactions upon hospital admission: dimensions and consequences of a dilemma. *Drug Safety*, 26(5), 353–362.

Fick D.M., Cooper J.W., Wade W.E., Waller J.L., Maclean J.R. & Beers M.H. (2003). Updating the Beers criteria for potentially inappropriate medication use in older adults: results of a US consensus panel of experts. *Archives of Internal Medicine*, 163(22), 2716–2724.

Forster, A.J., Murff, H.J., Peterson, J.F., Gandhi, T.K. & Bates D.W. (2003). The incidence and severity of adverse events affecting patients after discharge from the hospital. *Annals of Internal Medicine*, 138(3), 161–167.

Ghezzi, E.M. & Ship, J.A. (2003). Aging and secretory reserve capacity of major salivary glands. *Journal of Dental Research*, 82(10), 844–848.

Ghezzi, E.M., Wagner-Lange, L.A., Schork, M.A., Metter, E.J., Baum, B.J., Streckfus, C.F. et al. (2000). Longitudinal influence of age, menopause, hormone replacement, and other medications on parotid flow rates in healthy women. *Journal of Gerontology: Series A, Biological and medical sciences*, 55, M34–M42.

Gurwitz, J.H., Field, T.S., Judge, J., Rochon, P., Harrold, L.R., Cadoret, C. et al. (2005). The incidence of adverse drug events in two large long-term care facilities. *American Journal of Medicine*, 118, 251–258.

Janket, S.J., Jones, J.A., Rich, S., Meurman, J., Garcia, R. & Miller, D. (2003). Xerostomic medications and oral health: the Veterans Dental Study (part I). *Gerodontology*, 20(1), 41–19.

Levey, A.S., Bosch, J.P., Lewis, J.B., Greene, T., Rogers, N. & Roth, D. (1999). A more accurate method to estimate glomerular filtration rate from serum creatinine: a new prediction equation. Modification of Diet in Renal Disease Study Group. *Annals of Internal Medicine*, 130(6), 461–470.

Murray, M.D. & Callahan, C.M. (2003). Improving medication use for older adults: an integrated research agenda. *Annals of Internal Medicine*, 139, 425–429.

National Center for Health Statistics (2006). *Health, United States, 2006 with chartbook on trends in the health of Americans*. U.S. Department of Health and Human Services, Centers for Disease Control and Prevention, National Center for Health Statistics, Hyattsville, MD: 34–35.

Ness, J., Hoth, A., Barnett, M.J., Shorr, R.I. & Kaboli, P.J. (2006). Anticholinergic medications in community-dwelling older veterans: prevalence of anticholinergic symptoms, symptom burden and adverse drug events. *American Journal of Geriatric Pharmacotherapy*, 4(1), 42–51.

Seeman, T.E., McEwen, B.S., Rowe, J.W. & Singer, B.H. (2001). Allostatic load as a marker of cumulative biological risk: MacArthur studies of successful aging. *Proceedings of the National Academy of Sciences*, 98(8), 4770–4775.

Shenkin, J.D. & Baum, B.J. (2001). Oral health and the role of the geriatrician. *Journal of the American Geriatrics Society*, 49(2), 229–230.

Ship, J.A. (1999). The oral cavity. In: *Principles of geriatric medicine and gerontology, Hazzard W.R., Blass, J.P., Ettinger, W.H., Halter, J.B. & Ouslander, J.G. eds., McGraw-Hill, New York*, 591–602.

Ship, J.A. & Fischer, D.J. (1997). The relationship between dehydration and parotid salivary gland function in young and old healthy adults. *Journal of Gerontology (Series A, Biological sciences and medical sciences)*, 52(5), M310–319.

Ship, J.A., Nolan, N.E. & Puckett, S.A. (1995). Longitudinal analysis of parotid and submandibular salivary flow rates in healthy, different-aged adults. *Journal of Gerontology (Series A, Biological sciences and medical sciences)*, 50(5), M285–289.

Stagnitti, M.N., Miller, G.E., Moeller, J.F. (2003) *Outpatient prescription drug expenses, 1999*. Rockville, MD: Agency for Healthcare Research and Quality.

Tsuji-Hayashi, Y., Fukuhara, S., Green, J. & Kurokawa, K. (1999). Use of prescribed drugs among older people in Japan: association with not having a regular physician. *Journal of the American Geriatrics Society*, 47(12), 1425–1429.

Vestal, R.E. (1997). Aging and pharmacology. *Cancer*, 80(7), 1302–10.

Yeh, C.K., Johnson, D.A. & Dodds, M.W. (1998). Impact of aging on human salivary gland function: a community-based study. *Aging (Milano)*, 10(5), 421–428.

Chapter 10
Management of Alcohol and Tobacco Dependence in Older Adults

David A. Albert

Introduction

The elderly face unique risks from the use of alcohol because of their increased incidence of chronic illness and their use of multiple medications. Aging changes the way bodies metabolize alcohol (Smith, 1995). Concomitant alcohol and medication use is potentially dangerous and can result in fatal consequences. This can occur if alcohol is used with tranquilizers, sleeping pills, painkiller or antihistamines. Alcohol and prescription drug misuse affects as many as 17 percent of older Americans (Blow, 1998). It is estimated that as many as 2.5 million older adults in America have problems related to alcohol use, and this age group experiences more than half of all reported adverse drug reactions leading to hospitalization (Schonfeld & Dupree, 1995). Additionally, problems older adults face with alcohol use are likely to be under-identified, under-diagnosed, and under-treated (Begun & Manwell, 2004). Alcohol abuse in older adults is often not recognized by health professionals, and these adults do not typically seek treatment from specialized facilities (Barry & Blow, 2004).

Alcohol abuse, like smoking increases the risk of oral cancer (Robb & Smith, 1996). Alcohol and drug abusers are more likely to be heavy smokers and to have nutritional impairment, compounding their risk for poor oral health (Harris, Warnakulasuriya, Gelbier, Johnson, & Peters, 1997). They also are more likely to neglect their oral hygiene, increasing their risk of caries, dental erosion and periodontal disease.

Alcoholism among the aged is treatable. Greater awareness of the issues involved with alcohol in the older generation can help clinicians to identify problems accurately and to provide the best possible care. With the increasing interest in cost containment and preventive care in the health care sector, it is important that

D.A. Albert
Director, Division of Community Health; Associate Professor of Clinical Dentistry Columbia University College of Dental Medicine Associate Professor of Public Health, Columbia University Mailman School of Public Health 601 W168th Street, Suite 32, New York, NY 10032,
Tel: 212-342-8588, Fax: 212-342-8558
e-mail: daa1@columbia.edu

I.B. Lamster, M.E. Northridge (eds.), *Improving Oral Health for the Elderly*,
© Springer Science+Business Media, LLC 2008

practitioners are aware of tobacco and alcohol use and the problems resulting from use and/or misuse of these products in this population.

Tobacco cessation programs frequently do not address smoking in the elderly because there exists an incorrect assumption that seniors will not benefit from quitting and/or that they will not be receptive to cessation counseling or programs. While many think that those who quit at age 65 or older will fail to reap the health benefits of abstinence from tobacco, the benefits of cessation do extend to those who quit at an older age. Smoking cessation in older adults leads to significant risk reduction and other health benefits, even in those who have smoked for years (Dietrich, Maserejian, Joshipura, Krall, & Garcia, 2007). Tobacco-related diseases are responsible for significant morbidity in older Americans. Smoking is a major risk factor for premature death and can limit a person's longevity by a decade or more. Smoking increases the risk for oral and pharyngeal cancer and periodontitis (Sheiham & Watt, 2000; Tomar & Asma, 2000). The Centers for Disease Control and Prevention (CDC) estimated in 2002 that 57 percent of smokers age 65 and over reported a desire to quit (CDC, 2002). Currently, about 10 percent of elderly smokers quit each year, with 1 percent relapsing. Research has shown that given adequate support, older adults suffering from disease conditions related to smoking and tobacco use can successfully quit. Brief interventions by dentists and physicians advising patients to quit have been shown to have a small beneficial effect (Folsom & Grimm, 1987) but a somewhat more intensive intervention is more effective – about 10–15 percent of smokers are induced to abstain for at least a year (Chapman, 1993).

Alcohol Prevalence

The Surgeon General's report on mental health identifies alcohol misuse as a common problem among older adults (U.S. Department of Health and Human Services, 1999). Studies have found that although substance use is more common among adults aged 18–49 years than older adults (50 years and older), the misuse of alcohol is increasing among older adults (Blow, 2000; Korper & Council, 2002). Depending on the definition of at-risk problem, drinking as many as 15 percent of older adults can be classified as problem drinkers (Barry & Blow, 2004). The 2003 National Survey on Drug Use and Health (NSDUH) reports 44 percent alcohol use in those aged 50 and older, and a rate of 12 percent for binge alcohol use in this group (The NSDUH Report, 2005; Gfroerer, 2004). In addition, males 50 and over were more likely to report alcohol use than females in this age group. The rate of past month binge alcohol use was three times greater among men than women, and the rate of past month heavy alcohol use was more than seven times greater in men than women (The NSDUH Report, 2005). Additionally, past month alcohol use by older adults was greater among non-Hispanic Whites, than among Hispanics, and non-Hispanic Blacks, with rates of 48.3 percent, 33.6 percent, and 30.2 percent, respectively (The NSDUH Report, 2005). An earlier studies found that

African-American males had higher rates of alcoholism than Hispanic and White males, respectively; African-American females had higher alcoholism rates than White and Hispanic females, respectively (Helzer, Burnam, & McEvoy, 1991).

There a number of issues involved in aging that can make this population particularly susceptible to alcohol use and abuse. These issues include loss of family and friends, loss of job or retirement, diminished health, social isolation, financial problems, housing changes, reduced mobility, and impaired self-care that is often coupled with the loss of independence (Barry & Blow, 2004). Older women, compared to their male counterparts, are also at greater risk for alcohol problems because they are more likely to outlive their spouses and face other losses that can result in depression and feelings of loneliness (Blow & Barry, 2002).

Even with low levels of alcohol consumption use, older adults can experience impaired motor skills resulting in poor driving, and injuries from falls and accidents (Barry & Blow, 2004; Dufour & Fuller, 1995). A 1993 analysis of the National Health Interview Survey (NHIS) found that older individuals have a dramatically higher risk of being alcohol dependent at a given level of consumption than do younger individuals (Dawson & Archer, 1993). Results of a study using the Current Population Survey II (CPS-II) data found that alcohol consumption was related to increased rates of death from cirrhosis, and cancers of the mouth, esophagus, pharynx, larynx and liver. These rates were three to seven times as high in participants reporting at least four drinks per day as among nondrinkers (Thun et al., 1997). Male drinkers in this study also experienced 30 percent higher mortality from external causes such as unintentional injuries and suicide than in nondrinkers; among women, drinkers also experienced a 30 percent higher rate of death from breast cancer than do nondrinkers (Thun et al., 1997).

Tobacco Prevalence

The 2005 National Health Interview Survey (NHIS) reported that approximately 20 percent of U.S. adults were current cigarette smokers (CDC, 2006). The American Lung Association further estimates that over 42 percent of adult smokers are 45 years and older (American Lung Association, 2006). The 2003 National Survey on Drug Use and Health (NSDUH), a nationally representative survey of the U.S. civilian, noninstitutionalized population, reported a 12 percent rate of tobacco use in the past month in the over 50 population surveyed in the study (Gfroerer, 2004); combined 2002 and 2003 NSDUH data placed cigarette use in the past month among persons 50 years and older at approximately 17.1 percent (The NSDUH Report, 2005). The 2005 NHIS reported the prevalence of current cigarette smoking was 8.6 percent in adults 65 years and older indicating some decline in the use of cigarettes by older Americans (CDC, 2006).

Demographic data show little difference in smoking prevalence between older men and women. According to the data, 8.9 percent of male current smokers were 65 years and older compared to 8.3 percent of female smokers (CDC, 2006).

However, racial differences exist in cigarette use. Past month cigarette use by adults 50 years and older was significantly greater among non-Hispanic Blacks than non-Hispanic Whites and Hispanics, with rates of 22.6 percent, 17 percent and 13.8 percent, respectively (The NSDUH Report, 2005). Today's generation of older smokers are reported to have had some of the highest smoking rates when compared with previous U.S. generations (American Lung Association, 2006).

While the prevalence of current smoking among the elderly in the U.S. population is low, it has been reported that of the more than 430,000 U.S. deaths attributable to smoking annually, over 94 percent are of persons 50 years and older (The Center for Social Gerontology, 2001). Additionally, one-third of current smokers die prematurely from smoking-related diseases such as cancer, and respiratory illnesses, losing approximately 12–15 years of life versus normal life expectancy (U.S. Department of Health and Human Services, 2004; The Center for Social Gerontology, 2001). Male smokers over 65 years and older are twice as likely to die from stroke when compared to male nonsmokers of the same age (American Lung Association, 2006). Smoking is also related to a number of other debilitating diseases such as heart disease, high blood pressure, reductions in taste and smell, diabetes, oral health problems, impotence, dementia, and Alzheimer's (The Center for Social Gerontology, 2001; Rimer, Orleans, Keintz, Cristinzio, & Fleisher, 1990). Cigarette smokers are more than twice as likely as nonsmokers to develop dementia and Alzheimer's disease (Ott et al., 1998); smokers also have 2–3 times the risk of developing cataracts as nonsmokers (U.S. Department of Health and Human Services, 2004). Older smokers have an increased risk of developing smoking-related diseases due to the fact that they are likely to have smoked longer, and to be heavier smokers.

Survey results of a sample of 3,147 members of the American Association of Retired Persons (AARP) throughout the United States found that older smokers reported smoking for approximately 46 years. Of the sample, 66 percent reported smoking within 30 minutes of waking up, a strong indicator of addiction. Smokers in the 50- to 69- year-old group appeared to be more heavily addicted than those over 70 years, as they reported that they were more likely to smoke their first cigarette within 15 minutes of rising (Rimer et al., 1990). Current smokers were more likely to have trouble breathing, experience frequent coughing, and to tire easily when compared with former smokers, and never smokers. When compared to former and never smokers, current smokers were also less likely to attend to their overall health. They had fewer visits than nonsmokers to the physician, and received fewer mammograms, blood pressure checks, stool blood tests, Pap smears, digital rectal examinations, and electrocardiograms (Rimer et al., 1990).

A more recent study of 95 residents of a long-term care facility in Rochester, New York aged 51 years and over consisted of 26 percent current smokers, 39 percent former smokers, and 35 percent never smokers (Carosella, Ossip-Klein, Watt, & Podgorski, 2002). Current smokers reported having smoked for an average of 37 years; also, 36 percent of smokers consumed their first cigarette within 30 minutes of waking (Carosella et al., 2002).

The Cancer Prevention Study II (CPS-II) (an ongoing prospective cohort of approximately 1.2 million U.S. adults begun in 1982, when participants were at least 30), found that current and former pipe smokers were more likely to report alcohol consumption than never users of tobacco. Current pipe smokers also had significantly higher death rates than never users. This mortality was attributed to tobacco-related diseases, including cancers of the larynx, lung, pancreas, oropharynx, esophagus, and rectum; chronic obstructive pulmonary disease; cerebrovascular disease; and coronary heart disease (Henley et al., 2004).

Research has shown that quitting smoking can result in health improvement at any age, even in adults 65 years and older. Some health benefits can be immediate (The Center for Social Gerontology, 2001). Improved circulation occurs when an older person quits smoking; the lungs also begin to repair damage, risk of heart disease is halved, and the risk of stroke and lung cancer diminishes. Among smokers who quit at age 65, men gained 1.4–2.0 years of life, and women 2.7–3.4 years of life (Taylor, Hasselblad, Henley, Thun, & Sloan, 2002). A recent study on middle-aged smokers and former smokers with mild or moderate lung function impairment found that both groups breathed easier after smoking cessation; women in the study who were sustained quitters experienced greater improvement in lung function when compared to their male counterparts (Connett et al., 2003).

Oral Manifestations of Alcohol Use and Misuse

The effect of alcohol on periodontal disease can be due to the poor oral hygiene that is associated with alcohol users or from the independent effect of alcohol on periodontal tissues. Alcohol impairs neutrophil, macrophage, and T-cell functioning, resulting in an increased predilection for infection (Pitiphat, Merchant, Rimm, & Joshipura, 2003; Tezal, Grossi, Ho, & Genco, 2001). Hemorrhage of the liver, which can result from alcohol use, has been shown to lead to gingival inflammation, bluish-red discoloration, and excessive bleeding; moreover, protein metabolism and tissue healing are affected by the consumption of alcohol (Friedlander, Marder, Pisegna, & Yagiela, 2003; Tezal et al., 2001). In vitro studies have suggested that ethanol stimulates bone resorption and blocks the stimulation of bone formation (Tezal et al., 2001; Farley, Fitzsimmons, Taylor, Jorch, & Lau, 1985). Alcohol may also have a direct toxic effect on the periodontal tissues (Tezal et al., 2001; Gottsegen, 1993).

An Erie County, New York cross-sectional study of 1371 subjects ages 25–74 found that individuals reporting high alcohol consumption experienced significantly higher levels of calculus, gingival bleeding, clinical attachment loss, and alveolar bone loss when compared to low alcohol consumers (Tezal et al., 2001). A moderate but consistent dose-dependent relationship between alcohol consumption and periodontal disease has also been found in the Third National Health and Nutrition Examination Survey sample (Tezal, Grossi, Ho, & Genco, 2004). The Health Professionals Follow-up Study of 51,529 male health professionals aged 40–75 years in 1986 found that after adjusting for age men who reported drinking from 0.1 to as much as 30 grams of alcohol per day had 18–27 percent higher risk of having periodontal disease than nondrinkers (Pitiphat et al., 2003). Moreover, compared to nondrinkers, men reporting regular alcohol consumption also were more likely to be smokers (Pitiphat et al., 2003).

Alcohol consumption is a risk factor for developing cancer of the mouth, pharynx, and esophagus (Sheiham & Watt, 2000). The Health Professionals Follow-up Study reported that the relative risk of oral premalignant lesions were higher for drinkers compared with nondrinkers (Maserejian, Joshipura, Rosner, Giovannucci, & Zavras, 2006). At baseline, average alcohol consumption was significantly related to oral premalignant lesions, increasing risk by approximately 22 percent with each additional drink per day (Maserejian et al., 2006). At 10-year follow-up, men who consumed at least 30 grams of alcohol per day at baseline had experienced a 3 times higher risk for oral premalignant lesions when compared with nondrinkers. Men with past or current tobacco use who consume alcohol had significantly increased risk of oral premalignant lesions (Maserejian et al., 2006).

Other oral conditions

Salivary gland enlargement can occur in patients with heavy alcohol consumption. This results in a condition known as sialadenosis (Friedlander et al., 2003). This is a result of peripheral autonomic neuropathy that causes disordered salivary metabolism and secretion (Friedlander et al., 2003; Mandel & Kastin, 2000; Mandel & Hamele-Bena, 1997). Sialadenosis is associated with decreased salivary flow. Individuals with reduced salivary flow often ingest sweetened candies or drinks; when coupled with neglect of oral hygiene that exists among persons with excessive alcohol consumption, an increase in dental plaque occurs. These individuals are at higher risk for dental caries and periodontal disease (Friedlander et al., 2003; Kampov-Polevoy, Tsoi, Zvartau, Neznanov, & Khalitov, 2001; Dutta, Orestes, Vengulekur, & Kwo, 1992; Dutta, Dukehart, Narang, & Latham, 1989).

Alcohol-induced nutritional deficiencies also include glossitis and angular cheilosis. (Friedlander et al., 2003). Glossitis manifests initially as swollen fungiform papillae with concomitant tongue pain. In a patient with chronic glossitis, a burning tongue is associated with frank redness and atrophy. Angular cheilosis is typified by ulcerations at the corners of the mouth (Friedlander et al., 2003; Schottenfeld & Pantalon, 1999; Dreizen, 1989).

Alcohol consumption may also result in excessive bleeding during oral surgery, and poor wound healing following oral surgery. Following extraction or alveolar surgery, alcohol abusers experience a higher incidence of osteomylitis (Friedlander et al., 2003; Tezal et al., 2001). Excessive bleeding may arise because long-term consumption of alcohol can result in the suppression of megakaryocyte maturation which leads to a decrease in the number of platelets, and thromboxane A and B release inhibition affecting platelet aggregation (Friedlander et al., 2003). Other complications of long-term alcohol ingestion are attributed to the suppression of T-lymphocyte activity, and the mobilization and phagocytic capability of monocytes, macrophages, and neutrophils (Tønnesen & Kehlet, 1999, Davies & Carr, 1990).

Fractures of the mandible are also more common in alcohol consumers. This is primarily due to falls, and to lifestyles associated with alcohol use (Smith, Shepherd, & Hodgson, 1998; Passeri, Ellis, & Sinn, 1993).

Oral Manifestations of Tobacco Use

In addition to being associated with a number of cancers and coronary conditions, tobacco plays a role in the etiology of a number of oral conditions – it is a primary risk factor for oral cancer as well as leukoplakia, periodontitis, and delayed wound healing (Mashburg & Samit, 1995; Day et al., 1993; Dietrich et al., 1992; Christen, 1992). Alcohol and tobacco use contribute to almost 75 percent of all oral cancer (i.e., cancer of the lip, tongue, floor of the mouth, palate, gingiva and alveolar mucosa, buccal mucosa, or oropharynx) incidence. Fifty percent of smokers will die from a smoking-related disease. Using any form of tobacco raises the risk for esophageal cancer. The longer tobacco is used the greater the risk, with the greatest risk among persons who combine alcohol use with tobacco use (Brown & Devesa, 2002). Ninety-five percent of cases of oral and throat cancer occur in persons aged 40 and over; and the average age at diagnosis is 60 years. Oral cancer accounts for 2 percent to 4 percent of cancers diagnosed each year in the United States, with about 2/3 of the cancers occurring in the oral cavity and 1/3 in the throat.

Oral mucosal changes are attributed to irritants such as temperature, the drying effects of smoke, tobacco toxins, carcinogens and changes in the local immune response. These changes include the following:

Leukoplakia is defined as a white patch, or plaque, on the oral mucosa that cannot be classified clinically as any other disease. Tobacco use is the primary cause of leukoplakic lesions. Tobacco users are more likely to have leukoplakia than nonusers. The frequency and length of tobacco use is directly related to the prevalence of leukoplakia.

Nicotinic stomatitis appears as a diffuse palatal keratosis with chronic inflammation of the palatal salivary glands. It does not become malignant and is reversible with cessation of tobacco use.

Smoker's melanosis is a melanin pigmentation stimulated by smoking that may occur in the attached gingiva of about 5–10 percent of smokers. It is more common in heavy smokers.

Chronic hyperplastic candidiasis is an adherent red or white plaque on the oral mucosa that may be flat or slightly elevated and may incorporate erythematous areas.

Leukoedema is a diffuse grayish-white, opalescent lesion of the buccal mucosa. It is often present bilaterally. This is a benign lesion and is present more frequently in smokers.

Hairy tongue is an overgrowth of the filiform papillae of the tongue that can trap plaque and tobacco residues, contributing to poor appearance and bad breath.

Chronic smoking can lead to increased prevalence and severity of periodontal disease, contributing to the loss of teeth and edentulism. Interestingly, studies have calculated that a substantial percentage of the variance of periodontitis in the population (as high as 50 percent) can be attributed to smoking alone (Tomar & Asma, 2000; Papapanou, 1996; Martinez Canut, Lorca, & Magan, 1995). Longitudinal studies of both treated and untreated periodontitis have shown higher progression of attachment loss or bone loss in smokers than nonsmokers (Bergström, Eliasson, & Dock , 2000). A dose–response relationship between exposure to smoking, measured in pack years, and extent and severity of progressive periodontitis has been demonstrated as well. Nonsmokers respond better to periodontal therapy than smokers (Christen, 1992). Smoking is the primary reason for loss of teeth among adults (Krall, Garvey, & Garcia, 1999). Tobacco use is associated with an increased risk for tooth loss. Cessation of tobacco use results in a reduction in risk for tooth loss (Dietrich et al., 2007).

Overall, smokers show less favorable response to conventional periodontal therapy than nonsmokers. The difference in response becomes particularly pronounced in more elaborate treatment procedures, such as regenerative periodontal therapies (guided tissue regeneration and grafting procedures), that have been shown to be significantly less successful and predictable in smokers (Tonetti, Pini Prato, & Cortellini, 1995). Finally, studies have demonstrated the beneficial effects of smoking cessation on periodontal health. Progression of bone loss was decreased in patients that quit smoking versus subjects that continued to smoke throughout the observation period (Bolin, Eklund, Frithiof, & Lavstedt 1993).

Recently, maternal tobacco use has been related to primary caries development in their children (Williams, Kwan, & Parsons, 2000). However, the link between dental caries and tobacco is not conclusive. Smokeless tobacco can contribute to increased acid attack on the enamel surface if the brand of tobacco contains high concentrations of sugar. Gingival recession often occurs in the location that the user habitually places his/her smokeless tobacco. There may, therefore be a higher incidence of cervical or root caries in smokeless tobacco users.

Smokeless tobacco use is associated with halitosis, loss of taste, periodontal disease, stained teeth, altered sense of smell, and intraoral lesions. Other dangers include gum recession that results in exposed roots and increased sensitivity to heat and cold, drifting and tooth loss from damage to gingival tissue, and abrasion to tooth enamel due to high levels of sand and grit contained in smokeless tobaccos (Tomar & Winn, 1999; Bowles, Wilkinson, Wagner, & Woody, 1995). Smokeless tobacco increases the risk for oral, pharyngeal, and esophageal cancer. Repetitive use of smokeless tobacco can cause a precancerous condition in the mouth called leukoplakia (Christen, 1985). Occurring on the lips or inside the cheek, leukoplakia is a white, leathery-appearing patch, which results in cancer diagnosis in 3–5 percent of cases. The risk of cancer in soft oral tissues is almost 50 times greater in long-term users than nonusers. Most smokeless tobaccos contain substantial quantities of nicotine, leading to a similar pattern of addiction as seen with cigarette smoking (Severson, 1993).

Cigar smoking is seen by many as an alternative to cigarette smoking. Occasional cigar smoking may pose serious health risks. There is increased risk for periodontal disease, which can lead to tooth and alveolar bone loss (Albandar, Streckfus, Adesanya, & Winn, 2000). Risk of lung cancer and heart disease may be the same as that of cigarette smokers. Cigar smokers also suffer from excessive tooth stain and chronic halitosis (bad breath) (Baker et al., 2000).

Cosmetic conditions such as tobacco stains are more difficult to treat successfully in smokers and smokeless tobacco users. Tobacco stains can penetrate into enamel and restorative materials, creating brown to yellow darkening of teeth, discoloration of nonmetallic restorations, and dark outlines around restorative margins. Tobacco staining of removable prosthetic appliances can be a problem; patients are frequently unable to remove tenacious stains.

Clinician's Role in the Assessment of Alcohol Use and Interventions

Alcohol misuse among older adults is a sizeable and growing concern. Problem drinking, and alcohol abuse or dependence, is notably higher among older adults seen in health care clinical settings (Oslin, 2004; Institute of Medicine, IOM, 1990; Callahan and Tierney, 1995; Barry et al., 1998; Joseph, Ganzini, & Atkinson, 1995). Problems related to alcohol use and abuse are said to be the largest class of substance use problems seen in older adults. Despite the increased susceptibility to substance abuse disorders in this population and the negative interactions that are possible between alcohol and psychoactive medications, health care clinicians often do not identify older adults who consume alcohol at risky levels. Most adults use medications and many of them may interact adversely with alcohol (Oslin, 2004). Alcohol misuse can be reduced or eliminated among many older adults through prevention and early intervention (Blow, Bartels, Brockmann, & Van Citters, 2005). Health care settings represent essential venues for the prevention of and early intervention with alcohol misuse among older adults. Identifying patients with alcohol problems can not only help reduce problem drinking but also reduce any negative health consequences. There are many signs and symptoms of alcohol use that can be identified in the health care setting, these include the following: (1) poor nutrition, (2) anxiety, (3) incontinence, (4) increased tolerance to alcohol or medications, (5) social isolation, (6) depression and mood swings, (7) headaches, (8) new difficulties in decision making, (9) poor hygiene, (10) falls, bruises, and burns, and (11) family problems (Barry, Oslin, & Blow, 2001). The American Geriatrics Society recommends that all patients 65 or older should be asked about their use of alcohol at least annually to identify possible alcohol use disorders (www.americangeriatrics.org). Research supports the use of early interventions or targeted prevention strategies such as brief advice by primary care physicians and other brief interventions in health care settings to reduce alcohol consumption among older adults (Blow et al., 2005).

A controlled clinical trial, Project GOAL (Guiding Older Adult Lifestyles), found that patients receiving two brief physician-delivered counseling sessions demonstrated a significant reduction in 7-day alcohol use, episodes of binge drinking, and frequency of excessive drinking at 3, 6, and 12 month follow-up compared with those just receiving a general health booklet (Fleming, Manwell, Barry, Adams, & Stauffacher, 1999). In a more recent study conducted by Fink et al., it was found that when physicians receive reports on their patients' alcohol use, risks, and problems, and their patients concomitantly receive personalized education based on these reports that harmful drinking was reduced in the patient group by 23 percent and nonhazardous drinking by 12 percent over a 12-month period when compared to control (Fink, Elliott, Tsai, & Beck, 2005). In the Health Profiles Project, older adults who screened positive for hazardous drinking were randomized either to a brief (20–25 minutes) alcohol intervention or control condition. Intervention group patients received an intervention appointment during which the clinician and patient review together a Brief Alcohol Intervention booklet that included the patient's self-reported drinking data and develop a contract to reduce at-risk drinking. Preliminary results show significantly more reduction in frequency and quantity of alcohol consumption for the brief intervention compared to the control condition. These results suggest that an easy-to-administer, elder-specific brief alcohol intervention is effective in reducing at-risk drinking among older adults and shows promise in improving long-term alcohol-related health outcomes for this population (Blow et al., 2005). Two studies that targeted alcohol-related health literacy in seniors demonstrated improvements in knowledge of alcohol misuse among older adults. (Fink, Beck, & Wittrock, 2001). Another study found that women age 54–90 years, particularly moderate to heavy drinkers, demonstrated improved knowledge regarding alcohol misuse and other health behaviors immediately after a 60-minute educational presentation (Eliason & Skinstad, 2001).

Quantity and frequency measures have been identified as essential screening tools among older adults, as recommended alcohol consumption levels for older adults are lower than those for adults under 65 years of age (Oslin, 2004; Blow, 1998; NIAAA, 1995a; NIAAA, 1995b). There are a number of screening tools that have been found valid and reliable in identifying patients with alcohol problems (U.S. Department of Health and Human Services, 2003). These screening tools are designed to integrate into the conventional clinical visit. The U.S. Department of Health and Human Services recommends the following four steps to screen and briefly intervene with patients having alcohol problems:

1. Ask

Ask involves inquiring how often and how much the patient drinks. This information is used to determine the weekly average alcohol intake by multiplying the number of days a week patient drinks by how many drinks they have on a typical day that they drink. If their weekly average exceeds 14 drinks for men or 7 for women, the patient is at risk for alcohol-related problems. An alternative risk calculation can be made by asking the patient how many drinks he or she has had on any given day in the past month. In this situation, the limits for men and women are 4 and 3 drinks, respectively. Additional questions are asked for patients whose alcohol intake puts them at risk and/or patients over 65 who are taking medications that may interact with alcohol. The second Ask step is to use a screening test. The commonly used CAGE assessment promoted by the USPHS does not have high validity with the elderly, particularly with women (Adams et al., 1996). The advantage of the CAGE is its short length and ease of use. If the CAGE is used, it should be complemented by an interview that includes questions about quantity and frequency of alcohol use, and questions about consequences. The CAGE series of questions to ask patients include the following:

1. Have you ever felt that you should *cut down* on your drinking?
2. Have people *annoyed* you by criticizing your drinking?
3. Have you ever felt *guilty* about your drinking?
4. Have you ever had a drink first thing in the morning to steady your nerves or get rid of a hangover (*eye-opener*)?

A 'no' to all questions indicates an at-risk patient; a 'yes' to 1 or 2 questions indicates alcohol-related problems; and 'yes' to 3 or 4 of the questions indicate alcohol abuse. Raised laboratory values for hepatic enzymes, gamma glutaryl transferase (gamma GT), or raised mean corpuscular volume are also indicative of alcohol abuse. Malnutrition, diabetes, insomnia, gastrointestinal problems, and confusion may also be indicative of alcohol dependence (Phillips & Katz, 2001). The Short Michigan Alcoholism Screening Test—Geriatric Version (SMAST-G) is an alternative assessment to the CAGE program and has been shown to have validity in a geriatric population (Blow, Gillespie, Barry, Mudd, & Hill, 1998). In this assessment instrument, two or more "yes" responses is indicative of alcohol problem (0–10 possible). The SMAST-G questions include the following:

1. When talking with others, do you ever underestimate how much you actually drink?
2. After a few drinks, have you sometimes not eaten or been able to skip a meal because you don't feel hungry?
3. Does having a few drinks help decrease your shakiness or tremors?
4. Does alcohol sometimes make it hard for you to remember parts of the day or night?
5. Do you usually take a drink to relax or calm your nerves?

6. Do you drink to take your mind off your problems?
7. Have you ever increased your drinking after experiencing a loss in your life?
8. Has a doctor or nurse ever said they were worried or concerned about your drinking?
9. Have you ever made rules to manage your drinking?
10. When you feel lonely, does having a drink help?

2. Assess

Assess is used to determine the course of action to be taken with the patient; this may result in advice to abstain or cut down alcohol consumption. Patients who are using alcohol and meditations that can interact with alcohol should be assessed for cessation advice. Patients who are alcohol abusers with a history of: (1) alcohol-related blackouts, (2) repeated failed attempts to cut down, (3) injuries related to alcohol use such as car-related injuries, (4) hypertension, trauma, depression, anxiety, sleep disorders, headaches, or sexual dysfunction, and (5) behavioral indicators such as problems at work, home or school, should be assessed for advice to abstain or cut down on alcohol use by their clinician. Patients considered at risk who do not have a significant medical history or social and behavioral manifestations of alcohol abuse should be directly advised to cut down on alcohol use. The process described is designed as a brief step. Clinicians can tailor their assessment using the U.S. Department of Health and Human Services guide.

3. Advise and Assist

The clinician states his or her concerns about the patient's drinking based on his or her, drinking patterns, and other factors such as preexisting conditions and family history. Direct advice is then provided to the patient to either abstain or cut down alcohol use. The patient's readiness to follow through is ascertained. If the patient is ready to cut down, the clinician should help him or her, to set a goal to lower his or her, drinking limit or abstain, and encourage him or her, to weigh the reasons he or she, should cut down against the reasons he or she has for drinking. If the patient is prepared to abstain, he or she should be counseled by the clinician or referred for additional evaluation or treatment. It is important to involve the patient in making these decisions.

4. Arrange Follow-Up

It is also important to arrange a follow-up visit to determine the patient's progress, offer additional support as needed, and monitor the patient for withdrawal symptoms. At these visits, it is important to determine and reassess goals and patient progress. The patient should be congratulated for positive changes and encouraged to make additional changes if warranted. Concern should be expressed for those not making positive changes. If patients require additional help, further follow-up visits should be scheduled.

Clinician's Role in Identifying Tobacco Use and Providing Cessation Advice

Smoking contributes to 7 of the top 14 causes of death for persons over 65 (Orleans, 1997). Approximately 70 percent of the smoking-attributable deaths discussed earlier in this chapter occur in persons over 65. Stopping smoking reduces overall risk for morbidity and mortality. Epidemiologic data suggest that more than 70 percent of the 50 million smokers in the United States today have made at least one prior quit attempt, and approximately 46 percent try to quit each year. Most smokers make several quit attempts before they successfully kick the habit.

Health care providers can play an important role in helping their patients attempt and accomplish cessation. Brief interventions by clinicians such as simply advising patients to quit have been shown to have a small beneficial effect, but a somewhat more intensive intervention is more effective resulting in about 10 percent of smokers being induced to abstain for at least a year (Fiore et al. 2000). Currently, physicians provide most tobacco cessation interventions, although it has been demonstrated that all health care providers can be effective. Clinical trials conducted with older patients reveal that they are responsive to standard smoking cessation programs and are equally or more likely than younger adults to succeed in quitting with a variety of evidence based behavioral and pharmacologic treatments (Morgan et al., 1996; Orleans 1997; Ossip-Klein, Carosella, & Krusch, 1997).

Older smokers are less likely than younger smokers to attempt quitting. Smokers are assessed using a stages of change model: (1) precontemplation (not currently considering a change), (2) contemplation (ambivalent about change), (3) preparation (some experience with change and are trying to change), (4) action (practicing new behavior), (5) maintenance (continued commitment to sustaining new behavior), and (5) relapse (resumption of old behaviors) (Prochaska, DiClemente, & Norcross, 1992). Older patients are more likely to be pre-contemplators than younger patients. This is because older patients have smoked longer and may have less interest in quitting. This group, however, has a greater likelihood of accomplishing a successful quit than younger smokers (Burns, 2000).

Clinical smoking cessation trials with older patients have reported increases in abstinence rates. Morgan et al. investigated the effectiveness of providing counseling for older smokers by trained health care workers using the National Cancer Institute (NCI) Clear Horizons pamphlet that was designed for older patient populations (Morgan et al. 1996; Glynn & Manley, 1989). The intervention group had a 15 percent abstinence rate, which was almost twice the rate in the usual care control group. In another study, smoking cessation rates in older patients (>60 years) were higher in those who received counseling by a primary care physician and nurse in comparison to routine primary care visits (Appel et al., 2003).

In the 1986 Adult Use of Tobacco Study, older smokers reported that although they had smoked for longer, they did not have a significantly greater number of quit attempts or different quitting intentions than younger smokers (Orleans, Jepson,

Resch, & Rimer, 1994). The most dramatic differences between the groups were in their beliefs on the benefits and harms of smoking. Older smokers underestimated the risks of smoking and more than their younger counterparts. Intention to quit was strongly related to the perceived health benefits of quitting. Although older adults in this study had a longer history of nicotine addiction, they were not significantly different from younger smokers on current smoking habits or past quitting histories. They also perceived the same general quitting barriers. Focus groups with older smokers revealed the belief that the damage caused by smoking had already been done and little could currently be done to reverse or slow the resulting disease. The similarities between older and younger smokers suggest that similar interventions for smoking cessation can be used on older and younger populations (Orleans et al., 1994).

It is important that clinicians provide a consistent and firm message to their patients that smoking can be stopped at any age. The older patients should be reassured that they will benefit from quitting. These benefits include improvements in lifestyle and overall health. Clinicians should provide information on how to quit and suggest pharmacotherapeutics to assist the nicotine-dependent patient in quitting. Tobacco dependence should be viewed as a chronic disease by the clinician, with quit attempts commonly followed by phases of remission and relapse before permanent abstinence. The USPHS guideline, "Treating Tobacco Use and Dependence", was implemented to provide clinicians with evidence based recommendations for assessment and treatment of tobacco dependence (Fiore et al., 2000). The key recommendations made by this document are summarized in five steps referred to as the 5As. These guidelines can be effectively implemented in most populations, and often require sessions as brief as 3 minutes (Fiore et al., 2000). The proper management of the patient requires an understanding of when it is appropriate to utilize the 5As in practice and alternatively when a patient's tobacco addiction requires referral and treatment within a more comprehensive setting. The 5As are (1) ask, (2) advise, (3) assess, (4) assist, and (5) arrange.

1. Ask – Identify and flag tobacco users

Before addressing a patient's tobacco use, the clinician should ask if he or she uses tobacco. This can be done by asking the patient directly when reviewing the patient's health history, or alternatively during the clinical exam. All it takes is four words, "Do you use tobacco?" Once it is established whether or not the patient uses tobacco, it is important to record the information in the patient's chart. This will make it easier to follow up when the patient returns for the next visit.

2. Advise – Give direct advice to quit

Clinicians should advise patients to quit at every visit. The patient should be urged to quit in a clear, strong, and personalized manner.

3. Assess – Is the patient ready to quit?

Clinicians often think that tobacco users do not want to discuss quitting. However, research has shown that the majority of smokers would like to quit. Even with patients who are not ready to quit using tobacco, it has been found that they are receptive to the clinician's advice. By getting patients to talk about their tobacco use, they may move closer to a decision to quit.

4. **Assist – Help patients to quit, using behavioral and pharmacological approaches**

   When patients express an interest in quitting, clinician's should assist them by giving them information that they can use that will help them quit. They can provide self-help materials, make referrals to local resources, and they may also want to discuss the use of pharmacotherapy, such as nicotine gum or patches.

5. **Arrange – Provide follow-up contact and encouragement**

   For those patients who make a commitment to quit, a call from the office on or before the patient's quit date has been proved to be a key factor in patients successfully quitting. For those who are not quite ready to quit, it is essential to discuss their tobacco use at every visit – each time it is discussed, the patient may move closer to making a decision to quit.

It is significant to recognize that stopping tobacco use is a process, and there are a number of stages of quitting – every patient a clinician counsels will not be able to quit immediately (Prochaska, 1992). The clinician should be persistent, and supportive of patients, regardless of stage of quitting.

Pharmacotherapies for Tobacco Cessation

At any level of supportive care, effective pharmacotherapy generally doubles the cessation rate compared to placebo (Fiore et al., 2000). Every smoker should be encouraged to use pharmacotherapies endorsed in the USPHS guideline, except in the presence of special circumstances (Fiore et al., 2000). The clinician should explain how these medications increase smoking cessation success and reduce withdrawal symptoms. First line pharmacotherapy agents include bupropion SR (Zyban® or Wellbutrin® SR), nicotine replacement therapy [nicotine gum, nicotine lozenge (Commit®) nicotine inhaler, nicotine nasal spray (Nicotrol NS®), nicotine patch], and Varenicline (Chantix®). Nicotine replacement therapy (NRT) is the most common type of pharmacotherapy. Side effects from NRTs include insomnia, headache and hypertension. Nicotine patch can cause skin irritation, and nicotine spray can cause nasal irritation. Bupropion SR is an antidepressant. The drug's mechanism of action in relation to smoking cession is thought to be mediated by noradrenergic and dopaminergic mechanisms, however, the exact mechanism has not been determined (Henningfield, Fant, Buchhalter, & Stitzer, 2005). A clinical trial with bupropion found that older patients (>50 years old) were more likely to be abstinent from smoking when using this medication than younger smokers (Dale et al., 2001). Side effects of bupropion include dry mouth, headache, insomnia, nausea, constipation and tremors. Bupropion has a long history of safe use in the elderly as an antidepressant. Seizures are reported as a rare side effect. The FDA approved Varenicline in 2006. It is a nicotinic receptor partial agonist. Side effects associated with Varenicline include nausea, constipation, vivid dreams, vomiting, sleep disturbance, and flatulence.

Tobacco use has profound oral and systemic effects. Treatment of tobacco users is cost-effective. Smoking cessation interventions are less costly than other routine medical interventions such as treatment of mild to moderate high blood pressure and preventive medical practices such as periodic mammography. Reimbursement for tobacco cessation treatment is limited. Most private insurance programs do not reimburse clinicians for tobacco cessation counseling interventions. Many State Medicaid programs now cover pharmacologic treatments. Medicare now covers two types of tobacco cessation counseling: (1) intermediate cessation counseling which is 3–10 minutes per session and (2) intensive cessation counseling which is greater than 10 minutes per session. Medicare will cover two quit attempts per year (http://www.cms.hhs.gov/SmokingCessation/).

Acknowledgments The author acknowledges the assistance of Ms. Sharifa Barracks who assisted with research and manuscript preparation.

References

Adams, W. L., Barry, K. L., & Fleming, M. F. (1996). Screening for problem drinking in older primary care patients. *Journal of the American Medical Association, 276(24)*, 1964–1967.

Albandar, J. M., Streckfus, C. F., Adesanya, M. R., & Winn, D. M. (2000). Cigar, pipe, and cigarette smoking as risk factors for periodontal disease and tooth loss. *Journal of Periodontology, 71(12)*, 1874–1881.

American Lung Association (2006). Smoking among older adults fact sheet. Retrieved January 29, 2007 from http://www.lungusa.org

Appel, D. W., & Aldrich, T. K. Smoking cessation in the elderly (2003). *Clinics in Geriatric Medicine, 19(1)*, 77–100.

Baker, F., Ainsworth, S. R., Dye, J. T., Crammer, C., Thun, M. J., & Hoffmann, D. (2000). Health risks associated with cigar smoking. *Journal of the American Medical Association, 284(6)*, 735–740.

Barry, K. L., & Blow, F. C. (2004), Older adults and alcohol problems. NIAAA Social Work Education module 10C. In A. Begun (Ed.), *Social Work Curriculum on Alcohol Use Disorders*. Bethesda, MD: NIH Publication No. 03-5386.

Barry, K. L., Blow, F. C., Walton, M. A., Chermack, S. T., Mudd, S. A., & Coyne, J. C. (1998). Elder-specific brief alcohol intervention: 3-month outcomes. *Alcoholism, Clinical and Experimental Research, 22*, 32A.

Barry, K. L., Oslin, D. W., & Blow, F. C. (2001). *Alcohol Problems in Older Adults*. New York: Springer Publishing Company.

Begun, A., & Manwell, L. B. (2004). Epidemiology of alcohol problems in the United States. NIAAA Social Work Education module 1. In A. Begun (Ed.), *Social Work Curriculum on Alcohol Use Disorders*. Bethesda, MD: NIH Publication No. 03-5386.

Bergström, J., Eliasson, S., & Dock, J. (2000). A 10-year prospective study of tobacco smoking and periodontal health. *Journal of Periodontology, 71*, 1338–1347.

Blow, F. C. (1998). *Substance abuse among older adults. Treatment Improvement Protocol (TIP) series no. 26*. Rockville, MD: U.S. Department of Health and Human Services, Public Health Service, Substance Abuse and Mental Health Services Administration, Center for Substance Abuse Treatment.

Blow, F. C. (2000). Substance use among older adults: an invisible epidemic. In F.C. Blow, (Ed. Consensus Panel Chair), *Substance abuse among older adults* (DHHS Publication No. SMA 98–3179, (TIP) Series 26, Chapter 1). Rockville, MD: Office of Applied Studies, Substance Abuse and Mental Health Services Administration.

Blow, F. C., & Barry, K. L. (2002). Use and misuse of alcohol among older women. *Alcohol Research & Health, 26(4)*, 308–315.

Blow, F. C., Gillespie, B. W., Barry, K. L., Mudd, S. A., & Hill, E. M. (1998). Brief screening for alcohol problems in elderly populations using the Short Michigan Alcohol Screening Test-Geriatric Version (SMAST-G). Alcoholism, *Clinical and Experimental Research, 22(Suppl)*, 131A.

Blow, F. C., Bartels, S. J., Brockmann, L. M., & Van Citters, A. D. (2005). Evidence-based practices for preventing substance abuse and mental health problems in older adults. Retrieved May 16, 2007 from http://www.samhsa.gov/OlderAdultsTAC/EBPLiteratureReviewFINAL.pdf.

Bolin, A., Eklund, G., Frithiof, L., & Lavstedt, S. (1993). The effect of changed smoking habits on marginal alveolar bone loss. A longitudinal study. *Swedish Dental Journal, 17*, 211–216.

Bowles, W. H., Wilkinson, M. R., Wagner, M. J., & Woody, R. D. (1995). Abrasive particles in tobacco products: a possible factor in dental attrition. *Journal of the American Dental Association, 126(3)*, 327–332.

Brown, L. M., & Devesa, S. S. (2002). Epidemiologic trends in esophageal and gastric cancer in the United States. *Surgical Oncology Clinics of North America, 11(2)*, 235–256.

Burns, D. M. (2000). Cigarette smoking among the elderly: Disease consequences and the benefits of cessation. *American Journal of Health Promotion, 14(6)*, 357–361.

Callahan, C. M., & Tierney, W. M. (1995). Health services use and mortality among older primary care patients with alcoholism. *Journal of the American Geriatrics Society, 43(12)*, 1378–1383.

Carosella, A. M., Ossip-Klein, D. J., Watt, C. A., & Podgorski, C. (2002) Smoking history, knowledge, and attitudes among older residents of a long-term care facility. *Nicotine & Tobacco Research, 4*, 161–169.

Centers for Disease Control (2002). Cigarette smoking among adults – United States – 2000. *Morbidity and Mortality Weekly Report, 51(29)*, 642–645.

Centers for Disease Control (2006). Tobacco use among adults—United States, 2005. *Morbidity and Mortality Weekly Report, 55(42)*, 1145–1148.

Centers for Medicare and Medicaid Services (2007). Smoking Cessation. Retrieved May 16, 2007 from: http://www.cms.hhs.gov/SmokingCessation/

Chapman, S. (1993). The role of doctors in promoting smoking cessation. *British Medical Journal, 307*, 518–519.

Christen, A. G. (1992). The impact of tobacco use and cessation on oral and dental diseases and conditions. *American Journal of Medicine, 93(1A)*, 25S–31S.

Christen, A. G. (1985). The four most common alterations of the teeth, periodontium and oral soft tissues observed in smokeless tobacco users: a literature review. *Journal of Indiana Dental Association, 64(3)*, 15–18.

Connett, J. E., Murray, R. P., Buist, A. S., Wise, R. A., Bailey, W. C., Lindgren, P. G., et al. (2003). Changes in smoking status affect women more than men: results of the lung health study. *American Journal of Epidemiology, 157*, 973–979.

Dale, L. C., Glover, E. D., Sachs, D. P., Schroeder, D. R., Offord, K. P., Croghan, I. T., et al. (2001). Bupropion for smoking cessation: Predictors of successful outcome. *Chest, 119*, 1357–1364.

Davies, H. T., & Carr, R. J.(1990). Osteomyelitis of the mandible: a complication of routine dental extractions in alcoholics. *British Journal of Oral Maxillofacial Surgery, 28*, 185–188.

Dawson, D. A., & Archer, L. D. (1993). Relative frequency of heavy drinking and the risk of alcohol dependence. *Addiction, 88(11)*, 1509–1518.

Day, G. I., Blot, W. J., Austin, D. F., Bernstein, L., Greenberg, R. S., Preston-Martin, S., et al. (1993). Racial differences in risk of oral and pharyngeal cancer: alcohol, tobacco and other determinants. *Journal of the National Cancer Institue, 85*, 465–473.

Dietrich, A. J., O'Connor, G. T., Keller, A., Carney, P. A., Levy, D., & Whaley,F. S. (1992). Cancer: improving early detection and prevention. *British Medical Journal, 304*, 687–691.

Dietrich, A. J., Maserejian, N. N., Joshipura, K. J., Krall, E. A., & Garcia, R. I. (2007). Tobacco use and incidence of tooth loss among US male health professionals. *Journal of Dental Research, 86(4)*, 373–377.

Dreizen, S. (1989). Dietary and nutritional counseling in the prevention and control of oral disease. *Compendium, 10*, 558–564.

Dufour, M., & Fuller, R. K. (1995). Alcohol in the elderly. *Annual Review of Medicine, 46*, 123–132.

Dutta, S. K., Dukehart, M., Narang, A., & Latham, P. S. (1989). Functional and structural changes in parotid glands of alcoholic cirrhotic patients. *Gastroenterology, 96*, 510–518.

Dutta, S. K., Orestes, M., Vengulekur, S., & Kwo, P. (1992). Ethanol and human saliva: effect of chronic alcoholism on flow rate, composition, and epidermal growth factor. *American Journal of Gastroenterology, 87*, 350–354.

Eliason, M. J., & Skinstad, A. H. (2001). Drug & alcohol intervention for older women: a pilot study. *Journal of Gerontological Nursing, 27(12)*, 18–24; quiz 40–11.

Farley, J. R., Fitzsimmons, R., Taylor, A. K., Jorch, U. M., & Lau, K. H. (1985). Direct effects of ethanol on bone resorption and formation in vitro. *Achives of Biochemistry and Biophysics, 238*, 305–314.

Fink, A., Beck, J. C., & Wittrock, M. C. (2001). Informing older adults about non-hazardous, hazardous, and harmful alcohol use. *Patient Education and Counseling, 45(2)*, 133–141.

Fink, A., Elliott, M. C., Tsai, M., & Beck, J. C. (2005). An evaluation of an intervention to assist primary care physicians in screening and educating older patients who use alcohol. *Journal of the American Geriatrics Society, 53*, 1937–1943.

Fiore, M. C., Bailey, W. C., Cohen, S. J., Dorfman, S. F., Goldstein, M. G., Gritz, E. R., et al. (2000). Treating tobacco use and dependence: clinical practice guideline. US Department of Health and Human Services, Public Health Service. Retrieved January 20, 2007, from http://www.surgeongeneral.gov/tobacco/treating_tobacco_use.pdf.

Fleming, M. F., Manwell, L. B., Barry, K. L., Adams, W., & Stauffacher, E. A. (1999). Brief phycisian advice for alcohol problems in older adults: a randomized community-based trial. *The Journal of Family Practice, 48(5)*, 378–384.

Folsom, A. R., & Grimm, R. H. (1987). Stop smoking advice by physicians: A feasible approach? *American Journal of Public Health, 77*, 849–850.

Friedlander, A. H., Marder, S. R., Pisegna, J. R., & Yagiela, J. A. (2003). Alcohol abuse and dependence: Psycopathology, medical management and dental implications. *Journal of the American Dental Association, 134*, 731–740.

Gfroerer, J. (2004). Substance use among older adults (age 50+): current prevalence and future expectations. *Proceedings from Drug Abuse in the 21st Century: What Problems Lie Ahead for the Baby Boomers?* Bethesda, MD: National Institute on Drug Abuse.

Glynn T. J., & Manley, M. W. (1989). *How to Help Your Patients Stop Smoking: A National Cancer Institute Manual for Physicians*. Washington D.C.: U.S. Department of Health and Human Services, National Institutes of Health NIH Publication No. 89: 3064.

Gottsegen, R. (1993). Diabetes mellitus, cardiovascular diseases, and alcoholism. In S. Schulger, R. Yuodelis, R. C. Page, & R. H. Johnson (Eds.), *Perdiontal Diseases*(pp. 273–282). Philadelphia, PA: Lea & Febiger.

Harris, C., Warnakulasuriya, K. A., Gelbier, S., Johnson, N. W., & Peters, T. J. (1997). Oral and dental health in alcohol misusing patients. *Alcoholism: Clinical and Experimental Research, 21(9)*, 1707–1709.

Helzer, J. E., Burnam, A., & McEvoy, L. T. (1991). Alcohol abuse and dependence. In L. N. Robbins & D. A. Reiger (Eds.), *Psychiatric Disorders in America: The Epidemiologic Catchment Area Study*. New York: The Free Press, 81–115.

Henley, S. J., Thun, M. J., Chao, A., & Calle, E. E. (2004). Association between exclusive pipe smoking and mortality from cancer and other diseases. *Journal of the National Cancer Institute, 96(11)*, 853–861.

Henningfield, J. E., Fant, R. V., Buchhalter, A. R., & Stitzer, M. L. (2005). Pharmacotherapy for nicotine dependence. *Cancer Journal for Clinicians, 55(5)*, 281–299.

Institute of Medicine, IOM (1990). Who provides treatment? In Committee of the Institute of Medicine, Division of Mental Health and Behavioral Medicine (Ed.), *Broadening the Base of Treatment for Alcoholism*, 98–141. Washington D.C.: National Academy Press.

Joseph, C. L., Ganzini, L., & Atkinson, R. (1995). Screening for alcohol use disorders in the nursing home. *Journal of the American Geriatrics Society, 43(4)*, 368–373.

Kampov-Polevoy, A. B., Tsoi, M. V., Zvartau, E. E., Neznanov, N. G., & Khalitov, E. (2001). Sweet liking and family history of alcoholism in hospitalized alcohol and non-alcoholic patients. *Alcohol and Alcoholism, 36(2)*, 65–170.

Korper, S. P., & Council, C. L. (Eds.). (2002). Substance use by older adults: *Estimates of future impact on the treatment system*. Rockville, MD: Office of Applied Studies, Substance Abuse and Mental Health Services Administration (DHHS Publication No. SMA 03-3763, Analytic Series A-21).

Krall, E. A., Garvey, A. J., & Garcia, R. I. (1999). Alveolar bone loss in male cigar and pipe smokers. *Journal of the American Dental Association, 130*, 57–64.

Mandel, L., & Hamele-Bena, D. (1997). Alcoholic parotid sialadenosis. *Journal of the American Dental Association, 128*, 1411–1415.

Mandel L., & Kastin, B. (2000). *Alcoholic sialosis. New York State Dental Journal, 66*, 22–24.

Martinez Canut, P., Lorca, A., & Magan, R. (1995). Smoking and periodontal disease severity. *Journal of Clinical Periodontology, 22*, 743–749.

Maserejian, N. N., Joshipura, K. J., Rosner, B. A., Giovannucci, E., & Zavras, A. I. (2006). Prospective study of alcohol consumption and risk of oral premalignant lesions in men. *Cancer Epidemiology Biomarkers & Prevention, 15(4)*, 774–781.

Mashburg, A., & Samit, A. (1995). Early diagnosis of asymptotic oral and oropharyngeal squamous cancers. *Cancer Journal for Clinicians, 45*, 328–351.

Morgan, G. D., Noll, E. L., Orleans, C. T., Rimer, B. K., Amfoh, K., & Bonney, G. (1996). Reaching midlife and older smokers: tailored interventions for routine medical care. *Preventive Medicine, 25(3)*, 346–354.

National Institute on Alcohol Abuse and Alcoholism, (1995**a**). *The physician's guide to helping patients with alcohol problems*. Rockville, MD: US Department of Health and Human Services, Public Health Service, National Institutes of Health, NIAAA, NIH publication no. 95-3769.

National Institute on Alcohol Abuse and Alcoholism. (1995**b**). Diagnostic criteria for alcohol abuse. *Alcohol Alert, 30(PH359)*, 1–6.

Orleans, C. T. (1997). Reducing tobacco harms among older adults: a critical agenda for tobacco control. *Tobacco Control, 6(3)*, 161–163.

Orleans C. T., Jepson, C., Resch, N., & Rimer, B. K.(1994). Quitting motives and barriers among older smokers. The 1986 Adult Use of Tobacco Survey revisited. *Cancer, 74(7 Suppl)*, 2055–2061.

Oslin, D. W. (2004). Late-life alcoholism: Issues relevant to the geriatric psychiatrist. *American Journal of Geriatric Psychiatry, 12(6)*, 571–583.

Ossip-Klein, D. J., Carosella, A. M., & Krusch, D. A. (1997). Self-help interventions for older smokers. *Tobacco Control, 6(3)*, 188–193.

Ott, A., Slooter, A. J. C., Hofman, A., van Harskamp, F., Witteman, J. C., Van Broeckhaven, C., et al. (1998). Smoking and risk of dementia and Alzheimer's disease population-based cohort study: The Rotterdam Study. *The Lancet, 351(9119)*, 1840–1843.

Papapanou, P. N. (1996). Periodontal diseases: Epidemiology. *Annals of Periodontology, 1*, 36.

Passeri, L. A., Ellis, E., & Sinn, D. P. (1993). Relationship of substance abuse to complications with mandibular fractures. *Journal of Oral Maxillofacial Surgery, 51*, 22–25.

Phillips, P., & Katz, A. (2001). Substance misuse in older adults: an emerging policy priority. *Nursing Times Research, 6(6)*, 898–905.

Pitiphat, W., Merchant, A. T., Rimm, E. B., & Joshipura, K. J. (2003). Alcohol consumption increases periodontitis risk. *Journal of Dental Research, 82(7)*, 509–513.

Prochaska J. O., DiClemente, C. C. & Norcross, J. C. (1992). In search of how people change. Applications to addictive behaviors. *American Psychology, 47(9)*, 1102–1114.

Rimer B., Orleans T., Keintz, M., Cristinzio, S., & Fleisher, L. (1990) The older smoker. Status, challenges and opportunities for intervention. *Chest, 97(3)*, 547–553.

Robb N. D., & Smith, B. G., (1996). Chronic alcoholism: An important condition in the dentist-patient relationship. *Journal of Dentistry, 24(1–2)*, 17–24.

Schonfeld L., & Dupree, L. W. (1995). Treatment approaches for older problem drinkers. *International Journal of the Addictions, 30(13&14)*, 1819–1842.

Schottenfeld, R. S., & Pantalon, M. V. (1999). Assessment of the patient. In *Textbook of Substance Abuse Treatment*, Galanter, M. (Ed.). American Psychiatric Press: Washington, 109–119.

Severson, H. H. (1993). Smokeless tobacco: Risk, epidemiology and cessation. In C. T. Orleans & J. Slade (Eds.) *Nicotine addiction; principals and management* (pp. 262–278). New York: Oxford University Press.

Sheiham, A., & Watt, R.G. (2000). The common risk factor approach: a rational basis for promoting oral health. *Community Dentistry and Oral Epidemiology, 28*, 399–406.

Smith A. J., Shepherd, J. P., & Hodgson, R. J. (1998), Brief interventions for patients with alcohol-related trauma. *British Journal of Oral Maxillofacial Surgery, 36*, 408–415.

Smith J. W. (1995) Medical manifestations of alcoholism in the elderly. *International Journal of the Addictions 30(13&14)*, 1749–1798.

Taylor, D., Hasselblad, V., Henley, J., Thun, M. D., & Sloan, F. A. (2002). Benefits of smoking cessation for longevity, *American Journal of Public Health, 92*, 990–996.

Tezal, M., Grossi, S. G., Ho, A. W., & Genco, R. J., (2001). The effect of alcohol consumption on periodontal disease. *Journal of Periodontology, 72*, 183–189.

Tezal, M., Grossi, S. G., Ho, A. W., & Genco, R. J. (2004). Alcohol consumption and periodontal disease: The Third National Health and Nutrition Examination Survey. *Journal of Clinical Periodontology, 31*, 484–488.

The Center for Social Gerontology. (2001). Fact sheet on tobacco & older persons. Retrieved January 29, 2007 from http://www.tcsg.org/tobacco/facts.htm.

The NSDUH Report. (2005). Substance use among older adults: 2002 and 2003 update. Retrieved January 30, 2007 from http://www.oas.samhsa.gov/2k5/olderadults/olderadults.htm.

Thun, M. J., Peto, R., Lopez, A. D., Monaco, J. H., Henley, J., Heath,C., et al. (1997). Alcohol consumption and mortality among middle-aged and elderly U.S. adults. *The New England Journal of Medicine, 337(24)*, 1705–1714.

Tomar, S. L., & Winn, D. M. (1999). Chewing tobacco use and dental caries among U.S. men. *Journal of the American Dental Association, 30(11)*, 1601–1610.

Tomar, S. L., & Asma, S. (2000). Smoking-attributable periodontitis in the United States: 0findings from NHANES III. *Journal of Periodontology, 71*, 743–751.

Tonetti, M. S., Pini Prato, G., & Cortellini, P. (1995). Effect of cigarette smoking on periodontal healing following GTR in infrabony defects. A preliminary retrospective study. *Journal of Clinical Periodontology, 22*, 229–234.

Tønnesen, H., & Kehlet, H. (1999). Preoperative alcoholism and postoperative morbidity. *British Journal of Surgery, 86*, 869–874.

U.S. Department of Health and Human Services. (1999). *Mental health: a report of the Surgeon General*. Rockville, MD: U.S. Department of Health and Human Services, Substance Abuse and Mental Health Services Administration, Center for Mental Health Services, National Institute of Mental Health.

U.S. Department of Health and Human Services. (2003). *Helping patients with alcohol problems: a health practitioner's guide*. Rockville, MD: National Institute on Alcohol Abuse and Alcoholism, National Institutes of Health, U.S. Department of Health and Human Services. NIH Publication No. 03-3769.

U.S. Department of Health and Human Services. (2004). *Health consequences of smoking: a report of the surgeon general*. Rockville, MD: U.S. Department of Health and Human Services.

Williams, S. A., Kwan, S. Y., & Parsons, S. (2000). Parental smoking practices and caries experience in pre-school children. *Caries Research, 34(2)*, 117–122.

Part III
Oral Health and Dental Considerations

Chapter 11
Normal Oral Mucosal, Dental, Periodontal, and Alveolar Bone Changes Associated with Aging

Stefanie L. Russell and Jonathan A. Ship

Introduction

Importance of Oral Hard and Soft Tissues in Maintaining Oral and Systemic Health

The oral hard and soft tissues assist in three essential functions in human physiology: (1) the initiation of alimentation, (2) protection of the host, and (3) communication. The teeth, the periodontium, the alveolar supporting bone, and the mucosal soft tissues exist to prepare food for deglutition. The oral cavity is exposed to the external world and is potentially vulnerable to a limitless number of environmental insults. Accordingly, oral mucosal tissues in addition to saliva and a complex array of neuro- and chemo-sensory tissues provide host defense against a plethora of potential dangerous microbes and noxious compounds. They also contribute to the enjoyment of food and alert a person to potential problems. The tongue, muscles of facial expression and mastication, and oral mucosal tissues enable speech and communication. Importantly, the activities of the oral hard and soft tissues, muscles of mastication and facial expression, and neuro- and chemo-sensory tissues are finely coordinated, and a disturbance in any one function can significantly compromise speech, alimentation, host defense, and diminish the quality of a patient's life.

With the increased longevity of many older populations in the world, there has arisen greater risk for developing oral disorders. Furthermore, significant increases in the retention of teeth have occurred in recent decades (Beltrán-Aguilar et al., 2005), which has resulted in a greater number of tooth surfaces at risk for dental decay and periodontal diseases in older populations. Therefore, there is a greater burden on health care practitioners to prevent, identify and expeditiously treat oral hard and soft tissue disorders in older adults. Prompt treatment and identification of these disorders will prevent the development of problems with

S.L. Russell
Assistant Professor, Department of Epidemiology and Health Promotion, New York University College of Dentistry
e-mail: stefanie.russell@nyu.edu

I.B. Lamster, M.E. Northridge (eds.), *Improving Oral Health for the Elderly*,
© Springer Science+Business Media, LLC 2008

pain, mastication and deglutition, communication, and host defense, and ultimately protect and enhance a person's quality of life.

Importance of Differentiating Aging from Effects of Disease and Its Treatment

Both aging *and* systemic diseases and their treatments can influence the health and function of the oral soft and hard tissues, and it is important that one identify whether changes are due to one process or the other. Age-related changes of the oral tissues are summarized in Table 11.1. For example, while teeth naturally undergo time (age)-associated deterioration, soft tissues can remain remarkably resistant to clinically significant disorders in older healthy adults. In general, healthy older adults will not necessarily experience significant destruction of oral hard and soft tissues in the absence of oral and/or systemic pathology. Rather oral changes associated with these oral pathology (e.g., dental caries, periodontal attachment loss, salivary dysfunction), systemic conditions (e.g., diabetes, stroke, Alzheimer's disease, cancer), and treatments of these diseases (prescription and non-prescription medications, head and neck radiotherapy) predispose older persons to either initiation or progression of oral soft and hard tissue disease (Ciancio 2005; Tsai et al., 2002; Ship and Puckett 1994). Furthermore, the effects of *oral* diseases are likely not limited to the oral cavity: recent evidence suggests that bacterial infections of the oral cavity, including periodontal disease, can disseminate systemically via the blood or via aspiration, and lead to severe, even life-threatening consequences (Yoneyama et al., 2002; Shay 2002). Systemic mucocutaneous and dermatological diseases can also manifest in the oral cavity, which can predispose older individuals to additional oral and pharyngeal problems.

Oral Mucosal Tissues

Effects of Aging on Oral Mucosal Tissues

Clinical Effects

The primary function of the oral mucosa is to act as a barrier to protect the underlying structures from desiccation, noxious chemicals, trauma, thermal stress, and infection. The oral mucosa plays a key role in the defense of the oral cavity, and contributes to chewing, speaking, and swallowing. Aging is frequently associated with changes in the oral mucosa similar to those in the skin, with the epithelium becoming thinner, less hydrated (Shklar 1966) and thus supposedly more susceptible to injury. Clinically, however, studies have found that the appearance of the oral mucosa does not change with age (Wolff et al., 1991; Ship and Baum 1993) and aging *per se* does not appear to increase risk for oral mucosal lesions (MacEntee et al., 1998). The tongue becomes smoother with loss of filiform papillae, and other sites develop extravasated venules or varices (Ettinger, Manderson 1974). However,

Table 11.1 Age-Related Changes* in the Oral Tissues

Tissue	Histological Changes	Clinical Appearance	Clinical Implications
Oral Mucosa			
Epithelium	• **Loss of elasticity** • **Decreased width** • **Diminished keratinization**	• **Thinning** • **Loss of hydration (especially if there is loss of salivary output)** • **Satin-like**	• **May be more susceptible to trauma** • **If desiccated, more likely to develop fissures, abrasions, traumatic ulcers**
Tongue	• **loss of filiform papillae** • **increased varices**	• **increased smoothness** • **increased varices**	none
Periodontium			
Gingival Connective Tissue	• **increase in density** • **decreased fibroblasts** • **increased collagen content** • **increased stability of collagen fibers**	**NA**	none
Periodontal Ligament	• **possible increase in width** • **reduced number of epithelial cell rests**	**NA**	none
Alveolar Bone	• **increase in width of periosteum** • **decreased width of the cortical plate**	**NA**	• **possible increased fragility**
Teeth			
Enamel	• **decreased width**	• **change in color and form** • **loss of translucency**	• **esthetic considerations**
Dentin	• **increased width** • **obturation of dentinal tubules** • **decrease in number and length of odontoblasts** • **decreased regenerative capacity**	**NA**	• **decreased tooth sensitivity** • **increased, or decreased likelihood of need for endodontic therapy**
Cementum	• **increased width**	**NA**	none
Pulp	• **decreased vascularity** • **increased fiber cross-linking** • **increased likelihood of pulp stone formation**	**NA**	• **decreased tooth sensitivity**

* In many cases the evidence is inconclusive as to whether these changes are due entirely to aging, or whether they are disease-related.

these mucosal changes do not necessarily result in clinically important effects on mucosal function. In the presence of reduced salivary output, the mucosa becomes desiccated and more likely to develop fissures, abrasions, and traumatic lesions. Use of removable prostheses, ill-fitting fixed and removable prostheses, and salivary hypofunction are local conditions that affect the health and function of the oral mucosal tissues in the elderly (Janket et al., 2007; Shulman et al., 2004). The oral mucosa is also a common site for vesiculobullous, desquamative, ulcerative, lichenoid, infectious, and malignant lesions, and many of these lesions present with greater frequency in the elderly (Shulman et al., 2004). In general, regularly scheduled head, neck, and oral examinations are required to diagnose oral mucosal diseases at an early stage and to intervene with appropriate therapy. Importantly, even edentulous older adults should be seen annually to evaluate for benign and malignant oral mucosal lesions.

Histopathological Effects

Stratified squamous epithelium has been found to become thinner, lose elasticity, and atrophy with age (Shklar 1966). In addition, age-associated declines in immunological responsiveness are likely to increase susceptibility to infection and trauma (Kay 1979). There are multiple reasons for these age-related changes, including alterations in protein synthesis and responsiveness to growth factors and other regulatory mediators. Cell renewal and protein synthesis associated with oral mucosal keratinization occur at a slower rate in aging individuals. Alternatively, normal tissue architecture and patterns of histodifferentiation do not display any changes with age. There are changes in the oral mucosal vascularity that impair mucosal integrity due to reductions in cellular access to nutrients and oxygenation. Mucosal, alveolar, and gingival arteries demonstrate the effects of arteriosclerosis.

Pathological Conditions of Oral Mucosal Tissues in Older Adults

Oral Cancer

The oral mucosal disease with the greatest potential morbidity and mortality is cancer. Nearly 30,000 cases of head and neck cancer are diagnosed each year in the United States, resulting in nearly 8000 deaths per year (Jemal et al., 2007). The three greatest risk factors for developing oral cancer are older age, alcohol, and tobacco use. Nearly half of all oral cancers occur in persons older than 65 years of age with 5-year survival of only 30%–50%, depending upon age, race/ethnicity and sex (Morse and Kerr 2006). Neoplasms may arise in all oral soft and hard tissues and in the oropharyngeal and salivary gland regions. There is a diverse appearance of these cancers (ulcerative, erythematous, leukoplakic, papillary), which can be asymptomatic (Mashberg and Samit 1995). If a patient presents with an unusual and suspicious lesion with no readily apparent etiology (such as a denture sore), the patient should be referred to a specialist more familiar with the appearance of the oral mucosa. Carcinoma should be considered part of the differential diagnosis of any oral lesion.

Vesicullo-bullous, Ulcerative, and Erosive Diseases

There are numerous oral mucosal disorders that affect the elderly population, ranging from benign (e.g., recurrent aphthous ulcers, and traumatic lesions) to malignant (e.g., squamous cell carcinomas). A simple three-item classification is helpful: (1) acute multiple lesions (e.g., erythema multiforme, herpes simplex, herpes zoster, allergic reaction), (2) recurring oral ulcers (e.g., recurrent aphthous stomatitis, traumatic ulcer), and (3) chronic multiple lesions (e.g., pemphigus vulgaris, mucous membrane pemphigoid, lupus erythematosus, lichen planus, dysplasia, squamous cell carcinoma). If a lesion does not resolve after 2–3 weeks, a tissue biopsy is required. For lesions that are suspected to be oral manifestations of autoimmune connective tissue disorders (e.g., pemphigus, pemphigoid, lichen planus), biopsies should also include specimens for direct immunofluorescence.

Oral Mucosal Infections (Bacterial, Viral, Fungal)

A host of microbial infections occur in the elderly and can be life threatening in the severely immunocompromised older adult when disseminated to pharyngeal, pulmonary, and vascular tissues. Common bacterial infections are found in dental caries (e.g., *Streptococcus mutans*), while uncommonly *Staphylococcus* infections can occur in perioral tissues. Herpes simplex vesicles occur on labial (herpes labialis) and intraoral mucosal locations, particularly in immunocompromised adults. Herpes zoster (shingles) affects the dermatomes of the 1st, 2nd, and 3rd divisions of the trigeminal nerve in a unilateral fashion, and can cause long-term intractable pain and permanent neurosensory dysfunction. Oral fungal infections are common in older adults (e.g., *Candida albicans*) and have a wide variety of presentations, ranging from leukoplakic pseudomembraneous and removable plaques to non-removable hyperplastic and erythematous nodules. Precipitating factors include salivary hypofunction; use of antibiotics, corticosteroids, and other immunomodulating drugs; and wearing removable prostheses.

Pathological Conditions of Oral Mucosal Tissues Due to Common Conditions

Salivary Hypofunction

Salivary hypofunction and complaints of a dry mouth (xerostomia) are not considered to be normal sequelae of aging. Rather, many medications taken by older persons, radiation for head and neck neoplasms, cytotoxic chemotherapy, and a host of medical disorders (most commonly being Sjögren's syndrome), cause salivary hypofunction. Without adequate salivary output, mucosal tissues become desiccated and cracked, leaving the host more susceptible to microbial infection. Furthermore, salivary hypofunction can lead to difficulty in swallowing or speaking at length, pain (arising from either the teeth or oral soft tissues), impaired denture use, altered taste, and diminished food enjoyment.

Denture Use

The denture-bearing mucosa of aged maxillary and mandibular ridges shows significant morphologic changes. Ill-fitting dentures can produce mechanical trauma to the oral tissues as well as cause mucosal hyperplasia (MacEntee et al. 1998). Oral candidiasis frequently is found on denture-bearing areas in an edentulous individual, often occurring with angular cheilitis (deep fissuring and ulceration of the epithelium at the commissures of the mouth) (Lyon et al., 2006).

Radiotherapy

External beam radiotherapy treatment for head and neck cancer causes a host of short-term and permanent head and neck complications. Desiccated and ulcerated mucosal tissues, dysphagia, skin burns, fibrotic head and neck muscles, dental caries, microbial infections, impaired use of dentures, and dysgeusia are all common sequelae.

Medications

Numerous medications have been associated with oral mucosal changes. For example, long-term use of antibiotics frequently results in oral candidal infections, while drugs with xerostomic side effects increase the potential for mucosal injury. Drugs commonly used in older patients for arthritic conditions, hypertension, cardiac arrhythmias, seizures, and dementia are associated with lichenoid mucosal reactions.

The Periodontium

Effects of Aging on the Periodontium

Clinical and Histopathological Effects

The periodontium comprises those structures that support the teeth; it includes the gingival connective tissue, the periodontal ligament, the cementum, and the alveolar (i.e., tooth-supporting) bone. As is the case with other body tissues, there are limitations in the knowledge of what constitutes "normal aging." Results of many studies which attempt to answer this question are limited in their ability to define tissue changes that result from aging, since comparisons of older and younger cohorts might represent changes that occur for reasons other than age, for example, increased disease prevalence in the older cohort, or period or birth effects. In general, however, studies of age-associated changes of the periodontium have failed to identify clinical changes that appear to be solely related to age as opposed to diseases that are age-associated. Histopathological, as opposed to clinical changes, however, have been found to occur with age. Age-associated changes in the gingival connective tissue are comparable to changes in similar tissues found elsewhere in the body. The number of fibroblasts in the gingival connective tissue and the periodontal ligament decreases with age (Ryan et al., 1974) and the collagen content of the gingival connective tissue appears to increase with age (Hill 1984). In addition, the stability and biomechanical strength of the gingival collagen increases with age, and a greater proportion of collagen is insoluble, as opposed to soluble, and there is an overall decrease in the rate of collagen turnover (Johnson et al., 1986). Age-associated changes in the periodontal ligament include a decrease in overall fiber content (Severson et al., 1978). In addition, periodontal ligament cell repair appears to be impaired with aging due to a decrease in proliferative ability (Shiba et al., 2000). Studies that have examined the width of the periodontal ligament over time are inconclusive; changes in the periodontal ligament are closely related to the continuous apposition of cementum that has been seen to occur over time. Like other bones in the body, the regenerative capacity of the alveolar bone appears to be unrelated to age, *per se*. However, loss of the alveolar bone with age is implied in studies that have shown an increase in tooth loss, and a decrease in alveolar bone height (as well as a decrease in mandibular and maxillary bone height in edentulous persons) over time as populations age. Bone loss that occurs over time due to chronic periodontal disease should not be seen, however, as a natural aging process; while loss periodontal attachment in older persons is common, periodontal disease, be it in young or older persons, is an infectious disease caused by oral bacteria.

Pathological Changes as a Result of Common Conditions in the Elderly

Increased Plaque Retention and Gingivitis

Gingivitis, which manifests clinically as edema and erythema of the marginal gingival, is an inflammatory response of the gingival tissues to bacterial plaque, an oral biofilm that collects along the tooth surface at the gingival margin and comprises bacteria and their by-products. Classic studies have shown that in the absence of oral hygiene, gingivitis will develop more rapidly in older (65–78 year old) persons compared to younger (20–24 year old) persons (Holm-Pedersen et al., 1975). The reason for the difference seen is most likely related to the concomitant increased plaque accumulation seen in the older group. Most importantly, however, while gingivitis developed faster in the older group, when oral hygiene was resumed, both older and younger groups returned to a clinically healthy state in a matter of days. While reasons for the difference in experimental gingivitis rate seen may be attributed to both differences in the oral flora that developed over the experimental time (that were seen to vary by age group) (Holm-Pedersen et al., 1980) and/or an overall reduced capacity of older persons to adapt to the bacterial insult, it appears more likely, however, that the greater amount of plaque that accumulated in the older group over time (and the concomitant increase in gingivitis) was related to a greater oral surface area available for plaque retention due to greater amounts of gingival recession seen in the older persons.

Recession

In Western populations who have access to, and who utilize, dental care frequently, gingival recession has been closely linked to aging (Albandar, Kingman 1999; Beck et al., 1994a). In fact, much attachment loss is the result of increased gingival recession and not of increasing pocket depth (Holm-Pedersen et al., 2006; Thomson et al., 2004; Beck et al., 1994b). Whether attachment loss that increases with age manifests as increased recession, pocket depth, or a combination of both is related to tooth (e.g., surface) and patient characteristics. The increased recession seen occurs as a result of a combination of factors over time: a predisposition to develop recession due to tissue morphology, combined with periodontal disease, periodontal treatment, and oral hygiene practices may contribute to recession seen in elderly persons.

Periodontal Disease

Periodontal disease is a bacterial infection that affects the tooth-supporting structures, resulting in loss of clinical periodontal attachment, periodontal pocket depth and radiographic alveolar bone destruction. Periodontal disease is generally irreversible, and since its measurement reflects the cumulative effects of the disease over time, older populations manifest greater levels of disease (Miller et al., 1987), although the amount of disease measured may be an underestimation of the actual disease experience because of teeth that have been lost due to periodontal disease. In addition, while in general it has been found that periodontal disease is prevalent in older populations, the prevalence of disease in the study population depends largely on the level of disease used to define a "case." In older adults, if a case is defined by one or more tooth sites with greater than or equal to 4 mm of clinical attachment loss, then periodontal disease in older adults is almost universal, while if a more conservative definition is used, for example, one or more sites with greater than or equal to 6 mm of attachment loss, then the prevalence is far lower. Population based studies of periodontal disease prevalence in the United States have estimated that anywhere from 68% to 91% of those over the age of 65 have at least one site with at least 4 mm of attachment loss, and between 30% and 71% have at least one site with at least 6 mm of attachment loss (Katz et al., 1996). As in younger populations, however, severe pocketing and severe bone loss is uncommon, although in older populations, the relative rarity of severe periodontal disease likely reflects survivorship of those teeth with less disease.

The Dentition

Effects of Aging on the Dentition

Unlike the soft tissues of the oral cavity, the teeth are fully formed early in life, and most of the tissues that comprise tooth structure (enamel, dentin, and cementum) exhibit no or limited turnover later in life. The exception is the dental pulp, where cellular activity remains high throughout life. As is the case with the periodontium, what constitutes "normal aging" of the dentition is ill-defined, as teeth are subject to both physiologic and pathologic changes over years, and it is often difficult or impossible to distinguish between these two processes.

Clinical Effects of Aging

Teeth are affected by attrition (wear caused by tooth-to-tooth contact), abrasion (wear caused by other physical factors, e.g., a toothbrush), and erosion (wear caused by liquids, e.g., acids) over time, beginning soon after eruption into the oral cavity. Tooth color and form change with aging (Valenzuela et al., 2002); teeth become more yellow due to the altered surface thickness of enamel (Atsu et al., 2005) and in the quality and increased thickness of the underlying dentin (Nitzan et al., 1986). In addition, a loss of translucency with age has been reported (Mjör 1996). Pathologic processes such as caries and inadequate oral hygiene can also affect tooth color. Gingival recession, common in older persons, can make the teeth appear larger (longer) with age, and the cementum that previously covered the cervical area of the tooth, if exposed to the oral cavity, can wear away as a result of erosion or abrasion, further altering the color of the tooth.

Histopathological Effects of Aging

Age-associated histopathological changes in the dentition are apparent in all its structures. In general, it appears that fluoride concentration of both tooth enamel and cementum increases with age (Tsuboi et al., 2000; Brudevold et al., 1960). While many argue that enamel becomes more brittle and less permeable with age, there is scant scientific evidence to support this view. Age-associated changes in the dentin are largely related to the continuous apposition of dentin over time that occurs in the pulp chamber (secondary dentin formation) (Cameriere et al., 2004) and within the dentinal tubules, leading to obstruction of the tubules (Murray et al., 2002) and a concomitant increase in highly mineralized peritubular dentin and sclerotic dentin (Kinney et al., 2005). Obturation of the tubules serves to make the dentin more translucent. In addition, the mechanical properties of dentin vary by age of the tooth; specifically, the endurance strength of dentin from older persons is decreased, in comparison to younger persons (Arola and Reprogel 2005). Cementum is both deposited and resorbed on different areas of the roots of the teeth over time; apposition of cementum in the apical portion compensates for occlusal wear of the tooth; the width of the cementum has been shown to triple between the ages of 10 and

75 years (Zander and Hürzeler 1958) while at the same time, the susceptibility to cemental resoprtion increases with age (Shay 2002). In addition, in the presence of gingival recession, the cervical cementum is often lost as a result of exposure to the oral environment. The dental pulp, which is composed of the blood and nerve supply of the tooth as well as collagen fibers and other cells, is profoundly affected by both normal function of the tooth and pathological processes over time (Murray et al., 2002), and it is difficult to determine to what extent these two factors contribute to pulp change with aging. The blood supply decreases with age, as does the cross-linking of the collagen fibers in the pulp. In addition, there is an overall decrease in the number of cells present (Murray et al., 2002; Nishimura et al., 1997) and an increased likelihood of pulp stone formation. These histopathologic changes of the teeth result in an overall decreased sensitivity of teeth with age, as the pulp chamber grows smaller and less innervated over time and the dentinal tubules close, causing a decrease in the number and length of the odontoblasts. In addition, the reparative capacity of the dentin diminishes with age, as the blood supply decreases. However, because of the additional amounts of dentin that have formed in the pulp chamber in older persons, untreated caries in such persons is more likely to be a self-limiting disease, unlike in younger persons (Shay 2002).

Pathological Conditions of the Dentition in Older Adults

Diseases and pathologic conditions of the dentition, including tooth loss and edentulism (loss of all natural teeth), caries, tooth fractures, tooth abrasion and tooth erosion, are more likely to be seen in older adults due to the irreversible and cumulative nature of these conditions (Morse et al., 2002; Douglass et al., 1993; Graves et al., 1992;). Tooth loss in older adults is most commonly caused by either dental caries (decay) or periodontal disease, but is also influenced greatly by patterns of dental utilization, as well as access to care and treatment recommendations by the treating dentist. Rates of edentulousness in western populations have declined drastically over the past 40 years; in the United States, between just two national surveys, there was a significant reduction in edentulousness in adults over the age of 60, from 31% in 1988–1994 to 25% in 1999–2002 (Beltrán-Aguilar et al., 2005); this downward trend in edentulism has also been seen in other populations, including Sweden (Hugoson et al., 2005) and Australia (Sanders et al., 2004).

It is likely that this trend toward increased tooth retention, combined with longer life spans seen globally, will lead to increased rates of tooth decay and periodontal disease in older adults as more teeth are retained and therefore are likely to experience these oral diseases. Like periodontal disease measures, caries measures reflect cumulative disease experience, and therefore older persons will have greater caries levels. Indeed, DMFT (decayed, missing, and filled teeth) scores reflect high levels of disease experience in most populations: recent studies show that coronal caries is almost universal among older adults. The most recent U.S. study has demonstrated that 93% of all persons above the age of 60 have at least one lesion (Beltrán-Aguilar et al., 2005). The mean DMFT for populations of older adults ranges from a low of 13 to a high of 29 in older adults in studies conducted between 1965 and the present (Katz et al, 1996). Recent estimates show that approximately 30%–50%

of adults age 60 and older have experienced root caries (Graves et al., 1992) and although U.S. studies have demonstrated that the prevalence of both coronal and root caries has decreased in the older adult population in the past 15 years, both age-related structural changes in the oral cavity and disease-related factors, such as xerostomia caused by medications, salivary hypofunction, the increased tendency to collect supragingival plaque, compromised memory and dexterity, having more physical health problems and restorative factors may make some older adults more susceptible to recurrent or new disease. Indeed, older individuals have been shown to have a high caries incidence (Drake et al., 1997; Lawrence et al., 1996) except in cases where compliance with personal hygiene is very high (DePaola et al., 1989).

The increased prevalence of systemic disease seen in older persons may place these individuals at higher risk for oral disease. Periodontal disease has been shown to be more likely to occur in those with unstable diabetes (Tsai et al., 2002) and oral changes, including gingival hyperplasia, have been seen with medications used to treat systemic disease, such as hypertension and angina, in older persons. In general, there is a tendency for studies to show that older adults who are systemically less healthy exhibit more oral disease than the healthy older adults (Maupome et al, 2006; Maupome et al., 2003; Lin et al., 1999). Reasons for the positive association between systemic and corresponding oral disease may include direct cause, as is the case for unstable diabetes, or be related to a common factor, for example, smoking, which is a risk factor for both osteoporosis and periodontal disease. Most would argue that the relationship between underlying systemic and oral disease in older persons in not uni-dimensional but instead is related to a mixture of behavioral, age-related, and systemic disease factors.

In conclusion, the health and function of the oral hard and soft tissues is absolutely critical to maintaining oral and general health and quality of life of any older person. An understanding of changes that occur with aging, and those that occur because of disease processes, is essential in treating oral diseases and maintaining oral health of elderly persons. The combination of oral and systemic disease and their treatments are likely to affect adversely the function of the oral cavity. While advanced age does increase the likelihood of developing oral hard and soft tissue disorders, it is more likely that oral neglect, concomitant systemic conditions, and their treatments will lead to impaired oral function in older adults.

References

Albandar JM, Kingman A. (1999). Gingival recession, gingival bleeding, and dental calculus in adults 30 years of age and older in the United States, 1988–1994. *Journal of Periodontology* 70:30–43.

Arola D, Reprogel RK. (2005). Effects of aging on the mechanical behavior of human dentin. *Biomaterials* 26(18):4051–61.

Atsu SS, Aka PS, Kucukesmen HC, Kilicarslan MA, Atakan C. (2005). Age-related changes in tooth enamel as measured by electron microscopy: implications for porcelain laminate veneers. *Journal of Prosthetic Dentistry* 94(4):336–41.

Beck JD, Koch GG. (1994a). Characteristics of older adults experiencing periodontal attachment loss as gingival recession or probing depth. *Journal of Periodontal Research* 29(4):290–8.

Beck JD, Koch GG, Offenbacher S. (1994b). Attachment loss trends over 3 years in community-dwelling older adults. *Journal of Periodontology* 65(8):737–43.

Beltrán-Aguilar ED, BarkerLK, Canto MT, Dye BA, Gooch BF, Griffin SO, et al. (2005). Surveillance for Dental Caries, Dental Sealants, Tooth Retention, Edentulism, and Enamel Fluorosis-United States, 1988–1994 and 1999–2002 *Morbidity and Mortality Weekly Report* 54(03): 1–44.

Brudevold F, Steadman LT, Smith FA. (1960) Inorganic and organic components of tooth structure. *Annals of the New York Academy of Sciences* 85:110–32.

Cameriere R, Ferrante L, Cingolani M. (2004). Variations in pulp/tooth area ratio as an indicator of age: a preliminary study. *Journal of Forensic Sciences* 49(2):317–9.

Jemal A, Siegel R, Ward E, Murray T, Xu J, Thun MJ. (2007). Cancer Statistics, 2007. *CA: A Cancer Journal for Clinicians* 57:43–66.

Ciancio SG. (2005). Medications: a risk factor for periodontal disease diagnosis and treatment. *Journal of Periodontology* 76(11 Suppl):2061–5.

DePaola PF, Soparkar PM, Tavares M, Kent RL. (1989). The clinical profiles of individuals with and without root surface caries. *Gerodontology* 8:9–15.

Drake CW, Beck JD, Lawrence HP, Koch GG. (1997).Three-year coronal caries incidence and risk factors in North Carolina elderly. *Caries Research* 31:1–7.

Douglass CW, Jette AM, Fox CH, Tennstedt SL, Joshi A, Feldman HA, et al. (1993). Oral health status of the elderly in New England. *Journal of Gerontology* 48:M39–46.

Ettinger RL, Manderson RD. (1974). A clinical study fo sublingual varices. *Oral Surgery Oral Medicine Oral Pathology* 38:540–45.

Graves RC, Beck JD, Disney JA, Drake CW. (1992). Root caries prevalence in black and white North Carolina adults over age 65. *Journal of Public Health Dentistry* 52:94–101.

Hill MW. (1984). The influence of aging on skin and oral mucosa. *Gerodontol-ogy* 3:35–45.

Holm-Pedersen P, Agerbæk N, Theilade E. (1975).Experimental gingivitis in young and elderly individuals. *Journal of Clinical Periodontology* 2:14–24.

Holm-Pedersen P, Gawronsski TH, Folke LEA. (1980). Composition and metabolic activity of dental plaque from young and elderly individuals. *Journal of Dental Research* 59:771–76.

Holm-Pedersen P, Russell SL, Avlund K, Viitanen M, Winblad B, Katz RV. (2006). Periodontal disease in the oldest-old living in Kungsholmen, Sweden: findings from the KEOHS project. *Journal of Clinical Periodontology* 33: 376–384.

Hugoson A, Koch G, Gothberg C, Helkimo AN, Lundin SA, Norderyd O, et al. (2005). Oral health of individuals aged 3–80 years in Jonkoping, Sweden during 30 years (1973–2003). II. Review of clinical and radiographic findings. *Swedish Dental Journal* 29(4):139–55.

Janket SJ, Jones J, Rich S, Miller D, Wehler CJ, Van Dyke TE, et al. (2007). The effects of xerogenic medications on oral mucosa among the Veterans Dental Study participants. *Oral Surgery Oral Medicine Oral Pathology Oral Radiology and Endodontics* 103(2):223–30.

Johnson BD, Page RC, Narayanan AS, Pieters HP. (1986). Effects of donor age on protein and collagen synthesis in vitro by human diploid fibroblasts. *Lab Investigations* 55(4):490–6.

Katz RV, Neely AL, Morse DE. (1996). The epidemiology of oral diseases in older adults. In P. Holm-Pedersen & H. Löe (Eds.), *Textbook of Geriatric Dentistry* (pp. 263–301). Copenhagen: Munksgaard.

Kay MMB. (1979). An overview of immune aging. *Mechanisms of Ageing and Development* 9 (1–2):39–59.

Kinney JH, Nalla RK, Pople JA, Breunig TM, Ritchie RO. (2005). Age-related transparent root dentin: mineral concentration, crystallite size, and mechanical properties. *Biomaterials* 26(16):3363–76.

Lawrence HP, Hunt RJ, Beck JD. (1996).Five-year incidence rates and intraoral distribution of root caries among community-dwelling older adults. *Caries Research* 30(3):169–79.

Lin BP, Taylor GW, Allen DJ, Ship JA. (1999). Dental caries in older adults with diabetes mellitus. *Special Care in Dentistry* 19(1):8–14.

Lyon JP, da Costa SC, Totti VM, Munhoz MF, de Resende MA. (2006). Predisposing conditions for Candida spp. carriage in the oral cavity of denture wearers and individuals with natural teeth. *Canadian Journal of Microbiology* 52(5):462–7.

MacEntee, M I. Glick, N. Stolar, E. (1998). Age, gender, dentures and oral mucosal disorders. *Oral Diseases* 4(1):32–6.

Mashberg A, Samit A. (1995). Early diagnosis of asymptomatic oral and oropharyngeal squamous cancers. *Cancer Journal for Clinicians* 45(6):328–51.

Maupome G, Peters D, Rush WA, Rindal DB, White BA. (2006) The relationship between cardiovascular xerogenic medication intake and the incidence of crown/root restorations. *Journal of Public Health Dentistry* 66(1):49–56.

Maupome G, Gullion CM, White BA, Wyatt CC, Williams PM. (2003) Oral disorders and chronic systemic diseases in very old adults living in institutions. *Special Care in Dentistry* 23(6): 199–208.

Miller AJ, Brunelle JA, Carlos JP, Brown LJ, Löe H. (1987). Oral health of United States adults. The national survey of oral health in US employed adults and seniors: 1985–1986. Washington, CD: US Department of Health and Human Services (NIH publication number 87–28–68).

Mjör IA. (1996). Changes in the Teeth with Aging. In P. Holm-Pedersen & H. Löe (Eds.), *Textbook of Geriatric Dentistry* (pp. 94–102). Copenhagen: Munksgaard.

Morse DE, Kerr AR. (2006). Disparities in oral and pharyngeal cancer incidence, mortality and survival among black and white Americans. *Journal of the American Dental Association* 137(2):203–12.

Morse DE, Holm-Pedersen P, Holm-Pedersen J, Katz RV, Viitanen M, von Strauss E et al. (2002). Dental caries in persons over the age of 80 living in Kungsholmen, Sweden: findings from the KEOHS project. *Community Dental Health* 19:262–7.

Murray PE, Stanley HR, Matthews JB, Sloan AJ, Smith A. (2002).Age-related odontometric changes of human teeth. *Journal of Oral Surgery Oral Medicine Oral Pathology Oral Radiology & Endodontics* 93(4):474–82.

Nishimura F, Terranova VP, Braithwaite M, Orman R, Ohyama H, Mineshiba J, et al. (1997). Comparison of in vitro proliferative capacity of human periodontal ligament cells in juvenile and aged donors. *Oral Disease* 3:162–6.

Nitzan DW, Michaeli Y, Weinreb M, Azaz B. (1986) The effect of aging on tooth morphology: a study on impacted teeth. *Oral Surgery, Oral Medicine, Oral Pathology* 61(1):54–60.

Ryan EJ, Toto PD, Garguilo AW. (1974). Aging in human attached gingal epithelium. *Journal of Dental Research* 53:74–75.

Sanders AE, Slade GD, Carter KD, Stewart JF. (2004). Trends in prevalence of complete tooth loss among Australians, 1979–2002. *Australian and New Zealand Journal of Public Health* 28(6):549–54.

Severson JA, Moffett BC, Kokich V, Selipsky H. (1978). A histologic study of age changes in the adult human periodontal joint (ligament). *Journal of Periodontology* 49:189–200.

Shay K. (2002). Infectious Complications of Dental and Periodontal Diseases in the Elderly Population. *Clinical Infectious Diseases* 34:1215–1223.

Shiba H, Nakanishi K, Sakata M, Fujita T, Uchida Y, Kurihara H. (2000). Effects of ageing on proliferative ability, and the expressions of secreted protein, acidic and rich in cysteine (SPARC) and osteoprotegerin (osteoclastogenesis inhibitory factor) in cultures of human periodontal ligament cells. *Mechanisms of Ageing and Development* 117(1–3):69–77.

Ship JA, Puckett SA. (1994). Longitudinal study on oral health in subjects with Alzheimer's disease. *Journal of the American Geriatrics Society* 42(1):57–63.

Ship, JA, Baum, BJ. (1993). Old age in health and Disease. Lessons from the oral cavity. *Oral Surgery, Oral Medicine, Oral Pathology* 76(1):40–4.

Shklar G. (1966). The effects of aging upon oral mucosa. *Journal of Investigations in Dermatology* 47:115–120.

Shulman JD, Beach MM, Rivera-Hidalgo F. (2004). The prevalence of oral mucosal lesions in U.S. adults: data from the Third National Health and Nutrition Examination Survey, 1988–1994. *Journal of the American Dental Association* 135(9):1279–86.

Thomson WM, Slade GD, Beck JD, Elter, JR, Spencer AJ, Chalmers JM. (2004). Incidence of periodontal attachment loss over 5 years among older South Australians. *Journal of Clinical Periodontology* 31(2):119–125.

Tsai C, Hayes C, Taylor GW. (2002). Glycemic control of type 2 diabetes and severe periodontal disease in the US adult population. *Community Dentistry and Oral Epidemiology* 30(3):182–92.

Tsuboi S, Nakagaki H, Takami Y, Eba H, Kirkham J, Robinson C. (2000).Magnesium and fluoride distribution in human cementum with age. *Calcified Tissue International* 67(6):466–71.

Valenzuela A, Martin-De Las Heras S, Mandojana JM, De Dios Luna J, Valenzuela M, Villanueva E. (2002). Multiple regression models for age estimation by assessment of morphologic dental changes according to teeth source. *American Journal of Forensic and Medical Pathology* 23(4):386–9.

Wolff A, Ship JA, Tylenda CA, Fox PC, Baum BJ. (1991). Oral mucosal appearance is unchanged in healthy, different-aged persons. *Oral Surgery, Oral Medicine, Oral Pathology* 71(5):569–72.

Yoneyama T, Yoshida M, Ohrui T, Mukaiyama H, Okamoto H, et al. (2002). Oral care reduces pneumonia in older patients in nursing homes. *Journal of the American Geriatric Society* 50(3):430–3.

Zander HA, Hürzeler B. (1958). Continuous cementum apposition, *Journal of Dental Research* 37:1035–44.

Chapter 12
The Relationship Between Periodontal Disease and Systemic Disease in the Elderly

Dana L. Wolf and Panos N. Papapanou

Introduction

Periodontitis is a chronic inflammatory disease caused by the bacteria of the dental plaque that results in the progressive destruction of the tissues that support the teeth, i.e., the gingiva, the periodontal ligament and the alveolar bone (Pihlstrom, et al., 2005). Signs and symptoms of periodontitis include gingival redness and swelling, deepening of the gingival crevice surrounding the teeth resulting in the formation of a pathological periodontal pocket, root exposure due to gingival recession, and increased tooth mobility. Severe forms of the disease may lead to tooth migration, compromised esthetics, impaired masticatory function and, ultimately, tooth loss. Among several identified risk factors affecting the onset and progression of periodontitis, colonization by specific pathogenic bacteria, environmental exposures such as cigarette smoking and a number of systemic conditions, such as diabetes mellitus, are of primary importance [for review see Borrell & Papapanou (2005)].

Periodontitis is an infection of global prevalence and affects individuals of all ages, but the disease is more common in elderly individuals (Papapanou, 1996). This increased prevalence, extent and severity in older age cohorts is not necessarily thought to represent an increased susceptibility of the elderly, but rather to reflect the cumulative affect of a prolonged exposure to the established risk factors (Papapanou, et al., 1991; Borrell & Papapanou, 2005). As a result, periodontitis is a major reason for tooth loss in elderly subjects, second only to tooth caries that remains the primary cause across all ages. Nevertheless, more recent epidemiologic data suggest that increasing proportions of subjects do retain their natural dentition throughout their entire lifetime, in sharp contrast to the common occurrence of edentulism among individuals over the age of 60 years, observed only a few decades ago (Sanders, et al., 2004; Beltran-Aguilar, et al., 2005).

Over the past 20 years, literature evidence suggests a possible link between chronic inflammatory periodontitis and a number of systemic diseases including

D.L. Wolf
Division of Periodontics, Section of Oral and Diagnostic Sciences, Columbia University College of Dental Medicine, New York, NY
e-mail: dlw2004@columbia.edu

I.B. Lamster, M.E. Northridge (eds.), *Improving Oral Health for the Elderly*,   247
© Springer Science+Business Media, LLC 2008

diabetes mellitus, atherosclerosis and respiratory diseases. The trend for an increased mean life expectancy primarily in the developed world, coupled with the growing proportion of dentate elderly, calls for special consideration of the impact of a possible periodontitis–systemic health link in elderly populations. For example, given the increased prevalence of periodontitis, diabetes and cardiovascular disease in older cohorts, a possibility for an accentuated association between periodontitis and systemic disease cannot be ruled out, and the impact of multiple co-existing morbidities needs to be further explored. In this chapter, we will first review some key elements of the pathogenesis of periodontal disease that are relevant to the study of a periodontitis–systemic disease association. Next, we will explore the biologically plausible mechanisms supporting a relationship between periodontitis and specific systemic diseases and evaluate the strength of the epidemiologic evidence in support of such an association. In this context, we will adopt a general tiered approach according to ascending level of evidence. We will thus report data from cross-sectional or case–control studies, followed by findings from prospective cohort studies and, whenever available, from intervention studies that have as primary outcomes clinical events or, more commonly, surrogate markers of the disease under investigation. Lastly, we will discuss findings from studies particularly pertaining to the elderly, whenever available.

Key Elements of Pathogenesis

The pathogenesis of periodontal disease is complex and a complete review of this topic is beyond the scope of this chapter. Some key aspects of importance for our understanding of the potential association between periodontal disease and systemic diseases are highlighted below.

Dental plaque is a biofilm that adheres to the tooth surfaces in close contact with the epithelial lining of the gingival crevice. Currently, more than 600 species have been found to colonize the oral cavity (Marsh, 2004). In periodontal health, the dental plaque is composed of mostly gram-positive, aerobic, cocci. The development of gingival inflammation is paralleled by a marked shift in bacterial profiles characterized by an absolute and proportional increase in gram-negative, anaerobic rods (Theilade, et al., 1966). The microbiota of established periodontitis have been characterized in detail, and several clusters of pathogenic bacteria that are frequently encountered in deep or progressive periodontal lesions have been identified (Haffajee & Socransky, 1994). In response to several pathogenic bacteria including *Porphyromonas gingivalis, Tanerella forsythia, Treponema denticola* and *Aggregatibacter actinomycetemcomitans*, as well as to bacterially derived antigenic structures such as lipopolysaccharide (LPS), a cellular and humoral immuno-inflammatory response is mounted locally in the periodontal tissues in close proximity to the bacterial biofilm, aiming at the containment of the infectious stimulus and the prevention of a bacterial invasion into the tissue. The local secretion of pro-inflammatory, catabolic cytokines and the accumulation of tissue-degrading enzymes adjacent to the apical extent of the plaque biofilm result in an ulceration of the epithelial lining of the periodontal pocket, perturbation of its barrier function and subsequent damage of the tooth-supporting soft and hard tissues. It is noteworthy that although several pathogenic periodontal bacteria possess potent proteolytic and tissue-degrading properties, it is the host's inflammatory response to the bacterial challenge, rather than the bacteria themselves, which is responsible for most of the tissue breakdown associated with periodontitis (Offenbacher, 1996). Hence, periodontitis reflects an imbalance of the host homeostasis promoting destructive, catabolic processes following a failure to contain the apical propagation of the inflammatory, microbially induced lesion (Kornman, et al., 1997). The goal of periodontal therapy is the removal of the pathogenic bacterial biofilm from the tooth surface, the reduction/elimination of the gingival inflammation and the creation of a periodontal tissue anatomy that is conducive with the re-establishment of health-associated microbiota.

There are three aspects of the pathogenesis of periodontal disease which lend biologic plausibility to a periodontitis–systemic disease connection. First, the ulcerated epithelial barrier lining of the periodontal pocket may involve a substantial surface area (Hujoel, et al., 2001) and serves as a potential port of entry for bacteria and bacterially derived antigenic structures (Loos, 2005). Indeed, transient bacteremias have been reported to occur not only after episodes of active periodontal therapy, but also after minor manipulation of the gingival tissues such as chewing and toothbrushing (Baltch, et al., 1982; Daly, et al., 1997). After gaining entry into the bloodstream, oral bacteria may reach and seed distant sites. For example, Haraszthy, et al. (2000) have demonstrated the presence of bacterial DNA from periodontal pathogens in carotid endarterectomy specimens while recently Kozarov, et al. (2005) recovered viable periodontal pathogens from human atherosclerotic plaques.

A second potential pathway may be mediated by the systemic dissemination of inflammatory mediators that are produced locally in the periodontal tissues, including several pro-inflammatory cytokines such as IL-1, IL-6, IL-8 and TNF, that are known to be elevated in periodontal lesions (De Nardin, 2001). These may, in turn, induce subsequent systemic responses including the production of acute-phase reactants, such as C-reactive protein (CRP) (Ramadori & Christ, 1999), and the activation of vascular endothelium (Huang & Vita, 2006). Indeed, several investigators have found elevated serum CRP and IL-6 in subjects with periodontitis when compared to individuals with healthy periodontal tissues (Ebersole, et al., 1997; D'Aiuto, et al., 2004a; Loos, 2005). High levels of pro-inflammatory mediators are associated with increased risk for the development of a number of chronic systemic diseases, such as cardiovascular disease (Ridker, et al., 2000), inflammatory bowel disease (Forrester & Bick-Forrester, 2005), rheumatoid arthritis (Pasceri & Yeh, 1999) and dementia (Schmidt, et al., 2002).

Another potential link is thought to be mediated through a process termed molecular mimicry, i.e., an autoimmune response occurring due to homology between antigenic bacterial peptides and mammalian proteins. Bacterial heat-shock proteins, for example, have been conserved during evolution and are highly homologous among prokaryotic and eukaryotic cells. One particular bacterial heat-shock protein, hsp60, is highly immunogenic and has been implicated in the pathogenesis of a number of chronic inflammatory diseases such as systemic lupus erythematosus (Zampieri, et al., 2005) and coronary heart disease (Rothenbacher, et al., 2001). In the context of periodontitis, Tabeta, et al. (2000) have demonstrated significantly higher antibody titers to hsp60 in periodontitis patients vs. healthy controls. Additionally, the data from this study suggested cross-reactivity between antibodies to hsp60 and GroEL, a protein of the hsp60 family expressed by periodontal pathogens such as *P. gingivalis.*

In conclusion, several elements of the pathobiology of human periodontitis may provide biologically plausible links with systemic disease. In the following text, we will provide an overview of data supporting such a link for a number of conditions.

Diabetes Mellitus

The link between diabetes mellitus and periodontitis is one of the more extensively studied, with research being conducted over the past several decades. The association is considered to be bi-directional: diabetes as a risk factor for periodontitis and periodontitis as a possible severity factor for diabetes. Potential mechanisms accounting for the former association include impaired neutrophil function in response to the bacterial challenge; an upregulated pro-inflammatory monocyte response leading to enhanced secretion of inflammatory cytokines; impaired collagen synthesis; exaggerated response of proteolytic enzymes; and genetic predisposition [for review, see Lalla, et al. (2001)]. Recent research has focused on the consequences of hyperglycemia and the development of advanced glycation end products (AGEs). AGEs are compounds formed from the irreversible glycation of proteins and lipids that accumulate in the tissues and have been linked to the development of diabetic complications (Lalla, et al., 2001). Receptors for AGEs have been shown to be expressed on many cell types in the gingival tissues including endothelial cells and macrophages. Activation of the receptor for AGEs results in an exaggerated, sustained inflammatory response which, as discussed above, accounts for most of the periodontitis-associated tissue breakdown (Lalla, et al., 2001).

A plethora of epidemiologic studies have demonstrated that both gingivitis and periodontitis are more prevalent and severe in individuals with type 1 and 2 diabetes vs. non-diabetics (Nelson, et al., 1990; Emrich, et al., 1991; Grossi, et al., 1995; Cutler, et al., 1999). In a meta-analysis performed in conjunction with the last World Workshop in Periodontics, Papapanou (1996) reviewed studies published prior to 1996 that examined the association between non-insulin-dependent diabetes mellitus and periodontal disease. The analysis included over 3,500 adults and demonstrated a statistically significant association between diabetes and periodontitis. It has further been reported that the risk for periodontitis among diabetic individuals may be related to the duration of diabetes and the degree of diabetic control (Tervonen & Knuuttila, 1986; Tsai, et al., 2002). In a longitudinal study of Pima Indians, patients with poorly controlled type 2 diabetes had an 11-fold increased risk of progressive bone loss compared to non-diabetic controls, while individuals with well-controlled diabetes had no significant increase in risk (Taylor, et al., 1998). However, controlled studies assessing the response to non-surgical periodontal therapy in diabetics vs. non-diabetics have generally demonstrated a comparable periodontal healing capacity in the two groups (Tervonen, et al., 1991; Christgau, et al., 1998). Tervonen & Karjalainen (1997) evaluated the 4-week, 6- and 12-month response to non-surgical periodontal therapy among patients with type 1 diabetes of good, moderate or poor metabolic control vs. control subjects with periodontitis but no diabetes. At no time point was there any statistically significant difference observed among patients with diabetes as a whole and non-diabetic controls. Nevertheless, subjects with poor metabolic control were found to suffer from more bone loss at baseline and a faster recurrence over the course of the study.

There is a relative paucity of literature that specifically addresses the association between diabetes and periodontitis in the elderly. Zielinski, et al. (2002) compared the oral health of subjects over 60 years of age with and without non-insulin-dependent diabetes mellitus (NIDDM); 34 subjects with NIDDM and good metabolic control and 40 controls received an examination of their oral and periodontal status. No statistically significant differences were found in oral health parameters between the two groups. A study of a larger sample size (1,101 subjects aged 60–75 years) was published by Persson, et al. (2003). These authors addressed two questions: (i) to what extent is diabetes associated with periodontitis and (ii) how does periodontitis rank as a co-morbidity among other diseases in patients with diabetes. Their findings did not demonstrate statistically significant differences in periodontal conditions among subjects with and without type 1 or 2 diabetes, but the authors speculated that older subjects may approach similar levels of periodontitis regardless of whether or not they have diabetes. In this context, it is important to bear in mind that the prevalence of periodontitis increases with age, due to the cumulative effect of a prolonged exposure to risk/causative factors. Of note, the study reported that diabetes was more closely associated with cardiovascular disease than periodontal disease.

With respect to the potential of a compromised periodontal status to impact diabetic status, it should be remembered that infections are generally considered to contribute to a state of insulin resistance (McGuinness, 2005). Inflammatory mediators produced in response to infection have been shown to play a role in the development of insulin resistance. For example, high levels of TNF-α may cause the downregulation of genes necessary for the normal action of insulin (Moller, 2000) and have a negative effect on insulin's signal transduction pathway (Bastard, et al., 2006). IL-6 has been shown to impair insulin signaling by down-regulation of the insulin receptor and upregulation of a negative regulator of insulin signaling (Yu & Ginsberg, 2005). Thus, it is conceivable that periodontitis patients with elevated systemic pro-inflammatory cytokines are prone to a chronic state of insulin resistance.

This concept is supported by data from epidemiologic studies. Taylor, et al. (1996) reported that among individuals with diabetes of good to moderate glycemic control, patients with severe periodontitis at baseline were six times more likely to have poor glycemic control at follow-up than those with a better periodontal status. A recent longitudinal study has found periodontitis to be a significant predictor of the development of overt nephropathy and end stage renal disease in individuals with type 2 diabetes (Shultis, et al., 2007). Additionally, some studies have demonstrated improvements in glycemic control following conservative periodontal therapy (Miller, et al., 1992; Grossi, et al., 1997). Janket, et al. (2005) published a meta-analysis of intervention studies which assessed whether non-surgical periodontal treatment improves glycemic control in diabetic patients. Ten intervention studies with a total of 456 patients were included in the analysis which suggested a trend toward a decrease in levels of hemoglobin A1c (HbA1c) after periodontal therapy, with an overall weighted average decrease of 0.38%. The decrease amounted to 0.66% when restricted to type 2 diabetics and to 0.71% when adjunctive antibiotics were used. It is generally accepted that even 0.5–1% changes in HbA1c is clinically significant (UKPDS, 1998); nonetheless, none of these reductions were statistically significant.

Few studies have examined the effect of periodontitis as an exposure of significance for diabetes in the elderly. Taylor, et al. (2000) used data from the third National Health and Nutrition Examination Survey (NHANES III) and determined that periodontal disease represents an unmet treatment need in older adults. However, when reviewing clinical and epidemiologic evidence supporting the concept of periodontal infection as a risk factor for poor glycemic control in type 2 diabetes, they found limited representation of older adults in studies of this relationship. The lack of data on older adults is also reflected by the meta-analysis discussed above (Janket, et al., 2005). A majority of the 10 studies involved age cohorts below 65 years, and only one report (Stewart, et al., 2001) included subjects that were somewhat older. In this study, diabetic subjects in the treatment group had a mean age of 67 ± 10.8, while the controls who received no periodontal treatment had a mean age of 62 ± 8.4. Of note, this study demonstrated a significant improvement in HbA1c with periodontal therapy, but there was a significant improvement over time in control subjects as well.

In recognition of the need to specifically address the relationship between periodontitis and diabetes in the elderly, a group of investigators from Thailand examined the effect of periodontal therapy on type 2 diabetes in older adults (age 55–80, mean age 61 years) (Promsudthi, et al., 2005). Study subjects included individuals with poorly controlled diabetes and severe periodontitis. The treatment group ($N = 27$) received mechanical, non-surgical periodontal therapy and systemic doxycyline while the control group ($N = 25$) received no treatment. After 3 months, patients in the treatment arm showed an improvement in periodontal status and a trend toward decreased HbA1c; however, the difference did not reach statistical significance. The authors recommended further studies on older subjects that include larger sample sizes.

Despite the paucity of specific data examining the relationship of periodontal disease and systemic disease in the elderly, it is conceivable that such a relationship may be enhanced with older age, parallel to increases in insulin resistance (Perry, 1999) and the incidence and severity of both diabetes (Meneilly, 2006) and periodontitis (Papapanou, 1996). Therefore, older adults may be particularly impacted by the association. In the absence of adequate access to oral health care, elderly diabetic patients may experience accelerated periodontitis, increased tooth loss and, as a consequence, impaired masticatory function. Conversely, older individuals with periodontitis may be increasingly susceptible to the development of insulin resistance and diabetes. Future well-powered studies exploring the relationship between periodontal disease and diabetes in the elderly are clearly needed. In the meanwhile, health care professionals need to be aware of these particular co-morbidities and their potential synergism in elderly populations.

Cardiovascular and Cerebrovascular Diseases

A number of infectious inflammatory conditions have been hypothesized to promote atherogenesis and/or the progression of atherosclerosis (Zebrack & Anderson, 2002; Hansson, 2005), including infections by *Chlamydia pneumoniae*, human cytomegalovirus or herpes simplex viruses. As stated above, periodontal disease can directly or indirectly contribute to atherogenesis/atherosclerosis through a number of biologically plausible mechanisms. Consistent with the possibility of bacterial translocation from the oral cavity to the systemic circulation, DNA from periodontal pathogens has been recovered from atherosclerotic plaques removed from carotid or femoral arteries (Fiehn, et al., 2005). In response to bacterial antigens and inflammatory mediators produced locally in the periodontal lesion and entering the systemic circulation, acute-phase reactants including C-reactive protein are elevated (Wu, et al., 2000; Slade, et al., 2003). These mediators may play a role in the progression of atherosclerosis (Verma, et al., 2006; Wilson, et al., 2006; de Ferranti & Rifai, 2007). Heat-shock proteins (HSP) have been found to have a specific role in the pathogenesis of atherosclerosis. Being expressed both on oral bacterial membranes and human endothelial cells, they stimulate an immune response resulting in high levels of cross-reactive antibodies and aggressive T-helper cells. Endothelial cells that express HSPs are susceptible to anti-HSP antibody-mediated complement-dependent lysis, resulting in endothelial injury that promotes atherogenesis (Ludewig, et al., 2004).

Since the 1980s, a large number of studies assessing the relationship between periodontitis and cardiovascular diseases have been published. These studies have varied widely in terms of both their definition of exposures (i.e., periodontitis) and outcomes (i.e., inflammatory surrogate markers of disease; subclinical disease, such as atheromatic plaque thickness; or clinical events such as coronary heart disease, fatal myocardial infarction or stroke). Rather than attempting a comprehensive review, we will summarize (i) the findings of some large epidemiologic studies, (ii) the existing limited data from intervention studies and (iii) the literature that pertains to this association in elderly subjects in particular.

A report from the third National Health and Nutrition Examination Survey (NHANES III) included 5,564 subjects over the age of 40 with available data on periodontal status and information on heart attacks (Arbes, et al., 1999). In this study, the independent variable was the percent of periodontal sites per person with loss of periodontal attachment ≥ 3 mm, i.e., the extent of periodontitis (categorized as 0%, >0–33%, >33–67% and >67%), while the dependent variable was the self-reported history of myocardial infarction (MI). The analyses revealed extent of attachment to be associated with increased risk of MI. After adjustments for established cardiovascular risk factors and socio-demographic variables, the odds of heart attack were 3.8 times higher in subjects with >67% of sites with attachment loss compared to those with no attachment loss ($p = 0.02$).

The Atherosclerosis Risk in Communities (ARIC) study sampled cohorts of community-dwelling adults from four locations in the United States. Subjects were recruited between 1987 and 1989 and examined at three follow-up visits at intervals of approximately 3 years, with the final follow-up visit occurring between 1996 and 1998 (Beck, et al., 2001; Slade, et al., 2003; Beck, et al., 2005b). Slade et al. analyzed data from a sample of 5,552 subjects in ages 52–75 years, to assess the association between periodontitis and levels of C-reactive protein (CRP). Individuals with extensive periodontal disease (>30% sites with pocket depth ≥ 4 mm) had 30% higher CRP than subjects with no or localized periodontitis. In a multivariate linear regression model controlling for age, sex, diabetes mellitus, cigarette use and non-steroidal anti-inflammatory drug use, the association between extensive periodontal disease and CRP was modified by body mass index. Extensive periodontal pocketing was predictive of high CRP in individuals of low BMI only. However, in another report on a sub-sample of 5,002 subjects from this cohort, Beck et al. failed to demonstrate an association between incipient or severe periodontitis, defined by clinical measurements, and coronary heart disease (Beck, et al., 2005a). The authors did, however, find that serum IgG antibodies to specific periodontal pathogens (*T. denticola, Prevotella intermedia, Capnocytophaga ochracea* and *Veillonella parvula* in smokers and *Prevotella nigrescens, A. actinomycetemcomitans* and *C. ochracea* in never-smokers) were associated with prevalent heart disease in multivariate models.

The Oral Infection and Vascular Disease Epidemiology Study (INVEST) is a prospective cohort study investigating the relationship between oral infections, carotid atherosclerosis and stroke in subjects from Northern Manhattan in New York City. The study involved a cohort of 1,056 subjects over 55 years of age with no baseline history of stroke, myocardial infarction or chronic inflammatory disease. Study subjects received full-mouth periodontal evaluation as well as a Doppler ultrasound examination to assess the thickness of atherosclerotic plaques in the common (CCA) and internal (ICA) carotid arteries (Desvarieux, et al., 2003; Desvarieux, et al., 2005; Engebretson, et al., 2005). Additionally, intima-media thickness (IMT) of the CCA and ICA were assessed, since IMT of these vessels has been strongly associated with the risk of myocardial infarction and stroke in asymptomatic older adults (O'Leary, et al., 1999). The first publication from INVEST reported on a subset of 711 patients (Desvarieux, et al., 2003). Although the prevalence of carotid artery plaque was not associated with measurements of current or cumulative periodontal disease, i.e., probing depth and attachment level, respectively, tooth loss was associated with an increased prevalence of atherosclerotic plaque in a multivariate model adjusted for age, sex, smoking, diabetes, systolic blood pressure, LDL, HDL, ethnicity, education, toothbrushing, social isolation, physical activity and years of residence (OR 1.9, CI 1.2–3.0). In this cohort, an increased number of lost teeth correlated with increased severity of periodontal disease at the remaining teeth. It was therefore assumed that tooth loss reflected, to some degree, current or cumulative periodontal disease. In a radiographic study from the same cohort, Engebretson, et al. (2005) reported on a sub-sample of 203 subjects with available panoramic radiographs. Severe radiographic periodontal bone loss, defined as whole mouth average bone loss of $\geq 50\%$ of the root length, was associated with the presence of carotid plaques after adjustment in a multivariate model (OR 3.64, $p = 0.01$). Finally, data from a third INVEST publication demonstrated that carotid IMT and white blood cell count increased significantly in a fully adjusted model with increasing levels of subgingival colonization by a pre-defined complex of periodontal bacterial pathogens (*A. actinomycetemcomitans, P. gingivalis, T. forsythia* and *T. denticola*; Desvarieux, et al., 2005). Interestingly, the positive association was present only for the specific bacterial cluster and not for other tested putative periodontal pathogens or health-associated species. Overall, the data from INVEST suggest a strong association between periodontal disease and subclinical markers of atherosclerotic vascular diseases (ASVD).

In a systematic review of the literature that addressed the focused question "Does periodontal disease influence the initiation/progression of atherosclerosis?", Scannapieco, et al. (2003a) carried out a meta-analysis of 25 studies and concluded that periodontal disease is moderately associated with atherosclerosis-induced diseases such as CAD, stroke and peripheral vascular disease.

There are several difficulties in the design of a randomized control trial that may prospectively assess the effect of periodontal therapy on clinical events related to ASVD, including the relatively low incidence of such events necessitating inclusion of large samples to afford adequate power, the fact that the time period between initial exposure to a causative/risk factor and clinical manifestation of disease may amount to decades in the context of ASVD and the ethical issues associated with the follow-up of an untreated control group over prolonged time periods. As a result, the intervention studies dealing with the periodontitis–ASVD association available to date are limited to observations of the effect of periodontal therapy on surrogate markers for cardiovascular disease. D'Aiuto, et al. (2004b) published a report on 94 systemically healthy individuals with generalized severe periodontitis who were treated with non-surgical periodontal therapy and extractions. The goal of the study was to determine the impact of periodontal therapy on CRP-associated CVD risk, as defined at the American Heart Association (AHA) consensus conference (Pearson, et al., 2003). The findings showed that subjects with more severe periodontitis at baseline had an increased probability of having a higher CRP-associated CVD risk (OR 5.6, 95% CI 1.2–27.4). Additionally, after a 6-month follow-up, patients who had a better response to periodontal therapy were also more likely to have decreased their inflammatory risk category after adjustments for age, gender, ethnicity and cigarette smoking (OR 4.8, 95% CI 1.4–15.8). Another report from the same group of investigators focused on the short-term (i.e., 2 months post-therapy) impact of "standard" vs. "intensive" periodontal therapy on serum inflammatory markers and cholesterol levels in patients with severe periodontitis (D'Aiuto, et al., 2005). "Intensive" therapy included adjunctive use of locally delivered minocycline in addition to standard non-surgical periodontal therapy. Both modes of therapy resulted in significant reduction in median CRP levels compared to untreated controls. The findings held true in a multivariate model analysis adjusted for age, gender, body mass index, ethnicity and cigarette smoking status. A post hoc analysis revealed a more pronounced effect in non-smokers vs. smokers. IL-6 levels were significantly reduced in the intensive therapy group only, but no significant changes in cholesterol levels were observed. Findings on the effects of standard vs. intensive therapy after a 6-month follow-up (D'Aiuto, et al., 2006) revealed a significant reduction in white blood cell count, CRP levels, IL-6 levels, total cholesterol, LDL and systolic blood pressure in the intensive treatment group compared to the standard therapy group. The intensive treatment group also displayed a higher reduction in cardiovascular risk than the one observed in standard therapy.

Another surrogate marker of subclinical CVD that has been investigated in intervention studies of periodontal disease is endothelial dysfunction (ED). ED is characterized by a reduction in vasodilatory capability of peripheral blood vessels (Verma, et al., 2003), may precede the development of atheromatous plaques and has been associated with increased risk of atherosclerosis in healthy individuals. Assessments of ED are commonly made by measuring the brachial artery diameter prior to and after induction of reactive hyperemia (Celermajer, et al., 1992). Case–control studies have shown that endothelial dysfunction is more pronounced in subjects with chronic periodontitis than in periodontally healthy controls (Amar, et al., 2003; Mercanoglu, et al., 2004). Four prospective studies have reported improvements in endothelial function following periodontal therapy: two studies used mechanical periodontal treatment alone (Mercanoglu, et al., 2004; Elter, et al., 2006), one study used adjunctive local antibiotics (Tonetti, et al., 2007) while one study used adjunctive systemic antibiotics (Seinost, et al., 2005).

Few studies have specifically addressed the association between periodontitis and ASVD in the elderly. In a study examining surrogate markers for CVD, Bretz, et al. (2005) examined the association between the extent of deep pockets ($\geq$ 6 mm), the presence of periodontal pathogens and the levels of a number of plasma inflammatory mediators, in a sample of 1,131 subjects with a mean age of 73 years. In this study, colonization by *P. gingivalis, T. denticola* and *T. forsythia* was indirectly assessed using a microbial test based on the ability of these species to hydrolyze a synthetic trypsin-like substrate (BANA test). The authors reported that plasma levels of IL-6 and TNF-α were significantly higher in participants with more extensive periodontal disease (having deep pockets at $>10\%$ of their sites) and significantly higher CRP plasma levels in BANA-positive subjects after controlling for other factors.

Investigating clinical events, Lee, et al. (2006) analyzed data from elderly (over 60 years) NHANES III participants and explored the association between periodontal disease and stroke. Due to the large proportion of edentulous subjects in the examined age cohorts (1,563 out of the available 5,123; 30.5%), the authors developed a new index termed "periodontal health status", to also account for the role of periodontal disease as a major cause of tooth loss. Fully edentulous and partially edentulous subjects with appreciable periodontal attachment loss (subjects who had over the median value of percent of sites with $\geq$ 2 mm of attachment loss) were significantly more likely to have a history of stroke compared to dentate subjects without periodontal attachment loss ($p = 0.03$). This association remained significant after adjustment for age and smoking but not in a fully adjusted model including additional explanatory variables. It is important to consider that this study did not differentiate between ischemic and hemorrhagic stroke, i.e., two types of stroke with very different etiology. Considering potential biologic mechanisms linking periodontal disease and stroke, associations are more plausible between periodontal disease and ischemic stroke.

Loesche, et al. (1998) assessed the relationship between dental disease and coronary disease in elderly U.S. veterans. Subjects aged 60 years and older were recruited from an outpatient VA clinic and from a long-term care facility. The subjects were stratified into two groups (those with 1–14 teeth and with 15–28 teeth) and were examined with respect to oral health-related variables such as: the number of teeth, the number of restorations, amount of decay, probing depths, attachment levels, gingival recession, plaque index, papillary bleeding index, salivary levels of certain bacteria and BANA test for periodontal bacteria. The authors reported a statistically significant association between a diagnosis of heart disease and the salivary levels of *Streptococcus sanguis*, number of missing teeth, complaints of xerostomia and high BANA scores. The oral parameters were more strongly associated with coronary heart disease than established risk factors such as serum cholesterol, body mass index (BMI), diabetes and smoking. However, the authors cautioned that the reported findings may not be extrapolated to other populations, due to the fact that a convenience sample was studied.

Ajwani, et al. (2003) investigated the relationship between periodontitis and mortality in a cohort of home-dwelling individuals over the age of 75, a subset of the Helsinki Ageing Study cohort. A total of 364 subjects with medical and dental examinations in 1990 were followed for 5 years and were included in the analysis. Periodontitis was found to increase the risk of cardiovascular disease mortality after controlling for common risk factors (HR 2.28, CI 1.03–5.05). Among subjects with periodontitis, baseline CRP above 3 mg/l was associated with high mortality.

The question of how age influences the strength of the association between periodontitis and ASVD is rather complex and yet to be conclusively determined. Some studies have found the association to be stronger in younger individuals. For example, DeStefano, et al. (1993) using data from 9,760 subjects found a more pronounced increase in risk for CVD among men with periodontitis under the age of 50 years. In a case–control study involving subjects with a mean age of 56 years (cases 56.8 years and controls 56.3 years), Mattila, et al. (2000) reported a statistically insignificant higher prevalence of "dental infection" (a composite definition including clinical and radiographic measures of periodontitis) among subjects with diagnosed CVD and speculated that the lack of statistical significance could be attributed to the older age of the participants. Assuming that periodontitis is indeed a true risk factor for CVD albeit one of relatively moderate importance in relation to more powerful risk factors, one can envision a scenario whereby the relative contribution of periodontitis to overall CVD risk may become increasingly difficult to detect in older subjects, given that the prolonged exposure to and cumulative impact of other more decisive factors may account for increasing proportions of the variance in incident CVD. Of note, this increasing attributable risk to other factors may still neutralize a potential mounting role for periodontitis due to its increased prevalence with age. To further complicate the issue, the age-related differential role of periodontitis as a potential exposure of interest for CVD may likely differ across populations, as a function of their varying exposure to additional risk factors and co-morbidities.

In the context of co-morbidities, it is important to realize that cardiovascular disease is the leading cause of death in type 2 diabetes, and that an estimated 79% of diabetic patients die of cardiac complications after having had a myocardial infarction (Bax, et al., 2007). These disorders have common risk factors including smoking, obesity and hyperlipidemia. Importantly, smoking and diabetes are established risk factors for periodontitis and obesity has been recently reported to increase the risk for periodontitis. Investigators from Japan (Saito, et al., 2001) studied 643 healthy, dentate adults and demonstrated that in subjects with a high waist–hip ratio, a higher body mass index significantly increased the risk of periodontitis. An analysis based on NHANES III data revealed a significant association between body fat and periodontal disease in younger adults (18–34 years old), but not in middle aged (35–59 years old) or older adults (60–90 years old) (Al-Zahrani, et al., 2003). Genco, et al. (2005) examined the relationship between obesity and periodontal disease and evaluated to what extent insulin resistance and systemic levels of TNF-α may explain this relationship. Analyzing data from NHANES III, the authors found that BMI was significantly related to the severity of bone loss and that this relationship was likely mediated by insulin resistance. Overweight individuals who were in the highest quartile of insulin resistance had significantly elevated odds ratio for severe bone loss while those with high BMI and low insulin resistance did not. Plasma levels of and soluble receptors for TNF-α were assessed in a subset of patients from the MI Life Study of Erie and Niagara County conducted at the University at Buffalo (Noack, et al., 2001). Individuals over 50 years and those with a higher BMI had statistically significant higher levels of plasma TNF-α and TNF-α receptor. The authors proposed a mechanism linking obesity and diabetes whereby obesity leads to increased secretion of pro-inflammatory cytokines, including TNF-α, from adipocytes. In turn, high plasma levels of TNF-α contribute to insulin resistance and diabetes, and the hyper-inflammatory state associated with diabetes may lead to increased periodontal breakdown in response to the periodontal bacterial challenge. Although the precise time sequence and interplay between these events have yet to be elucidated, clinicians must consider the synergistic potential of co-morbidities and how this may affect both the oral and systemic health of the elderly patients.

Respiratory Diseases

Respiratory diseases such as chronic obstructive pulmonary disease (COPD) and pneumonia are among the systemic conditions that have been linked to periodontitis. Pneumonia is of special relevance in the elderly population. Nursing home-acquired pneumonia (NAP) and hospital-acquired pneumonia (HAP) result in significant increases in morbidity, mortality and health care costs, particularly in older adults (Sopena, et al., 2005). NAP is the leading cause of death among nursing home patients and the second most common cause for hospitalization (Shay, et al., 2005). Some of the risk factors for NAP include swallowing dysfunction, requirement of help feeding and poor oral care (Terpenning, 2005). HAP usually occurs within 48 hours of hospital admittance and is more common in infants, individuals over the age of 65 and people with underlying serious illnesses (Azarpazhooh & Leake, 2006). The incidence is also higher among patients in the intensive care unit (ICU) and those undergoing mechanical ventilation, where the mortality rates are high (Sopena, Sabria, & the Neunos Study, 2005). While the main causes of community-acquired pneumonia are viral and pneumococcal pathogens, NAP and HAP are almost always caused by anaerobic gram-negative bacilli (Shay, et al., 2005). The most common route of lower airway infection is by aspiration of oropharyngeal secretions. However, aspiration of gastric contents, inhalation of infectious aerosols, spread of infection from contiguous sites and hematogenous spread from extrapulmonary sources are also considered possible modes of infection.

Different mechanisms have been proposed to explain how oral bacteria may be involved in the pathogenesis of respiratory infection (Scannapieco, 1999). One possibility is that oral bacteria are released from the dental plaque into the saliva and are then aspirated into the lower respiratory tract. Indeed, a variety of anaerobes implicated in periodontal disease pathogenesis such as *P. gingivalis* and *Fusobacterium nucleatum* have been cultured from infected lung fluids. Another possibility is that periodontal disease-associated enzymes, especially proteases, cause mucosal alterations that foster colonization by respiratory pathogens. Additionally, some oral bacteria possess hydrolytic enzymes capable of destroying protective salivary pellicles thus hindering bacterial clearance from mucosal surfaces. Finally, cytokines from inflamed periodontal tissues may upregulate the expression of adhesion molecules on mucosal surfaces, thereby promoting adhesion of respiratory pathogens.

Patients in hospitals or nursing homes tend to have poorer oral hygiene than ambulatory community-dwelling individuals (Scannapieco, 1999). As dental plaque increases in mass, it increases in complexity and may also be colonized by respiratory pathogens. In this case, dental plaque may effectively serve as a reservoir for respiratory pathogens (Scannapieco, 1999). A number of epidemiologic studies have implicated oral health status in the development of pneumonia (Terpenning, et al., 1993; Fourrier, et al., 1998; Terpenning, et al., 2001). Fourrier, et al. (1998) studied consecutively admitted patients to the ICU and prospectively assessed the relationship between dental plaque and the subsequent development of nosocomial infection. Semi-quantitative assessment of plaque levels was made using the plaque index of Silness & Löe (1964) after which plaque samples were aerobically cultured. Plaque culture was considered positive when the concentration was $\geq 10^3$ colony-forming units. Dental plaque colonization at day 0 and day 5 of admission was significantly associated with the risk for nosocomial pneumonia and bacteremia.

Several intervention studies have been conducted to determine whether an improvement in the oral health of hospital or nursing home patients reduces the occurrence of pneumonia (Fourrier, et al., 2000; Bergmans, et al., 2001; Yoneyama, et al., 2002; Fourrier, et al., 2005). Fourrier, et al. (2000) conducted a study on 60 consecutively admitted adult patients with a medical condition requiring mechanical ventilation and suggesting an ICU stay of 5 days. Treatment consisted of antiseptic decontamination of the oral cavity using a 0.2% chlorhexidine gel three times a day during the entire stay in the ICU. The control group received oral rinsing with bicarbonate isotonic serum followed by suctioning four times a day. There was a 53% relative risk reduction for nosocomial infection in the treatment group suggesting that interference with oral bacterial colonization may reduce the incidence of nosocomial infections in ICU patients.

In 2003, Scannapieco et al. performed a meta-analysis of randomized controlled trials evaluating oral interventions to reduce incidence of pneumonia (Scannapieco, et al., 2003b). The evaluated treatment regimens ranged broadly from topical antimicrobial prophylaxis in the oropharynx (Bergmans, et al., 2001), to toothbrushing by nurses or caregivers (Yoneyama, et al., 2002), and daily professional dental care by a dentist and dental hygienist (Yoneyama, et al., 1996). Nevertheless, the results of the analysis supported the notion that treatment aimed at reducing the oral microbial burden reduces the risk of pneumonia in high-risk subjects. A more recent review by Azarpazhooh & Leake (2006) concurred that there is good evidence that oropharyngeal decontamination using antimicrobials may reduce the progression or occurrence of respiratory infection.

Seniors in nursing homes may require aid with routine oral hygiene procedures due to factors such as impaired visual acuity, decreased manual dexterity and arthritic conditions. However, it has been reported that oral health is of low priority to nursing home aides, who receive at best limited training in performing oral hygiene practices, and little or no rebuke if oral care is overlooked (Terpenning & Shay, 2002). Considering the substantial impact of pneumonia on morbidity, mortality and health care spending, it appears necessary to educate both hospital nurses and nursing home attendants on the value of oral health and to provide the patients with the necessary means to maintain good oral health practices. Particular attention should be given to patients with prevalent periodontal disease whose significant oral bacterial burden may put them at increased risk for the development of pneumonia.

Osteoporosis

Osteoporosis is a disorder characterized by low bone mass, bone fragility and increased susceptibility to fracture. Since bone mass decreases with age, osteoporosis is more prevalent in older adults and affects a sizeable portion of the population worldwide (Lane, 2006). In the United States, osteoporosis is projected to impact approximately 14 million individuals over the age of 50 by the year 2020. Since a hallmark of periodontal disease is loss of alveolar bone support, it is conceivable that the osteoporosis would have an impact on the development and/or progression of periodontitis. It has been postulated that low bone density in the jaw bones due to osteoporosis may result in more rapid bone resorption upon challenge by bacterial pathogens (Wactawski-Wende, 2001). In addition, individuals with systemic bone loss have been shown to display increased systemic production of inflammatory cytokines that may, in turn, impact resorption of maxillary and mandibular bone s(Smith, et al., 2006). Finally, osteoporosis and periodontitis share smoking as a risk factor. The literature that explores the relationship between osteoporosis and periodontitis is difficult to interpret due to wide variability in the methodology for assessments of both osteoporosis and periodontitis. Most of the studies are cross-sectional, uncontrolled and of small sample size.

Mandibular bone density, tooth loss, alveolar crestal bone height and loss of periodontal attachment are among the outcome measures that have been used to measure the effect of systemic bone loss or osteoporosis on oral health status. A series of classic articles by Kribbs et al. demonstrated a significant relationship between skeletal bone mass and mandibular bone mass (Kribbs, et al., 1983; Kribbs, et al., 1989; Kribbs, et al., 1990). Low bone density or bone mass in the mandible, however, does not necessarily indicate the presence of periodontal disease. Similarly, tooth loss may be the result of factors other than periodontal disease. Therefore, our focus will be on studies that use outcome measures that are more specific for periodontitis such as probing depth, loss of clinical attachment or loss of alveolar crestal bone height.

In a study of 30 postmenopausal women Mohammad, et al. (2003) investigated the association between osteoporosis and periodontitis as measured by tooth loss, plaque index, probing depths and clinical attachment levels. Lower bone mineral density (BMD) was found to be associated with increased clinical attachment loss and tooth loss. In contrast, in a study of 292 dentate women with a mean age of 75.5 years, Weyant, et al. (1999) failed to confirm such an association. This study explored several alternative periodontal outcome measures (mean attachment loss, number of sites with attachment loss of $\geq$ 4 mm and $\geq$ 6 mm, number of sites with bleeding on probing and the deepest probing depth per person) but failed to find statistically significant associations between any measure of periodontal disease and systemic BMD after controlling for age, smoking and the number of remaining natural teeth.

One of the larger studies investigating the association between osteoporosis and alveolar crestal height was conducted by Wactawski-Wende, et al. (2005). A subsample of 1,341 postmenopausal women from the Buffalo Clinical Center of the Observational Study of the Women's Health Initiative (Langer, et al., 2003) with a mean age of 66.7 were included and evaluated for radiographic alveolar bone loss and tooth loss due to periodontal disease. A significant association was observed between osteoporosis and alveolar bone loss after adjusting for possible confounders and was found to be stronger in women over the age of 70 years.

A longitudinal study by Yoshihara et al. assessed the relationship between systemic BMD and longitudinal loss of periodontal attachment (Yoshihara, et al., 2004). The 179 participants were divided into an osteopenia and a non-osteopenia group, each of which had periodontal assessments at baseline and 3-year follow-up. In a multivariate analysis, bone mineral density was found to be significantly associated with the number of sites with progressing periodontitis, defined as longitudinal loss of attachment of ≥ 3 mm. In contrast, other longitudinal studies failed to demonstrate a relationship between osteoporosis and progressive periodontitis (von Wowern, et al., 1992; Klemetti, et al., 1993).

Assuming an association between osteoporosis and periodontitis, one might expect that hormone replacement therapy (HRT) would improve periodontal status. Norderyd, et al. (1993) studied the relationship between HRT and periodontal status in 228 women of age 50–64 years. Periodontal status included assessments of supragingival plaque, subgingival calculus, gingival bleeding, probing pocket depth, clinical attachment level, alveolar bone height and number of remaining teeth. Women receiving HRT had less plaque, lower levels of colonization by *Capnocytophaga* species and significantly less gingival bleeding than controls. However, there were no associations between HRT and the remaining periodontal variables.

While most studies have considered the effect of osteoporosis on periodontal status, there is also biologic plausibility for a bi-directional relationship. Inflammatory cytokines are known to promote bone resorption via osteoclast activation (Manolagas, 1995), and increased levels of systemic inflammatory cytokines as a result of periodontitis may conceivably enhance the susceptibility to systemic bone loss. In an attempt to test this assertion, Famili, et al. (2005) conducted a longitudinal study that evaluated 398 women >65 years of age who were enrolled in the Pittsburgh Clinical Center Study of Osteoporotic Fractures. Patients had assessments of systemic BMD as well as a periodontal examination, and repeat assessments of systemic BMD were performed 2 years later. The findings indicated no difference in BMD or percentage change in BMD among those with and without periodontitis.

In conclusion, while some evidences suggest an association between osteoporosis and periodontitis, the data are conflicting. Future studies with appropriate design, sample size and adjustment for potential confounders are needed to clarify this relationship.

Other Conditions

As mentioned in the introduction, periodontal disease remains a significant cause of tooth loss and the ramification of tooth loss in the elderly population should not be underestimated. As the topic of impaired mastication and nutrition is covered in depth in another chapter of this textbook, we will briefly summarize here some evidence suggesting that tooth loss has a negative impact on diet. Joshipura, et al. (1996) examined the role of edentulism on food and nutrient intake in a sample of 49,501 health professionals, aged 40–80 years (mean age of 55), who provided data on their dietary intake and number of teeth. Subjects who were edentulous consumed fewer vegetables, less fiber and carotene and more saturated fat and calories than subjects who had 25 or more teeth. A longitudinal interdisciplinary study on aging by a group of investigators in Japan examined the relationship between the number of teeth present and nutrient intake in 57 subjects who were 74 years old (Yoshihara, et al., 2005). In a stratified analysis based on the number of remaining teeth ($1–19$ or ≥ 20), significant associations were found between number of teeth and intake of several nutrients including total protein, animal protein, sodium, vitamins D, B1, B6, niacin and pantothenic acid, while subjects with fewer teeth consumed fewer vegetables, fish and shellfish than those with more teeth. Lastly, a recent study by Ogawa, et al. (2006) reported on the relationship between nutritional status, overall health and periodontal disease in the elderly. Nutritional status and overall health were assessed using levels of serum albumin, since low serum albumin is associated with inflammation and malnutrition (Don & Kaysen, 2004) and is a predictor of mortality in the elderly (Phillips, et al., 1989). The study sample consisted of 600 community-dwelling elders (over 70 years of age) with roughly equal numbers of men and women. The periodontal examination consisted of assessments of number of teeth present and percent of sites with loss of attachment of $\geq 6\,mm$. A significant association was reported between the percent of sites with $\geq 6\,mm$ attachment loss and serum albumin, after adjustment for additional co-variates. The authors speculated that the observed inverse relationship between periodontal disease status and levels of serum albumin was related to nutritional factors in the study population.

Conclusions

The present review concludes that the link between periodontitis and systemic disease in the general population and in elderly individuals in particular is both biologically plausible and supported by epidemiologic data. We have discussed the role of periodontal bacteria as systemic health stressors and the contribution of periodontitis to the individual aggregate pathogen/inflammatory burden. Systemic inflammation has been known to impact the development and/or progression of a number of conditions including geriatric frailty (Walston, et al., 2006). Frailty is currently considered a syndrome that includes unintentional weight loss, weakness, slow walking speed and low physical activity (Fried, et al., 2001). Importantly, serum inflammatory markers have been shown to be predictive of mortality rates and functional decline in community-dwelling elders (Reuben, et al., 2002). Other systemic conditions such as diabetes, and perhaps osteoporosis, that may put the elderly at increased risk for periodontitis may also contribute to a cycle of expanded, and possibly synergistic, co-morbidity. As discussed above, the exact sequence of events in the pathobiology of the periodontitis/systemic health interaction are not fully appreciated, and it is often difficult to differentiate between exposures and outcomes. Irrespectively, it is clear that periodontitis occupies a central position in a foul circle of co-morbidities affecting the elderly and its role in the successful, holistic, management of their health care cannot and should not be overlooked. As pointed out by Jepsen & Kuchel (2006) in a recent editorial, the current fragmentation of health care services among different specialists may explain why oral health may be overlooked by physicians and why there has been little intersection between dental and geriatric research. Physicians and dentists need to work together to develop research initiatives that will better clarify the relationship between periodontal disease and systemic disease in the elderly. As a result, the administration of appropriate health care interventions in the elderly will be enhanced and the quality of life in this ever-growing segment of the population will be improved.

References

Ajwani, S., Mattila, K. J., Tilvis, R. S. & Ainamo, A. (2003). Periodontal disease and mortality in an aged population. *Special Care in Dentistry*, 23, 125–130.

Al-Zahrani, M. S., Bissada, N. F. & Borawskit, E. A. (2003). Obesity and periodontal disease in young, middle-aged, and older adults. *Journal of Periodontology*, 74, 610–615.

Amar, S., Gokce, N., Morgan, S., Loukideli, M., Van Dyke, T. E. & Vita, J. A. (2003). Periodontal disease is associated with brachial artery endothelial dysfunction and systemic inflammation. *Arteriosclerosis, Thrombosis, and Vascular Biology* 23, 1245–1249.

Arbes, S. J., Jr., Slade, G. D. & Beck, J. D. (1999). Association between extent of periodontal attachment loss and self-reported history of heart attack: an analysis of NHANES III data. *Journal of Dental Research*, 78, 1777–1782.

Azarpazhooh, A. & Leake, J. L. (2006). Systematic review of the association between respiratory diseases and oral health. *Journal of Periodontology*, 77, 1465–1482.

Baltch, A. L., Schaffer, C., Hammer, M. C., Sutphen, N. T., Smith, R. P., Conroy, J. & Shayegani, M. (1982). Bacteremia following dental cleaning in patients with and without penicillin prophylaxis. *American Heart Journal*, 104, 1335–1339.

Bastard, J. P., Maachi, M., Lagathu, C., Kim, M. J., Caron, M., Vidal, H., Capeau, J. & Feve, B. (2006). Recent advances in the relationship between obesity, inflammation, and insulin resistance. *European Cytokine Network*, 17, 4–12.

Bax, J. J., Inzucchi, S. E., Bonow, R. O., Schuijf, J. D., Freeman, M. R. & Barrett, E. (2007). Cardiac imaging for risk stratification in diabetes. *Diabetes Care*, 30(5), 1295–304.

Beck, J. D., Eke, P., Heiss, G., Madianos, P., Couper, D., Lin, D., Moss, K., Elter, J. & Offenbacher, S. (2005a). Periodontal disease and coronary heart disease: a reappraisal of the exposure. *Circulation*, 112, 19–24.

Beck, J. D., Eke, P., Lin, D., Madianos, P., Couper, D., Moss, K., Elter, J., Heiss, G. & Offenbacher, S. (2005b). Associations between IgG antibody to oral organisms and carotid intima-medial thickness in community-dwelling adults. *Atherosclerosis*, 183(2), 342–8.

Beck, J. D., Elter, J. R., Heiss, G., Couper, D., Mauriello, S. M. & Offenbacher, S. (2001). Relationship of periodontal disease to carotid artery intima-media wall thickness: The atherosclerosis risk in communities (ARIC) study. *Arteriosclerosis, Thrombosis, and Vascular Biology*, 21, 1816–1822.

Beltran-Aguilar, E. D., Barker, L. K., Canto, M. T., Dye, B. A., Gooch, B. F., Griffin, S. O., Hyman, J., Jaramillo, F., Kingman, A., Nowjack-Raymer, R., Selwitz, R. H. & Wu, T. (2005). Surveillance for dental caries, dental sealants, tooth retention, edentulism, and enamel fluorosis–United States, 1988–1994 and 1999–2002. *MMWR Surveillance Summaries*, 54, 1–43.

Bergmans, D. C., Bonten, M. J., Gaillard, C. A., Paling, J. C., van der Geest, S., van Tiel, F. H., Beysens, A. J., de Leeuw, P. W. & Stobberingh, E. E. (2001). Prevention of ventilator-associated pneumonia by oral decontamination: a prospective, randomized, double-blind, placebo-controlled study. *American Journal of Respiratory and Critical Care Medicine*, 164, 382–388.

Borrell, L. N. & Papapanou, P. N. (2005). Analytical epidemiology of periodontitis. *Journal of Clinical Periodontology*, 32 Suppl 6, 132–158.

Bretz, W. A., Weyant, R. J., Corby, P. M., Ren, D., Weissfeld, L., Kritchevsky, S. B., Harris, T., Kurella, M., Satterfield, S., Visser, M. & Newman, A. B. (2005). Systemic inflammatory markers, periodontal diseases, and periodontal infections in an elderly population. *Journal of the American Geriatrics Society*, 53, 1532–1537.

Celermajer, D. S., Sorensen, K. E., Gooch, V. M., Spiegelhalter, D. J., Miller, O. I., Sullivan, I. D., Lloyd, J. K. & Deanfield, J. E. (1992). Non-invasive detection of endothelial dysfunction in children and adults at risk of atherosclerosis. *Lancet*, 340, 1111–1115.

Christgau, M., Palitzsch, K.-D., Schmalz, G., Kreiner, U. & Frenzel, S. (1998). Healing response to non-surgical periodontal therapy in patients with diabetes mellitus: clinical, microbiological, and immunological results. *Journal of Clinical Periodontology*, 25, 112–124.

Cutler, C. W., Machen, R. L., Jotwani, R. & Iacopino, A. M. (1999). Heightened gingival inflammation and attachment loss in type 2 diabetics with hyperlipidemia. *Journal of Periodontology*, 70, 1313–1321.

D'Aiuto, F., Nibali, L., Parkar, M., Suvan, J. & Tonetti, M. S. (2005). Short-term effects of intensive periodontal therapy on serum inflammatory markers and cholesterol. *Journal of Dental Research*, 84, 269–273.

D'Aiuto, F., Parkar, M., Andreou, G., Suvan, J., Brett, P. M., Ready, D. & Tonetti, M. S. (2004a). Periodontitis and systemic inflammation: Control of the local infection is associated with a reduction in serum inflammatory markers. *Journal of Dental Research*, 83, 156–160.

D'Aiuto, F., Parkar, M., Nibali, L., Suvan, J., Lessem, J. & Tonetti, M. S. (2006). Periodontal infections cause changes in traditional and novel cardiovascular risk factors: results from a randomized controlled clinical trial. *American Heart Journal*, 151, 977–984.

D'Aiuto, F., Ready, D. & Tonetti, M. S. (2004b). Periodontal disease and C-reactive protein-associated cardiovascular risk. *Journal of Periodontal Research*, 39, 236–241.

Daly, C., Mitchell, D., Grossberg, D., Highfield, J. & Stewart, D. (1997). Bacteraemia caused by periodontal probing. *Australian Dental Journal*, 42, 77–80.

de Ferranti, S. D. & Rifai, N. (2007). C-reactive protein: a nontraditional serum marker of cardiovascular risk. *Cardiovascular Pathology*, 16, 14–21.

de Nardin, E. (2001). The role of inflammatory and immunological mediators in periodontitis and cardiovascular disease. *Annals of Periodontology*, 6, 30–40.

de Stefano, F., Anda, R. F., Kahn, H. S., Williamson, D. F. & Russell, C. M. (1993). Dental disease and risk of coronary heart disease and mortality [see comments]. *British Medical Journal*, 306, 688–691.

Desvarieux, M., Demmer, R. T., Rundek, T., Boden-Albala, B., Jacobs, D. R., Jr., Papapanou, P. N. & Sacco, R. L. (2003). Relationship between periodontal disease, tooth loss, and carotid artery plaque: The oral infections and vascular disease epidemiology study (INVEST). *Stroke*, 34, 2120–2125.

Desvarieux, M., Demmer, R. T., Rundek, T., Boden-Albala, B., Jacobs, D. R., Jr., Sacco, R. L. & Papapanou, P. N. (2005). Periodontal microbiota and carotid intima-media thickness: The oral infections and vascular disease epidemiology study (INVEST). *Circulation*, 111, 576–582.

Don, B. R. & Kaysen, G. (2004). Serum albumin: Relationship to inflammation and nutrition. *Seminars in Dialysis*, 17, 432–437.

Ebersole, J. L., Machen, R. L., Steffen, M. J. & Willmann, D. E. (1997). Systemic acute-phase reactants, C-reactive protein and haptoglobin, in adult periodontitis. *Clinical and Experimental Immunology* 107, 347–352.

Elter, J. R., Hinderliter, A. L., Offenbacher, S., Beck, J. D., Caughey, M., Brodala, N. & Madianos, P. N. (2006). The effects of periodontal therapy on vascular endothelial function: a pilot trial. *American Heart Journal*, 151, 47.e1–47.e6.

Emrich, L. J., Shlossman, M. & Genco, R. J. (1991). Periodontal disease in non-insulin-dependent diabetes mellitus. *Journal of Periodontology*, 62, 123–131.

Engebretson, S. P., Lamster, I. B., Elkind, M. S., Rundek, T., Serman, N. J., Demmer, R. T., Sacco, R. L., Papapanou, P. N. & Desvarieux, M. (2005). Radiographic measures of chronic periodontitis and carotid artery plaque. *Stroke*, 36(3), 561–6.

Famili, P., Cauley, J., Suzuki, J. B. & Weyant, R. (2005). Longitudinal study of periodontal disease and edentulism with rates of bone loss in older women. *Journal of Periodontology*, 76, 11–15.

Fiehn, N. E., Larsen, T., Christiansen, N., Holmstrup, P. & Schroeder, T. V. (2005). Identification of periodontal pathogens in atherosclerotic vessels. *Journal of Periodontology*, 76, 731–736.

Forrester, J. S. & Bick-Forrester, J. (2005). Persistence of inflammatory cytokines cause a spectrum of chronic progressive diseases: Implications for therapy. *Medical Hypotheses*, 65, 227–231.

Fourrier, F., Cau-Pottier, E., Boutigny, H., Roussel-Delvallez, M., Jourdain, M. & Chopin, C. (2000). Effects of dental plaque antiseptic decontamination on bacterial colonization and nosocomial infections in critically ill patients. *Intensive Care Medicine*, 26, 1239–1247.

Fourrier, F., Dubois, D., Pronnier, P., Herbecq, P., Leroy, O., Desmettre, T., Pottier-Cau, E., Boutigny, H., Di Pompeo, C., Durocher, A. & Roussel-Delvallez, M. (2005). Effect of gingival and dental plaque antiseptic decontamination on nosocomial infections acquired in the intensive care unit: a double-blind placebo-controlled multicenter study. *Critical Care Medicine*, 33, 1728–1735.

Fourrier, F., Duvivier, B., Boutigny, H., Roussel-Delvallez, M. & Chopin, C. (1998). Colonization of dental plaque: A source of nosocomial infections in intensive care unit patients. *Critical Care Medicine*, 26, 301–308.

Fried, L. P., Tangen, C. M., Walston, J., Newman, A. B., Hirsch, C., Gottdiener, J., Seeman, T., Tracy, R., Kop, W. J., Burke, G. & McBurnie, M. A. (2001). Frailty in older adults: Evidence for a phenotype. *Journals of Gerontology Series A: Biological Sciences and Medical Sciences*, 56, M146–M156.

Genco, R. J., Grossi, S. G., Ho, A., Nishimura, F. & Murayama, Y. (2005). A proposed model linking inflammation to obesity, diabetes, and periodontal infections. *Journal of Periodontology*, 76, 2075–2084.

Grossi, S. G., Genco, R. J., Machtei, E. E., Ho, A. W., Koch, G., Dunford, R., Zambon, J. J. & Hausmann, E. (1995). Assessment of risk for periodontal disease. II. Risk indicators for alveolar bone loss. *Journal of Periodontology*, 66, 23–29.

Grossi, S. G., Skrepcinski, F. B., DeCaro, T., Robertson, D. C., Ho, A. W., Dunford, R. G. & Genco, R. J. (1997). Treatment of periodontal disease in diabetics reduces glycated hemoglobin. *Journal of Periodontology*, 68, 713–719.

Haffajee, A. D. & Socransky, S. S. (1994). Microbial etiological agents of destructive periodontal diseases. *Periodontology 2000*, 5, 78–111.

Hansson, G. K. (2005). Inflammation, atherosclerosis, and coronary artery disease. *New England Journal of Medicine*, 352, 1685–1695.

Haraszthy, V. I., Zambon, J. J., Trevisan, M., Zeid, M. & Genco, R. J. (2000). Identification of periodontal pathogens in atheromatous plaques. *Journal of Periodontology*, 71, 1554–1560.

Huang, A. L. & Vita, J. A. (2006). Effects of systemic inflammation on endothelium-dependent vasodilation. *Trends in Cardiovascular Medicine*, 16, 15–20.

Hujoel, P. P., White, B. A., Garcia, R. I. & Listgarten, M. A. (2001). The dentogingival epithelial surface area revisited. *Journal of Periodontal Research*, 36, 48–55.

Janket, S. J., Wightman, A., Baird, A. E., Van Dyke, T. E. & Jones, J. A. (2005). Does periodontal treatment improve glycemic control in diabetic patients? A meta-analysis of intervention studies. *Journal of Dental Research*, 84, 1154–1159.

Jepsen, R. & Kuchel, G. A. (2006). Nutrition and inflammation: The missing link between periodontal disease and systemic health in the frail elderly? *Journal of Clinical Periodontology*, 33, 309–311.

Joshipura, K. J., Willett, W. C. & Douglass, C. W. (1996). The impact of edentulousness on food and nutrient intake. *Journal of the American Dental Association*, 127, 459–467.

Klemetti, E., Vainio, P., Lassila, V. & Alhava, E. (1993). Trabecular bone mineral density of mandible and alveolar height in postmenopausal women. *Scandinavian Journal of Dental Research*, 101, 166–170.

Kornman, K. S., Page, R. C. & Tonetti, M. S. (1997). The host response to the microbial challenge in periodontitis: assembling the players. *Periodontology 2000*, 14, 33–53.

Kozarov, E. V., Dorn, B. R., Shelburne, C. E., Dunn, W. A., Jr. & Progulske-Fox, A. (2005). Human atherosclerotic plaque contains viable invasive *Actinobacillus actinomycetemcomitans* and *Porphyromonas gingivalis*. *Arteriosclerosis, Thrombosis, and Vascular Biology*, 25, e17–e18.

Kribbs, P. J., Chesnut, C. H., Ott, S. M. & Kilcoyne, R. F. (1989). Relationships between mandibular and skeletal bone in an osteoporotic population. *Journal of Prosthetic Dentistry*, 62, 703–707.

Kribbs, P. J., Chesnut, C. H., Ott, S. M. & Kilcoyne, R. F. (1990). Relationships between mandibular and skeletal bone in a population of normal women. *Journal of Prosthetic Dentistry*, 63, 86–89.

Kribbs, P. J., Smith, D. E. & Chesnut, C. H. (1983). Oral findings in osteoporosis. Part I: Measurement of mandibular bone density. *Journal of Prosthetic Dentistry*, 50, 576–579.

Lalla, E., Lamster, I. B., Stern, D. M. & Schmidt, A. M. (2001). Receptor for advanced glycation end products, inflammation, and accelerated periodontal disease in diabetes: Mechanisms and insights into therapeutic modalities. *Annals of Periodontology*, 6, 113–118.

Lane, N. E. (2006). Epidemiology, etiology, and diagnosis of osteoporosis. *American Journal of Obstetrics and Gynecology*, 194, S3–S11.

Langer, R. D., White, E., Lewis, C. E., Kotchen, J. M., Hendrix, S. L. & Trevisan, M. (2003). The Women's Health Initiative Observational Study: baseline characteristics of participants and reliability of baseline measures. *Annals of Epidemiology*, 13, S107–S121.

Lee, H. J., Garcia, R. I., Janket, S. J., Jones, J. A., Mascarenhas, A. K., Scott, T. E. & Nunn, M. E. (2006). The association between cumulative periodontal disease and stroke history in older adults. *Journal of Periodontology*, 77, 1744–1754.

Loesche, W. J., Schork, A., Terpenning, M. S., Chen, Y. M., Dominguez, B. L. & Grossman, N. (1998). Assessing the relationship between dental disease and coronary heart disease in elderly U.S. veterans. *Journal of the American Dental Association*, 129, 301–311.

Loos, B. G. (2005). Systemic markers of inflammation in periodontitis. *Journal of Periodontology*, 76, 2106–2115.

Ludewig, B., Krebs, P. & Scandella, E. (2004). Immunopathogenesis of atherosclerosis. *Journal of Leukocyte Biology*, 76, 300–306.

Manolagas, S. C. (1995). Role of cytokines in bone resorption. *Bone*, 17, 63S-67S.

Marsh, P. D. (2004). Dental plaque as a microbial biofilm. *Caries Research*, 38, 204–211.

Mattila, K. J., Asikainen, S., Wolf, J., Jousimies-Somer, H., Valtonen, V. & Nieminen, M. (2000). Age, dental infections, and coronary heart disease. *Journal of Dental Research*, 79, 756–760.

McGuinness, O. P. (2005). Defective glucose homeostasis during infection. *Annual Review of Nutrition* 25, 9–35.

Meneilly (2006). Diabetes in the Elderly. *Medical Clinics of North America*, 90, 909–923.

Mercanoglu, F., Oflaz, H., Oz, O., Gokbuget, A. Y., Genchellac, H., Sezer, M., Nisanci, Y. & Umman, S. (2004). Endothelial dysfunction in patients with chronic periodontitis and its improvement after initial periodontal therapy. *Journal of Periodontology*, 75, 1694–1700.

Miller, L. S., Manwell, M. A., Newbold, D., Reding, M. E., Rasheed, A., Blodgett, J. & Kornman, K. S. (1992). The relationship between reduction in periodontal inflammation and diabetes control: a report of 9 cases. *Journal of Periodontology*, 63, 843–848.

Mohammad, A. R., Hooper, D. A., Vermilyea, S. G., Mariotti, A. & Preshaw, P. M. (2003). An investigation of the relationship between systemic bone density and clinical periodontal status in post-menopausal Asian-American women. *International Dental Journal*, 53, 121–125.

Moller, D. E. (2000). Potential role of TNF-alpha in the pathogenesis of insulin resistance and type 2 diabetes. *Trends in Endocrinology and Metabolism*, 11, 212–217.

Nelson, R. G., Shlossman, M., Budding, L. M., Pettitt, D. J., Saad, M. F., Genco, R. J. & Knowler, W. C. (1990). Periodontal disease and NIDDM in Pima Indians. *Diabetes Care*, 13, 836–840.

Noack, B., Genco, R. J., Trevisan, M., Grossi, S., Zambon, J. J. & De Nardin, E. (2001). Periodontal infections contribute to elevated systemic C-reactive protein level. *Journal of Periodontology*, 72, 1221–1227.

Norderyd, O. M., Grossi, S. G., Machtei, E. E., Zambon, J. J., Hausmann, E., Dunford, R. G. & Genco, R. J. (1993). Periodontal status of women taking postmenopausal estrogen supplementation. *Journal of Periodontology*, 64, 957–962.

O'Leary, D. H., Polak, J. F., Kronmal, R. A., Manolio, T. A., Burke, G. L. & Wolfson, S. K., Jr. (1999). Carotid-artery intima and media thickness as a risk factor for myocardial infarction and stroke in older adults. Cardiovascular Health Study Collaborative Research Group. *New England Journal of Medicine*, 340, 14–22.

Offenbacher, S. (1996). Periodontal diseases: Pathogenesis. *Annals of Periodontology*, 1, 821–878.

Ogawa, H., Yoshihara, A., Amarasena, N., Hirotomi, T. & Miyazaki, H. (2006). Association between serum albumin and periodontal disease in community-dwelling elderly. *Journal of Clinical Periodontology*, 33, 312–316.

Papapanou, P. N. (1996). Periodontal diseases: Epidemiology. *Annals of Periodontology*, 1, 1–36.

Papapanou, P. N., Lindhe, J., Sterrett, J. D. & Eneroth, L. (1991). Considerations on the contribution of ageing to loss of periodontal tissue support. *Journal of Clinical Periodontology*, 18, 611–615.

Pasceri, V. & Yeh, E. T. H. (1999). A Tale of Two Diseases: Atherosclerosis and Rheumatoid Arthritis. *Circulation*, 100, 2124–2126.

Pearson, T. A., Mensah, G. A., Alexander, R. W., Anderson, J. L., Cannon, R. O., 3rd, Criqui, M., Fadl, Y. Y., Fortmann, S. P., Hong, Y., Myers, G. L., Rifai, N., Smith, S. C., Jr., Taubert, K., Tracy, R. P. & Vinicor, F. (2003). Markers of inflammation and cardiovascular disease: application to clinical and public health practice: A statement for healthcare professionals from the Centers for Disease Control and Prevention and the American Heart Association. *Circulation*, 107, 499–511.

Perry, H. M., 3rd (1999). The endocrinology of aging. *Clinical Chemistry*, 45, 1369–1376.

Persson, R. E., Hollender, L. G., MacEntee, M. I., Wyatt, C. C. L., Kiyak, H. A. & Persson, G. R. (2003). Assessment of periodontal conditions and systemic disease in older subjects. Focus on diabetes mellitus. *Journal of Clinical Periodontology*, 30, 207–213.

Phillips, A., Shaper, A. G. & Whincup, P. H. (1989). Association between serum albumin and mortality from cardiovascular disease, cancer, and other causes. *Lancet*, 2, 1434–1436.

Pihlstrom, B. L., Michalowicz, B. S. & Johnson, N. W. (2005). Periodontal diseases. *Lancet*, 366, 1809–1820.

Promsudthi, A., Pimapansri, S., Deerochanawong, C. & Kanchanavasita, W. (2005). The effect of periodontal therapy on uncontrolled type 2 diabetes mellitus in older subjects. *Oral Diseases*, 11, 293–298.

Ramadori, G. & Christ, B. (1999). Cytokines and the hepatic acute-phase response. *Seminars in Liver Disease*, 19, 141–155.

Schmidt, R., Schmidt, H., Curb, J. D., et al. (2002). Early inflammation and dementia: A 25-year follow-up of the Honolulu-Asia aging study. *Annals of Neurology*, 52, 168–174.

Reuben, D. B., Cheh, A. I., Harris, T. B., Ferrucci, L., Rowe, J. W., Tracy, R. P. & Seeman, T. E. (2002). Peripheral blood markers of inflammation predict mortality and functional decline in high-functioning community-dwelling older persons. *Journal of the American Geriatrics Society*, 50, 638–644.

Ridker, P. M., Hennekens, C. H., Buring, J. E. & Rifai, N. (2000). C-Reactive protein and other markers of inflammation in the prediction of cardiovascular disease in women. *New England Journal of Medicine*, 342, 836–843.

Rothenbacher, D., Hoffmeister, A., Bode, G., Miller, M., Koenig, W. & Brenner, H. (2001). Helicobacter pylori heat shock protein 60 and risk of coronary heart disease: a case control study with focus on markers of systemic inflammation and lipids. *Atherosclerosis*, 156, 193–199.

Saito, T., Shimazaki, Y., Koga, T., Tsuzuki, M. & Ohshima, A. (2001). Relationship between upper body obesity and periodontitis. *Journal of Dental Research*, 80, 1631–1636.

Sanders, A. E., Slade, G. D., Carter, K. D. & Stewart, J. F. (2004). Trends in prevalence of complete tooth loss among Australians, 1979–2002. *The Australian & New Zealand Journal of Public Health*, 28, 549–554.

Scannapieco, F. A. (1999). Role of oral bacteria in respiratory infection. *Journal of Periodontology*, 70, 793–802.

Scannapieco, F. A., Bush, R. B. & Paju, S. (2003a). Associations between periodontal disease and risk for atherosclerosis, cardiovascular disease, and stroke. A systematic review. *Annals of Periodontology*, 8, 38–53.

Scannapieco, F. A., Bush, R. B. & Paju, S. (2003b). Associations between periodontal disease and risk for nosocomial bacterial pneumonia and chronic obstructive pulmonary disease. A systematic review. *Annals of Periodontology*, 8, 54–69.

Seinost, G., Wimmer, G., Skerget, M., Thaller, E., Brodmann, M., Gasser, R., Bratschko, R. O. & Pilger, E. (2005). Periodontal treatment improves endothelial dysfunction in patients with severe periodontitis. *American Heart Journal*, 149, 1050–1054.

Shay, K., Scannapieco, F. A., Terpenning, M. S., Smith, B. J. & Taylor, G. W. (2005). Nosocomial pneumonia and oral health. *Special Care in Dentistry*, 25, 179–187.

Shultis, W. A., Weil, E. J., Looker, H. C., Curtis, J. M., Shlossman, M., Genco, R. J., Knowler, W. C. & Nelson, R. G. (2007). Effect of periodontitis on overt nephropathy and end-stage renal disease in type 2 diabetes. *Diabetes Care*, 30, 306–311.

Silness, J. & Loee, H. (1964). Periodontal Disease in Pregnancy. Ii. Correlation between Oral Hygiene and Periodontal Condition. *Acta Odontologica Scandinavica*, 22, 121–135.

Slade, G. D., Ghezzi, E. M., Heiss, G., Beck, J. D., Riche, E. & Offenbacher, S. (2003). Relationship between periodontal disease and C-reactive protein among adults in the Atherosclerosis Risk in Communities study. *Archives of Internal Medicine*, 163, 1172–1179.

Smith, B. J., Lerner, M. R., Bu, S. Y., Lucas, E. A., Hanas, J. S., Lightfoot, S. A., Postier, R. G., Bronze, M. S. & Brackett, D. J. (2006). Systemic bone loss and induction of coronary vessel disease in a rat model of chronic inflammation. *Bone*, 38, 378–386.

Sopena, N., Sabria, M. & the Neunos Study, G. (2005). Multicenter Study of Hospital-Acquired Pneumonia in Non-ICU Patients. *Chest*, 127, 213–219.

Stewart, J. E., Wager, K. A., Friedlander, A. H. & Zadeh, H. H. (2001). The effect of periodontal treatment on glycemic control in patients with type 2 diabetes mellitus. *Journal of Clinical Periodontology*, 28, 306–310.

Tabeta, K., Yamazaki, K., Hotokezaka, H., Yoshie, H. & Hara, K. (2000). Elevated humoral immune response to heat shock protein 60 (hsp60) family in periodontitis patients. *Clinical and Experimental Immunology*, 120, 285–293.

Taylor, G. W., Burt, B. A., Becker, M. P., Genco, R. J. & Shlossman, M. (1998). Glycemic control and alveolar bone loss progression in type 2 diabetes. *Annals of Periodontology*, 3, 30–39.

Taylor, G. W., Burt, B. A., Becker, M. P., Genco, R. J., Shlossman, M., Knowler, W. C. & Pettitt, D. J. (1996). Severe periodontitis and risk for poor glycemic control in patients with non-insulin-dependent diabetes mellitus. *Journal of Periodontology*, 67, 1085–1093.

Taylor, G. W., Loesche, W. J. & Terpenning, M. S. (2000). Impact of oral diseases on systemic health in the elderly: Diabetes mellitus and aspiration pneumonia. *Journal of Public Health Dentistry*, 60, 313–320.

Terpenning, M. (2005). Geriatric oral health and pneumonia risk. *Clinical Infectious Diseases*, 40, 1807–1810.

Terpenning, M., Bretz, W., Lopatin, D., Langmore, S., Dominguez, B. & Loesche, W. (1993). Bacterial colonization of saliva and plaque in the elderly. *Clinical Infectious Diseases*, 16 Suppl 4, S314–316.

Terpenning, M. & Shay, K. (2002). Oral health is cost-effective to maintain but costly to ignore. *Journal of the American Geriatrics Society*, 50, 584–585.

Terpenning, M. S., Taylor, G. W., Lopatin, D. E., Kerr, C. K., Dominguez, B. L. & Loesche, W. J. (2001). Aspiration pneumonia: dental and oral risk factors in an older veteran population. *Journal of the American Geriatrics Society*, 49, 557–563.

Tervonen, T. & Karjalainen, K. (1997). Periodontal disease related to diabetic status. A pilot study of the response to periodontal therapy in type 1 diabetes. *Journal of Clinical Periodontology*, 24, 505–510.

Tervonen, T. & Knuuttila, M. (1986). Relation of diabetes control to periodontal pocketing and alveolar bone level. *Oral Surgery Oral Medicine Oral Pathology*, 61, 346–349.

Tervonen, T., Knuuttila, M., Pohjamo, L. & Nurkkala, H. (1991). Immediate response to nonsurgical periodontal treatment in subjects with diabetes mellitus. *Journal of Clinical Periodontology*, 18, 65–68.

Theilade, E., Wright, W. H., Jensen, S. B. & Loe, H. (1966). Experimental gingivitis in man. II. A longitudinal clinical and bacteriological investigation. *Journal of Periodontal Research*, 1, 1–13.

Tonetti, M. S., D'Aiuto, F., Nibali, L., Donald, A., Storry, C., Parkar, M., Suvan, J., Hingorani, A. D., Vallance, P. & Deanfield, J. (2007). Treatment of Periodontitis and Endothelial Function. *New England Journal of Medicine*, 356, 911–920.

Tsai, C., Hayes, C. & Taylor, G. W. (2002). Glycemic control of type 2 diabetes and severe periodontal disease in the US adult population. *Community Dentistry and Oral Epidemiology*, 30, 182–192.

UK Prospective Diabetes Study (UKPDS) Group (1998). Intensive blood-glucose control with sulphonylureas or insulin compared with conventional treatment and risk of complications in patients with type 2 diabetes (UKPDS 33). *The Lancet*, 352, 837–853.

Verma, S., Buchanan, M. R. & Anderson, T. J. (2003). Endothelial function testing as a biomarker of vascular disease. *Circulation*, 108, 2054–2059.

Verma, S., Devaraj, S. & Jialal, I. (2006). Is C-reactive protein an innocent bystander or proatherogenic culprit? C-reactive protein promotes atherothrombosis. *Circulation*, 113, 2135–2150; discussion 2150.

von Wowern, N., Klausen, B. & Olgaard, K. (1992). Steroid-induced mandibular bone loss in relation to marginal periodontal changes. *Journal of Clinical Periodontology*, 19, 182–186.

Wactawski-Wende, J. (2001). Periodontal diseases and osteoporosis: Association and mechanisms. *Annals of Periodontology*, 6, 197–208.

Wactawski-Wende, J., Hausmann, E., Hovey, K., Trevisan, M., Grossi, S. & Genco, R. J. (2005). The association between osteoporosis and alveolar crestal height in postmenopausal women. *Journal of Periodontology*, 76, 2116–2124.

Walston, J., Hadley, E. C., Ferrucci, L., Guralnik, J. M., Newman, A. B., Studenski, S. A., Ershler, W. B., Harris, T. & Fried, L. P. (2006). Research agenda for frailty in older adults: Toward a better understanding of physiology and etiology: summary from the American Geriatrics Society/National Institute on Aging Research Conference on Frailty in Older Adults. *Journal of the American Geriatrics Society*, 54, 991–1001.

Weyant, R. J., Pearlstein, M. E., Churak, A. P., Forrest, K., Famili, P. & Cauley, J. A. (1999). The association between osteopenia and periodontal attachment loss in older women. *Journal of Periodontology*, 70, 982–991.

Wilson, A. M., Ryan, M. C. & Boyle, A. J. (2006). The novel role of C-reactive protein in cardiovascular disease: Risk marker or pathogen. *International Journal of Cardiology*, 106, 291–297.

Wu, T., Trevisan, M., Genco, R. J., Falkner, K. L., Dorn, J. P. & Sempos, C. T. (2000). Examination of the relation between periodontal health status and cardiovascular risk factors: serum total and high density lipoprotein cholesterol, C-reactive protein, and plasma fibrinogen. *American Journal of Epidemiology*, 151, 273–282.

Yoneyama, T., Hashimoto, K., Fukuda, H., Ishida, M., Arai, H., Sekizawa, K., Yamaya, M. & Sasaki, H. (1996). Oral hygiene reduces respiratory infections in elderly bed-bound nursing home patients. *Archives of Gerontology and Geriatrics*, 22, 11–19.

Yoneyama, T., Yoshida, M., Ohrui, T., Mukaiyama, H., Okamoto, H., Hoshiba, K., Ihara, S., Yanagisawa, S., Ariumi, S., Morita, T., Mizuno, Y., Ohsawa, T., Akagawa, Y., Hashimoto, K. &

Sasaki, H. (2002). Oral care reduces pneumonia in older patients in nursing homes. *Journal of the American Geriatrics Society*, 50, 430–433.

Yoshihara, A., Seida, Y., Hanada, N. & Miyazaki, H. (2004). A longitudinal study of the relationship between periodontal disease and bone mineral density in community-dwelling older adults. *Journal of Clinical Periodontology*, 31, 680–684.

Yoshihara, A., Watanabe, R., Nishimuta, M., Hanada, N. & Miyazaki, H. (2005). The relationship between dietary intake and the number of teeth in elderly Japanese subjects. *Gerodontology*, 22, 211–218.

Yu, Y.-H. & Ginsberg, H. N. (2005). Adipocyte Signaling and Lipid Homeostasis: Sequelae of Insulin-Resistant Adipose Tissue. *Circulation Research*, 96, 1042–1052.

Zampieri, S., Iaccarino, L., Ghirardello, A., Tarricone, E., Arienti, S., Sarzi-Puttini, P., Gambari, P. & Doria, A. (2005). Systemic Lupus Erythematosus, Atherosclerosis, and Autoantibodies. *Annals of the New York Academy of Sciences*, 1051, 351–361.

Zebrack, J. S. & Anderson, J. L. (2002). The role of inflammation and infection in the pathogenesis and evolution of coronary artery disease. *Current Cardiology Reports*, 4, 278–288.

Zielinski, M. B., Fedele, D., Forman, L. J. & Pomerantz, S. C. (2002). Oral health in the elderly with non-insulin-dependent diabetes mellitus. *Special Care in Dentistry*, 22, 94–98.

Chapter 13
Caries, Tooth Loss, and Conventional Tooth Replacement for Older Patients

Ejvind Budtz-Jørgensen and Frauke Müller

Introduction

During the recent decades, industrialized countries have shown an important decline in edentulism and a corresponding increase in the mean number of teeth present among elderly people (Atchieson & Andersen, 2000; Morse, Holm-Pedersen, & Holm-Pedersen, 2002). However, studies still show rather large populations of older with few or no teeth (Kiyak, 2000; Avlund, Holm-Pedersen, & Schroll, 2001). This implies that prevention of oral health problems should be aimed at the growing number of older adults at risk of oral diseases and that caries therapy and prosthetic therapies should be considered and implemented in order to maintain and restore oral function and aesthetics. Because any restorative caries or prosthetic therapies have a short-term or long-term biologic price, such therapies should only be implemented when there is clear evidence that function or aesthetics is invalidated.

When considering the indications for prosthetic therapy and the choice of treatment modality, professional considerations as well as the patient's demand and socio-economic situation are key factors. However, treatment planning for the medically compromised or dependent geriatric patient is even more complex, as it also includes an assessment of the patient's general physical and cognitive state and the patient's perceived need for prosthetic treatment as well as the realistic need (Vigild, 1989). The latter is based on a professional assessment of the normative need, the perceived need, and the expressed demand for treatment, taking into account the general mental and physical state of each individual.

Finally, dental and prosthodontic treatment planning is dependent on the allocation of resources, and hence is a political decision. Socio-economic factors are particularly important in the prosthetic treatment of older patients because restricted financial means often limits the possibilities to very simple treatments, such as treatment with conventional complete dentures (Mojon, Thomason, & Walls, 2004; Palmqvist, Söderfeldt, & Vigild, 2001).

E. Budtz-Jørgensen
Professor emeritus, Division of Gerodontology and Removable Prosthodontics, University of Geneva, Rue Barthélely-Menn, 19, 1205 Geneva, Switzerland
e-mail: budtz@bluewin.ch

I.B. Lamster, M.E. Northridge (eds.), *Improving Oral Health for the Elderly*,
© Springer Science+Business Media, LLC 2008

When cohorts of 70-year-old Swedish subjects were compared, it appeared that the prevalence of edentulism, which was 51% in 1971, had declined to 7% in 2001 (Österberg & Carlsson 2007). On the contrary, the prevalence of FPD had increased from 26% to 68% and subjects having 20 remaining teeth or more from 13% to 65% during the same period. In another study, carried out in Pomerania, Germany, tooth loss among older individual was more important than in the Swedish study (Mack et al., 2003; Mack et al., 2004). In this study, tooth loss and the risk of wearing complete dentures were primarily associated with old age but also factors such as low income, low education level, and smoking.

When considering restorative caries or prosthetic therapies for older patients, it is important to identify major risk factors associated with progression of periodontal disease, caries activity, residual ridge resorption, and functional problems (Budtz-Jørgensen, 1999). In this context, it should be taken into account that a high incidence of secondary caries and root caries was found, especially among the very old, and that the caries-promoting factors were most unfavourable among the subjects in the oldest age groups (Fure, 2004). This indicates that the causal treatment of caries had not been successful and that there is an unmet need for an increased implementation of caries-preventive measures with an increasing age of the patients.

Caries and Restorative Caries Therapy

Dental Caries and Tooth Loss in the Elderly

The prevalence of dental caries in older populations is available in many recent studies indicating that untreated caries is an increasing problem, particularly among institutionalized patients, but to a lesser extent among free-living elderly (Chapter 2).

Root surface caries is a major problem due to gingival recession. Clinically, root surface caries comprises changes from small, softened, and discoloured spots on the root to extensive, brownish, or very dark, soft areas encircling a part or the entire root surface, which are usually covered by plaque (Fig. 13.1) (Fejerskov & Nyvad, 1996). On the contrary, inactive lesions are typically dark-brown, while the surface is frequently shiny, smooth, hard on probing and usually plaque-free. Inactive lesions are often prevalent among free-living elderly, whereas active lesions are prevalent among elderly living in long-term institutional care (Fejerskov, Luan, Nyvad, Budtz-Jørgensen, & Holm-Pedersen, 1991; Galan & Lynch, 1993; Katz, Neely, & Morse, 1996).

The major associated predisposing conditions for caries development are impaired cognitive function and functional ability, decreased salivary secretion rates, diabetes mellitus, number of exposed root surfaces, poor oral hygiene, high sugar consumption, and poor socio-economic conditions (Avlund, Holm-Pedersen, Morse, Viitanen, & Winblad, 2004; Budtz-Jørgensen, Mojon, Rentsch, Roerich, von der Muehll, & Baehni, 1996a; Fure, 2004; Guivante-Nabert, Berenholc, &

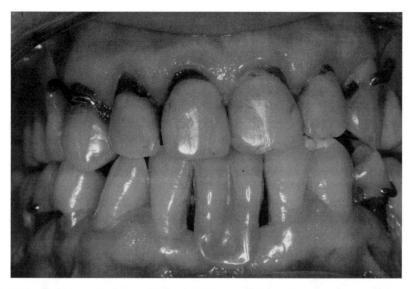

Fig. 13.1 Active root surface caries lesions exhibiting a typical location along the cemento-enamel junction (*See* Color Plate 1)

Berdal, 1999; Lundgren, 1997; Mojon et al., 2004). Caries is the major cause for tooth extraction among both free-living and institutionalized elderly (Fure, 2003; Hämäläinen, Meurman, Keskinen, & Heikkinen, 2004).

That the increment in caries can take place very fast was shown in a study on 76 nursing home residents of whom the majority had moderate to severe cognitive impairment (Chalmers Carter, & Spencer, 2005). After 1 year, 54% of the residents could be examined, and they showed an incidence of coronal caries of 64% and of root surface caries of 49%, respectively. In fact, 72% of the residents had coronal and/or root surface caries increment between base-line and 1 year.

In a recent study, an evaluation of caries risk factors in the elderly was carried out using a computer program, the Cariogram (Petersson, Fure, & Bratthall, 2003); thus, the aim of the study was to compare the risk assessment using the program with that of the actual caries increment in a group of 208 persons (55-, 65-, and 75-year-olds) over a period of 5 years. The parameters, which were introduced in the Cariogram, were information about the participants' general health status and dietary habits; data on oral hygiene and use of fluoride; saliva analyses with respect to mutans streptococci, lactobacilli, buffering capacity, and secretion rate. Overall, a significant proportion of the participants had a high risk of caries according to the Cariogram. The mean increment (DMFS) after 5 years was 12.8% in the high/rather high risk group, which included 43% of the individuals. In the low/rather low risk group, it was 5.2%, and 21% of the participants were sorted to this group.

Although elderly individuals may suffer coronal caries, usually as recurrent caries around existing restorations, it is arguably the condition of root caries that most concerns gerodontologists (Mojon, Rentsch, & Budtz-Jørgensen, 1995).

Recently, a German oral health survey revealed a significant increase in the prevalence of root caries in the population between 65 and 74 years (Schiffner & Reich, 1999; Schiffner, 2006). From 1999 to 2006, the prevalence of root caries increased from 15.5% to 45%.

In future, the number of people aged 65 years and older is expected to increase substantially in highly industrialized countries. Moreover, advances in dental treatment and prevention of caries and periodontal diseases will result in reduced levels of the edentulous condition; as a consequence, there will be more elderly people in need of various dental services. It is assumed that a combination of natural teeth and fixed or removable dentures will still be common for the next couple of decades, and that the management of this situation among older adults will be an important issue for dentists for many years to come. Even today, there is an unmet need for all types of dental care among old people living in institution.

Prevention of caries and tooth loss in the elderly is based around accurate risk assessment (which can be difficult) and the institution of an appropriate regime of dietary advice, oral hygiene measures, the management of plaque retentive factors, and topical fluoride therapy (Curzon & Preston, 2004). Oral hygiene must be considered the major disease determinant compared to other determinants such as diet, saliva secretion rate, buffer capacity, and the composition of the oral micro flora (Fejerskov & Nyvad, 1996). Thus, frequent plaque removal carried out by professionals in conjunction with daily use of fluoride toothpaste almost totally prevented root surface caries development (Lindhe & Nyman, 1975). In a longitudinal study carried out in a nursing home, the effects of the introduction of an oral health program reduced caries incidence and mutans streptococci colonization (Mojon, Rentsch, Budtz-Jørgensen, & Baehni, 1998). However, untreated caries remained a problem in spite of the oral hygiene program. Therefore, adequate restorative caries therapy remains a frequent treatment option to control caries progression to avoid pulp complications or tooth fractures. This is supported by a recent study on 719 institutionalized subjects, who were followed for 6 years (Shimzaki, Soh, Koga, Miyazaki, & Takehara, 2004). Those who had had dental treatments during the 6-year period needed fewer extractions and presented less caries than the non-treated. The outcome of the study is, however, not quite clear since the general health status was better among the treated patients.

Caries Therapy

The optimal but not always efficient way of treating caries in the elderly is to institute oral hygiene measures, including treatment with fluoride and chlorhexidine. Indeed, clinical observations suggest that caries lesions can be arrested at any stage of lesion development, provided that clinically plaque-free conditions are obtained (Fejerskov & Nyvad, 1996). Treatment with fluorides can prevent and arrest caries by inhibiting bacterial metabolism, by inhibiting demineralization of the tooth, and by enhancing remineralization of initial caries lesions (Featherstone, 2000). For patients predisposed to caries and with high levels of cariogenic bacteria in the oral cavity, treatment with chlorhexidine rinse, gel, or varnish at 3 months' intervals is indicated to control bacterial levels (Banting et al., 2000; Featherstone, 2000). However, in elderly patients with distinct carious lesions, it may be impossible to maintain a low bacterial level, even by regular application of fluoride or chlorhexidine. Therefore, restorative caries therapy is often indicated to prevent caries progression and restore aesthetics and function.

The atraumatic restorative treatment (ART) technique has been developed particularly for treatment of people in rural and subrural areas in less industrialized countries (Frencken, Songpaisan, Phantumvanit, & Pilot, 1994). The concept is a minimal intervention based on removing infected tooth material using hand instruments only; after cleaning of the exposed dentine, the cavity is subsequently filled with glass ionomer cement. The success rate of ART fillings in the permanent dentition for single surface fillings was 93% after 1 year (Frencken et al., 1994). In a study on 119 old people (mean age 72.5 years), ART-fillings were provided for 33 of the patients (Honkala & Honkala, 2002). After 1 year, 68% of the fillings were assessed as good, 11% as having a slight material defect, and 16% for having unacceptable marginal defects. Thus, the ART technique might also be applied in restorative caries therapy of the elderly patients, but to obtain the most reliable results and good aesthetics it seems more appropriate to use a conventional operative treatment technique.

Treatment with amalgam restorations is a realistic option in the posterior region of the mandible and the maxilla, as they are less sensitive to moisture control; however, this technique is often less appropriate since it is usually necessary to remove more tooth structure to obtain a retentive cavity.

Today, composite resins and polyacid-modified composite resins are widely used to restore carious lesions, particularly of the anterior and premolar teeth. Such restorative procedures require adequate technical skill and optimal conditions, such as absence of saliva, to secure retention and integrity of the margins of the restorations. These conditions are rarely present when restorative caries therapy is implemented on frail, physically or mentally handicapped residents of long-term care facilities.

Recently, operative caries treatment was applied in nursing home residents when the carious lesions had reached a depth at which maintenance of a plaque-free cavity surface by proper oral hygiene was no longer possible (Molinari et al., 2007). In 25 consecutive patients, a total of 42 restorations were placed of which 23 were in composite resin and 19 in compomer. The restorations were placed without the use of rubber dam, as the patients refused the dam mostly based on their compromised health situation. The working conditions such as patient cooperation, quantity of saliva, location of the cavity margins, size of the cavities, and absence or presence of gingival inflammation were evaluated prior to treatment. The quality of the restorations was evaluated at baseline, after 6 months and after 12 months, respectively (Lutz, Lüscher, Ochsenbein,& Mühlemann, 1976). The results showed that all examined restorations were clinically acceptable after 12 months; however, six patients had diseased and the plaque scores increased significantly during the study period, reflecting that the patients' general health situation deteriorated. Thus, the placement of adhesive restorations seems to be a realistic treatment in elderly, medically compromised patients in order to restore aesthetics and function and prolong the longevity of the teeth in the anterior and the premolar regions.

The extraction of carious teeth should not take place if other treatment options are possible. Particularly, in a population of dependent or frail elderly, it is important to avoid the psychological trauma of tooth extractions. In addition, mastication, swallowing, and speech disorders may be the consequence of tooth extraction and subsequent replacement with a removable denture (Budtz-Jørgensen, Chung & Mojon, 2000).

Controlling caries is a major issue for successful aging of elderly individuals (MacEntee, 2000). To obtain this, carious teeth should be restored and appropriate oral hygiene measures including regular mouth wash with chlorhexidine with or without fluoride supplement should be introduced. However, today educational strategies to reduce the threat of caries in this population are focused mainly on oral hygiene with almost no attention paid to control of sugar abuse (MacEntee, 2000). In future, much more effort should be used to reduce ingestion of refined carbohydrates, which is not a very well-recognized factor of caries among residents of long-term care facilities.

Prosthetic Treatment of the Elderly

Indications

The primary indications for instituting prosthetic therapy in the elderly are to restore aesthetics, oral comfort, and masticatory function. The minimum number of teeth needed to guarantee sufficient aesthetics and function depends on both local and systemic factors, but these requirements are poorly defined. Some studies support a minimal functional level concept based on data from cross-sectional and longitudinal studies (Käyser, 1981; Leake, Hawkins, & Locker, 1994). According to this concept, eight occluding pairs of teeth in the anterior and the premolar region seem to be sufficient to satisfy elderly patients' aesthetic and functional demand. However, in future, older individuals might be more demanding in this respect. Based on a series of studies concerning the need of prosthetic treatment, it was concluded that there does not exist any true subjective or objective need (Narby, Kronström, Söderfeldt, & Palmqvist, 2005). Thus, need is established only in a communicative dialogue with mutual respect between the professional and the patient, an approach that can be difficult to follow when treating elderly with cognitive impairment.

To age successfully, we assume that it is important for older individuals to be able to comminute food during mastication for swallowing and further processing in the digestive tract, to have a pleasant appearance, and an unimpaired faculty of speech (Budtz-Jørgensen et al., 2000). In the following, aspects of prosthetic treatment planning for the partially or completely edentulous elderly patient will be considered.

Treatment Planning

The primary objectives of prosthetic treatment planning for the partially edentulous patient are, if possible, to secure stable occlusal conditions by natural tooth contacts; to maintain or restore a functional vertical dimension of occlusion; to apply biological principles of prosthetic therapy to minimize direct treatment sequels and long-term negative effects; to apply simple treatment procedures that result in comfort and good aesthetics; and to choose a financially acceptable treatment plan (Budtz-Jørgensen, 1999).

Partially Edentulous Patients

The need for prosthetic rehabilitation in the partially edentulous elderly patient may be due to functional disturbances of the masticatory system, poor masticatory performance, aesthetic or phonetic problems, or a risk of developing functional disturbances. The main functional indications for replacement of missing posterior teeth are complaints of reduced masticatory ability, overt symptoms in the masticatory system, or a reduced occlusal face height. It should be realized, however, that symptoms from the masticatory system (temporo-mandibular joints, jaw muscles) in the elderly are usually not severe and that there is seldom a direct association between the severity of the symptoms and the extent of tooth loss (Budtz-Jørgensen et al., 1985a). Furthermore, cross-sectional studies indicate that if tooth loss and occlusal changes occur at a slow rate, acceptable oral function can be maintained by the premolar and the anterior teeth (Käyser, 1981; Meuwissen, van Waas, Meuwissen, & Käyser, 1995).

Complaints of reduced masticatory ability may be the effect of a reduction of the occlusal contact area but may also be associated with factors such as old age, poor general health, living alone, and low income (Österberg, Carlsson, Tsuga, Sundh, & Steen, 1996; Ow, Loh, Neo, & Khoo, 1997). Masticatory performance (the capacity to reduce test food particles) is related linearly with the number of teeth present and can be restored by fixed or removable partial dentures in patients with extensive loss of posterior teeth (Gunne, 1985). However, masticatory ability with regard to whether the daily and normal food intake is felt to be hindered is generally sufficient as long as at least 20 well-distributed teeth remain (Aukes, Käyser, & Felling, 1988). Further tooth loss in such situations may have a negative effect on food selection (Ekelund, 1989). Indeed, reported difficulty in chewing as a result of tooth loss or problems of wearing dentures was associated with poor diet, impaired food choice, and lower MNA (Mini Nutritional Assessment) scores (Daly et al., 2003).

The risk of developing signs and symptoms of temporo-mandibular disorders is increased in older patients with extremely shortened dental arches, that is, fewer than two occlusal units in each jaw. However, a functional adaptation usually is most likely to take place if tooth loss and occlusal changes occur at a slow rate (Kalk, Käyser, & Witter, 1993). On the other hand, adaptive capacity is reduced if occlusal instability develops suddenly, either by tooth extraction or placement of a poorly designed prosthesis. It is a merely mechanical and not a biological approach to replace posterior tooth loss in older individuals only to prevent functional problems, when there are no overt signs or symptoms of temporo-mandibular disorders. Instead, the situation should be followed and treatment postponed until symptoms appear.

Loss of posterior teeth can promote severe tooth wear in the elderly to a degree that the occlusal face height may be reduced (Dahl, Carlsson, & Ekfeldt, 1993). The main problem is to control further tooth wear and to resolve the aesthetic complaints. The strategy for these patients should be limited treatment with the aim of preventing further tooth wear; this is often difficult as it is unrealistic to anticipate that the anterior functional pattern will change markedly, even after replacement of missing posterior teeth.

Edentulous patients

A number of epidemiologic studies have yielded information about the prevalence of oral mucosal lesions in wearers of complete dentures of which denture stomatitis, i.e. inflammation of the mucosa covered by the denture, is of particular relevance. Denture stomatitis is often associated with a heavy colonization by *Candida*, particularly among patients in long-term hospital care (Budtz-Jørgensen, Mojon, Banon-Clément, & Baehni, 1996b; Vigild, 1987; Wilkieson, Samaranayake, MacFarlane, Lamey, & MacKenzie, 1991). The infection is essentially due to a colonization of the fitting denture surface by *Candida* but tends to spread to involve the tongue and the angles of the mouth. The predisposing conditions are essentially the same as for caries such as institutionalization, medications, frequent carbohydrate intake, reduced salivary flow, poor oral hygiene, and denture wearing (Budtz-Jørgensen, 2000). In fact, the lesions will often clear up by institution of meticulous oral and denture hygiene or if the dentures are not worn during 2 weeks. Traumatic ulcers associated with wearing removable dentures is particularly a problem among patients in psychiatric hospitals compared with nursing homes, probably due to the fact that psychiatric patients often are unable to inform the staff about their oral situation or that the pain threshold may be increased due to intake of psychopharmacologic drugs (Vigild, 1987).

The primary objective of prosthetic therapy in the elderly edentulous patient is to restore the occlusal face height and to provide stable occlusal conditions, acceptable aesthetics, and good oral comfort. In elderly edentulous patients, treatment with complete dentures frequently involves replacement of existing complete dentures that are broken or poor fitting due to wear of the acrylic resin, the denture teeth, or resorption of the underlying residual ridge. It is often difficult to diagnose the underlying reason for the patients' complaints and to establish a safe treatment plan. Thus, one of the great challenges, particularly in treatment with conventional complete dentures, is the discrepancy between the patient's demands and his or hers treatment ability and the objective treatment needs (Mojon & MacEntee, 1992). In this situation, it is important to use the patient's existing dentures to assess which changes of the existing prosthetic situation the patient may accept. A comprehensive prosthetic treatment with complete dentures should not be considered if there is evidence of underlying mental disorders, if the existing dentures do not have major faults, or if the person does not accept the diagnostically modified dentures (Budtz-Jørgensen, 1999).

Quality of Life and Prosthodontics

In a recent study, data about impaired Oral Health Related Quality of Life (OHRQoL) were provided in 107 patients seeking prosthodontic treatment and receiving fixed or removable prostheses (Mike, Slade, Szentpétery, & Setz, 2004). The patients had a considerably impaired level of OHPQoL before treatment. However, OHRQoL improved rapidly within 1 month after treatment and continued to improve the following 6–12 months. The largest improvement was observed in patients treated with fixed partial dentures and the smallest one in patients treated with complete dentures. Thus, this study confirms previous observations that older patients often have difficulty to adapt to and attain a comfortable and efficient oral function with removable dentures (Agerberg & Carlsson, 1981). Use of osseo-integrated implants is an important means to secure retention and stability of a complete denture as well as comfort during denture-wearing. This subject will be treated extensively in the subsequent chapter of this textbook.

Risk Factors for Prosthetic Therapy

Partially Edentulous Patients

The main risk factors to consider in the partially edentulous patient are associated with caries activity and the progression of periodontal disease. A summary of the various risk indicators for caries, which include various oral, medical, mental, behavioural, and psychosocial conditions, are found in Table 13.2, based on the observations by Galan & Lynch (1993) and Katz et al., (1996).

The increased risk of root caries in the elderly is a major problem, which is essentially the result of gingival retraction due to age and/or periodontal disease with subsequent exposure of the root surface. Additional risk factors are poor oral hygiene, frequent carbohydrate intake, high levels of mutans streptococci in saliva, the wearing of removable dentures, and reduced salivary flow (Galan & Lynch, 1993; Keltjens, Schaeken, & van der Hoeven, 1993, Lundgren, 1997; Närhi, Ainamo, & Meurman, 1994). Caries is particularly a problem in wearers of removable partial dentures or overdentures due to increased accumulation of plaque on tooth surfaces in contact with the dentures (Budtz-Jørgensen, 1996a; Budtz-Jørgensen & Isidor, 1990; Jepson, Moynihan, Kelly, Watson, & Thomason, 2001). Progression of root caries in older individuals is generally a larger problem than progression of periodontal disease and requires intense preventive measures. Because root caries in older adults seldom provokes severe pain, untreated and uncontrolled root caries will often result in fracture of the teeth. Thus, root remnants are found in about 40%–70% of dependent dentate adults. Rapidly progressing root caries is a serious problem in frail or dependent elderly, calling for institution of rigorous hygiene measures immediately after institutionalization or hospitalization.

The elderly partially edentulous patient is normally expected to have a reasonable periodontal prognosis due to the fact that there are natural teeth left. In a 10-year longitudinal study, it was shown that the predictors of further tooth loss due to periodontal disease were few teeth at baseline, higher periodontal scores, need for extraction, a history of smoking, and low ascorbic acid intake (Ekelund & Burt, 1994). Furthermore, teeth having shown attachment loss during one follow-up period were also more likely to show progression of periodontal disease or to become extracted in the subsequent period (Beck, Kock, & Offenbacher, 1994; Katz et al., 1996). However, progression of periodontal disease in the elderly may be controlled by conservative and surgical periodontal therapy and by instituting strict hygiene measures (Isidor & Budtz-Jørgensen, 1990). Thus, it was possible to establish stable periodontal conditions prior to and after prosthetic treatment with fixed or removable partial dentures.

In a 5-year follow-up study on prosthetic therapy carried out in 113 of 364 patients aged 76–86 years at baseline, significant modifications of the dental/prosthetic status were observed (Nevalinen, Närhi, & Ainamo, 2004). The mean number of teeth decreased from 14.9 to 13.5, and the prosthetic status had changed in 40% of the elderly people: 25% had received new prostheses, whereas 15% had not been replaced. New fixed partial dentures had been made in nine mandibles and five maxillas. The authors concluded that fixed rather than removable prostheses should be used in elderly patients.

Edentulous Patients

Normally, older well-adapted denture wearers will not seek prosthodontic treatment because of overt denture problems, or marked symptoms from the underlying mucosa, muscles, or the temporo-mandibular joints. They are rather satisfied with existing dentures although, when using objective criteria, these seem to be highly insufficient with respect to occlusion, fit, and maintenance of the vertical dimension of occlusion. Therefore, there is an obvious risk of poor adaptation if the new dentures have been modified in several aspects compared to the old dentures in order to "restore" function and aesthetics.

In fact, adaptation to new complete dentures is a complex process, and it is difficult to anticipate the result of such treatment (van Waas, 1990a; van Waas, 1990b). It has been suggested that oral awareness and pronounced tactile sensibility of the oral mucosa may limit the habituation process that ultimately should lead to adaptation (Landt & Fransson, 1975). By means of an oral sterognosis test, testing the ability to identify different objects placed in the oral cavity, elderly subjects were found to have less tactile sensitivity, and as a consequence might tolerate new dentures better in spite of the continuous retrogressive oral changes with age (Landt & Fransson, 1975). Generally, however, there is no relationship between oral sterognosis ability and patients' satisfaction with complete dentures (Müller, Link, Fuhr, & Utz, 1995). On the contrary, the adaptive capacity to new dentures tends to decrease with age probably because of the progressive loss of neurons from the central nervous system, leading to a decreased ability to form new reflex arcs. Therefore, to reduce the risk of poor adaptation, it is important to use the design of the existing dentures as a guide for designing the new ones.

Important risk factors of poor treatment outcome with complete dentures include chewing problems, localized pain reactions, burning mouth syndrome, dissatisfaction with existing dentures, and reduced salivary flow (Budtz-Jørgensen, 1999). Chewing problems are frequent among wearers of conventional complete dentures and may result in a less ideal food selection, which, however, did not improve by provision of new dentures (Allen, 2005). Thus, further efforts are required to promote a health diet in older age groups than just providing new dentures.

Localized pain reactions are often the consequence of severe resorption of the residual ridge. In order to reduce the symptoms and the risk of further resorption of the residual ridge placement of dental implants to relive the pressure exerted by the denture on the oral mucosa and underlying structures is today the treatment of choice rather than extensive pre-prosthetic surgery (Widmark, Andersson, Carlsson, Ivanoff, & Lindvall, 1998).

A particular risk group among denture wearers is patients who complain of burning and itching in the mucosa, underlying the dentures (burning mouth syndrome). This condition is not necessarily associated with the wearing of complete dentures but is rather due to psychiatric disorders such as anxiety, depression, obsession, or hostility (Rojo, Silvestre, Bagan, & De Vicente, 1994). If there is suspicion of this condition, the patient should imperatively be referred to a specialist before any prosthetic treatment is considered.

Patients who are unable to adapt to "objectively" well-fitting dentures or diagnostically modified dentures constitute another risk group. These patients may have underlying psychiatric disorders, or they may not be able psychologically to accept the wearing of complete dentures. Major pre-prosthetic surgery or treatment with implants should not be considered before the mental/psychiatric status of the patient has been clarified and before the actual dentures have been evaluated (Budtz-Jørgensen, 1999). In this context, it should be emphasized that pre-prosthetic surgery should be restricted to patients with poor anatomic conditions and not be applied in patients with underlying psychiatric disorders. Treatment with implant-retained complete dentures in older patients with poor anatomic conditions or difficulties in adapting to complete dentures remains the gold standard.

The factors that favour good retention of complete dentures are a well-developed border seal and a thin saliva film covering the entire denture surface, i.e. a tight contact between the denture and the mucosa and the presence of saliva. Thus, in patients with impaired salivary secretion, retention of the dentures relies entirely on the patient's ability to maintain the dentures by muscular control. In addition to poor retention, denture wearers with dry mouth often complain of burning or itching oral mucosa, chewing problems, and that food tends to stick to the polished denture surfaces.

Restoration of the Partially Edentulous Mouth

Fixed Partial Denture (FPD)

If given the option, most patients with a shortened dental arch and the need for additional molar and premolar support prefer a FPD to a removable partial denture (RPD). There are two options of treatment: an extension cantilever FPD or an implant-supported FPD. In this chapter, the tooth-borne solution will be considered. In a systematic review of the literature, it was shown that the probability of survival of conventional FPDs with end-abutments was 89.1% (Tan, Petjurrson, Lang, & Chan, 2004) and that for cantilever FPDs, 82% (Petjursson et al., 2004). Thus, the survival and success rates of cantilever FPDs were lower than that for end-abutment supported FPDs and the technical complications were also more frequent with cantilever FPDs.

Cross-Arch FPDs

Cross-arch cantilever FPDs with distal extensions in one or both sides have yielded good results in patients with loss of many teeth and severely reduced periodontal support and mobility of the presumptive abutment teeth (Nyman & Lindhe, 1979; Decock, De Nayer, & De Boever, 1996). Provided that periodontal health can be maintained and the bridgework has been designed to preclude undue stress concentrations, these dentures can also be applied successfully in the elderly (Glantz, Ryge, Jendresen, & Nilner, 1984). However, if these reconstructions are applied using abutment teeth without significant loss of periodontal attachment, the risk of fracture of the abutment teeth or loss of retention is important, particularly if the denture includes long pontic spans and long free-end segments (Randow, 1986). Treatment with cross-arch cantilever FPDs has limited indications in older adults because a decline in oral hygiene resulting in caries of the abutments may give serious complications. Treatment with several smaller FPDs or placement of implants is a more safe solution when the patients' ability to cooperate cannot be guaranteed on long term.

Small Cantilever FPDs

Small unilateral or bilateral extension FPDs were originally conceived for treatment of older patients who were edentulous in the maxilla and had fewer than 10 teeth left in the mandible in order to create at least a premolar occlusion that might be sufficient for function and stability of the maxillary denture (Budtz-Jørgensen, Isidor,

& Karring, 1985b). Preparation of the abutment teeth was minimal as retention was secured by parallel pin restorations whenever this was possible and the dentures were designed with open embrasure spaces to permit mechanical cleansing of the under surface and interproximal surfaces of the pontics and the abutments. The restorations were cemented using zinc-phosphate cement.

Altogether, 27 patients with an average age of 70 years (range 61–83 years) were provided with a total of 41 FPDs, of which 8 were cross-arch cantilever FPDs, 12 were 3–4 unit dentures with 2 abutments, and 21 were 2–3 unit dentures with 1 abutment (Budtz-Jørgensen & Isidor, 1990). The extension of the cantilever in one or both sides of the mandible corresponded to the width of a premolar tooth (Fig. 13.2).

To assess small cantilever extension FPDs as a treatment modality in older patients, an additional group of 26 patients, within the same age range and with a similar distribution of remaining teeth and periodontal situation (case control study), was treated with RPDs in the mandible, and both groups of patients were provided with a new complete denture in the maxilla. The RPDs were designed with a cobalt chromium framework, a dental or a sublingual bar as major connector, mesially placed occlusal rests, a distally place minor connector, and two retentive clasps (Fig. 13.3). The patients in both groups were followed regularly by a dental hygienist for the 5-year study period in order that an appropriate oral hygiene could be maintained.

Immediately following treatment, improvements in chewing function and stability of the maxillary denture were reported in the FPD group, even among patients who had adapted well to wearing a RPD (Budtz-Jørgensen et al., 1985b). Generally, a good oral hygiene and unchanged periodontal conditions were maintained in both

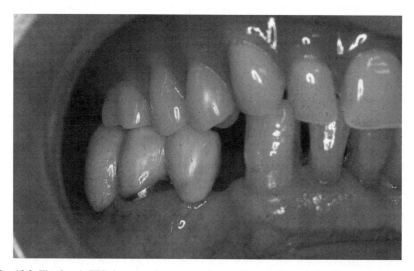

Fig. 13.2 The 3-unit FPD has one abutment and extends mesially and distally to provide stable occlusal conditions with the complete upper denture (*See* Color Plate 2)

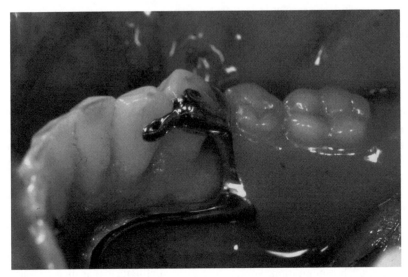

Fig. 13.3 Extension denture base with a mesial occlusal rest, a lingual bracing arm (lingual and distal guide planes have been prepared), and a proximal minor connector. Note the open embrasure space (*See* Color Plate 3)

groups of patients during the 5-year study period (Isidor & Budtz-Jørgensen, 1990). However, caries was observed six times more frequently in the group of patients wearing RPDs, and occlusal and functional conditions deteriorated only in this group (Budtz-Jørgensen & Isidor, 1990). Of the FPDs 97% were in service after 5 years, while 38% of the RPDs had been replaced or had undergone major modifications. Consequently, the need for dental and prosthetic follow-up treatment was more pronounced in the group treated with RPDs than in the group treated with FPDs.

That the wearing of RPDs is associated with an increased risk of caries and, to a lesser extent, periodontal disease, especially in the long term was confirmed in a double blind study comprising 30 patients treated with resin-bonded FPDs in the mandible and 30 treated with cobalt-chromium RPDs (Jepson et al., 2001). The incidence of caries was also six times higher among the patients wearing RPDs according to this study. There was also a reported superiority of FPDs with respect to patient satisfaction (Jepson, Allen, Moynihan, Kelly, & Thomason, 2003).

In a recent study, the survival of 3-unit fixed–fixed and 2-unit cantilevered FPDs was compared in 168 patients receiving a total of 210 FPDs (Chai, Chu, Newsome, & Chow, 2005). At 48 months, the cumulative survival rate was 82% for the fixed–fixed veneer FPDs, 81% for the 2-unit resin bonded cantilevered FPDs, 77% for the 2 unit full veneer cantilevered FPDs, and 63% for the 3-unit fixed–fixed resin bonded FPDs.

Thus, treatment with one or two small cantilever FPDs bonded to the enamel may be a favourable alternative to RPDs in older patients if the occlusal forces can be controlled and the abutment teeth are vital (Table 13.1). Apparently, the

Table 13.1 Replacement of posterior tooth loss in elderly patients with FPDs or RPDs (Wöstmann et al., 2005)

	FPD	RPD
Masticatory function	++	++
Patient satisfaction	++	(+)
Risk of caries	(+)	++
Risk of periodontal disease	(+)	+
Prevention of TMD symptoms	No evidence	No evidence
Occlusal stability	++	(+)
Cost / benefit short term	−	++
Cost / benefit long term	+	+
Esthetics	++	+

economic advantages of treatment with RPDs are fewer when the long-term need for various follow-up treatments is evaluated against those needed after treatment with cantilever FPDs.

Removable Partial Denture (RPD)

Treatment with RPDs is a non-invasive and low-cost solution for the prosthetic rehabilitation of patients who have functional or aesthetic need for replacement of anterior and/or posterior teeth. In patients with shortened dental arches, a major benefit from wearing RPDs is improved masticatory performance (Gunne, 1985; Kapur, Garrett, Dent, & Hasse, 1997). However, unless the patients have fewer than three occluding pairs of posterior teeth, there seems to be no socio-functional benefit to be gained from replacing missing posterior teeth (Locker, Clarke, & Payne, 2000). In addition, the wearing of removable dentures may be associated with complaints related to impaired aesthetics or oral comfort (Witter, van Elteren, Käyser, & van Rossum, 1989). This may be to a degree that patients often decide not to wear the denture (Cowan, Gilbert, Elledge, & McGlynn, 1991). Furthermore, the comfort of wearing a FPD largely surpasses that of wearing a RPD (Holm, 1994; Jepson et al., 2003). Constructional or design aspects that can explain low patient satisfaction have, however, not been identified (Öwall et al., 2002). It is assumed that complaints about wearing RPDs can be reduced if the framework for the dentures is designed according to simple and logical principles in order to secure the stability of the denture and best possible comfort when wearing it (Budtz-Jørgensen & Bochet, 1998). However, the basic design principles of force distribution, support, stability, and retention are founded on ideas that are not scientifically proven (Öwall et al., 2002.)

The use of RPDs is associated with an increased risk of caries and periodontal disease, but there is no evidence that RPDs per se cause damage. However, significantly more tooth sites adjacent to narrow embrasure spaces harboured plaque than those adjacent to wide embrasures (Yeung, Chow, & Clark, 2000). With appropriate design respecting the adjacent tissues and appropriate plaque control, long-term clinical use of RPDs has no detrimental effects on the periodontium of abutment teeth (Bergman, Hugoson, & Olsson, 1995; Vanzeveren, D'Hoore, & Bercy, 2002). By contrast, the development of root caries is often a problem (Budtz-Jørgensen & Isidor, 1990; Wright, Hellyer, Beighton, Heath, & Lynch, 1992). The reason is probably that the wearing of RPDs predisposes to high salivary levels of mutans streptococci and yeasts (Beigton, Hellyer, Lynch, & Heath, 1991).

Major complications to treatment with RPDs are mechanical failures, such as fracture of major or minor connectors, as well as occlusal rests and deformation or fracture of retentive clasps (Lewis, 1978; Vermeulen, Keltjens, van't Hof, & Käyser, 1996). Thus, the 50% survival time for clasp-retained metal framework RPDs was about 10 years and that for acrylic resin RPDs only 3 years. However, more recent longitudinal studies show very satisfactory results with RPDs after a period of 4–17 years, showing an average survival rate of about 75% (Vanzeveren, D'Hoore, Bercy, & Leloup, 2003a; Vanzeveren et al., 2003b). Most failures were attributable to RPDs with free-end saddles in the lower jaw.

The concept of design of RPDs seems to be of much less importance for periodontal health than post-insertion controls in order to maintain stable occlusal conditions and good oral hygiene (Berg, 1985). However, the coverage of the gingival tissues by the minor connectors has in particular a detrimental effect on periodontal health (Runov, Kroone, Stoltze, Maeda, El Ghamrawy, & Brill, 1980).

Based on a recent and extensive review of the literature, it was concluded that evidence for indications and contraindications for the prescription of RPDs was not clearly defined (Wöstmann et al., 2005). However, there appears to be a trend in favour of applying the shortened dental arch concept or implant-supported restorations in stead of conventional RPDs, given the evidence that on long-term removable, dentures are associated with increased risk of caries, periodontal disease, and lower patient acceptance than FPD (Table 13.1). When there are sound abutment teeth or if socio-economic factors influence the decision-making process, RPDs are often chosen.

The basic principles of the open design or "hygenic design" for RPDs in order to reduce the negative effects of denture wearing have been described in details elsewhere (Budtz-Jørgensen, 1999; Budtz-Jørgensen & Bochet, 1998; Öwall et al., 2002). The following guidelines for denture design can be used (Budtz-Jørgensen, 1996a):

1. The dentures should be designed with embrasure spaces between abutment teeth and saddles (Fig. 13.3) and a 6–8 mm open space between the abutments and the major connector (Figs. 13.4–13.6) to reduce plaque accumulation in the dentogingival areas and the risk of caries and periodontal disease.
2. To prevent technical failures and in order to distribute the occlusal forces, the dentures should be designed with rigid major and minor connectors, reciprocating clasp arms, and occlusal rests, the latter placed in well-prepared rest seats.
3. In distal extension RPDs, occlusal rests should be placed in a way that they create reciprocation for the retentive clasp arm, i.e. usually mesially as it is an

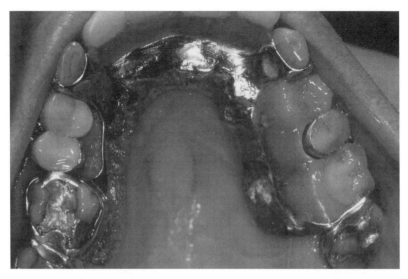

Fig. 13.4 Existing RPD with a horse-shoe-shaped major connector in close relation with the abutment teeth (*See* Color Plate 4)

advantage to place the retentive clasp arm disto-buccally for aesthetic reasons. Minor connectors, connecting the occlusal/lingual rest with the major connector (Fig. 13.3) should be extended directly from the base onto the proximal aspects of the abutment tooth, allowing an open embrasure to be created.

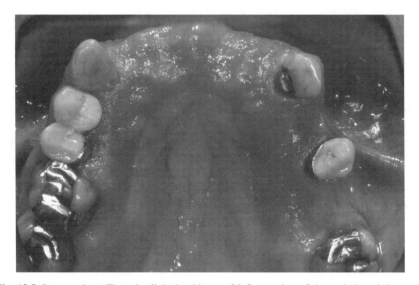

Fig. 13.5 Same patient. There is clinical evidence of inflammation of the periodontal tissues as well as the palatal mucosa (*See* Color Plate 5)

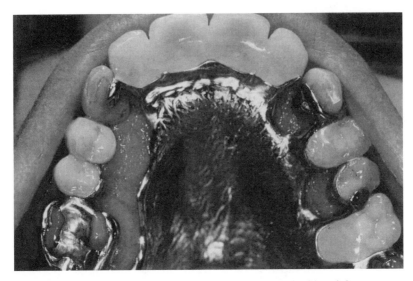

Fig. 13.6 Same patient. The replacement RPD has been designed with a 6–8 mm open space between the natural teeth and the major connector. Note that periodontal health has improved (*See* Color Plate 6)

4. In distal extension RPDs, the denture should be designed, for aesthetic and mechanical reasons, in such a way that appropriate retention is achieved with two retentive clasps on the distal abutments.

The prosthetic rehabilitation of patients with shortened dental arches and tooth wear with or without reduction of the occlusal face height may include rehabilitation with extensive FPDs, crowns, and RPDs. However, an acceptable result can frequently be obtained by less complicated treatment procedures, including RPDs with occlusal overlay rests and restoration of anterior teeth with composite resin (Budtz-Jørgensen, 1986). Such treatment procedures have the advantage of being less expensive, reversible, and not involving extensive preparation of tooth structure.

There does not exist any consensus how to design RPDs for frail and dependent elderly (Budtz-Jørgensen, 1999). An acrylic resin denture is often recommended because it is faster and easier to work with, less expensive, and amenable to repair or alter (Iacopino & Wathen, 1993). However, this type of prosthesis has serious drawbacks regarding prognosis for the remaining teeth and patient comfort. Thus, if the patient's oral hygiene can be maintained appropriately with help of the caregivers or family, other treatment solutions may become realistic.

Overdentures

Overdentures supported by tooth abutments are a preferable alternative to treatment with conventional complete dentures in patients with few remaining teeth, which are considered inadequate to serve as abutments for fixed or removable partial dentures (Ettinger, 1988; Toolson & Taylor, 1989). The advantages of overdentures over conventional complete dentures are better preservation of neuromuscular function, perceptive ability and proprioception, improved masticatory performance, mainte-nance of the residual ridge, improved stability of the denture, stable occlusion, and psychological benefits for the patient (Table 13.2) (Budtz-Jørgensen, 1999).

Simple Overdentures

In the elderly partially edentulous patient, treatment with a complete overdenture is indicated if there are few remaining teeth or teeth with an unfavourable distribution in the jaw or a heterogeneous prognosis, severe loss of periodontal attachment, and complicated functional or aesthetic conditions due to tooth migration or occlusal tooth wear (Fig. 13.7). Thus, support from the abutments will be mainly axial due to the improved relationship between abutment/root length, and the denture can readily be modified if one or several abutments are lost. Treatment with an overdenture in the maxilla supported by two or three abutments is particularly indicated, if an implant-supported complete denture is provided for the mandible in order to keep stable occlusal conditions and reduce resorption of the residual ridge of the anterior part of the maxilla.

Longitudinal studies over 5–10 years of overdenture wearers with controlled oral hygiene indicate a rate of loss of overdenture abutments of 5–20%, and that the original prostheses can, to a large extent, be maintained by minor modifications (Budtz-Jørgensen, 1994; Ettinger, 1988; Toolson & Taylor, 1989). The conditions for these excellent results were good patient cooperation and regular recalls. In this respect, initial oral hygiene was not a good predictor of a patient's cooperation and the long-term prognosis of the abutments. Thus, patients who initially had poor oral hygiene and poor dental and periodontal status were able to maintain an improved oral hygiene for 5 years after the denture treatment had been completed.

The wearing of overdentures may be associated with caries and progression of periodontal disease in relation to the tooth abutments, even if preventive measures are introduced (Budtz-Jørgensen, 1995; Ettinger, 1988). One of the reasons is that bacterial colonization of the fitting denture surface and the underlying abutments

Table 13.2 Advantages and disadvantages of treatment with overdentures compared with conven-tional complete dentures

	Overdentures	Conventional complete dentures
Masticatory function	++	+
Neuromuscular function	++	+
Maintenance of residual ridge	+	−
Maintenance of occlusal stability	+	−
Maintenance of denture stability	+	−
Comfort (lower denture)	+	−
Esthetics (upper denture)	−	+
Repairs	−	+

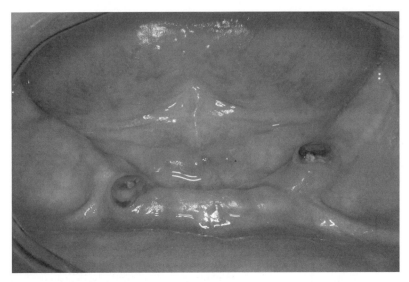

Fig. 13.7 Teeth 34 and 43 have been maintained as abutments for a lower overdenture. Note plaque and superficial caries (*See* Color Plate 7)

are enhanced by micro-organisms from saliva and the mucosa (Theilade & Budtz-Jørgensen, 1988). This plaque is composed mainly of gram-positive facultative anaerobic bacteria quite similar to plaque located at dento-gingival areas and associated with caries and gingivitis. Plaque formation is enhanced by high sugar consumption, inflammation of the mucosa, continuous wearing of the dentures, and poor hygiene. Bleeding on probing is a reliable clinical indicator of periodontal problems adjacent to overdenture abutments (Ettinger & Jacobsen, 1996).

In order to improve stability of the overdenture, the abutments should be reduced in height to a level not inferior of 2–3 mm above the gingival margin. To reduce the risk progression of periodontal disease and caries of the abutments, it is important to eradicate existing periodontal pockets before or in association with the placement of the overdenture, and to have the patient abstain from wearing the denture during night (Budtz-Jørgensen, 1994).

Attachment-Retained Overdentures

Treatment with attachment-retained overdentures may be an alternative to conventional RPDs if crowning of the abutment teeth is necessary, and an alternative to a simple overdenture to improve retention and stability of the denture and in order to avoid covering the palate with a plate of acrylic resin. Such treatment is particularly indicated if there is existing attachment loss adjacent to the abutment teeth, which precludes treatment with a FPD or an RPD. Longitudinal data on clinically documented overdentures with attachments are sparse. In one study on 109 periodontally treated patients who were followed for up to 10 years (average 5.9 years), failures were observed in 24% of the abutments, half of which had to be extracted (Mericske & Mericske-Stern, 1993). The survival rate of the abutments was, however, not influenced by the initial periodontal support or the denture wearing period.

Telescopic or double crown system may provide advantages with insertion or removal of the denture for older people with decreased manual dexterity (Igarashi & Goto, 1997; Widbom, Löfquist, Widbom, Söderfeldt, & Kronström, 2004). According to retrospective studies, a relatively satisfactory outcome was found for tooth-supported telescopic crown-retained dentures with loss of 7%–16% of the abutments after 4–10 years (Widbom et al., 2004). In both studies, the incidence of loss of abutments was particularly high, up to 35%, in patients who had few remaining teeth and mucosa-tooth born denture saddles. Thus, in elderly patients with few remaining teeth as abutments for an attachment or conical crown retained denture treatment with an implant-supported denture should rather be considered.

Restoration of the Edentulous Mouth with Conventional Complete Dentures

In elderly people, treatment with complete dentures most frequently involves replacing existing complete dentures. Thus, patients may seek prosthetic treatment because the existing dentures have broken, because of excessive wear of the denture teeth or for aesthetic reasons. Most frequently denture wearers seeking treatment are satisfied with the old dentures in spite of poor fit, loss of the vertical dimension of occlusion, and occlusal instability. Today, the restoration with implant-supported complete dentures is an obvious alternative to conventional complete dentures to secure long-term stability and patient comfort. However, seen in a global perspective, the costs make implants quite unrealistic for the great majority of edentulous people (Owen, 2004). Furthermore, when costs were removed as a limiting factor for the choice of implants, 36% of older edentulous patients still refused the offer of free implants to retain their lower dentures (Walton & MacEntee, 2005). Thus, restoration of the edentulous mouth with conventional complete dentures will remain a frequent choice of treatment, also for the nearest future.

The clinical procedures to follow in treatment with complete dentures are poorly supported by scientific evidence and principally rely on clinical experience. Recently, a consensus among 41 international experts was elaborated on the principles to be followed when constructing complete dentures, a Minimum Acceptable Protocol (MAP) (Owen, 2006). The guidelines for the MAP include the initial preparatory phase (patient's specific goals with treatment and experience with complete dentures, insurance of healthy oral mucosa); the treatment phase (impressions, centric relation, vertical dimension of occlusion, tooth arrangement, aesthetics, final adjustment of occlusion, and instruction of the patient); and the post-treatment phase with control of hygiene, occlusion, and function.

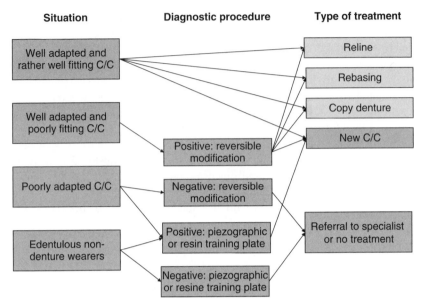

Fig. 13.8 Diagnostic procedures and types of treatment with conventional complete dentures according to the clinical situation of the edentulous patient

When considering elderly, it seems relevant to distinguish between three groups of patients: those who are well-adapted to existing dentures, poorly adapted denture wearers, and edentulous patients with no experience in wearing dentures (Fig. 13.8) (Budtz-Jørgensen, 1996b).

Existing Denture Wearers

Well-Adapted Denture Wearers

Relining or rebasing of the existing dentures is the treatment of choice if the existing dentures are relatively well-fitting, the vertical dimension of occlusion satisfactory, and the occlusion relatively stable. With reduced vertical dimension of occlusion, poor fit, and unstable occlusal conditions, it is important to use the existing dentures diagnostically, e.g. by using them to make a diagnostic reline, which restores occlusal face height, occlusion, and fit. If the patient accepts the modified dentures after having worn them for 1–2 weeks, they could be rebased or used as individual trays for a functional impression and as a guide to determine the vertical dimension of occlusion (Budtz-Jørgensen, 1996b).

The copy denture technique could also be applied by which the features of the existing dentures are reproduced as closely as possible by provision of new appliances, with alterations limited to those aspects of the existing dentures that are causing problems (Heath & Johnson, 1981). This is done with copies of the existing dentures, which are used as impression trays, as occlusion rims, and for mounting the denture teeth. With this technique, the treatment is limited to a clinical diagnostic stage; a laboratory stage for accomplishing the copy denture; a second clinical stage for impression-taking and recording of the inter-maxillary relationship in centric relation and at an appropriate vertical dimension of occlusion; a second laboratory stage for mounting in articulator, mounting of the denture teeth at the planned vertical dimension of occlusion and processing of the denture in acrylic resin; at the third clinical stage, the denture copy is delivered.

Non-adapted Denture Wearers

In elderly people who have had a number of unsuccessful prosthetic treatments, a careful interview and examination of the existing dentures should be carried out. Prosthetic treatment should rather not be carried out if there are no major disorders of the existing dentures, if the person does not accept the diagnostically modified dentures, or if there is evidence of an underlying mental disorder (Fig. 13.8). In this case, it is preferable to refer the patient to a specialist for diagnosing the cause of the patient's complaint and eventually carrying out the treatment (Hammond & Thomson, 1982).

Edentulous Patients Without Existing Dentures

In older patients who are mentally disabled, it is wise to provide the maxillary denture first, which may be satisfactory to a degree that a lower complete denture can be avoided. If a lower denture is indicated, two different procedures can be employed (Budtz-Jørgensen, 1999).

By one technique, a functional impression is obtained using an occlusion rim, which is adapted to the existing maxillary denture, providing a convenient vertical dimension of occlusion. With the impression in situ, the patient can give valuable information regarding the extension, outline, and fit of the occlusion rim, the vertical dimension of occlusion, and comfort. Indeed, if the functional impression does not satisfy the patient, there is no reason to believe that the denture will do so either.

The other procedure consists in constructing a try-in denture to determine a comfortable vertical dimension of occlusion and outline of the lower denture. This can be accomplished in a simple way by making a replica in acrylic resin of a functional impression obtained using a piezographic occlusion rim, which has been adapted to the upper denture, the tongue, and the buccal musculature. The replica in acrylic resin is subsequently adjusted occlusally against the existing upper denture to provide a stable occlusion and relined with tissue-conditioning material. The replica is worn during daytime only and adjusted regularly until the patient finds it satisfactory. Finally, the replica is used as individual tray and occlusion rim in the lower jaw against the existing upper denture, and the denture is constructed with a shape, similar to that of the replica.

It is evident that treatment with implant-retained complete dentures is an excellent alternative to overcome or reduce the risk of complications following treatment with complete dentures if there are no medical contraindications.

Conclusions

In a society where older adults are often denture wearers, the appropriate care for these patients is relatively simple, including provision with new RPDs, transformation of existing RPDs to overdentures or conventional complete dentures, or reline and re-adaptation of existing complete dentures. As mentioned previously, recent studies indicate that the dental and prosthetic status of older adults is changing radically and rapidly. Still, important differences in the oral health status exist even among highly industrialized countries, partly depending on to which degree oral health services for the elderly are publicly financed. Clearly, old age and poor socio-economic conditions will have a negative impact on patients' oral health status and their drive to seek dental professional care.

New generations of elderly people may have different oral health care attitudes and may be more demanding with respect to more sophisticated dental and prosthetic therapy. Today, oral health interventions are mostly performed individually rather than community based and often occur only in emergency situations (De Visschere & Vanobbergen, 2006). However, if adequate oral health service is not developed for frail and dependent elderly, their oral health situation will become quite unmanageable and require multiple extractions followed by conventional prosthetic treatment. It is unlikely that such treatment will meet the patient's requirements on short or long terms and secure acceptable function and oral comfort.

References

Agerberg, C., & Carlsson, G. E. (1981). Chewing ability in relation to dental and general health: Analyses of data obtained from a questionnaire. *Acta Odontologica Scandinavica, 39*, 147–153.

Allen, P. F. (2005). Association between diet, social resources and oral health related quality of life in edentulous patients. *Journal of Oral Rehabilitation, 32*, 623–628.

Atchieson, K. A., & Andersen, R. M. (2000). Demonstrating successful ageing using the international collaborative study for oral health outcomes. *Journal of Public Health Dentistry, 60*, 282–288.

Aukes, J. N. S. C., Käyser, A. F., & Felling, A. J. A. (1988). The subjective experience of mastication in subjects with shortened dental arches. *Journal of Oral Rehabilitation, 15*, 321–324.

Avlund, K., Holm-Pedersen, P., Morse, D. E., Viitanen, M., & Winblad. (2004).Tooth loss and caries prevalence in very old Swedish people: The relationship to cognitive function and functional ability. *Gerodontology, 21*, 17–26.

Avlund, K., Holm-Pedersen, P., & Schroll, M. (2001). Functional ability and oral health among older people: A longitudinal study from age 75 to 80. *Journal of American Geriatric Society, 49*, 954–962.

Banting, D. W., Papas, A., Clark, D. C., Proskin, H. M., Schultz, M., & Perry, R. (2000). The effectiveness of 10% chlorhexidine varnish treatment on dental caries incidence in adults with dry mouth. *Gerodontology, 17*, 67–76.

Beck, J. D., Kock, G. G., & Offenbacher, S. (1994). Attachment loss trends over 3 years in community-dwelling older adults. *Journal of Periodontology, 65*, 737–743.

Beigton, P. S., Hellyer, P. H., Lynch, E., & Heath, M. R. (1991). Salivary levels of mutans streptococci, lactobacilli and root caries prevalence in non- institutionalized elderly patients. *Community Dentistry and Oral Epidemiology, 19*, 302–307.

Berg, E. (1985). Periodontal problems associated with the use of distal extension removable partial dentures – a matter of construction? *Journal of Oral Rehabilitation, 12*, 369–379.

Bergman, B., Hugoson, A., & Olsson, C. O. (1995). A 25 year longitudinal study of patients treated with removable partial dentures. *Journal of Oral Rehabilitation, 22*, 595–599.

Budtz-Jørgensen, E. (2000). Ecology of *Candida*-associated denture stomatitis. *Microbial Ecology in Health and Disease, 12*, 170–185.

Budtz-Jørgensen, E. (1999). Prosthodontic treatment planning in older adults. In E. Budtz-Jørgensen (Ed.), *Prosthodontics for the Elderly* (pp. 75–106). Chicago: Quintessence Publishing Co, Inc.

Budtz-Jørgensen, E. (1996a). Restoration of the partially edentulous mouth – a comparison of overdentures, removable partial dentures, fixed partial dentures and implant treatment. *Journal of Dentistry, 24*, 237–244.

Budtz-Jørgensen, E. (1996b). Prosthetic consideration in geriatric dentistry. In P. Holm-Pedersen & H. Loe (Eds.), *Textbook of Geriatric Dentistry* (pp. 446–466). Copenhagen: Munksgaard.

Budtz-Jørgensen, E. (1995). Prognosis of overdenture abutments in elderly patients with controlled oral hygiene: A 5-year study. *Journal of Oral Rehabilitation, 22*, 3–8.

Budtz-Jørgensen, E. (1994). Effect of denture-wearing habits on periodontal health of abutment teeth in patients with overdentures. *Journal of Clinical Periodontology, 22*, 265–269.

Budtz-Jørgensen, E. (1986). Restoration of the occlusal face heightby removable dentures in elderly patients. *Gerodontics, 2*, 67–71.

Budtz-Jørgensen, E., & Bochet, G. (1998). Alternate framework designs for removable partial dentures. *Journal of Prosthetic Dentistry, 80*, 58–66.

Budtz-Jørgensen, E., & Isidor, F. (1990). A 5-year longitudinal study of cantilevered fixed partial dentures compared with removable partial dentures in a geriatric population. *Journal of Prosthetic Dentistry, 64*, 42–47.

Budtz-Jørgensen, E., Chung, J.-P., & Mojon, P. (2000). Successful aging – the case for prosthetic therapy. *Journal of Public Health Dentistry, 60*, 326–329.

Budtz-Jørgensen, E., Mojon, P., Rentsch, A., Roerich, N., von der Muehll, D., & Baehni, P. (1996a). Caries prevalence and associated predisposing conditions in recently hospitalized persons. *Acta Odontologica Scandinavica, 54*, 251–256.

Budtz-Jørgensen, E., Mojon, P., Banon-Clément, J. M., & Baehni, P. (1996b). Oral candidosis in long-term hospital care: Comparison of edentulous and dentate subjects. *Oral Diseases, 2*, 285–290.

Budtz-Jørgensen, E., Luan, W.-M., Holm-Pedersen, P., & Fejerskov, O. (1985a). Mandibular dysfunction related to dental, occlusal and prosthetic conditions in a selected elderly population. *Gerodontics, 1*, 28–33.

Budtz-Jørgensen, E., Isidor, F., & Karring, T. (1985b). Cantilevered fixed partial dentures in a geriatric population: preliminary report. *Journal of Prosthetic Dentistry, 54*, 467–473.

Chai, J., Chu, F. S. C., Newsome, P. R. H., & Chow, T. W. (2005). Retrospective survival analysis of 3-unit fixed-fixed and two-unit cantilevered fixed partial dentures. *Journal of Oral Rehabilitation, 32*, 759–765.

Chalmers, J. M., Carter, K. D., & Spencer, A. J. (2005). Caries incidence and increments in Adelaide nursing home residents. *Special Care in Dentistry, 25*, 96–105.

Cowan, R. D., Gilbert, J. A., Elledge, D. A., & McGlynn, F. D. (1991). Patients' use of removable partial dentures: Two- and four-year telephone interviews. *Journal of Prosthetic Dentistry, 65*, 668–670.

Curzon, M. E. J., & Preston, A. J. (2004). Risk groups: Nursing bottle caries/ caries in the elderly. *Caries Research, 38 (suppl. 1)*, 24–33.

Dahl, B. L., Carlsson, G. E., & Ekfeldt, A. (1993). Occlusal wear of teeth and restorative materials: A review of classification, etiology, mechanisms of wear, and some aspects of restorative procedures. *Acta Odontologica Scandinavica, 51*, 299–613.

Daly, R. M., Elsner, R. J. F., Allen, P. F., & Burke, F. M. (2003). Associations between self-reported dental status and diet. *Journal of Oral Rehabilitation, 30*, 964–970.

Decock, V., De Nayer, K., & De Boever, J. A. (1996). 18-year longitudinal study of cantilevered fixed restorations. *International Journal of Prosthodontics, 9*, 331–340.

De Visschere, L. M., & Vanobbergen J. N. (2006). Oral health care for frail elderly people: Actual state and opinions of dentists towards a well-organised community approach. *Gerodontology, 23*, 170–176.

Ekelund, T. (1989). Dental state and subjective chewing ability of institutionalized elderly people. *Community Dentistry and Oral Epidemiology, 17*, 24–27.

Ekelund, T & Burt, B. A. (1994). Risk factors for total tooth loss in the United States: Longitudinal analyses of national data. *Journal of Public Health Dentistry, 54*, 5–14.

Ettinger, R. L. (1988). Tooth loss in an overdenture population. *Journal of Prosthetic Dentistry, 60*, 459–462.

Ettinger, R. L., & Jacobsen, J. (1996). Periodontal consideration in an overdenture population. *International Journal of Prosthodontics, 9*, 230–238.

Featherstone, J. D. B. (2000). The science and practice of caries prevention. *Journal of American Dental Association, 131*, 887–899.

Fejerskov, O., & Nyvad, B. (1996). Dental caries in the aging individual. In P. Holm-Pedersen, & H. Loe (Eds.), *Textbook of Geriatric Dentistry* (pp. 338–372). Copenhagen: Munksgaard.

Fejerskov, O., Luan, W.-M., Nyvad, B., Budtz-Jørgensen, E., & Holm-Pedersen, P. (1991). Active and inactive root surface caries lesions in a selected group of 60-to-80-year- old Danes. *Caries Research, 25*, 385–391.

Frencken, J. E., Songpaisan, Y., Phantumvanit, P., & Pilot, T. (1994). An atraumatic restorative treatment (ART) technique: Evaluation after one year. *International Dental Journal, 44*, 460–464.

Fure, S. (2004). Ten-year cross-sectional and incidence study of coronal and root caries and some related factors in elderly Swedish individuals. *Gerodontology, 21*, 130–139.

Fure, S. (2003). Ten-year incidence of tooth-loss and dental caries in elderly Swedish individuals. *Caries Research, 37*, 462–469.

Galan, D., & Lynch, E. (1993). Epidemiology of root caries. *Gerodontology, 10*, 59–71.

Glantz, P. O., Ryge, G., Jendresen, M. D., & Nilner, K. (1984). Quality of extensive fixed prosthdontics after five years. *Journal of Prosthetic Dentistry, 52*, 475–479.

Guivante-Nabert, C., Berenholc, C., & Berdal, A. (1999). Caries activity and associated risk factors in elderly hospitalised populations – 15 months follow-up in French institutions. *Gerodontology, 16*, 47–58.

Gunne, H. J. (1985). The effect of removable partial dentures on masticatory function and dietary intake. *Acta Odontologica Scandinavica, 43*, 269–278.

Hammond, J., & Thomson, J. C. (1982). Diagnosis of complete denture difficulties. *Dental Update, 9*, 35–40.

Heath, J. R., & Johnson, A. (1981). The versatility of the copy denture technique. *British Dental Journal, 150*, 189–193.

Holm, B. (1994). Muscular activity and chewing ability before and after treatment with extension bridges or removable partial dentures (Doctoral dissertation, University of Copenhagen, Denmark, 1994).

Honkala, S., & Honkala, E. (2002). Atraumatic dental treatment among Finnish elderly persons. *Journal of Oral Rehabilitation, 29*, 435–440.

Hämäläinen, P., Meurman, J. H., Keskinen, M., & Heikkinen, E. (2004). Changes in dental status over 10 years in 80-year-old people: A prospective cohort study. *Community Dentistry and Oral Epidemiology, 32*, 374–384.

Iacopino, A. M., & Wathen, W. F. (1993). Geriatric prosthdontics: An overview. Part II. Treatment considerations. *Quintessence International, 24*, 253–261.

Igarashi, Y., & Goto, T. (1997). Ten-year follow-up study of conical crown retained dentures. *International Journal of Prosthodontics, 10*, 149–155.

Isidor, F., & Budtz-Jørgensen, E. (1990). Periodontal conditions following treatment with distally extending cantilever bridges or removable partial dentures in elderly patients. A 5-year study. *Journal of Periodontology, 61*, 21–26.

Jepson, N. J., Allen, F., Moynihan, P. J., Kelly, P. J., & Thomason, J. M. (2003). Patient satisfaction following restoration of shortened dental arches in a randomized controlled study. *International Journal of Prosthodontics, 16*, 409–414.

Jepson, N. J., Moynihan, P. J., Kelly, P. J., Watson, G. W., & Thomason, J. M. (2001). Caries incidence following restoration of lower shortened dental arches in a randomized controlled study. *British Dental Journal, 191*, 140–144.

Kalk, W., Käyser, A. F., & Witter, D. J. (1993). Needs for tooth replacement. *International Dental Journal, 43*, 41–49.

Kapur, K. K., Garrett, N. R., Dent, R. J., & Hasse, A. L. (1997). A randomized clinical trial of two basic removable partial denture designs. Part II: Comparisons of masticatory scores. *Journal of Prosthetic Dentistry, 78*, 15–21.

Katz, R. V., Neely, A. L., & Morse, D. E. (1996). The epidemiology of oral diseases in older adults. In P. Holm-Pedersen & H. Loe (Eds.), *Textbook of Geriatric Dentistry* (pp. 263–301). Copenhagen: Munksgaard.

Keltjens, H., Schaeken, T., & van der Hoeven, H. (1993). Preventive aspects of root caries. *International Dental Journal, 43*, 143–148.

Kiyak, H. A. (2000). Successful ageing: Implications for oral health. *Journal of Public Health Dentistry, 60*, 276–281.

Käyser, A. F. (1981). Shortened dental arches and oral function. *Journal of Oral Rehabilitation, 8*, 457–468.

Landt, H., & Fransson, B. (1975). Oral ability to recognize forms and muscular coordination ability in dentulous young and elderly adults. *Journal of Oral Rehabilitation, 2*, 125–138.

Leake, J. L., Hawkins, R., & Locker, D. (1994). Social and functional impact of reduced posterior functional units in older adults. *Journal of Oral Rehabilitation, 21*, 1–10.

Lewis, A. J. (1978). Failure of removable partial denture castings during service. *Journal of Prosthetic Dentistry, 39*, 147–149.

Lindhe, J., & Nyman, S. (1975). The effect of plaque control and surgical pocket elimination on the establishment and maintenance of periodontal health. A longitudinal study on periodontal therapy in cases of advanced disease. *Journal of Clinical Periodontology, 2*, 67–69.

Locker, D., Clarke, M., & Payne, B. (2000). Self-perceived oral health status, psychological well-being, and life satisfaction in older adult population. *Journal of Dental Research, 79*, 970–975.

Lundgren, M. (1997). On dental caries and related factors in old age (Doctoral dissertation, Faculty of Odontology, Göteborg, Sweden).

Lutz, F., Lüscher, B., Ochsenbein, H., & Mühlemann, H. R (1976). *Adhäsive Zahnheilkunde.* (ISBN3-260-04047-1): Zürich.

MacEntee, M. (2000). Oral care for successful aging in long-term care. *Journal of Public Health Dentistry, 60*, 326–329.

Mack, F., Mojon, P., Budtz-Jørgensen, E., Kocher, T., Splieth, C., Schwan, C. et al. (2004). Caries and periodontal disease of the elderly in Pomerania, Germany: Results of the Study of Health in Pomerania. *Gerodontology, 21*, 27–36.

Mack, F., Mundt, T., Budtz-Jørgensen, E., Mojon, P., Schwan, C., Bernhardt, O. et al. (2003). Prosthodontic status among old adults in Pomerania, related to income, education level, and general health (results of the Study of Health in Pomerania, SHIP). *International Journal of Prosthodontics, 16*, 313–318.

Mericske, E. A., & Mericske-Stern, R. (1993). Overdenture abutments and reduced periodontium in elderly patients. *Schweizerische Monatsschrift fürZahnmedizin, 103*, 1245–1251.

Meuwissen, J. H., van Waas, M. A. J., Meuwissen, R., & Käyser, A. F. (1995). Satisfaction with reduced dentitions in elderly people. *Journal of Oral Rehabilitation, 22*, 397–401.

Mike, T. J., Slade, G. D., Szentpétery, A., & Setz, J. M. (2004). Oral health-related quality of life in patients treated with fixed, removable, and complete dentures 1 month and 6 to 12 months after treatment. *International Journal of Prosthodontics, 17*, 503–511.

Mojon, P., & MacEntee, M. I. (1992). Discrepancy between need for prosthodontic treatment and complaints in an elderly edentulous population. *Community Dentistry and Oral Epidemiology, 20*, 48–52.

Mojon, P., Thomason, J. M., & Walls, A. W. (2004). The impact of falling rates of edentulism. *International Journal of Prosthodontics, 17*, 434–440.

Mojon, P., Rentsch, A., Budtz-Jørgensen, E., & Baehni, P. C. (1998). Effects of an oral health program on selected clinical parameters and salivary bacteria in a long-term care facility. *European Journal of Oral Sience, 106*, 827–834.

Mojon, P., Rentsch, A., & Budtz-Jørgensen, E. (1995). Relationship between prosthodontic status, caries, and periodontal disease in a geriatric population. *International Journal of Prosthodontics, 8*, 564–571.

Molinari, C., Pazos, E., Grundman, M., Bartolotto, T., Krejci, T., & Budtz-Jørgensen, E. (2007). Restorative caries therapy in nursing home residents using composite resins and compomers without rubberdam. *Quintessence International, 38*, 60–66.

Morse, D. E., Holm-Pedersen, P., & Holm-Pedersen, J. (2002). Dental caries in persons over the age of 80 living in Kungsholmen, Sweden: Findings from the KEOHS project. *Community Dental Health, 19*, 262–269.

Müller, F., Link, I., Fuhr, K., & Utz, K. H. (1995). Studies on adaptation to complete dentures. Part II: Oral sterognosis and tactile sensitivity. *Journal of Oral Rehabilitation, 22*, 759–767.

Narby, B., Kronström, M., Söderfeldt, B., & Palmqvist, S. (2005). Prosthodontics and the patient: What is oral rehabilitation need? Conceptual analysis of need and demand for prosthetic treatment. Part 1: A conceptual analysis. *International Journal of Prosthodontics, 18*, 75–79.

Nevalinen, M. J., Närhi, T. O., & Ainamo, A. (2004). A 5-year follow-up study on the prosthetic rehabilitation of the elderly in Helsinki, Finland. *Journal of Oral Rehabilitation, 31*, 647–652.

Nyman, S., & Lindhe, J. (1979). A longitudinal study of combined periodontal and prosthetic treatment of patients with advanced periodontal disease. *Journal of Periodontology, 50*, 163–169.

Närhi, T. O., Ainamo, A., & Meurman, J. H. (1994). Mutans streptococci and lactobacilli in the elderly. *Scandinavian Journal of Dental Research, 102*, 97–102.

Ow, R. K. K., Loh, T., Neo, J., & Khoo, J. (1997). Perceived masticatory function among elderly people. *Journal of Oral Rehabilitation, 24*, 131–137.

Owen, C. P. (2006). Guidelines for a minimum acceptable protocol for the construction of complete dentures. *International Journal of Prosthodontics, 19*, 467–474.

Owen, C. P. (2004). Appropriatech: Prosthodontics for the many, not just the few. *International Journal of Prosthodontics, 17*, 261–262.

Österberg, T., & Carlsson, G. E. (2007). Dental state, prosthodontic treatment and chewing ability: A study of five cohorts of 70-year-old subjects. *Journal of Oral Rehabilitation, 34*, 553–559.

Österberg, T., Carlsson, G. E., Tsuga, K., Sundh, V., & Steen, B. et al. (1996). Associations between self-assessed masticatory ability and some general health factors in a Swedish population. *Gerodontology, 13*, 110–117.

Öwall, B., Budtz-Jørgensen, E., Davenport, J., Mushimoto, E., Palmqvist, S., Renner, R., (2002). Removable partial denture design: A need to focus on hygienic principles? *International Journal of Prosthodontics, 15*, 371–378.

Palmqvist, S., Söderfeldt, B., & Vigild, M. (2001). Influence of dental care systems on dental status: A comparison between different systems but similar living standards. *Community Dental Health, 18*, 16–19.

Petersson, G. H., Fure, S., & Bratthall, D. (2003). Evaluation of a computer- based caries risk assessment program in an elderly group. *Acta Odontologica Scandinavica, 61*, 164–171.

Petjursson, B. E., Tan, K., Lang, N. P., Brägger, U., Egger, M., & Zwalen, M. (2004). A systematic review of the survival and complicaton rates of fixed partial dentures (FPDs) after an observation period of at least 5 years. Part IV: Cantilever or extension FPDs. *Clinical Oral Implant Research, 15*, 667–676.

Randow, K. (1986). On the functional deformation of extensive fixed partial dentures. An experimental clinical and epidemiological study. *Swedish Dental Journal, 34(Suppl. 1)*, 1–164.

Rojo, L., Silvestre, F. J., Bagan, J. V., & De Vicente V. (1994). Prevalence of psychopathology in burning mouth syndrome. A comparative study of patients with and without psychiatric disorders and controls. *Oral Surgery, Oral Medicine and Oral Pathology, 78*, 312–316.

Runov, J., Kroone, H., Stoltze, K., Maeda, T., El Ghamrawy, E., & Brill, N. (1980). Host response to two different designs of minor connectors. *Journal of Oral Rehabilitation, 3*, 147–153.

Schiffner, U. (2006). Krankheits- und Versorgungsprävalenzn bei Senioren (65–74 Jahre). In W. Micheelis & U. Schiffner (Eds.), *Vierte Deutsche Mundgesundheitsstudie (DMS IV)* (pp 207–337). Deutscher Zahnärzte Verlag, Köln.

Schiffner, U., & Reich, E. (1999). Prävalenzen zu ausgewählten klinischen Variablen bei den Senioren (65–74 Jahre). In W. Micheelis & E. Reich (Eds.), *Dritte Deutsche Mundgesundheitsstudie (DMS III)* (pp 337–431). Deutscher Ärzteverlag, Köln.

Shimzaki, Y., Soh, I., Koga, T., Miyazaki, H., & Takehara, T. (2004). Relationship between dental care and oral health in institutionalized elderly people in Japan. *Journal of Oral Rehabilitation, 31*, 837–842.

Tan, K., Petjurrson, B. E., Lang, N. P., & Chan, E. (2004). A systematic review of survival and complication rates of fixed partial dentures (FPDs) after an observation period of at least 5 years. III. Conventional FPDs. *Clinical Oral Implant Research, 15*, 654–666.

Theilade, E., & Budtz-Jørgensen, E. (1988). Predominant cultivable microflora of plaque on removable dentures in patients with denture-induced stomatitis. *Oral Microbiology and Immunology, 3*, 8–13.

Toolson, L. B., & Taylor, T. D. (1989). A 10-year report of longitudinal recall of overdenture patients. *Journal of Prosthetic Dentistry, 62*, 179–181.

van Waas, M. A. J. (1990a). The influence of clinical variables on patients' satisfaction with complete dentures. *Journal of Prosthetic Dentistry, 63*, 307–310.

van Waas, M. A. J. (1990b). The influence of psychologic factors on patients' satisfaction with complete dentures. *Journal of Prosthetic Dentistry, 63*, 545–548.

Vanzeveren, C., D'Hoore, W., Bercy, P., & Leloup, G. (2003a). Treatment with removable partial dentures: A longitudinal study. Part II. *Journal of Oral Rehabilitation, 30*, 459–469.

Vanzeveren, C., D'Hoore, W., Bercy, P., & Leloup, G. (2003b). Treatment with removable partial dentures: A longitudinal study. Part. I. *Journal of Oral Rehabilitation, 30*, 447–458.

Vanzeveren, C., D'Hoore, W., & Bercy, P. (2002). Influence of removable partial denture on periodontal indices and dental indices and dental status. *Journal of Oral Rehabilitation, 22*, 232–239.

Vermeulen, A. H., Keltjens, H. M., van't Hof, M. A., & Käyser, A. F. (1996). Ten-year evaluation of removable partial dentures: Survival rates based on retreatment, not wearing and replacement. *Journal of Prosthetic Dentistry, 76*, 267–272.

Vigild, M. (1989). Dental caries and the need for treatment among institutionalized elderly in Denmark. *Community Dentistry and Oral Epidemiology, 17*, 102–105.

Vigild, M. (1987). Oral mucosal lesions among institutionalized elderly in Denmark. *Community Dentistry and Oral Epidemiology, 15*, 309–313.

Walton, J. E., & MacEntee, M. I. (2005). Choosing or refusing oral implants: A prospective study of edentulous volunteers for a clinical trial. *International Journal of Prosthodontics, 18*, 483–488.

Widbom, T., Löfquist, L., Widbom, C., Söderfeldt, B., & Kronström, M. (2004). Tooth-supported telescopic crown-retained dentures: An up to 9-year retrospective clinical follow-up study. *International Journal of Prosthodontics, 17*, 29–34.

Widmark, G., Andersson, B., Carlsson, G. E., Ivanoff, C.-J., & Lindvall, A. M. (1998). Rehabilitation of patients with severely resorbed maxillae by means of implants with or without bone grafts. A 1-year follow-up study. *International Journal of Oral and Maxillofacial Implants, 13*, 474–482.

Wilkieson, C., Samaranayake, L. P., MacFarlane, T. W., Lamey, P.-J., & MacKenzie, D. (1991). Oral candidosis in the elderly in long term hospital care. *Journal of Oral Pathology and Medicine, 20*, 13–16.

Witter, D. J., van Elteren, P., Käyser, A. F., & van Rossum, M. J. M. (1989). The effect of removable partial dentures on the oral function in shortened dental arches. *Journal of Oral Rehabilitation, 16*, 27–33.

Wöstmann, B., Budtz-Jørgensen, E., Jepson, N., Mushimoto, E., Palmqvist, S. et al. (2005). Indications for removable partial dentures: A literature review. *International Journal of Prosthodontics, 18*, 139–145.

Wright, P. S., Hellyer, P. H., Beighton, D., Heath, R., & Lynch, E. (1992). Relationship of removable partial denture use to root caries in an older population. *International Journal of Prosthodontics, 5*, 39–46.

Yeung, A. L. P., Chow, T. W., & Clark, R. K. F. (2000). Oral health status of patients 5–6 years after placement of cobalt-chromium removable partial dentures. *Journal of Oral Rehabilitation, 27*, 183–189.

Chapter 14
Implant Dentistry as an Approach to Tooth Replacement for Older Adults

Hans-Peter Weber

Indications for Dental Implants in the Older Patient and Types of Implant-Supported Prostheses

Modern comprehensive dental care for older patients needs to include the consideration of dental implants. Since the initial description of osseointegration in experimental studies (Brånemark et al., 1969, 1977; Schroeder et al., 1976, 1981), scientific evidence has been established through human clinical studies that dental implants will serve as long-term predictable anchors for fixed and removable prostheses in fully and partially edentulous patients and that patient satisfaction with dental implant therapy is high (Adell et al., 1990; Fritz, 1996; Buser et al., 1997; Lindh et al., 1998; Feine & Carlsson, 2003; Moy et al., 2005; Pjetursson et al., 2005; Iqbal & Kim, 2007). The occurrence of biological and technical complications with dental implants, implant restorative components, and prosthetic superstructures has been documented (Bragger et al., 2005). While they need to be recognized as part of the long-term management of implant patients, they are more likely to affect components and prostheses (technical complications) than the implants per se (Salinas & Eckert, 2007; Weber & Sukotjo, 2007). Overall, the pool of information on contributing factors enhancing or compromising treatment success with dental implants continues to grow and is becoming more and more valuable despite its diversity and scientific inconsistency. This is possible through a focused interpretation of the published information, for instance via systematic reviews on specific questions related to implant therapy (Iacono & Cochran, 2007; Proskin et al., 2007).

The indications for dental implants in the older adult are in general not different from the rest of the population. Chronological age is not a contraindication for dental implants. Bryant and Zarb (1998) compared osseointegration of oral implants in older and younger adults. In a comparison of two closely matched groups of completely edentulous younger and older patients with dental implants after

H.-P. Weber
Raymond J. and Elva Pomfret Nagle Professor of Restorative Dentistry and Biomaterials Sciences, Harvard School of Dental Medicine, 188 Longwood Avenue, Boston, MA 02115, USA,
Tel: 617-432-1286, Fax: 617-432-0901
e-mil: hpweber@hsdm.harvard.edu

I.B. Lamster, M.E. Northridge (eds.), *Improving Oral Health for the Elderly,*
© Springer Science+Business Media, LLC 2008

follow-up times of 4–16 years, they found a cumulative success rate of 92% in the older and 86.5% in the younger group. Even more importantly, the prosthesis success rate was 100%, and the original prosthesis was in place throughout the respective observation periods for 41 of 45 of the older patients. The remaining prostheses needed repair at some point in the follow-up. The same authors found that older individuals responded to oral implants in the same manner as younger adults, despite their tendency for systemic illness (Bryant & Zarb, 2002). The main factors for reduced implant treatment success were unfavorable jawbone quantity and quality, specifically the atrophied maxilla. Nevertheless, since the risk for systemic conditions, which may primarily affect the surgical phase of implant treatment, increases with older age, it is especially important to perform a careful patient evaluation in this segment of the population as it will be outlined in this chapter.

Implants in the older individual are useful as anchors for single crowns, fixed and removable partial or full arch prostheses to improve function (mastication, speech), esthetics, and overall well-being. It has to be emphasized today that dental implants offer many advantages in the oral rehabilitation of older patients. (Chiappelli et al., 2002; Douglass et al., 2002a, b; Feine & Carlsson, 2003). Especially for individuals who are or will become edentulous, the use of dental implants for support and/or retention of fixed or removable prostheses has shown to be a tremendous opportunity to enhance prosthodontic treatment outcomes and quality of life for patients suffering from this predicament (Bryant & Zarb, 2002; Feine & Carlsson, 2003). The catalogue of treatment options (and related treatment cost) is almost unlimited, and it would go beyond the scope of this text to elaborate on them in detail. They range from fixed full arch prostheses to overdentures assisted by only two implants as illustrated in Figs. 14.1–14.10.

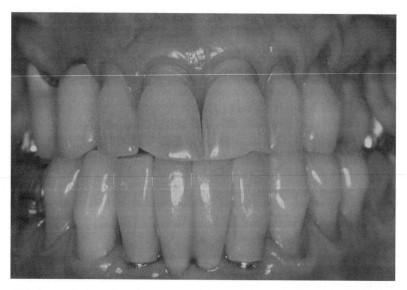

Fig. 14.1 Intraoral view of implant supported single crown # 6 and implant supported FPD #23xx26 in 78 year old male patient; status 12 years after insertion of prosthesis (*See* Color Plate 8)

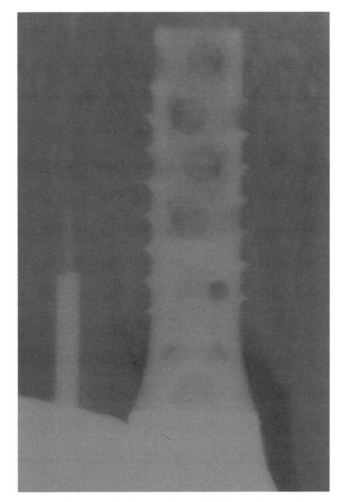

Fig. 14.2 Periapical radiograph of implant #6; 12-year follow-up

It is important for the clinician to understand the advantages implant therapy may offer and to strongly recommend it to the patients who may be candidates for it. And there are many. While the prevalence of edentulism has dropped substantially over the past two decades, for the year 2000 it was estimated that still about 33% of Americans age 65 and older were completely edentulous (Doundoulakis et al., 2003). There were significant disparities in the rate of edentulism among racial and ethnic groups. Available state-specific data also revealed a wide geographic variation for adults without teeth over age 65. They were lowest in Hawaii with 13.9% and highest in West Virginia with 47.9% (Doundoulakis et al., 2003).

Especially for patients with mandibular edentulism, implants can offer significant improvement over conventional dentures. Several studies have documented that masticatory function, overall satisfaction, and well-being of the edentulous patient

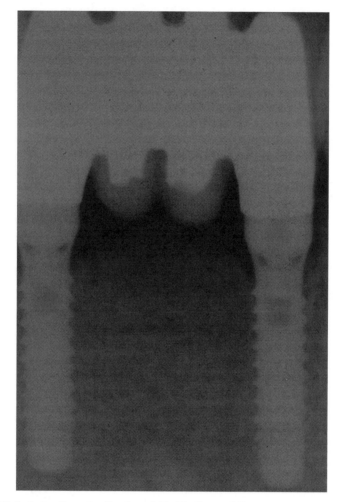

Fig. 14.3 Periapical radiograph of implants # 23, 26; 12-year follow-up

were significantly enhanced when at least two implants with retention anchors were added to support an overdenture in the edentulous mandible compared to conventional complete denture treatment to the level that the profession has embraced it as a new standard of care (Feine & Carlsson, 2003). This recommendation is, however, not unequivocal. Fitzpatrick (2006) found in a systematic review that there is no sufficient evidence for a single, universally superior treatment modality for the edentulous mandible. Better-designed, long-term studies are needed to further explore differences in patient acceptance to each treatment intervention for the edentulous mandible. The author also found from this review that the functional demands of edentulous patients are highly variable and that patient treatment responses are individual, vary significantly, and are influenced by psychosocial forces. Furthermore,

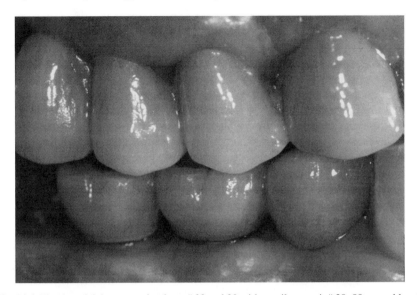

Fig. 14.4 Fixed partial denture on implants # 29 and 30 with cantilever unit # 28; 89-year old male patient; 13-year follow-up visit. The cantilever solution was chosen at the time of planning because tooth #28 had to be extracted and the present alveolar bone deficiency would had required grafting and longer healing, which the patient could not accept (*See* Color Plate 9)

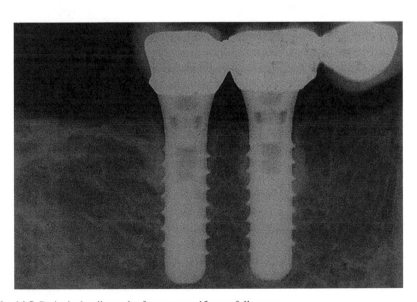

Fig. 14.5 Periapical radiograph of same case; 13-year follow-up

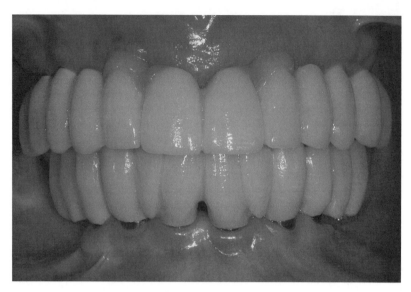

Fig. 14.6 Intraoral view of upper and lower full-arch fixed prostheses, ceramo-metal, with distal cantilevers in 60-year old female patient at time of delivery of prosthesis (*See* Color Plate 10)

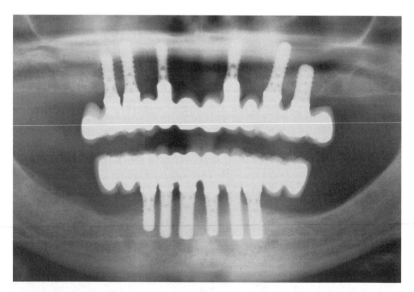

Fig. 14.7 Panoramic radiograph of case at time of delivery. Implants were placed at time of extraction of remaining teeth and immediately loaded with provisional prostheses approximately one year prior to delivery of the final prostheses

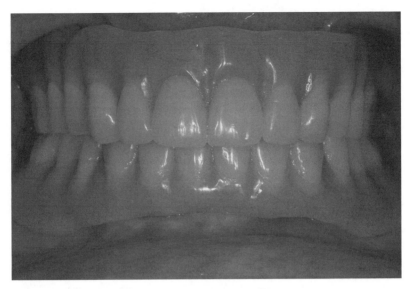

Fig. 14.8 Intraoral view of upper and lower overdentures placed two years ago in 58-year old female patient (*See* Color Plate 11)

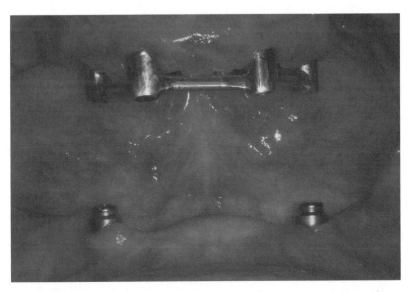

Fig. 14.9 Intraoral view of upper bar supported by 4 implants and two single implants with Locator® abutments for overdenture support and retention (*See* Color Plate 12)

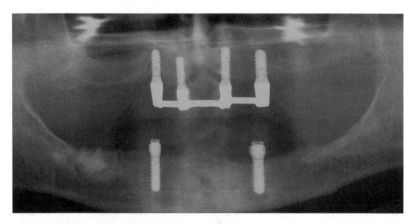

Fig. 14.10 Panoramic radiograph of case at two-year follow-up

it demonstrated that patient acceptance of specific treatment modalities is modified by social and cultural influences, financial means, and individual adaptive capacity. Patient acceptance of a particular treatment modality is also influenced by her/his educational background, knowledge, objective experience of the dental health-care provider and a number of other socioeconomic, regional, cultural, age, and gender influences.

If scientific evidence for a specific best treatment for the edentulous mandible is insufficient, it is even less satisfactory for the implant prosthetic rehabilitation of the edentulous maxilla (Bryant et al., 2007). The edentulous maxilla is considerably more complex due to various factors, most importantly lesser bone quality and more unfavorable alveolar bone resorption, which stand in direct opposition to the esthetic and phonetic demands of proper (anterior) tooth positioning and biomechanical requirements. It has been documented that bone quantity, reflected by implant length, had a significant impact on implant failure risk (Jemt & Häger, 2006). There is also convincing scientific evidence that the survival rates can be significantly improved when using implants with a rough surfaced bone contact area especially in sites with bone of lower quality and quantity or sites where bone grafting was performed (Gallucci et al., 2007; Lambert et al., 2007). At this point, it is foremost left to the experience of the treating clinician to choose the presumably best option for an individual patient. Based on clinical evidence, the placement of at least four implants to be connected with a bar for support of a maxillary overdenture is frequently proposed as the minimal treatment option with a favorable long-term prognosis in the edentulous maxilla (Figs. 14.8–14.10).

While the impact of implant-assisted prosthodontics in the edentulous patient may intuitively be perceived as more substantial than in the partially edentulous, dental implants have also substantially widened the range of restorative options in the latter group. Implants offer the possibility of leaving unrestored teeth or teeth with existing, intact restorations such as inlays, onlays, or crowns adjacent to edentulous spaces untouched. They also facilitate treatment decisions, which are more typically needed for the older patient: teeth with reduced periodontal support, endodontic, or structural deficiencies, which may have a good to fair prognosis if left alone, but would not make predictable abutments for prosthetic devices, can be maintained without compromising the prognosis of the planned restorations (Figs. 14.1–14.3).

The decision whether to use the remaining natural teeth as abutments for conventional fixed prostheses or to add dental implants for the replacement of diseased natural teeth is influenced by a number of factors such as the location in the dental arches, strategic value and treatment prognosis for such teeth, subjective and objective need for tooth replacement, dimensions of the alveolar process, esthetic impact, as well as access for treatment. As mentioned earlier, equally important in the planning process is assessment of the patient's systemic condition and ability to undergo implant surgery.

In the edentulous arches, implants supporting fixed or removable prostheses will more frequently be inserted in the anterior regions where more favorable alveolar bone dimensions and quality are found. In the partially edentulous patients, implants as anchors for tooth replacements are needed just as much in posterior regions. In these areas, anatomical conditions are often less favorable. Especially in dentitions where teeth have been lost due to periodontal disease, the volume of the alveolar process may be substantially reduced (Fig. 14.7). This brings about a number of concerns related to the longevity of implant anchorage, function, and esthetics.

In the posterior areas of the jaw, such concerns may primarily be of biomechanical nature due to the resulting unfavorable "crown-root ratios" in regions of greatest masticatory forces. Treatment alternatives include the use of multiple short implants splinted together with the fixed partial denture they support (Weber, 2003), external or internal sinus floor elevation (Wallace & Froum, 2003), ridge augmentation with various bone grafting and regeneration techniques or osseous distraction (Esposito et al., 2006; Aghaloo & Moy, 2007), distal extension fixed prostheses anchored on remaining natural teeth (Nyman & Lindhe, 1976), or premolar occlusion without replacement of the failed molars (shortened dental arch concept; Kayser, 1989; Kanno & Carlsson, 2006).

Prior to the availability of dental implants and bone augmentation techniques for the replacement of lost posterior teeth, cantilevered fixed partial dentures were used as an alternative to extend dental arches distally to spare the patient from removable partial dentures (Nyman & Lindhe, 1976). Whereas this type of periodontal prostheses performed admirably when designed and maintained properly, the biological and biomechanical risks associated with such reconstructions have shown to be considerable (Hammerle et al., 2000, Pjetursson et al., 2004). In the patient with a substantially compromised anterior dentition and a lack of sufficient posterior bone volume for dental implants, the extraction of the remaining compromised anterior dentition for the purpose of placing implants in combination with cantilevered full-arch prostheses as originally described by Brånemark et al. (1985) may be the prognostically most favorable treatment approach (Adell et al., 1990) (Figs. 14.6–14.7).

In this regard, the question of whether the presence of periodontal disease will reduce the long-term outcome of implant therapy is of specific interest and has been addressed in recent studies (Ellegaard et al., 1997; Baelum & Ellegaard, 2004). The authors found that after 5 years of function, there was no difference between implants in patients free of periodontal disease versus those in patients with disease. After 10 years of follow-up, a slightly greater increased risk for peri-implantitis including bone loss and subsequent implant failure was observed for some implants. Despite this finding, the authors proposed that dental implants are still a good treatment option for patients with periodontal disease. Similarly, the outcome with implants placed in combination with sinus floor elevation in patients with periodontal disease was no different from subjects free of periodontal disease (Ellegaard et al., 2006). A recent systematic review was confirmatory to the above in that a history of treated periodontitis did not seem to adversely affect implant survival but may reduce implant success rates (greater bone loss) over longer observation periods (Klokkevold & Han, 2007).

In the anterior region, the loss of periodontal hard and soft tissues and the subsequent "lengthening" of teeth brings along esthetic concerns, which can become complex, especially in patients with high expectations and smile lines. It is important to envision such problems and carefully analyze local conditions at time of examination so that expected outcomes can be appropriately discussed with the patient prior to the initiation of therapy (Figs. 14.1–14.3).

Patient Evaluation

Patient History

Implant therapy is part of a comprehensive treatment plan. This is also true for older patients, who more likely to have a longer history of oral-dental diseases, such as periodontal and endodontic pathology, caries, root caries, traumatic lesions including those of iatrogenic nature, and, consequently, various amounts of "aged" restorative dentistry. An understanding of the patient's needs, social and economic background, and general medical condition is a prerequisite for successful therapy. In order to expedite history taking, the patient should fill out a health questionnaire prior to the initial examination visit. Such questionnaires are best constructed in a way that the professional immediately realizes compromising factors that may modify the treatment plan and may have to be discussed in detail with the patient during the initial visit or may require medical consults to enable proper treatment planning. The assessment of the patient's history should include (a) chief complaint and expectations, (b) social and family history, (c) dental history, (d) motivation and compliance (e.g., oral hygiene), (e) habits (smoking, recreational drugs, bruxism), and (f) medical history and medications.

Chief Complaint and Expectations

To facilitate a successful treatment outcome, it is of critical importance to recognize and understand the patient's needs and ability for treatment. Patients usually have specific desires and expectations regarding treatment and outcomes. These may not mesh with the attainable outcome projected by the clinician after assessment of the specific clinical situation. Optimal individual treatment results may only be achieved if the patient's demands are in balance with the objective evaluation of the condition and the projected treatment outcomes. Therefore, the patient's expectations have to be taken seriously and must be incorporated in the evaluation. Especially in regard to dentofacial esthetics, a clear understanding of the patients' views is essential. Esthetic compromises often need to be made when implant restorations are performed in the periodontally compromised dentition because of the loss of hard and soft tissues. If a patient has been referred for specific treatment, the extent of the desired treatment has to be defined and the referring dentist informed of the intentions for treatment and the expectations regarding outcomes.

Social and Family History

Before assessing the clinical condition in detail, it is helpful to interview the patient on her/his professional and social environment and on his/her priorities in life, especially when extensive, time consuming, and costly dental treatment is envisioned as it is often the case with dental implant treatment. Likewise, a family history may reveal important clues with respect to time and cause for tooth loss, systemic or local diseases such as aggressive forms of periodontitis or other genetic predispositions, habits, compliance, and other behavioral aspects.

Dental History

It is important that previous dental care including prophylaxis and maintenance is explored with the patient if not stated by a referring dentist. Information regarding cause for tooth loss, signs, and symptoms of dental problems noted by the patient such as pain, migration, and increasing mobility of teeth, bleeding gums, food impaction, and difficulties in chewing have to be explored in this context. Patient comfort in regards to function and esthetics and the subjective need for tooth replacement is assessed at this time.

Motivation and Compliance

In this part of the communication, an assessment is made on the patient's interest and motivation for extended and costly therapy. The patient's view on oral health, her/his last visit to a dentist and/or hygienist, frequency and regularity of visits to the dentist, and detailed information on home-care procedures are helpful pieces of information in this regard.

Habits

Smoking is considered a risk factor for implant failure (Bain & Moy, 1993; Chuang et al., 2002; McDermott et al., 2003). Smoking affects healing and tissue health in several ways, including impaired neutrophil function, altered blood flow, and diminished oxygen perfusion. A recent systematic review by Klokkevold & Han (2007) confirmed that smoking has the potential to adversely affect the outcome of implant treatment as measured by implant survival or success. In the context of outcome assessment of implant therapy, implant survival means simply that an implant is stable and continues to support a prosthetic device securely and without causing discomfort to the patient. To assess implant success, other more stringent evaluation criteria are used, such as stability of radiographic bone levels adjacent to an implant, absence of infection, absence of hard and/or soft peri-implant tissue defects, including recession, as well as objective and subjective criteria regarding function and esthetics. Consequently, implant success rates in long-term studies are most often lower than survival rates because of the more stringent criteria applied. In the mentioned review by Klokkevold & Han (2007), implant survival rates for various studies with observation periods from 1 to 12 years ranged from 78.13% to 100% with a pooled estimate of 89.7% for smokers and 93.3% for non-smokers. The difference, although lower than generally expected, was statistically significant. When assessing survival rates for maxilla and mandible separately, the pooled estimates for implant survival in the maxillae of smokers was 86.1% and in non-smokers 92.4%, indicating that the effect of smoking on implant survival was predominantly related to areas of sparse trabecular bone. With this being the case, the use of implants with rough surfaces is recommended in these indications as they enhance quality and quantity of bone-implant contact and tend to lead to better outcomes. While there is sufficient evidence to support this statement for implants placed in trabecular bone in general, the body of the literature assessing this specifically for smokers is too limited to make scientifically evidenced conclusions (Klokkevold & Han, 2007). The above-mentioned data indicate, though, that smoking cannot be seen as a contraindication for dental implants. However, implant candidates need to be informed about the increased risk and certainly should be encouraged to stop smoking not only for the purpose of treatment with dental implants but even more importantly as part of a comprehensive approach to improving a patient's health.

Bruxism is a condition, which is considered a biomechanical risk factor for implant failure, especially if it is severe. While the scientific evidence for this correlation is lacking, reports indicated that prosthetic complications such as fractures of the veneering material appear to be more frequent. Reports in the literature support the value of including precautionary measures in the implant treatment plan such as the use of implants of sufficient length and diameter, splinting of multiple implants, use of retrievable restorations, and occlusal guards. Early recognition of bruxism or clenching is certainly beneficial for appropriate treatment planning (Lobbezoo et al., 2006). Unfortunately, it is often not possible to diagnose the condition appropriately at the outset of treatment.

Medical History Including Medications

A thorough review of the patient's medical history is important. Certain medical conditions may negatively affect the outcome of dental implant therapy (Hollender et al., 2003). Any condition, which has the potential to compromise normal wound healing, should be considered at least a conditional or temporary risk factor. Included are chemotherapy and radiation therapy for the treatment of cancers, antimetabolic therapy for the treatment of arthritis, seriously impaired cardiovascular function, and bleeding disorders including medication induced anticoagulation.

Of the chronic systemic diseases, uncontrolled or insufficiently controlled diabetes is considered a risk factor for implant failure. As a metabolic disease that alters tissue integrity, impairs wound healing, and increases susceptibility to infection, it appears to negatively affect peri-implant bone healing quantitatively and qualitatively compared to non-diabetic controls as shown in experimental studies in animals (Fiorellini et al., 1999). Results from clinical studies to date are, however, inconclusive (Klokkevold & Han, 2007). They tend to indicate that diabetes may not be a contraindication for dental implant treatment, after all, as long as it is adequately controlled through diet and/or medication. Treatment guidelines that are based on scientific evidence will need to be established on the basis of randomized controlled clinical trials, which include type and time of onset of diabetes, as well as the acceptable glucosylated hemoglobin levels for uncompromised peri-implant tissue healing (Kotsovilis et al., 2006)

In light of the increasing intake of medications in the aging population, an accurate assessment of the patient's prescribed and over-the-counter medications with their potential interactions and effects on therapeutic procedures has to be made. Most frequent are, in this content, anticoagulants such as coumadin and aspirin. Also to be recognized is the increased frequency for antibiotic prophylaxis for dental surgical procedures in the older patient, for instance after joint replacement.

Recently, the occurrence of ostoenecrosis of the jaw in patients on current long-term bisphosphonate therapy or a history thereof has been described. The occurrence of osteonecrosis has primarily been observed after oral surgical procedures in patients on long-term intravenous bisphosphonate therapy as used in the treatment of cancers but has also occurred in patients taking oral drugs of this kind, although with a much lower incidence (Marx et al., 2005; Woo et al., 2006; Koka et al., 2007, Dello Russo et al., 2007). Mortensen et al. (2007) concluded that the increasing number of reports about bisphosphonate associated osteomyelitis and the difficulty in treating these patients require further investigation to identify those patients who are at increased risk. Also, the optimal and safe duration of treatment with bisphonates remains to be determined. Due to the existing uncertainty in this area, recognition of patients on bisphosphonate therapy, communication with the treating physician(s) and a benefit/risk assessment have to be made for such patients, who are considered for implant therapy (Melo & Obeid, 2005). Koka et al. (2007) also found that the risk of bisphosphonate-induced osteonecrosis appears to be very small in patients taking oral bisphosphonates, mostly for treatment of osteoporosis. This small risk has to be put in perspective with the consequences of an osteoporotic fracture, which likely will have significantly greater mortality and morbidity than bisphoshonate-induced osteonecrosis.

Lack of patient compliance is another potential contraindication. This group may include patients with drug addictions including alcohol abuse. Also, patients with psychiatric conditions may not be good candidates for implant therapy. Unfortunately, they are often difficult to identify at the time of initial examination. If identified, these patients should be thoroughly examined by medical specialists before they are accepted for implant treatment (Hollender et al., 2003).

In summary, while most of this medical information can be extracted from a health questionnaire as mentioned earlier, it is important for the clinician to ask specific questions related to the patient's answers in the questionnaire to clarify their potential impact on treatment with dental implants. In many instances, it will be necessary to contact the patient's physician for detailed information relevant to the planned treatment.

Local Examination

Extraoral

An extraoral examination should be part of any initial patient examination. The clinician should look for asymmetries, lesions, or swellings of the head and neck areas. Observation of function and palpation of the head and neck musculature and temporo-mandibular joints are performed. Appropriateness of the height of the lower face (vertical dimension of occlusion) is assessed extraorally to determine if loss of vertical dimension of occlusion is present, as it is often the case in the older individual with a diminished or worn dentition. Angular cheilitis, as it is a quite frequent finding in this patient population, may be an indicator of loss of vertical tooth height. This is also the perfect time to take note of esthetic characteristics such as lip and cheek support, smile line, lip line, gingival line, and dento-facial composition.

General Intraoral Examination and Radiographs

The general intraoral examination includes the assessment of the condition of soft and hard tissues of the oral cavity. This also entails a careful cancer screening. Soft or hard tissue lesions will most likely require treatment prior to the placement of dental implants. Pathological soft tissue conditions include herpetic stomatitis, candidiasis, prosthesis-induced stomatitis, tumors, and forms of hyperplasia. Hard tissue pathoses, which most likely require treatment prior to implant therapy, include tooth impactions, bone cysts, root fragments, residual infections in the alveolar bone, e.g., caused by failed endodontic treatment, or tumors.

In the partially edentulous, dental hard tissues are equally carefully examined to determine the need for restorative treatment in the remaining dentition, most importantly those for teeth directly adjacent to edentulous spaces. The need for restoration of the latter may influence the treatment plan in terms of choosing a conventional fixed partial denture over an implant-supported restoration to replace a missing tooth. Pathologies such as caries, root caries, fractures, attrition, abrasion, abfraction, and tooth mobility or tooth misalignment are noted. Existing restorations are recorded and deficiencies such as open margins, open contacts, or fractures identified. Testing for vitality of teeth, especially of those adjacent to potential implant sites, will point to possible endodontic pathologies, which should be treated prior to implant placement. The examination of periodontal tissues includes the observation of plaque and calculus, inflammatory changes in the gingivae, probing depth, bleeding on probing and, of course, the assessment of the patient's oral hygiene.

Finally, static and dynamic aspects of the patient's occlusion are determined, including the adequacy of the patient's vertical dimension of occlusion, maxillomandibular relationship (Angle classification), overbite, overjet, stability in habitual occlusion, centric relation, slide in centric, lateral and anterior excursive contacts (canine guidance, group function, anterior guidance). In this context, it is also important to evaluate the opening amplitude of the mandible since instrumentation involved with dental implant therapy requires that the patient is able to open sufficiently wide. For the edentulous patient, current dentures – if existing – have to be assessed in regards to their adequacy of fulfilling the patient's esthetic and functional needs including denture stability in static and dynamic occlusion as well as the integrity of denture teeth and denture base.

The initial patient evaluation will include a radiographic survey. For the implant candidate with remaining teeth, a full-mouth set of periapical radiographs is needed to supplement the intraoral examination. In addition, a panoramic view is often required to sufficiently reveal structures surrounding the remaining teeth such as the infra-alveolar nerve canal, the mental foramina as well as the floor of the maxillary and nasal sinuses as well as pathological findings in the jaws. The initial radiographs will allow for a quick assessment if implant therapy is feasible. Especially the presence of sufficient bone height in potential implant sites is of importance. Minimal radiographic bone height requirements for implant placement depend on a number of factors such as recommended implant length for a single implant restoration, single vs. multiple adjacent implants, jaw location and ease and predictability of ridge augmentation in that location. For the fully edentulous patient, a panoramic film will be the initial radiograph of choice.

Implant Specific Diagnostics Including Radiographs

If the initial evaluation and discussion with the patient is in favor of implant therapy, more detailed planning steps are undertaken. These include the prosthetic plan ("restoratively driven implant treatment'), radiographic templates, and additional radiographs such as occlusal views, cephalometric images, lateral or computer tomograms. With the availability of cone beam computer tomography, which leads to a much lower radiation exposure than conventional CT technology and is also less expensive, the use of computer-aided tomography in implant treatment planning has increased substantially.

In the partially edentulous patient, an implant specific intraoral examination emphasizing the local characteristics of potential implant sites is important. Different locations in the oral cavity have varying requirements in this regard, primarily due to differing esthetic impact of implant treatment. Although the older patient maybe more focused on regaining function than ideal esthetics, an assessment of the projected esthetic outcome is still important.

The evaluation of the condition of the local mucosa needs to be part of the examination. The clinical width and height of the alveolar process in potential implant areas is examined. At the same time, pathological changes are noted including mucosal hyperplasia or hypertrophy. Probing of the local tissues may be indicated to assess tissue thickness and confirm the presence of sufficient alveolar bone. This can be done with a bone mapping procedure using a fine needle or explorer after local anesthesia has been applied.

Besides the above, local assessment of sites consists primarily of a three-dimensional space assessment and evaluation of the condition of the adjacent neighbor teeth and surrounding hard and soft tissues. It is strongly recommended to obtain diagnostic impressions and adequate bite records to produce articulator-mounted casts, on which these critical diagnostic steps can be properly performed, including a diagnostic tooth set-up or wax-up. This is especially important for extended edentulous spaces in the partially edentulous and for the completely edentulous arches where teeth are no longer available as reference.

From a restorative point of view, sites to be restored with implant crowns or fixed partial dentures should ideally have the mesio-distal width of the natural tooth (teeth) that would normally be there. In the older patient with a history of tooth loss over time, tooth movements have to be expected, which often compromise optimal space conditions. Orthodontic pretreatment may be desirable or even required even in the older individual.

From the perspective of implant placement, a mesio-distal width of 7 mm will allow the insertion of a regular platform or regular neck implant (3.75–5 mm). For spaces only 5–6 mm wide, narrow platform or narrow neck implants of $\sim$ 3.5 mm diameter are available. For single tooth spaces larger than 7 mm, wide platform or wide neck implants with a platform diameter of 6–7 mm may be the choice. It is important to note that wide neck or platform implants generally will also have a wider screw diameter. Thus, sufficient buccal–lingual bone for the placement of a wider diameter implant is important to not compromise long-term outcomes due to perforation of the alveolar bone buccal or lingual to the implant. The bucco-lingual width of the alveolar process at an implant site is assessed either by bone sounding or cross-sectional radiographs (see paragraph on radiographs below).

A minimum vertical distance from the crestal mucosa of the potential implant site(s) to the opposing dentition is needed for implant restorations. This space requirement may vary depending on the design of the restoration including the choice of abutments. As a general guideline, a vertical distance of at least 4 mm from top of the mucosa to the opposing tooth (teeth) is required for straightforward implant placement and restoration. In the patient with tooth loss due to periodontal disease, this does not usually pose a problem. Due to the concomitant bone loss, the distance is more likely greater than the original height of a natural tooth (teeth) so that the potential esthetic and biomechanical impacts of the resulting overlong implant restoration have to be taken in consideration as documented earlier.

Fully Edentulous

In addition to the extra- and intraoral examination steps outlined above for the dentate patient, in the edentulous individual the adequacy of existing removable prostheses has to be assessed in terms of their stability, function, esthetics, and material integrity. In the majority of cases, existing dentures are deficient and a new set has to be made to correctly determine the vertical dimension of occlusion, inter-arch relationship and tooth positioning for optimal esthetic, phonetic and functional effects. This diagnostic denture set-up will aid the clinician to a great extent with the assessment if a fixed implant borne prosthesis is feasible or if a removable approach promises to be more favorable. The latter may be advantageous because it allows the patient's demands for proper esthetics (lip support) and phonetics to be predictably fulfilled while maintaining easy access to the implants for daily maintenance measures. It has to be kept in mind that denture wearers may adapt to a fixed implant supported prostheses only with difficulty or not at all.

After the final try-in, the diagnostic denture set-up is used for a radiographic study. For that purpose, the diagnostic denture is duplicated in clear resin and radio-opaque markers are added to visualize tooth contours or tooth axes in the radiographs. If anatomical and other patient factors are complex, i.e., in the presence of advanced ridge resorption, superficial position of inferior alveolar nerve or mental foramen in relation to the crest of the alveolar ridge, and minimal thickness of maxillary or nasal sinus floor, a computer tomographic study is strongly recommended. The latter is also indicated if the prosthodontic plan foresees a fixed prosthesis, for which implant placement in precise relation to prosthetic tooth units is important.

If the prosthodontic plan is simpler such as for an overdenture with implant support in the front only, a simpler radiographic technique such as a panoramic radiograph with a trial denture and metal markers in the planned implant areas is often sufficient in addition to the clinical intraoral evaluation.

The diagnostic template is subsequently used as a surgical guide. Imaging technology today even allows the third party preparation of surgical guides and provisional restorations to fit on the implants placed with the guide. However, these exciting techniques are not flawless and as predictable as manufacturers try to make clinicians and patients believe in their promotion of new products and procedures. They can certainly not replace the experience and skill of the clinician experienced in implant dentistry.

Treatment Plan, Treatment Sequence, Informed Consent

After completion of the diagnostic evaluation, two to three treatment options of varying complexity are formulated in treatment plans for discussion with the patient. Benefits, risks, treatment time and sequence, number of visits, surgical interventions and postoperative expectations, and of course cost of treatment are discussed with the patient. Low cost option such as a removable partial denture vs. an implant supported fixed partial denture often has to be included in the treatment plan options as implant dentistry is expensive and many elderly patients may not be willing or able to afford it. As discussed earlier, multiple patient factors play a role in this decision-making process. The patient is then asked to sign a consent form for the treatment chosen.

A commonly followed treatment sequence for dental implants is listed in Table 14.1. There are many variations possible, and their detailed discussion would go beyond the range of this chapter. A few aspects are important for mentioning in this context, though, as discussed next.

The original "prescription" for successful osseointegration of dental implants was presented by Brånemark et al. (1969) and included placement of the "fixtures" under the oral mucosa for a 3–6 month healing time without attaching a prosthesis (unloaded healing). This is still considered the "conventional mode" (Cochran et al., 2004). However, subsequent studies have shown that implants can be placed in a one-stage surgical procedure (Buser et al., 1990) without reducing success. Similarly, more recent studies and reviews have shown that loading can occur much earlier or even immediately at time of placement without compromising the outcome (Chiapasco, 2004; Ganeles & Wismeijer, 2004; Jokstad & Carr, 2007). Careful choice of indication, clinician's experience and patient compliance are, however, important when more aggressive loading protocols are used. Primary implant stability at time of implant placement, sufficiently long implants (≥ 10 mm) and implants with rough surfaces are considered important cofactors for successful early or immediate loading. Also, the possibility of splinting multiple implants together around the alveolar arch as is the case in edentulous situations will substantially minimize the risk of too much force on an implant too early, i.e., before peri-implant bone healing has sufficiently progressed.

Table 14.1 Treatment sequence for implant assisted prosthodontics

- Examination, diagnosis and treatment planning (one or more visits)
- Presentation of treatment plan(s), patient consent
- Treatment of active disease including extractions (caries, periodontal, pulpal, other)
- Re-evaluation
- Orthodontic pre-treatment (if indicated)
- Surgical pretreatment (if indicated; e.g. bone or soft tissue augmentation)
- Implant surgery (single stage to multiple stages) and healing
- Prosthodontic phase:

    a. Provisional restoration (especially in complex cases and implants in the esthetic zone

    b. Permanent restoration

- Maintenance (long-term)

Regarding the question on how the timing of implant placement to tooth extraction will affect the outcome, the answer is unclear. Whereas in the early stages of osseointegration, it was expected that an extraction socket would need to heal completely before an implant was placed in the same location, immediate or only shortly delayed implant placement after extraction is regularly performed today. In a recent systematic review on this topic, Quirynen et al. (2007) found that because of the lack of long-term data, questions on whether peri-implant health, prosthesis stability, degree of bone loss, and esthetic outcome of immediate or early placed implants are comparable with implants in healed sites, remain unanswered. Implant loss after immediate placement was the major complication (4%–5% incidence). The incidence of implant loss was higher when immediate implant placement was combined with immediate loading.

The more aggressive implant placement and loading procedures described above have potentially great advantages especially for the older individual, who may be interested in a faster completion of treatment due the fact that her/his life expectancy may not be the same as for a younger person. Also, reducing the number of visits to the dentist to complete all treatment is valuable for many older patients, for whom multiple visits can become challenging. Today, not surprisingly, "teeth in a day" or even "teeth in an hour for everybody" are heavily promoted by some manufacturers, almost to the level that any other way of providing implant prosthodontic treatment appears antiquated. The experienced implant clinician knows that this is not so. Despite the potential attractive benefits of these more aggressive treatment protocols, one needs to carefully weigh benefits and risks of these procedures for each individual patient before proceeding.

Maintenance

Long-term maintenance is equally important for dental implants as for teeth (Lang, 1996) as oral microbiota and host response factors may pose a similar risk for dental implants as for natural teeth (Paquette et al., 2006). A well-organized recall program with a proper maintenance care protocol is essential to the long-term success of implant treatment. The person's home-care practices have to include mechanical plaque control with regular and power rotary toothbrushes, special brushes such as end-tufted brushes for interdental and interimplant cleaning. Elderly patients with impaired manual dexterity may perform better with power-driven brushes. Mechanical plaque removal may be supported by the use of antimicrobial agents such as chlorhexidine digluconate (0.12%, Peridex®). This may not only be recommended in the post surgical phase but also for intermittent application over longer periods of time. Older patients may benefit from a 1-month period of daily rinses with chlorhexidine followed by a 3-month period of regular home care, following which a professional tooth and implant cleaning is appropriate (Lang & Brecx, 1986).

Implant patients should be recalled every 6 months for examination and professional cleaning. At these visits, implants are checked for stability/mobility and sites inspected for local pathology (plaque, calculus, bleeding, suppuration) and need for treatment. If inflammation or infection is detected clinically, diagnostic radiographs are obtained as well. Implant mobility becomes only apparent when osseointegration, i.e., bony anchorage, is lost. Hence, the initial signs of peri-implant pathology should be diagnosed to provide early treatment. Usually the entire dentition should be treated prophylactically if inflammation is present. Implants are in general not instrumented with curettes except for the careful removal of mineralized deposits with special non-metal curettes, followed by polishing with a non- or minimally abrasive polishing paste and rubber cup.

Conclusion

Modern comprehensive dental care for older patients with structurally, functionally, and esthetically compromised dentitions has to include the consideration of dental implants. Implant assisted replacement of teeth that are missing or need to be extracted due to their condition and poor prognosis is an overall predictable treatment alternative for the older as much as for the younger patient. Esthetic and functional demands of older patients are highly variable as are their treatment responses, which are individual and with substantial variation. Multiple factors will affect patient acceptance of a specific implant treatment modality. In addition to the clinician's experience and skill, listening to and hearing the patient's chief complaint as well as adequate patient information, which are substantiated by a signed informed consent to treatment, are important components for successful therapy.

Acknowledgments I would like to thank Ms. Paula Anderson for her assistance in the preparation of this chapter.

References

Adell, R., Ericsson B., Lekholm, U, Brånemark P.-I. & Jemt, T.A. (1990). A long-term follow-up study of osseointegrated implants in the treatment of totally edentulous jaws. *International Journal of Oral and Maxillofacial Implants* **5**: 347–359.

Aghaloo, T.L & Moy, P.K. (2007). Which hard tissue aumentation techniques are the most successful in furnishing bony support for implant placement? *International Journal of Oral and Maxillofacial Implants* **22** (Supplement): 49–70.

Baelum, V. & Ellegaard, B. (2004). Implant survival in periodontally compromised patients. *Journal of Periodontology* **75**: 1404–1412.

Bain, C.A. & Moy, P.K. (1993). The association between the failure of dental implants and cigarette smoking. *International Journal Oral and Maxillofacial Implants* **8**: 609–615.

Bragger, U., Karoussis, I., Persson, R., Pjetursson, B., Salvi, G. & Lang, N. (2005). Technical and biological complications/failures with single crowns and fixed partial dentures on implants: a 10-year prospective cohort study. *Clinical Oral Implants Research* **16**: 326–324.

Brånemark, P.-I., Adell, R., Breine, U., Hansson, B.O., Lindstrom, J. & Ohlsson, A. (1969). Intraraosseous anchorage of dental prostheses. I. Experimental studies. *Scandinavian Journal of Plastic and Reconstructive Surgery* **3**: 81–100.

Brånemark, P.I., Hansson, B.O., Adell, R., Breine, U., Lindström, J., Hallén, O. & Ohman, A. (1977). Osseointegrated implants in the treatment of the edentulous jaw. Experience from a 10-year period. *Scandinavian Journal of Plastic and Reconstructive Surgery (Suppl.)* **16**: 1–132.

Brånemark, P.I., Zarb, G.A. & Albrektsson, T. (1985). *Tissue-Integrated Prostheses: Osseointegration in Clinical Dentistry*. Chicago: Quintessence Publishing, Co.

Bryant, S.R. & Zarb, G.A. (1998). Osseointegration of oral implants in older and younger adults. *International Journal of Oral and Maxillofacial Implants* **13**: 492–499.

Bryant, S.R. & Zarb, G.A. (2002). Outcomes of implant prosthodontic treatment in older adults. *Journal of the Canadian Dental Association* **68**: 97–102.

Bryant, S.R., MacDonld-Jankowski, D. & Kim, K. (2007). Does the type of implant prosthesis affect outcomes for the completely edentulous arch? *International Journal of Oral and Maxillofacial Implants* **22** (Supplement): 117–139.

Buser, D., Weber, H.P. & Lang, N.P. (1990). Tissue integration of non-submerged implants. 1-year results of a prospective study with 100 ITI hollow-cylinder and hollow-screw implants. *Clinical Oral Implants Research* **1**: 33–40.

Buser, D., Mericske-Stern, R., Bernard, J.P., Behneke, A., Behneke, N., Hirt, H.P., Belser, U.C. & Lang, N.P. (1997). Long-term evaluation of non-submerged ITI implants. Part 1: 8-year life table analysis of a prospective multi-center study with 2359 implants. *Clinical Oral Implants Research* **8**: 161–72.

Chiapasco, M. (2004). Early and immediate restoration and loading of implants in completely edentulous patients. *International Journal of Oral & Maxillofacial Implants* **19** (Supplement): 76–91.

Chiappelli, F., Bauer, J., Spackman, S., Prolo, P., Edgerton, M., Armenian, C., Dickmeyer, J. & Harper, S. (2002). Dental needs of the elderly in the 21st century. *General Dentistry* **50**: 358–363.

Chuang, S.K., Wei, L.J., Douglass, C.W. & Dodson, T.B. (2002). Risk factors for dental implant failure: a strategy for the analysis of clustered failure-time observations. *Journal of Dental Research* **81**: 572–577.

Cochran, D.L., Morton, D. & Weber, H.P. (2004). Consensus statements and recommended clinical procedures regarding loading protocols for endosseous dental implants. *International Journal of Oral & Maxillofacial Implants* **19** (Supplement): 109–113.

Dello Russo, N.M., Jeffcoat, M.K., Marx, R.E. & Fugazzotto, P. (2007). Osetonecrosis in the jaws of patients who are using oral bisphosphonates to treat osteoporosis. *International Journal of Oral & Maxillofacial Implants* **22**: 146–153.

Douglass, C.W., Shih, A. & Ostry, L. (2002a). Will there be a need for complete dentures in the United States in 2020? *Journal of Prosthetic Dentistry* **87**: 5–8.

Douglass, C.W. & Watson, A.J. (2002b). Future needs for fixed and removable partial dentures in the United States. *Journal of Prosthetic Dentistry* **87**: 9–14.

Doundoulakis, J.H., Eckert, S.E., Lindquist, C.C. & Jeffcoat, M.K. (2003). The implant supported overdenture as an alternative to the complete mandibular dentures. *Journal of the American Dental Association* **134**: 1455–1458.

Ellegaard, B., Baelum, V. & Karring T. (1997). Implant therapy in periodontally compromised patients. *Clinical Oral Implants Research* **8**: 180–188.

Ellegaard, B., Baelum, V. & Kølsen-Petersen J. (2006). Non-grafted sinus implants in periodontally compromised patients: a time-to-event analysis. *Clinical Oral Implants Research* **17**: 156–164.

Esposito, M., Grusovin, M.G., Coulthard, P. & Worthington, H.V. (2006). The efficacy of various bone augmentation procedures for dental implants: a Cochrane systematic review of randomized controlled clinical trials. *International Journal of Oral and Maxillofacial Implants* **21**: 696–710.

Feine, J.S. & Carlsson, G.E. (2003). *Implant Overdentures*. The Standard of Care for Edentulous Patients. Chicago: Quintessence Publishing, Co.

Fiorellini, J.P., Nevins, M.L., Norkin, A., Weber, H.P. & Karimbux, N.Y. (1999). He effect of insulin therapy on ossoeintegration in a diabetic rat model. *Clinical Oral Implants Research* **10**: 362–368.

Fitzpatrick, B. (2006). Standard of care for the edentulous mandible: a systematic review. *Journal of Prosthetic Dentistry* **95**: 71–78.

Fritz, M. (1996). Implant therapy II. *Annals of Periodontology* **1**: 796–815.

Gallucci, G.O., Susarla, S.M., Lambert, F.E., Belser, U.C. & Weber, H.P. (2007). Fixed implant rehabilitation of the edentulous maxilla: a systematic literature review. Part II: Prosthodontic survival rates. *Clinical Oral Implants Research* (submitted).

Ganeles, J. & Wismeijer, D. (2004). Early and immediately restored and loaded dental implants for single-tooth and partial-arch applications. *International Journal of Oral and Maxillofacial Implants* **19** (Supplement): 92–102.

Hammerle, C.H., Ungerer, M.C., Fantoni, P.C., Bragger, U., Burgin, W. & Lang, N.P. (2000). Long-term analysis of biologic and technical aspects of fixed partial dentures with cantilevers. *Intenational Journal of Prosthodontics* **13**: 409–415.

Hollender, L.G., Arcuri, M.R., & Lang, B.R. (2003). Diagnosis and treatment planning. In: *Osseointegration in Dentistry. An overview.* Chicago: Quintessence Publishing, pp. 19–29.

Iacono, V.J. & Cochran, D.L. (2007) State of the science on implant dentistry: a workshop developed using an evidence based approach. *International Journal of Oral & Maxillofacial Implants* **22** (Supplement): 7–10.

Iqbal, M.K. & Kim, S. (2007) For teeth requiring endodontic treatment, what are the differences in outcomes of restored endodontically treated teeth compared to implant-supported restorations? *International Journal of Oral & Maxillofacial Implants* **22** (Supplement): 96–116.

Jemt, T. & Häger, P. (2006). Early complete failures of fixed implant-supported prostheses in the edentulous maxilla: a 3-year analysis of 17 consecutive cluster failure patients. *Clinical Implant Dentistry and Related Research* **8**: 77–86.

Jokstad, A. & Carr, A.B. (2007) What is the effect on outcomes of time-to-loading of a fixed or removable prosthesis placed on implant(s). *International Journal of Oral & Maxillofacial Implants* **22** (Supplement): 19–48.

Kanno, T. & Carlsson, G.A. (2006). A review of the shortened dental arch concept focusing on the work by the Kayser/Nijmegen group. *Journal of Oral Rehabilitation* **33**: 850–862.

Kayser, A.F. (1989) Shortened dental arch: a therapeutic concept in reduced dentitions and certain high-risk groups. *International Journal of Periodontics and Restorative Dentistry* **9**: 426–449.

Klokkevold, P.R. & Han, T.J. (2007). How do smoking, diabetes, and periodontitis affect out-comes of implant treatment? *International Journal of Oral & Maxillofacial Implants* **22** (Supplement): 173–202.

Koka, S., Clarke, B.L., Amin, S., Gertz, M. & Ruggiero, S.L. (2007). Oral bisphosphonate therapy and osteonecrosis of the jaw: what to tell the concerned patient? *International Journal of Prosthodontics* **20**: 115–122.

Kotsovilis, S., Karoussis, I.K & Fourmoussis, I. (2006). A comprehensive and critical review of dental implant placement in diabetic animals and patients. *Clinical Oral Implants Research* **17**: 587–599.

Lambert, F.E., Weber, H.P., Susarla, S.M., Belser, U.C. & Gallucci, G.O. (2007). Fixed implant rehabilitation of the edentulous maxilla: a systematic literature review. Part I: Implant survival rates. *Clinical Oral Implants Research* (submitted).

Lang, N.P. (1996) Oral implants in elderly patients. In: Holm-Pedersen, P.H. & Loe, H. *Textbook of Geriatric Dentistry.* Munksgaard: Copenhagen, pp. 483–502.

Lang, N.P. & Brecx, M.C. (1986). Chlorhexidine digluconate – an agent for chemical plaque control and prevention of gingival inflammation. *Journal of Periodontal Research* **21** (Supplement 16): 23–32.

Lindh, T., Gunne, J. Tillberg, A. & Molin, M. (1998). A meta-analysis of implants in partial edentulism. *Clinical Oral Implants Research* **9**: 80–90.

Lobbezoo, F., Van Der Zaag, J. & Naeije, M. (2006). Bruxism: its multiple causes and its effects on dental implants – an updated review. *Journal of Oral Rehabilitation* **33**: 293–300.

Marx, R.E., Sawatari, Y., Fortin, M. & Broumand, V. (2005). Bisphosphonate-induced exposed bone (osteonecrosis/osteopetrosis) of the jaws: risk factors, recognition, prevention, and treatment. *Journal of Oral and Maxillofacial Surgery* **63**: 1567–1575.

McDermott, N.E., Chuang, S.K., Woo, V.V. & Dodson, T.B. (2003). Complications of dental implants: identification, frequency, and associated risk factors. *International Journal of Oral and Maxillofacial Implants* **18**: 848–855.

Melo, M.D. & Obeid, G. (2005). Osteonecrosis of the jaws in patients with a history of receiving bisphosphonate therapy: strategies for prevention and early recognition. *Journal of the American Dental Association* **136**:1675–1681.

Mortensen, M., Lawson, W. & Montazem, A. (2007). Osteonecrosis of the jaw associated with bisphosphonate use: presentation of seven cases and literature review. *Laryngoscope* **117**: 30–34.

Moy, P.K., Medina, D., Shetty, V. & Aghaloo, T.L. (2005). Dental implant failure rates and associated risk factors. *International Journal of Oral & Maxillofacial Implants* **20**: 569–577.

Nyman, S. & Lindhe, J. (1976). Prosthetic rehabilitation of patients with advanced periodontal disease. *Journal of Clinical Peridontology* **3**: 135–147.

Paquette, D.W., Brodala, N. & Williams, R.C. (2006). Risk factors for endosseous dental implant failure. *Dental Clinics of North America* **50**: 361–374.

Pjetursson, B.E., Tan K., Lang, N.P., Bragger, U., Egger, M. & Zwahlen M. (2004). A systematic review of the survival and complication rates of fixed partial dentures (FPDs) after an observation period of at least 5 years. *Clinical Oral Implants Research* **15**: 667–676.

Pjetursson, B.E., Karoussis, I., Burgin, W., Bragger, U. & Lang, N.P. (2005). Patients' satisfaction following implant therapy. A 10-year prospective cohort study. *Clinical Oral Implants Research* **16**: 185–193.

Proskin, H.M., Jeffcoat, R.L., Catlin, A., Campbell, J. & Jeffcoat, M.J. (2007). A meta-analytic approach to determine the state of the science on implant dentistry. *International Journal of Oral & Maxillofacial Implants* **22** (Supplement): 11–18.

Quirynen, M., Van Assche, N., Botticelli, D. & Berglundh, T. (2007). How does timing o implant placement to extraction affect outcome? *International Journal of Oral & Maxillofacial Implants* **22** (Supplement): 203–223.

Salinas, T.J. & Eckert, S.E. (2007). In patients requiring single tooth replacement, what are the outcomes of implant- as compared to tooth-supported restorations? *International Journal of Oral and Maxillofacial Implants* **22** (Supplement): 71–95.

Schroeder, A., Pohler, O. & Sutter, F. (1976). Tissue reaction to an implant of a titanium hollow cylinder with a titanium surface spray layer. *Schweizerische Monatsschrift für Zahnheilkunde* **86**: 713–27.

Schroeder, A., van der Zypen, E., Stich, H. & Sutter, F. (1981). The reactions of bone, connective tissue, and epithelium to endosteal implants with titanium-sprayed surfaces. *Journal of Maxillofacial Surgery* **9**: 15–25.

Wallace, S.S. & Froum, S.J. (2003). Effect of maxillary sinus augmentation on the survival of endosseous dental implants. *Annals of Periodontology* **8**: 328–343.

Weber, H.P. (2003) Restorative considerations in the treatment of the atrophic posterior mandible. *International Journal of Oral and Maxillofacial Implants* **18**: 764–765.

Weber, H.P. & Sukotjo, C. (2007). Does the type of implant prosthesis affect outcomes in the partially edentulous patient? *International Journal of Oral and Maxillofacial Implants* **22** (Supplement): 140–172.

Woo, S.B., Hellstein, J.W. & Kalmar, J.R. (2006). Systematic review: bisphosphonates and osteonecrosis of the jaws. *Annals of Internal Medicine* **144**: 753–761.

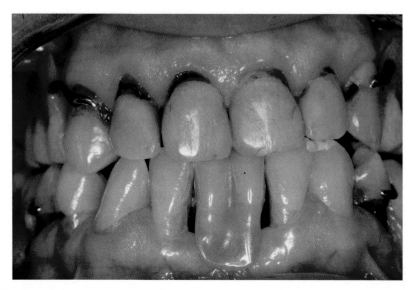

Color Plate 1 Active root surface caries lesions exhibiting a typical location along the cemento-enamel junction

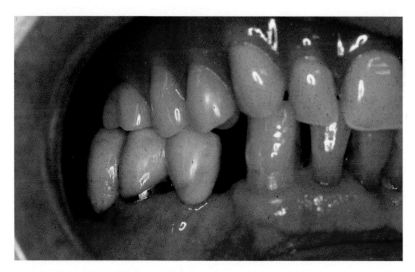

Color Plate 2 The 3-unit FPD has one abutment and extends mesially and distally to provide stable occlusal conditions with the complete upper denture

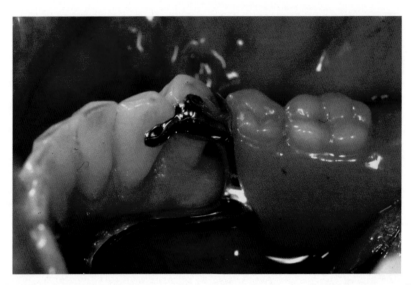

Color Plate 3 Extension denture base with a mesial occlusal rest, a lingual bracing arm (lingual and distal guide planes have been prepared), and a proximal minor connector. Note the open embrasure space

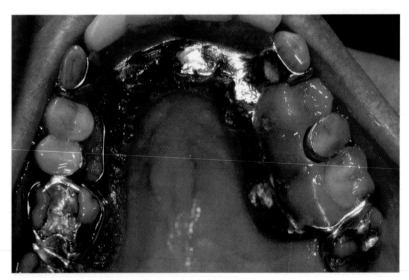

Color Plate 4 Existing RPD with a horse-shoe-shaped major connector in close relation with the abutment teeth

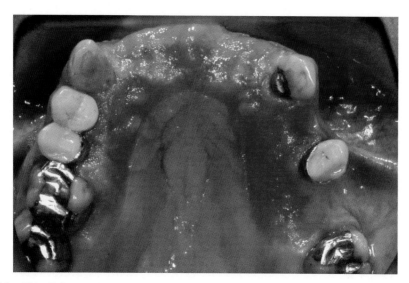

Color Plate 5 Same patient. There is clinical evidence of inflammation of the periodontal tissues as well as the palatal mucosa

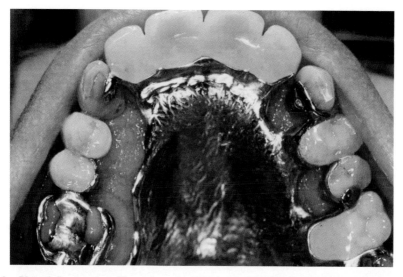

Color Plate 6 Same patient. The replacement RPD has been designed with a 6–8 mm open space between the natural teeth and the major connector. Note that periodontal health has improved

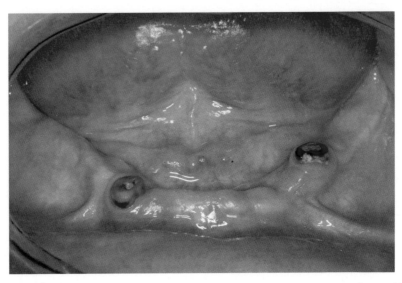

Color Plate 7 Teeth 34 and 43 have been maintained as abutments for a lower overdenture. Note plaque and superficial caries

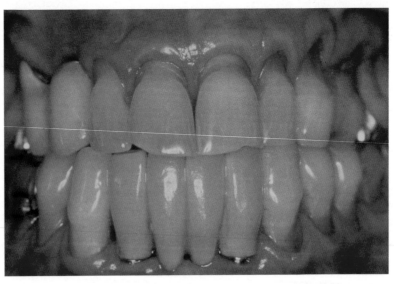

Color Plate 8 Intraoral view of implant supported single crown # 6 and implant supported FPD #23xx26 in 78 year old male patient; status 12 years after insertion of prosthesis

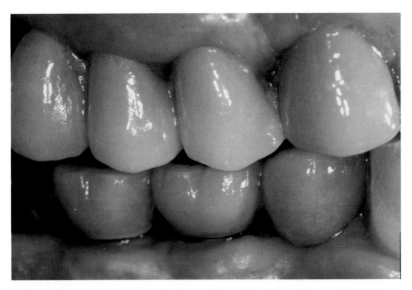

Color Plate 9 Fixed partial denture on implants # 29 and 30 with cantilever unit # 28; 89-year old male patient; 13-year follow-up visit. The cantilever solution was chosen at the time of planning because tooth #28 had to be extracted and the present alveolar bone deficiency would had required grafting and longer healing, which the patient could not accept

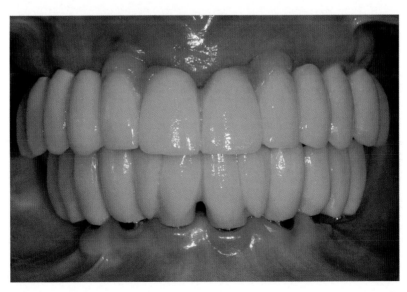

Color Plate 10 Intraoral view of upper and lower full-arch fixed prostheses, ceramo-metal, with distal cantilevers in 60-year old female patient at time of delivery of prosthesis

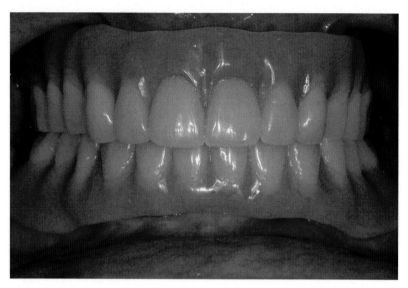

Color Plate 11 Intraoral view of upper and lower overdentures placed two years ago in 58-year old female patient

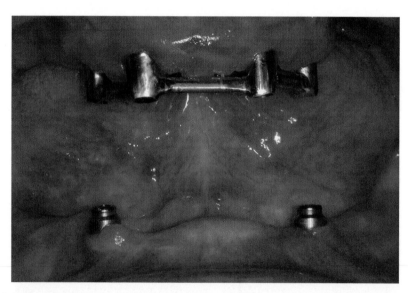

Color Plate 12 Intraoral view of upper bar supported by 4 implants and two single implants with Locator® abutments for overdenture support and retention

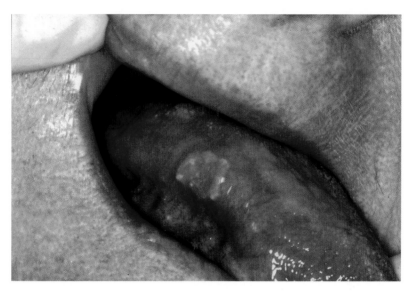

Color Plate 13 This is a 65-year-old white female with a one-pack-per-day cigarette habit for more than 40 years. She has this adherent flat white patch of the lateral tongue surface. It was firm and tender upon palpation. Biopsy revealed carcinoma in situ

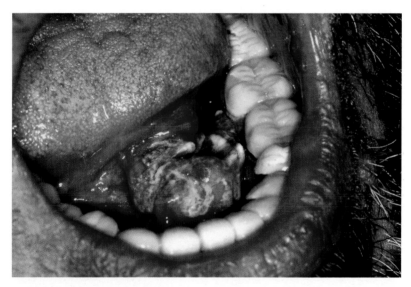

Color Plate 14 This is a 48-year-old white male with a five-cigar-per-day tobacco habit. He presented initially with this large firm-fixed painful mass of the anterior floor of mouth. Biopsy revealed squamous cell carcinoma. Despite treatment, he died of disease 6 months after initial biopsy procedures

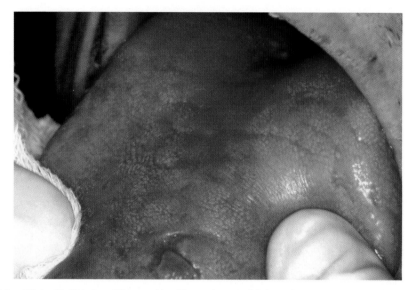

Color Plate 15 This is a 73-year-old white male complaining of a burning tongue. Note the atrophic red dorsal tongue surface with an ulcerative lesion at the inferior margin. A fungal culture was vividly positive in one week's time (candidiasis). The tongue appearance reversed itself to normal after one week of antifungal therapy

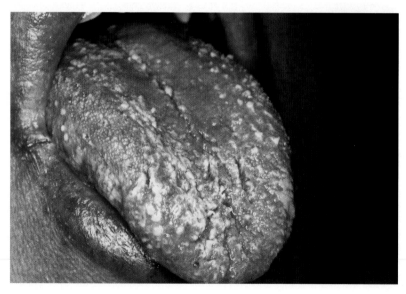

Color Plate 16 This is a 56-year-old white female with AIDS. She presented initially with a burning mouth and these moveable white "milk curds" of candidal microbes. A fungal culture was very positive in one week's time (candidiasis), and she improved dramatically with antifungal therapy

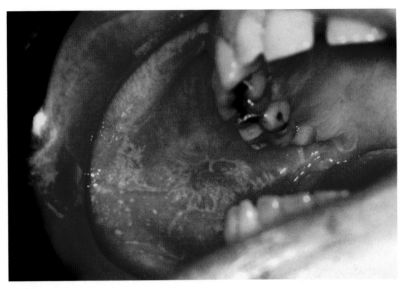

Color Plate 17 This is a 57-year-old patient with asymptomatic white papules and laces upon several oral mucosal sites as demonstrated here involving the buccal mucosa. A biopsy confirmed lichen planus and since the patient was symptom-free, no medications were prescribed initially

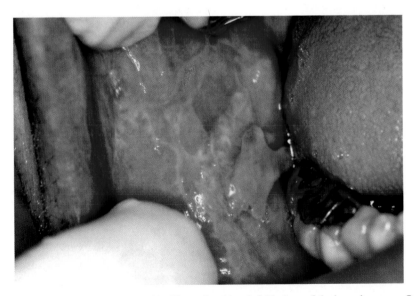

Color Plate 18 This is a 68-year-old white male with painful lesions of the buccal mucosa. Oral examination revealed painless white lacey lines and painful beige ulcers of lichen planus. Biopsy confirmed LP and the patient was given sublesional steroid injections which eliminated the painful ulcers

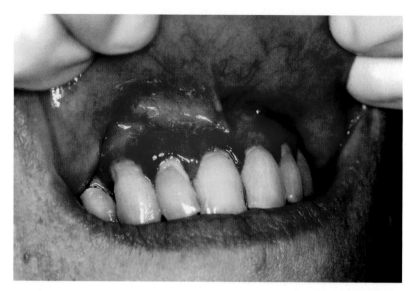

Color Plate 19 This is a 67-year-old white female with mildly uncomfortable "sloughing" lesions of the maxillary and mandibular gingival soft tissues. Examination revealed flat red lesions that dislodged with minimal pressure. Biopsy confirmed mucosal pemphigoid

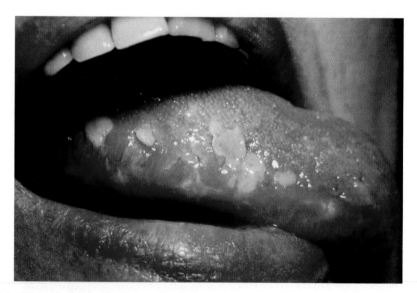

Color Plate 20 This is a 54-year-old white female with several months of painful oral mucosal lesions that began in her throat and " spread to my mouth". She lost 17 pounds due to an inability to eat. Although these white lesions appear leucoplakic, they were in fact classic painful focally ulcerated lesions of pemphigus vulgaris. A biopsy confirmed PV demonstrating intraepithelial clefting and acantholysis

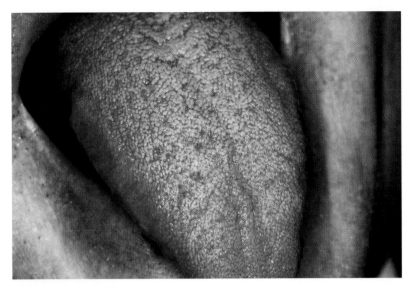

Color Plate 21 This is an 82-year-old white female concentration camp survivor who presented with an otherwise negative medical history, a normal appearing oral mucosa, and a several months history of a burning mouth. In part via the process of exclusion, the final diagnosis was recorded as burning mouth syndrome

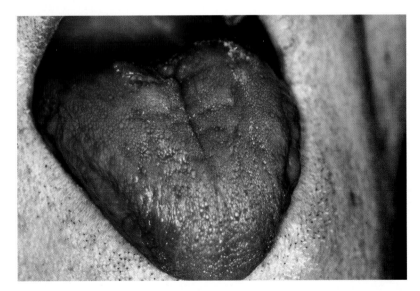

Color Plate 22 This is an 82-year-old white female concentration camp survivor who presented with an otherwise negative medical history, a normal appearing oral mucosa, and a several months history of a burning mouth. In part via the process of exclusion, the final diagnosis was recorded as burning mouth syndrome

Chapter 15
Saliva and the Salivary Glands in the Elderly

Louis Mandel

Salivary secretory dysfunction and/or salivary gland pathology are conditions that can be found in all segments of the population. The aged are uniquely susceptible to some of these entities which may reflect manifestations of local, systemic or even imagined disorders. Many other salivary gland disease processes, both local and systemic, do not particularly seek out the elderly nor do they discriminate against them. In this chapter, attention will be focused on the great variety of disorders that concern the older patients who present for diagnosis and treatment in the Salivary Gland Center (SGC) of Columbia University College of Dental Medicine. Clinical, pathophysiologic and therapeutic considerations will be highlighted.

Saliva is produced by three major paired salivary glands: the parotid, submandibular and sublingual glands. Small contributions are made by hundreds of accessory glands scattered throughout the oral cavity. These glands with their secretions are critical in maintaining both oral and systemic health. Saliva accomplishes this assignment by carrying out numerous functions.

A prime function of saliva is to buffer endogenous and exogenous acids and thus inhibit dental demineralization. A significant complementary function, remineralization, is facilitated by the availability of salivary calcium and phosphate ions. Antibacterial, antifungal and antiviral activities of saliva are mediated through salivary IgA, lactoferrin, lysozyme, peroxidase systems and histatins (Vissink, Spijkervet, & van nieuw Amerongen, 1996). Saliva also aids in mastication by softening foods while its role in lubrication is instrumental in the swallowing process. One simple measure of salivary hypofunction is observing the capacity of the patient to moisten and swallow a dry cracker. Futhermore, mucosal lubrication by saliva is important for a patient using a removable dental prosthesis. Saliva's lubricating presence also acts to prevent glossodynia. Food digestion begins in the oral cavity with the ability of salivary amylase to metabolize carbohydrates. Taste is expedited because saliva dissolves the chemical tastants within food and delivers these to taste

L. Mandel

Director, Salivary Gland Center; Assistant Dean and Clinical Professor of Dentistry Oral and Maxillofacial Surgery Columbia University College of Dental medicine, Columbia University, New York, USA

I.B. Lamster, M.E. Northridge (eds.), *Improving Oral Health for the Elderly*,
© Springer Science+Business Media, LLC 2008

bud receptors. Speech impairment will also become apparent without saliva moistening the oral mucosa.

It is generally accepted that approximately 1500 ml of saliva are produced in a 24 hour period by all of the salivary glands (Atkinson & Wu, 1994). When nothing is in the mouth and the glands are at rest, normal levels of whole saliva are calculated as 0.4 ml/min (Sreebny, 1989), mostly originating from the submandibular/sublingual gland complex. However, with stimulation, salivary volumes from the parotid glands equal that produced by the submandibular/sublingual glands. The normal level of stimulated whole saliva has been reported as 2.0 ml/min (Astor, Hanft, & Ciocon, 1999). Measured values that are above these normal resting and stimulated volumes represent salivary hyperfunction, while values below reflect salivary hypofunction. However, volumes can vary from individual to individual, are lower in women and dependent upon collection technique and time of day of the collection.

In the following discussion, xerostomia will be defined as a subjectively perceived complaint of dryness by a patient whose salivary volume, when measured, is within normal limits. Salivary hypofunction is the term that represents a decreased production of saliva substantiated by an objective measurement. The patient's awareness of a dry mouth develops when resting whole saliva falls below the range of 0.1–0.2 ml/min (Sreebny, 1989; Longman, Higham, Rai, Edgar, & Field, 1995). Nevertheless a complaint of dryness is frequently heard at the Columbia University College of Dental Medicine's Salivary Gland Center (SGC) when gland hypofunction does not exist.

Sialorrhea will be used to describe a patient's notion of the presence of excessive saliva when quantitative evaluation does not indicate salivary hyperfunction. If objective measurements testify to increased salivary volume, salivary hyperfunction is the appropriate description. Drooling represents the leakage of saliva on to the chin which may originate from hyperfunction. Where hyperfunction is not a factor, drooling may have its roots in disturbed neuromuscular swallowing mechanisms, mental retardation, habit or loss of oro-facial muscle tone.

With aging, a significant change occurs in the histologic features of the salivary glands. Parenchymal depletion develops with a corresponding increase in fibro-adipose tissue and the number of dilated ducts (Drummond & Chisholm, 1984). A 30%–40% decrease in parenchymal volume of individual salivary glands has been reported (Baum, Ship, & Wu, 1992). Besides the microscopic evidence, acinar loss has also been observed in CT scans of the parotid gland. A significant decrease in parotid gland density, reflecting loss of parenchyma and increased presence of fibro-adipose tissue, is seen (Drummond, Newton, & Abel, 1995).

Despite this age-related loss of secreting acini, no meaningful decrease in salivary production takes place (Fox, 1997; Ship, Pillemer, & Baum, 2002; Nagler, 2004). The probable explanation rests in the fact that both the parotid and submandibular glands have an idling non-functioning secretory reserve. The reserve is activated when the secreting parenchyma present in young individuals atrophies with age (Baum et al., 1992; Drummond et al., 1995; Baum, 1989). Aging does bring about modest decreases in submandibular/sublingual salivary volumes

(Atkinson & Wu, 1994; Fox, 1997; Nagler, 2004), but the magnitude is unlikely to cause symptomatology (Longman et al., 1995). Unfortunately when the glandular reserve is reduced in the elderly, their glands become more susceptible to the effects of medications, radiation and systemic disease, particularly autoimmune disease.

Hypersalivation is an infrequent finding in older patients. The antipsychotics (clozapine, lithium) and some antihypertensives (reserpine) are known causes of increased salivation (Sreebny & Schwartz, 1997). The cholinergic agents used in the treatment of Alzheimer's disease, myasthenia gravis and asthma also increase salivation. Patients who are exposed to mercury toxins or the cholinesterase inhibitors found in insecticides will produce high salivary volumes. The manic phase of bipolar affective disorder can also cause episodic salivary hyperfunction. Amelioration of symptoms may be attained with medications such as atropine and antihistamines and botulinum toxin injections. The sporadic excessive salivation caused by gastroesophageal reflux is best managed by treating the underlying cause.

More commonly, patients seen in the SGC are concerned about a dry mouth. The management of decreased salivation and its effects involve treating the specific etiologic cause plus the utilization of a variety of adjunctive therapeutic modalities. Cholinergic drugs, pilocarpine or cevimeline, may be prescribed. Increasing fluid intake and frequent rinsing are helpful. Sugarless gum or candy will stimulate salivary production. Artificial salivas are commercially available. Fluorides and remineralizing solutions are advocated to protect the teeth from caries.

In non-institutionalized 65 years and older patients, the high reported incidence of oral dryness varies from 16% to 30% while it is in the 44%–61% range for institutionalized patients (Atkinson & Wu, 1994; Vissink et al., 1996; Ship et al., 2002). The problem relates most often to the multitude of medications prescribed for the systemic illnesses associated with aging. Other sources of a dry mouth complaint include the systemic illness itself and radiation that may have been given for the treatment of head and neck cancers. Dehydration, an underdiagnosed condition in the aging population, will lead to decreased salivary volumes and can provoke an acute parotitis. In addition, patients with Alzheimer's disease are known to have submandibular salivary gland hypofunction. Often the complaint of dryness is not objectively present (Ship & Fischer, 1997) and represents somatoform disease, a perceptual condition associated with a psychiatric abnormality (Table 15.1).

Medications

With aging, the elderly inevitably require an increasing number of medications as a means of controlling illness. Among those that are 65 years of age or older, 75% are reported to be taking at least one medication (Ship et al., 2002). Many of these drugs, over 400 of them, decrease salivation usually through an anticholinergic activity. The psychotherapeutic agents, sedatives, many cardiovascular drugs, the antihistamines, diuretics and belladonnas are some of the medicinals that cause glandular hypofunction (Sreebny & Schwartz, (1997)).

Table 15.1 Outline of salivary and/or salivary gland abnormalities seen in the elderly patient

---

  I. Pathologic conditions with significant incidence in the elderly

     A Oral dryness

        1. Medications
        2. Sjogren's syndrome
        3. Radiation
        4. Dehydration
        5. Alzheimer's
        6. Oral sensorial complaint

     B Gastroesophageal reflux
     C Neuromuscular disease

        1. Parkinson's
        2. Amyotrophic lateral sclerosis

     D Loss of muscle tone

        1. Submandibular salivary gland prominence
        2. Drooling
        3. Mouth breathing

  II. Pathologic conditions with a wide age range that include the elderly

     E Manifestations of local disease

        1. Sialolithiasis
        2. Chronic parotitis

     F Manifestations of systemic disease

        1. Sialosis
        2. Sarcoidosis
        3. HIV

  III. Neoplasms

These drugs make their presence known by decreasing the volume, of resting saliva. Nevertheless, stimulation overcomes the medication's effect on resting parotid and submandibular salivary production, and when quantified normal returns are obtained (Vissink et al., 1996; Kagami, Hayashi, Shigetomi, & Ueda, 1995). Therein lies the ability to differentiate a drug-related decrease in saliva from one that is caused by a systemic illness such as Sjogren's syndrome (SS). The SS patients' complaint of both dryness at rest and when stimulated will be verified by objective volume measurements. This axiom has proven to be a most useful tool employed by the SGC for the differentiation of a salivary gland disease from a medication-related condition.

Saliva is a very significant factor in maintaining dental integrity and avoiding root caries to which the elderly are prone. The aged take many anticholinergic medications which cause a hypofunction of resting saliva. Kitamura, Kiyak, & Mulligan (1986) have reported that these medications are the cause of increased coronal and root caries in the elderly. Conversely, most reports indicate that caries incidence in the aged is in direct proportion to oral hygiene, sugar intake and periodontal breakdown, while the use of medications are poor predictors of increases in caries (Persson, Izutsu, & True-love, 1991; MacEntee, Clark, & Glick, 1993; Younger, Harrison, & Streckfus, 1998). A study by Saunders and Handelsman (1992) demonstrated no statistical increase in either coronal or root caries in patients 65 years or older, who are in a long-term care facility and are taking medications that induce hyposalivation when compared to a non-medicated control group.

Sjogren's Syndrome

Sjogren's syndrome (SS) is a debilitating systemic autoimmune exocrinopathy, with the elderly representing 20% of the patient cohort (Al-Hashimi, 2005). It is characterized by the presence of decreased salivation and lacrimation, and in this form it is referred to as the sicca complex, or primary SS. Primary SS predominates in the older age groups (Cassel, Leipzig, Cohen, Larson, & Meier, 2003). Systemic autoimmune diseases, usually rheumatoid arthritis, lupus erythematosus or scleroderma, are associated with the salivary and lacrimal hypofunction. This triad of symptoms represents secondary SS and its occurrence in the elderly is in direct relation to the age range of the accompanying systemic autoimmune disease. After rheumatoid arthritis, SS represents the second most common autoimmune disease, affecting approximately 1%–4% of the adult population (Ship et al., 2002) with more than 90% of the patients being post-menopausal women (Baum, 1992; Ship et al., 2002; Cassel et al., 2003).

The pathogenesis of SS involves a lymphocytic infiltration, predominantly CD4 cells, into exocrine glands and epithelia, while B cells represent approximately 20% of the total infiltrating cell population. With this lymphocytic invasion, acinar cell death ensues and results in diminished glandular secretions. The lymphoproliferation within the gland may become extensive and tumor-like in its appearance, but this pseudolymphoma stage does not meet the criteria for a true neoplasm. Regardless, it is well known that SS patients are susceptible to the development of a lymphomatous neoplasm (Vitali et al., 2002).

Patients are most frequently seen in the SGC with complaints of xerostomia and xerophthalmia, but because SS is a systemic disease, multiple organs and tissues can be involved. Approximately one-third of the patients present themselves with systemic extraglandular manifestations (Vitali et al., 2002). Dryness of the respiratory and gastrointestinal tracts can cause coughing and dysphagia, respectively. Vaginal dryness may develop and pulmonary, renal and neurologic involvement can be anticipated. Vasculitis is present in 20% of patients with primary SS (Vitali et al., 2002).

Diagnosis of SS is now based on the criteria established by the American–European Consensus Group (Vitali et al., 2002). The group has listed six criteria that must be used in reaching a diagnostic decision as to the presence of SS. In summary:

I. Ocular symptoms derived from the patient's positive response to complaints regarding the presence of eye dryness.
II. Oral symptoms associated with decreased salivation or a history of swollen salivary glands.
III. Ocular signs testifying to the objective presence of decreased lacrimation. A positive Schirmer test must demonstrate a decreased lacrimal wetting of a litmus strip, 5 mm or less, within a 5 minute period.
IV. Histopathologic evidence of a diagnostic focal lymphocytic infiltration into a minor salivary gland. A lymphocytic focus is defined as a dense aggregate of 50 or more lymphocytes in a $4\,mm^2$ section of glandular tissue. A focus score of 1 or more is required to establish the presence of SS.
V. Salivary gland involvement is determined by the objective measurement of decreased salivary flow. Positive evidence of decreased unstimulated whole saliva is acknowledged if 1.5 ml or less is collected in 15 minutes.
Additionally parotid sialography usually reveals sialectasis, a duct appearance that manifests itself as a punctuate, cavitary or destructive pattern.
VI. Autoantibodies will be found in the serum, specifically to the antigen SS-A and/or SS-B.

Classifying a patient as having primary SS is confirmed by the presence of any four of the six listed items, as long as either the histopathology (item IV) or the serology (item VI) is included. The existence of primary SS may also be defined by the presence of any three of the four objective criteria (items III, IV, V, VI). Secondary SS is indicated by the presence of item I or II plus any two among items III, IV or V.

In a clinical setting several diagnostic modalities can be used to establish the presence of SS. Questioning is helpful in determining the existence of hypofunction. Is there difficulty in swallowing dry foods, is there frequent drinking, does the mouth burn or is there decreased taste acuity? Visual examination of the oral cavity often reveals the presence of a dry mucosa, a high caries incidence with involvement of the cervical areas of the teeth and a cobblestone-like appearance of the tongue.

Both unstimulated whole saliva and stimulated parotid saliva can be quantitated and will be decreased in SS. Parotid sialography, the use of a radio-opaque dye to visualize the gland's ductal tree, is performed to determine the existence of sialectasis, a pattern representing multiple intralobular duct dilatations. Histopathologic evidence of SS, often considered the gold standard for diagnosis, is obtained by a biopsy of labial salivary glands.

Patients should be referred to the ophthalmologist for objective studies regarding signs of xerophthalmia and for any necessary treatment for a developing conjunctivitis. Referral to the internist/rheumatologist is also indicated for serologic study and for an evaluation regarding any related systemic manifestations. It is also the physician's responsibility to monitor the patient. Progression of SS is hallmarked by systemic involvement, particularly vasculitis, and the reported 44-fold increase in the occurrence of lymphoma (Ship et al., 2002).

Because there is no cure, SS can only be treated symptomatically. Hydroxychloroquine is prescribed because of its proven efficacious effect in other autoimmune diseases. Corticosteroids or other immunosuppressive agents are indicated in the presence of serious extraglandular manifestations. The cholinergic agonists pilocarpine and cevimeline have been of some value in increasing salivation. The use of sugarless chewing gum or sour candy is also helpful as a sialogogue. Artificial salivas and oral lubricants are available. Aggressive fluoride therapy, to abort the increased incidence of dental caries, should be instituted.

Radiation and Chemotherapy

Approximately 40,000 head and neck cancers develop each year in the United States with a high percentage occurring in the elderly. Surgery with or without radiation and/or chemotherapy is the treatment of choice. Cancericidal radiation doses involve treatments with 60 Gy or more. Such intensive dosages lead to a radiation sialadenitis and permanent salivary hypofunction if the beam inadvertently targets the salivary glands. Collateral salivary gland damage from the therapeutic use of dosages even as low as 25 Gy will cause an almost immediate decrease of 60%–90% in salivary volume. Some recovery can be expected with time if less than 25 Gy has been used (Ship et al., 2002).

The serous cells of the parotid gland are very susceptible to radiotherapy (RT) while the mucus cells of the submandibular salivary gland are less affected by the destructive effects of the RT. Clinical evidence for the relative resistance of the mucous cell to RT can be derived from the fact that the diminished saliva in patients who have received RT is very viscous. This reflects the relative proportional increase in viscous mucus over the decreased aqueous serous production of a RT-damaged parotid gland. However, with the higher RT cancericidal doses, total loss of all salivary gland secretions can be expected.

It is believed that even low doses of radiation have an effect on the secretory granules present in the serous cells (Nagler, Marmary, Golan, & Chevion, 1998). The RT interacts with the metallic ions present in the granules. Free oxygen radicals are produced and are thought to be the cause of the cell's destruction and the resultant decreased salivation (Bohuslavizki et al., 1998). Amifostine has been advocated as a radioprotector of salivary glands because it serves as a scavenger of these free radicals (Bohuslavizki et al., 1998).

Rampant radiation caries is an inevitable sequela of RT-induced hyposalivation. Effective prevention and control can be attained with aggressive fluoride therapy. Fluoride toothpastes, flouride mouthwashes, fluoride gels in individualized trays and topical flouride applications will inhibit the progression to radiation caries.

No effective treatment for radiation salivary hypofunction has been developed. Patients respond minimally to sialogogues (pilocarpine, cevimeline, sugarless gum/candy) with a very modest increase in resting saliva, probably from some residual submandibular gland cellular activity, but with little change in stimulated salivary flow (Kutta et al., 2005). Lubricants, artificial salivas and frequent use of mouthwashes are helpful symptomatic approaches to the problem.

The clinician should also be aware that elderly patients with thyroid cancer are treated with orally ingested radioactive iodine (^{131}I). As part of normal metabolism, the ^{131}I is picked up by any residual thyroid cells that have been left behind following surgical ablation of the thyroid gland and its malignancy. The beta radiation produced by the ^{131}I destroys normal and malignant thyroid tissues. Simultaneously a significant portion of the ^{131}I is secreted through the salivary glands. The result is radiation damage to both the parotid and the submandibular glands. Because the submandibular gland is more resistant to radiation, the radiation sialadenitis that develops will more frequently and extensively involve the parotid gland. However, any combination of symmetric or asymmetric unilateral or bilateral involvement of the parotid gland and/or the submandibular gland may be observed (Mandel & Mandel, 2003). Initially, ductal inflammation with obstructive symptoms manifests itself as glandular swellings associated with eating. The acinar damage will result in decreased salivary production, but its magnitude is in direct proportion to the ^{131}I dosage and the passage of time (Mandel & Mandel, 2003).

No distinct change in salivary flow rate has been confirmed following chemotherapy. The use of cytotoxic agents for cancer therapy may cause an early decrease in salivary production, but a quick return to normal volumes is expected within 14 days. Some long-term effect on salivary composition has been reported (Baum, Bodner, Fox, Izutsu, Pizzo, & Wright, 1985; Ship et al., 2002; Nagler, 2004; Meurman et al., 1997). Oral mucositis is an inevitable cytotoxic effect of certain chemotherapeutic agents on mucous membranes because of the rapid mitotic rate of mucosal epithelium.

Dehydration and Acute Parotitis

Dehydration is a common and underdiagnosed condition in the elderly. The hospital rate of dehydration per 10,000 discharges has been reported as 12.1 for the 55 to 64-year age category, but this rate increases to 287 per 10,000 for those in the 65 to 75-year age range (Ship & Fischer, 1997, Ship et al., 2002). In the ambulatory patient, dehydration is usually caused by a decreased fluid intake or excessive sweating. Hospitalized patients have an increased incidence for several reasons. Sweating from a febrile condition, loss of blood from surgery, vomiting, diarrhea, prescribed medications and inadequate intravenous fluid replacement are all contributing factors. Frequently the problem arises when the patient is forbidden oral nourishment following a gastrointestinal surgical procedure.

Salivary hypofunction becomes an inevitable consequence of dehydration. Decreased unstimulated and stimulated parotid salivary flow rates have been reported and cause lip dryness and complaints of thirst (Ship et al., 1997).

Additionally, the hypofunction leads to a loss of the protective aspects of saliva and encourages oral infections. Furthermore oral pain and problems with mastication, swallowing and digestion are encountered as saliva's abilities to lubricate, soften and digest food are compromised.

Acute parotitis (AP) represents a more severe outcome of dehydration. The associated decreased salivary production with its failure to flush the duct system can lead to an ascending duct infection and an acute parotid abscess. Many factors play a role in the development of the AP. Elderly patients use a variety of medications, many of which decrease salivary production. These patients, particularly the demented, often are not eating properly and lose the detergent action of foods and additionally they fail to maintain good oral hygiene. Oral bacterial levels increase precipitously and, when combined with a failure of adequate duct lavage, the groundwork is laid for an acute ascending duct infection. The SGC has examined several patients with Alzheimer's disease who have become dehydrated, disoriented and had poor oral hygiene. The combination of these conditions facilitated the development of AP. The process is encouraged by the fact that many in the elderly group have systemic diseases that make them more susceptible to the onset of an acute infection.

The diagnosis of a true AP is based largely upon the clinical recognition of the pre-existing conditions for its development. The AP is identified by the sudden onset of a painful parotid swelling. The overlying skin is erythematous and a fever is usually present. An intraoral examination will reveal pus exiting from the parotid duct orifice. Eating greatly accentuates pain as retained stimulated saliva adds to the already existing inflammatory pressure within the gland. Parotid swelling associated with the abscess is inhibited to some degree by the presence of the gland's dense fibrous capsule. The increased intracapsular pressure, exerting its force upon the sensory nerves within the gland, is the source of severe patient discomfort.

Therapeutic surgical intervention is usually not necessary because the duct system acts as a natural drainage mechanism. The key to successful therapy is rehydration and supportive therapy. Increased fluid intake will bring about increased salivary production and duct lavage. Supportive therapy includes oral nourishment, oral hygiene, bed rest and antibiotic therapy as indicated. Rapid amelioration of symptoms and regression of parotid swelling can be expected.

Alzheimer's Disease

Dementia is considered an important, usually progressive neurologic disorder of old age and is the fifth leading cause of death in the United States (Ship, DeCarli, Friedland, & Baum, 1990). It is characterized by a loss of cognitive abilities that impedes the performance of normal daily activities with loss of memory being the most prevalent sign. Alzheimer's disease (AD) is the most common variety of dementia. AD, or progressive dementia is an advancing degenerative disease occurring in an estimated 5%–20% of the 65 years or older population (Ship et al., 1990). Approximately 4.5 million people in the United States have AD.

The first features of AD are characterized not only by memory loss but by a gradual deterioration in personality and intellectual ability. Anxiety, problems with sleeping, depression and an aggressive or even an apathetic behavior are often present. Abstract reasoning, ability to learn, judgment and language skills are impaired (Somerman, 1987). Patients cannot care for themselves and eventually lose motor function with accompanying weakness and wasting from lack of food. Death usually results from a fatal pneumonia, probably caused by aspiration of food and oral microorganisms, facilitated by a developing salivary hypofunction and difficulty with swallowing (Friedlander, Norman, Mahler, Norman, & Yagiela, 2006).

The etiology of AD is unknown, but a familial relationship has been shown to exist in about 5% of the patients (Friedlander et al., 2006). Deposits of extracellular B-amyloid plaques and intracellular neurofibrillary tangles have been noted in the brain. These deposits probably disturb synaptic function and cause neuronal death where acetylcholine is the neurotransmitter. A variety of neurochemical abnormalities develop. Most consistently, deficiency in the cholinergic system results and is distinguished by decreased activity of choline acetyl-transferase, an enzyme needed for the synthesis of acetylcholine (Deville de Periere, Sanchez, Bertrand, & Gonzalez, 1987).

It can be anticipated that with the decrease in cholinergic activity, salivary hypofunction will result. However, when unstimulated and stimulated salivary volumes are measured, only the submandibular salivary gland demonstrated a decreased secretion. The parotid gland showed no changes in salivary volume (Ship et al., 1990). The cause for this selective effect on the submandibular gland is unknown.

Patients with AD receive numerous psychotherapeutic and mood-stabilizing medications to control symptoms of dementia. Most of the drugs are anticholinergic in their activity and will decrease the production of resting saliva. In addition, levodopa, a common neurotherapeutic agent for AD, has been reported to decrease salivary volume (Somerman, 1987). Treatment may also include cholinesterase inhibitors whose aims are to boost cholinergic transmission at the remaining functional synapses and bring about improved cognitive performance and ameliorate behavioral symptoms. Simultaneously the increased cholinergic activity causes an increased salivary volume. Consequently salivary production in patients with AD is varied and is the result of the interplay of two diametrically opposite therapeutic approaches. The psychotherapeutics and levodopa decrease the salivary production that is supplemented by the pre-existing hypofunction of the submandibular gland, while the cholinesterase inhibitors tend to increase salivary volume.

Oral Sensorial Complaints

Oral sensorial complaints (OSC) have been defined as a triad of symptoms that include dry mouth, burning mouth and a disturbed sense of taste (Nagler, 2004; Nagler & Hershkovich, 2005). The triad is often seen in the elderly who may also complain of a variety of bizarre salivary symptoms. Those concerns center around constant swallowing or expectoration, drooling, spraying during speech, thick viscous saliva, slimey saliva, granular saliva, saliva that forms a distressing film on the teeth and saliva that has become aerated and is foam-like and milky in appearance. Objective clinical investigation demonstrates no evidence of any salivary abnormality. These subjective complaints represent a common initiating request made for care by the elderly with xerostomia being the most frequent. It has been reported that as many as one-third of the elderly who complain of xerostomia have no discernible salivary hypofunction (Nagler, 2004).

The OSC patients represent a group whose triad of symptoms appear to be somatoform in origin, wherein the patients' psychological problems, frequently the depression seen in the aged, are manifested by a physical complaint. Prior to presentation in the SGC, they have visited numerous specialty offices and no satisfactory resolution has been achieved.

Common denominators in the somatoform patients include a history of emotional disturbances (depression/anxiety) and the use of psychotherapeutic medications. Frequently the patient traces the start of the problem to an oral event. The oral incident, whether it is a dental procedure, food irritation or even a medication-related dryness, only serves to focus the patient's attention on the mouth. Triggering factors also can include stressful work and family or social situations. Patients may bring an extremely detailed chronologic dossier of their symptoms, medical visits and medications. Questioning usually reveals that the salivary problem intensifies as the day progresses and there is difficulty sleeping. Concurrently clenching/bruxing, atypical facial pain patterns and temporomandibular problems may be present.

Volume measurements in patients with disturbed perceptions of oral dryness or even sialorrhea will be normal except for a decrease in resting salivary volume in those patients who are taking anticholinergic psychotherapeutics. However, when these patients are stimulated, normal salivary volumes are obtained because the stimulus overrides the anticholinergic effect the medication has on the resting salivary glands.

Accurate early categorization negates invasive complex and costly procedures. A sympathetic explanation and patient understanding can relieve symptoms. Psychiatric consultation may be recommended, but many patients resist all such suggestions and continue to have subjective salivary complaints. An underlying medical reason may exist for the sensorial complaints, but presently medical science has not defined the etiology.

Gastroesophageal Reflux Disease (GERD)

Gastroesophageal reflux disease (GERD) is a common condition affecting at least 30% of the elderly with an increased prevalence occurring with age (Cassel et al., 2003). Reflux of gastric contents into the esophagus, because of an incompetent lower esophageal sphincter, causes heartburn. The pyrosis is most pronounced after meals, particular after ingesting spicy foods. Gravity favors its occurrence with the problem becoming accentuated when the patient is prone while sleeping. Classically heartburn is recognized by a midline retrosternal burning sensation that may extend from the xiphoid process to the throat.

Repeated incursions of gastric acids into the esophagus over prolonged periods inevitably lead to esophageal erosions and ulcerations and dysphagia. Acid-mediated esophageal injury may cause the squamous epithelial lining of the lower esophagus to undergo a metaplastic change to a columnar lining. The metaplasia is considered a premalignant condition and is known as Barrett's esophagus. Oral corrosive damage to dental structures from regurgitated gastric acids reaching the oral cavity may also develop.

Clearance of most of the gastric acid from the esophagus is accomplished by physiologic peristalsis initiated by swallowing and/or local esophageal stimulation. However, peristalsis alone is not sufficient to clear the residual gastric acid affecting the lower esophageal wall, and further acid clearance is necessary (Helm, 1989). Final and effective clearance of the acid results from an esophagosalivary reflex (ESR) mechanism mediated through a vagal afferent innervation. Stimulation of the ESR causes a salivary hypersecretion known as "water brash". The ESR is intimately involved in the inhibition of the development of GERD symptomatology. With increased salivary production and the inevitable swallow, saliva with its buffering capacity neutralizes the residual gastric acids and simultaneously lavages and protects the esophageal wall from the irritative effect of the gastric acids (Helm, Dodds, & Hogan, 1987; Kahrilas, 1990).

Elderly patients frequently are seen in the SGC with a history of GERD and complaints of excessive salivation. When questioned, they characteristically relate the hypersecretion to episodes of heartburn. Often they state that their pillow is wet upon awakening in the morning. Their horizontal position during sleep favors regurgitation and a resulting salivary hypersecretion. Inevitably, the increased saliva tends to drool out of the corner of the mouth on the side that the head is turned during sleep. The chronic escape of saliva mixed with the regurgitated gastric acids displaced into the mouth results in excoriated and macerated soft tissue at the angle area of the mouth (Mandel & Tamari, 1995) and serves as a telltale marker of uncontrolled GERD.

There are many treatment options for the management of GERD. A variety of medications are available to inhibit gastric secretions. In addition, preparations are prescribed to neutralize the gastric acids or to form a protective coating on the esophageal wall. Elevating the head during sleep, avoiding large meals and not consuming substances such as alcohol, caffeine and spices will lessen GERD symptomatology. Clinical control of GERD will eliminate the drool that represents salivary hypersecretion and regurgitated contents. The oral clinical consequences, angular cheilitis and dental corrosion, are prevented.

Neuromuscular Disease

Management of accumulated saliva requires an intact functioning neuromuscular swallowing system. The inability to swallow causes saliva to flood the mouth floor. Because management of the volume of saliva can be difficult in neuromuscular disease, drooling of the saliva occurs. Parkinson's disease (PD) and amyotrophic lateral sclerosis (ALS) are examples of such conditions.

Parkinson's Disease

Although Parkinson's disease (PD) can occur in individuals in their thirties, the peak age of onset is generally in the seventh decade of life. This chronic slowly progressing degenerative neurologic disease is characterized by tremors, muscle rigidity, loss of postural reflexes and slowing of voluntary movement. A shuffling slow gait and a tendency to fall develop. Difficulty in initiating movement and a blank or staring facial appearance are features of PD. The salivary production in patients with PD is considered to be normal (Prouix, de Courval, Wiseman, & Panisset, 2005). Any dryness that may develop is a side effect of prescribed medications.

The neuromuscular dysfunction associated with PD causes a reduced rate and increased difficulty with swallowing. Salivary pooling in the mouth floor develops as a result of this dysphagia, which is not a result of salivary hyperfunction. Because there is an increased accumulation of saliva volume and because PD patients usually have their head in a bent forward position, saliva tends to drool out. This visible drooling of saliva has been interpreted in the past as excessive salivary production.

The therapeutic approach to PD includes the use of levodopa as well as several other medications that have a side effect of reducing salivary production (Prouix et al., 2005). Therapeutically, the anticholinergic agents can reduce the normal but unmanageable salivary volume. Recently Botox injections into the salivary glands to reduce salivary production have met with success (Lagalla, Millevolte, Capecci, Provinciali & Ceravolo, 2000).

Amyotrophic Lateral Sclerosis

Amyotrophic lateral sclerosis (ALS) has a peak incidence in the sixth or seventh decades of life with a slightly greater incidence among males. The clinical features of ALS, a progressive neuromuscular disease with a median survival of 3–5 years, result from a degeneration of both upper and lower motor neurons. The motor neuron loss is characterized by progressive voluntary muscle weakness with disorders of speech and swallowing becoming apparent. Inevitably respiratory failure, from costal muscle and diaphragm degeneration, leads to death.

Salivary dysphagia is a severe problem in the bulbar form of ALS with patients most concerned about drooling from what they believe is excessive salivation.

Again, the problem is not salivary hyperfunction but rather an inability to manage saliva. Poor oral transport and disturbances in the swallowing mechanism result from muscle dysfunction. Consequently saliva accumulates in the anterior mouth floor and with a developing labial muscle incompetence, the lips cannot seal adequately and saliva tends to drool out.

Occasionally ALS patients complain of thick saliva. Dehydration and a tendency to mouth breathe are the culpable factors. The aqueous serous element of saliva is most affected, thus raising the relative salivary concentration of the mucus content, resulting in increased viscosity. Dehydration can occur when patients avoid fluids because of their swallowing difficulties.

A variety of approaches has been advocated to manage the salivary problem. Papase, a proteolytic enzyme in tablet form, can be used to liquefy viscous saliva. Some success in the management of drooling can be attained with the use of anticholinergic medications. A more successful approach utilizes Botox injections into the major salivary glands (Giess et al., 2000).

Loss of Muscle Tone

Submandibular Prominence

What is first thought to be bilateral submandibular salivary gland enlargement is not an unusual finding in the aged population. In the 50 to 79-year age category, such prominences were noted extraorally in 22% of the patients (Scott, 1960). The incidence increases to 36% (Kelemen & Montgomery, 1958) when patients up to the age of 90 years are included.

When palpated extraorally, these glands are painless, normal in consistency and do not fluctuate in size over time. No intraoral signs of swelling are evident. Although initially interpreted as pathologic, in truth they represent an anatomic variation in the aged. With aging there is a loss of muscle tone, connective tissue support and skin elasticity. The result is that the submandibular gland takes a dependent position and appears to protrude bilaterally in the cervical region of both thin and obese elderly patients. Furthermore, the visibility of the glands becomes accentuated in the elderly as subcutaneous fat is lost and atrophy of the skin develops.

Angular Drooling

The SGC has examined many elderly patients whose chief complaint concerned drooling from the angles of the mouth. Salivary evaluations indicated the presence of normal flow rates and the absence of swallowing defects. These patients were not using any medications that could cause excessive salivation nor did they have any systemic disease that might lead to increased flow rates.

During the examinations, it became apparent that these patients had a lax perioral musculature which prevented a satisfactory oral seal. As normal volumes of saliva accumulate in the anterior mouth, leakage of saliva occurs extraorally on to the surface tissues because of loss of muscle tone with the angle of the lips representing the most susceptible location for the problem. The condition is exacerbated by gravity as the head tilts forward and inferiorly with age.

Mouth Breathing

Laxity of the peri-oral musculature not only causes angular drooling, but also plays a significant role in the patient's complaint of xerostomia. The loss of muscle tone that occurs with aging often leads to increased mouth breathing. The flow of air across the oral mucosa, as the patient inspires and expires, causes rapid evaporation of the aqueous serous element of saliva. Subjective dryness results from the loss of saliva's moisturizing effect.

The problem is further emphasized during sleep when gravity encourages an open mouth and snoring occurs. Snoring is commonly seen in the aged. These patients will state that the dryness is most severe upon awakening in the morning or if they awaken in the middle of the night. The dryness that develops during sleep is accentuated by the fact that only minimal amounts of saliva are produced during sleep because no oral stimuli are present. The sparse nocturnal secretions rapidly evaporate when mouth breathing is present.

Sialolithiasis

Sialoliths, or salivary stones are calcific concretions that develop within the ductal systems of major and minor salivary glands. Approximately 83% of the salivary stones form in the submandibular salivary gland, while 10% are found in the parotid system and 7% develop in the sublingual and minor salivary glands (Lustmann, Regev, & Melemed, 1990). Because they can develop in any age category, the elderly are not immune to their occurrence.

Although the exact evolution of a sialolith has not been determined, three prerequisites seem to be necessary. First, a subclinical retrograde infection from the oral cavity can develop and cause damage to the glycoprotein contained within the intraductal saliva. This results in the formation of a glycoprotein gel that then serves as a nidus (Mandel, 1980). The second prerequisite, salivary stasis, results from the blockage and is followed by a salt precipitation (the third requirement) into the glycoprotein matrix (Bodner & Fliss, 1995). With continued mineral deposition, a clinically apparent sialolith evolves and eventually manifests itself with obstructive subjective and objective symptoms.

The submandibular salivary gland is more vulnerable to the development of salivary stones than the parotid system for several reasons. Submandibular saliva includes a greater concentration of calcium and phosphate salts. It also contains a significant mucous element in its secretion, making submandibular saliva relatively viscous when compared to the aqueous serous secretion of the parotid gland. Viscosity favors stagnation and salt precipitation. Furthermore because the submandibular gland is at a lower level than its orifice, the secretions run uphill and stagnation with salt deposition is more likely to occur.

Usually, patients are seen with a history of recurrent tender salivary gland swellings that spontaneously resolve and are associated with eating. The increased salivary production during meals meets the stone blockage and the resultant retrograde salivary retention causes gland swelling and discomfort. This clinical picture often occurs intermittently over several years with the symptoms tending to become more severe with the passage of time.

During an acute attack, the patient will be seen with an extraoral gland swelling that palpation reveals to be painful and indurated. Intraorally, the floor of the mouth along the course of the submandibular duct is inflamed. Pus is often visible exiting from the duct's orifice when secondary infection is superimposed upon the blockage. If the floor of the mouth is not too swollen, careful palpation of the mouth floor will reveal the location of the hard sialolith. However, for diagnostic palpation to succeed, the stone must not be too small and must be located distal to the right angle bend that the duct makes posterior to the mylohyoid muscle as it exits the gland.

Imaging with computerized tomography (CT) confirms the diagnosis of a stone by visualizing it and identifying its exact location. The CT scan has proven to be exquisitely sensitive to the minute amounts of calcific salts present in relatively lucent stones (Mandel & Hatzis, 2000) and has become the imaging technique of choice. Radiography (particularly with occlusal films), sialography and ultrasound are other imaging modalities that can also be used for diagnosis.

Spontaneous delivery of a stone can occur but it is an uncommon occurrence. Intervention is usually necessary. A variety of approaches for the removal of a sialolith has been advocated. Intraoral surgical procedures are most commonly used when the stone is positioned near the orifice and can be reached. Frequently, extraoral surgery is required to remove both the gland and the stone. Non-surgical methods are beginning to be used. Endoscopic duct instruments are now available to remove smaller stones. Lithotripsy and laser techniques represent newer procedures that have been advocated in defined situations (Nahlieli, Nakar, Nazarian, & Turner, 2006).

Chronic Parotitis

The most common pathologic problem seen in the SGC is chronic parotitis. Usually the patients are over 50 years of age with an equal gender distribution. Chronic parotitis is a non-specific sialadenitis that has been present for many years and characterized by sporadic unilateral moderately painful parotid swellings with variable periods of remission. The swellings seem to be initiated by eating and tend to last from several hours to a week or two. The waxing and waning persist for years with each successive flare-up tending to be more intense and causing increased glandular damage. The etiology of chronic parotitis seems to be related to a decrease in salivary production and/or an impedance of its delivery (Sadeghi, Black, & Frenkiel, 1996). An ascending ductal infection from the oral cavity is thought to develop because of the resulting inadequate salivary lavage. Decreased salivation caused by many medications taken by the elderly may serve as the instigator of the infectious process.

Clinically the extraoral swelling follows the anatomic contour of the parotid gland. Palpation indicates that the swellings are painful and indurated. Fever may be present. Aggressive massage of the gland will produce a salivary flow, albeit diminished, from the duct orifice of the involved gland. The reduced return is cloudy, indicating the presence of pus. During periods of remission, normal volumes without suppurative contents will be present.

The cycle of inflammation and repair causes duct strictures and partial obstructions. Furthermore mucopus is produced leading to clogging of the duct lumen. The damming effect that ensues produces salivary retention and duct dilatation. The salivary stasis encourages further infection with more strictures and duct dilatations and the inevitable glandular swelling.

Imaging has proven to be essential to diagnosis. Sialography, the radio-opaque visualization of the duct system, demonstrates a "sausage-like" pattern. This pattern of duct delineation reflects the presence of alternating areas of duct wall dilatation and stricturing. Primarily the major duct is involved, but the secondary ducts will also show changes in direct proportion to the duration and severity of the chronic parotitis (Wang, Zou, Wu, & Sun, 1992).

The CT scan is useful in chronic parotitis because it provides positive diagnostic data concerning the gland's parenchyma. Increased density and enhancement of the parotid, representing the presence of the inflammatory infiltrate, will be noted. Furthermore because the major parotid duct is obstructed and engorged with retained saliva and inflammatory debris, it will be visualized by the CT scan as it traverses the lateral border of the masseter muscle.

Parotid stones, because of their obstructive nature, can mimic the symptomatology of chronic parotitis. In these cases, it must be emphasized that the parotitis that develops is secondary to the primary problem, the sialolith. Similarly, the Sjogren's syndrome (SS) patient will produce a decreased salivary volume and becomes susceptible to an ascending infection. Here again the parotitis that develops is secondary and results from the underlying SS and its associated salivary hypofunction.

Patients who have chronic parotitis are treated on the basis of symptomatology. The treatment can be conservative with observation being an acceptable approach because the pain and swelling are often self-limiting and transient. Sialogogues such as sugarless gum or sour candy are helpful in increasing salivary lavage. Increased fluid intake, parotid gland massage, duct probing, good oral hygiene and analgesics are helpful. Antibiotics may be utilized when indicated. Endoscopic techniques that lavage, balloon the duct and destroy strictures are relatively new and have proven to be successful (Nahlieli et al., 2006).

Frequent severe attacks may demand a more aggressive therapeutic approach. Retrograde duct injection of a sclerosing agent has met with success because it leads to duct fibrosis and atrophy of the parotid gland (Wang et al., 1998). If the symptoms are severe and do not respond to therapy, surgical removal of the superficial lobe of the parotid gland should be considered (Sadeghi et al., 1996).

Sialosis

Sialosis, or sialadenosis presents as a bilateral soft painless non-neoplastic persistent enlargement of the parotid glands with occasional involvement of the submandibular salivary glands. A variety of conditions has been associated with sialosis, particularly alcoholism and diabetes mellitus which are disorders often seen in the aged.

Chronic alcoholism usually leads to liver cirrhosis. When cirrhosis is present, as many as 80% of the patients develop sialosis. In patients with non-cirrhotic alcohol-damaged livers, only 10% develop these distinctive parotid swellings (Proctor & Shori, 1996). There are approximately 16 million patients in the United States with diabetes mellitus and, with the increasing obesity, the incidence is growing in the elderly. Unfortunately, no statistical survey have been made to establish the frequency of sialosis in diabetics.

The common denominator in these patients with sialosis is the presence of an autonomic neuropathy which manifests itself as a demyelinating polyneuropathy. The secreting acinar cells of the parotid gland have both parasympathetic and sympathetic innervation. The parasympathetic innervation is concerned with fluid and electrolyte secretion, while the sympathetic innervation is responsible for protein synthesis and protein secretion (Chilla, 1981). With a dysregulation of the autonomic nerve supply to the parenchymal cells, changes in intracellular protein synthesis occur. The neuropathy results in an excessive intracellular protein production and/or an inhibition of its secretion into the saliva. Cytoplasmic engorgement with zymogen granules, the protein precursor of salivary amylase, results in a distension of individual acinar cells (Chilla, 1981; Ascoli, Albedi, DeBlasiis, & Nardi, 1993). With expansion of the cell, parotid hypertrophy becomes clinically evident.

Initially, the CT scan in these patients will show an increased parotid density that approaches the density associated with muscle. The parotid gland normally has a high fat content which decreases the density of the gland. However, with the increase in acinar size, the fat is replaced and a denser gland is observed. On occasion the parotid gland will demonstrate a marked increase in fat content with the scan showing a lucent gland. It is not known whether such a fatty parotid represents an advanced expression or an alternate pathway of sialosis (Rabinov & Weber, 1985; Layfield, Glasgow, Goldstein, & Lufkin, 1991).

Increased salivary flow rates in patients with sialosis have been objectively confirmed by the SGC. In the presence of the gland's hypertrophy, such a determination should not be unexpected. Patients with a fatty infiltration rather than cellular hypertrophy probably have a decreased salivary volume, but no definitive studies have been reported.

Other than cosmetic changes, the parotid swellings associated with sialosis are asymptomatic. Regardless, diagnosis is imperative because differentiation from inflammatory or neoplastic disease is required to avoid unnecessary treatment. Early diagnosis is also important because the presence of sialosis points to the existence of an underlying disease which mandates appropriate referral to address the antecedent cirrhosis or diabetes. Medical therapy directed at the underlying problem results in some decrease in parotid gland size, but the long-term prognosis is variable. Unfortunately no treatment specifically aimed at the parotid enlargement has been established.

Sarcoidosis

Sarcoidosis is a multisystem non-caseating granulomatous disorder of unknown etiology. Typically bilateral hilar lymphadenopathy, pulmonary infiltrations and skin or eye lesions are present. Respiratory symptoms such as coughing or dyspnea often develop, and a linkage between sarcoidosis and lymphoma has been reported (Olewiecki, Kotecha, Kingston, & Rothera, 1992). Sarcoidosis usually affects young adults in the 30 to 40-year-old age range. However, as with most pathologic entities, the aged population is also affected.

Salivary glands are prone to the disease process but the pattern of glandular involvement varies. Usually bilateral parotid enlargement from granulomatous infiltration is seen in 4%–6% of the patients (James, Neville, & Siltzbach, 1976). The submandibular salivary glands are infrequently involved, but minor salivary glands may have granulomatous infiltrates. Because of the granulomatous infiltration into major and minor salivary glands, some decrease in salivary volume can be expected.

Diagnosis is mostly dependent on the radiologic identification of distinctive lung infiltrates and a hilar lymphadenopathy. Blood studies may show elevated calcium and alkaline phosphatase levels along with increases in angiotensin converting enzyme. Confirmation of a clinical diagnosis of sarcoidosis is based on the accumulated pathologic signs and symptoms and often substantiated by a labial gland biopsy. Because 58% of the labial gland biopsies have proven to be positive (Nessan & Jacoway, 1979), such an intervention is a reasonable part of the diagnostic approach.

Treatment of the disease is generally symptomatic because spontaneous resolution does occur. Corticosteroids and other immunosuppressives are prescribed for the more serious cases, especially in patients with ocular involvement. Blindness is a known complication, and its prevention may require aggressive pharmacologic management.

Human Immunodeficiency Virus

The human immunodeficiency virus (HIV) does not respect age. Although the SGC has seen this condition primarily in younger adults, older adults have also been seen. A multiorgan viral invasion results in a diverse symptomatology. Approximately

5%–10% of HIV patients develop parotid enlargement (Schioldt et al., 1989). The parotid swellings are usually bilateral, often cystic and are seen in association with cervical lymphadenopathy. Evidence also exists of a persistent circulating CD8 lymphocytosis with a diffuse visceral CD8 infiltration. This symptom complex has been defined as the diffuse infiltrative CD8 lymphocytosis syndrome (Itescu et al., 1990).

As the virus replicates, a florid response of intraparotid lymphocytes or an extraglandular lymphocytic infiltration into the parotid is the cause of the parotid swelling (Itescu et al., 1990; Schiodt, 1992). The lymphoproliferation probably is a reaction to the presence of a high virus concentration within the gland. Bilateral lymphoepithelial cysts have also been observed (Elliott & Oertel, 1990; Mandel & Reich, 1992). Hypothetically, both HIV-induced cytokines and the lymphoid hyperplasia may stimulate ductal epithelium to form these cysts (Uccini et al., 2000).

The parotids are often large and cosmetically disfiguring, but the submandibular salivary glands are only occasionally involved. The swellings are painless and do not fluctuate in size. Palpation indicates the swellings are either firm or soft, reflecting, respectively, massive lymphoproliferative activity or the presence of lymphoepithelial cysts.

Highly active antiretroviral therapy (HAART) has become the most effective treatment for HIV disease. The combination of antiviral medications in HAART aims to stop viral replication and produce some degree of immune restoration. With the decrease in viral load and improved immunity, HAART has succeeded in eradicating the parotid swellings (Craven et al., 1998; Mandel & Suratttanont, 2002). Maintenance therapy has proven successful in preventing recurrences of the swelling.

The long teem we of MAART has created collateral damage. A metabolic disorder, in the form of a lipodystroply syndrome (LDS), may develop. The LDS is characterized by the trend of fat redistribution, dyslipidemia and insulin resistance. Fat redistribution may manifest itself in the head and neck region as paraparotis fat depositem in the subcontineous tissues, a "buffalo" and a thick neck.

Neoplasms

Tumors of the salivary glands represent 3%–6% of all adult head and neck tumors, with an incidence in the United States of 1.5 cases per 100,000 (Ward & Levine, 1998). The mean age for malignant salivary tumors is reported to be between 55 and 65 years of age while the mean age of benign growths occur approximately 10 years earlier (Ward & Levine, 1998). Obviously both benign and malignant tumors can develop in those 65 years of age and older.

Most neoplasms (70%–85%) occur in the parotid gland while 8%–15% develop in the submandibular salivary gland and less than 1% occur in the sublingual gland (Spiro, 1986). The minor salivary glands are responsible for 5%–8% of the total salivary neoplasms (Spiro, 1986). Generally the smaller the salivary gland, the more likely it is to harbor a malignant growth. Only 15%–25% of the parotid tumors are malignant while 37%–43% of the tumors in the submandibular system are malignant (Spiro, 1986). The malignant incidence in the sublingual gland and the minor salivary glands increases to 80% (Spiro, 1986).

Accurate diagnosis of a neoplasm of a salivary gland is dependent upon a detailed history and clinical examination. This will differentiate these lesions from infectious, autoimmune and other salivary enlargements. Benign salivary neoplasms tend to be slow growing, localized and painless masses located within the salivary gland. A swelling is usually visible and is the impetus for the patient's desire to seek care. Palpation will reveal the mass to be circumscribed, movable and painless. Its feel can vary from soft to firm. No facial motor deficits will be present nor will there be any associated cervical lymphadenopathy. The salivary return from the involved gland is usually adequate and clear and serves to differentiate the swelling from an infection which produces a cloudy, pus-containing saliva.

Malignant salivary neoplasms usually present a much different history and clinical picture. The lesions tend to grow rapidly and can be painful. Palpation does not reveal theses masses to be circumscribed. Their outline is difficult to identify, they are firm, and as they infiltrate surrounding tissues they become fixed in position. Because the gland has an intimate relation to the facial nerve, invasion into the branches of the facial nerve can be anticipated. Inevitably facial motor loss will develop and can readily be observed when the activity of the facial musculature is examined. When a sensory nerve is involved, facial numbness can develop. Because of its ability to metastasize, cervical lymphadenopathy is a diagnostic sign.

Imaging studies (CT scan, MRI, PET, ultrasound) are key components in the diagnostic study. The imaged margins of the mass, the composition of the lesion and its location in the gland are very helpful in differentiating a benign lesion from a malignant one and is most useful in determining the surgical approach. Cervical lymph node metastases can be recognized, reflecting the spread of a malignancy and the need for a nodal dissection.

An exact pre-operative diagnosis is attained by examining tissue obtained from an incisional biopsy. A fine-needle aspiration biopsy can be used for cytology. The study can indicate whether the lesion is benign or malignant and may even identify the precise histologic variety. This aspiration biopsy procedure has proven to be most useful in pre-operative planning.

It is believed that salivary gland tumors arise from stem cells located in either the secretory duct or the intercalated duct (Johns & Harri, 2005). This theory would explain the many cell types seen in individual salivary neoplasms. The secretory duct stem cells are responsible for the development of the mucoepidermoid and squamous cell carcinomas while the pleomorphic adenoma, adenocarcinoma and adenoid cystic carcinoma arise from intercalated duct stem cells.

Histologically, the pleomorphic adenoma is the most common benign tumor that occurs in the salivary glands. This tumor can be lobulated and has a capsule which is usually thin and incomplete. In addition, the tumor may have small projections that perforate and extend beyond the capsule into the surrounding normal glandular parenchyma. The papillary cystadenoma lymphomatosum or Warthin's tumor is the second most common benign salivary tumor. It is unique in that it can occur bilaterally, occurs most frequently in men and smoking seems to increase its frequency. A third benign epithelial tumor occurring in the salivary glands is the oncocytoma that is characteristically found in older patients (Chahin, Kaufman, Abbarah, & Chahin, 2005).

The mucoepidermoid carcinoma is the most common malignant lesion of the parotid gland while the adenoid cystic carcinoma is the most common salivary malignancy involving the submandibular gland (Chahin et al., 2005). The low-grade mucoepidermoid carcinoma has a large mucoid cell element and is relatively non-aggressive. The high-grade variety of the mucoepidermoid carcinoma contains masses of malignant epidermoid cells and is quite aggressive. The adenoid cystic carcinoma is recognized by its basaloid epithelial elements that form cylindrical structures. This tumor is indolent and relentless in its growth pattern as it characteristically extends along the perineural lymphatics. The acinic cell carcinoma, the adenocarcinoma and the carcinoma ex-pleomorphic adenoma represent the majority of other salivary gland malignancies (Chahin et al., 2005).

Surgery is the treatment of choice for all salivary gland tumors. Superficial lobe parotidectomy represents the best approach for benign parotid tumors. The submandibular gland with a benign tumor lends itself to total gland removal. This gland has a well-defined capsule, which delineates the gland from its surroundings and facilitates the surgery.

Malignant lesions demand extensive surgery whose success is defined by adequate margins of normal tissue around the malignancy. Cervical lymph node dissection is performed as a therapeutic measure. Distant metastases predict a poor patient prognosis. Radiation and chemotherapy are employed when necessary.

Salivary gland surgery is always fraught with complications. Parotid surgery can lead to damage to the facial nerve as it courses through the gland and causes paralysis of some facial muscles. Often the loss of motor function is temporary but it can be permanent. In addition parotid surgery may result in the development of Frey's syndrome. The syndrome causes gustatory sweating when the auriculotemporal nerve and its parasympathetic secretory fibers are surgically damaged. Healing with regrowth of fibers will occur, but the fibers may be misdirected and end up supplying facial sweat glands. Stimulation of these secretory nerves during eating will then cause facial sweating. Botulinum toxin has proven to be successful in the management of this abnormal sweating. When the submandibular salivary gland is surgically removed, care must be taken to avoid injury to the lingual or hypoglossal nerves and the mandibular branch of the facial nerve.

With the aging of the population, an increased frequency of visits by the elderly to the dental practitioner's office can be expected. These patients will often bring a variety of complaints associated with salivary secretory dysfunction and/or salivary gland disease. Some problems may be unique to the aged while other conditions reflect pathologic entities that affect all age ranges. It is necessary for the profession to be cognizant of the manifestations of the diverse abnormalities which may develop in this patient group.

The purpose of this chapter is to alert the profession to the symptomatology, both subjective and objective, of these patients with salivary problems. Knowledge will result in prompt and accurate diagnoses. Needless investigative and therapeutic measures will be avoided.

References

Al-Hashimi, I. (2005). Xerostomia secondary to Sjogren's syndrome in the elderly: Recognition and management. *Drugs & Aging, 22*, 887–99.

Ascoli, V., Albedi, F. M., DeBlasiis R., & Nardi, F. (1993). Sialadenosis of the parotid gland; report of four cases diagnosed by fine-needle aspiration cytology. *Diagnostic Cytopathology, 9*, 151–5.

Astor, F. C., Hanft, K. L., & Ciocon, J. O. (1999). Xerostomia: A prevalent condition in the elderly. *Ear Nose & Throat Journal, 78*, 476–9.

Atkinson, J. G., & Wu, A. J. (1994). Salivary gland dysfunction: Causes, symptoms, treatment. *JADA, 125*, 409–16.

Baum, B. J., Bodner, L., Fox, P. C., Izutsu, K. T., Pizzo, P. A., & Wright (1985). Therapy induced dysfunction of salivary glands: Implications for oral health. *Special Care in Dentistry, 5*, 274–277.

Baum, B. J. (1989). Salivary gland aging: fluid secretion during aging. *Journal of the American Geriatrics Society, 37*, 453–8.

Baum, B. J. (1992). Age-related vulnerability. *Otolaryngology Head and Neck Surgery, 106*, 730–2.

Baum, B. J., Ship, J. A., & Wu, A. J. (1992). Salivary gland functions and aging: A model for studying the interaction of aging and systemic disease. *Critical Reviews in Oral Biology & Medicine, 4*, 53–64.

Bodner, L. & Fliss, D. M. (1995). Parotid and submandibular calculi in children. *International Journal of Pediatric Otorhinolaryngology, 31*, 35–42.

Bohuslavizki, K.-H., Brenner, W., Klutmann, S., Hubner, R. H., Lassmann, S., Feyerabend B., et al. (1998). Radioprotection of salivary glands by amifostine in high-dose radioiodine therapy. *Journal of Nuclear Medicine, 39*, 1237–42.

Cassel, C. K., Leipzig, R. M., Cohen, H. J., Larson, E. B., & Meier, D. B. (2003). *Geriatric medicine; an evidenced based approach* (4th ed., p. 838). New York: Springer.

Chahin, F., Kaufman, M. R, Abbarah, T., & Chahin C. (2005). Salivary gland tumors, major, benign. eMedicine, [cited February 21, 2007] http://www.emedicine.com/med/topic2789.htm.

Chilla, R. (1981). Sialadenosis of the salivary glands of the head. *Advances in Otorhinolaryngology, 26*, 1–38.

Craven, D. E., Duncan, R. A., Stram, J. R., O'Hara, C. J., Steger, K. A., Jhamb K., et al. (1998). Response of lymphoepithelial parotid cysts to antiretroviral treatment of HIV-infected adults. *Annals of Internal Medicine, 128*, 455–9.

Deville de Periere, D., Sanchez, J., Bertrand, L., & Gonzalez L. (1987). Dementia of the Alzheimer's type: An oral and biochemical study. *Gerodontology, 6*, 149–55.

Drummond, J. R., & Chisholm, D. M. (1994). A qualitative and quantitative study of the ageing human labial salivary glands. *Archives of Oral Biology, 29*, 151–5.

Drummond, J. R., Newton, J. P., & Abel, R. W. (1995). Tomographic measurements of age changes in the human parotid gland. *Gerodontology, 12*, 26–30.

Elliott, J. N., & Oertel, Y. C. (1990). Lymphoepithelial cysts of the salivary glands. *American Journal of Clinical Pathology, 93*, 39–43.

Fox, P. C. (1997). Management of dry mouth. *Dental Clinics of North America, 41*, 863–75.

Friedlander, A. H., Norman, D. C., Mahler M. E., Norman, K. M., & Yagiela, J. A. (2006). Alzheimer's disease: psychopathology, medical management and dental implications. *JADA, 137*, 1240–51.

Giess, R., Naumann, M., Werner, E., Riemann, R., Beck, M., Puls, I., et al. (2000). Injections of botulinum toxin type A into the salivary glands improve sialorrhea in amyotrophic lateral sclerosis. *Journal of Neurology Neurosurgery and Psychiatry, 69*, 121–3.

Helm, J. F. (1989). Role of saliva esophageal function and disease. *Dysphagia, 4*, 76–84.

Helm, J. F., Dodds, W. J., & Hogan, W. J. (1987). Salivary response to esophageal acid in normal subjects and patients with reflux esophagitis. *Gastroenterology, 93*, 1393–7.

Itescu, S., Brancato, L. J., Buxbaum, J., Gregersen, P. K., Rizk, C. C., Croxson, S., et al. (1990). A diffuse infiltrative CD8 lymphocytosis syndrome in human immunodeficiency virus (HIV) infection: a host immune response associated with HLA-DR5. *Annals of Internal Medicine, 112*, 3–10.

James, D., Neville, D., & Siltzbach L. (1976). A worldwide review of sarcoidosis. *Annals of the New York Academy of Sciences, 278*, 321–34.

Johns M. M., & Harri, P. A. (2005). Salivary Gland neoplasms. eMedicine, [cited February 21, 2007] http:// www. emedicine.com/Ent/topic679.htm.

Kagami, H., Hayashi, T., Shigetomi, T., & Ueda, M. (1995). Assessment of the effects of aging and medication on salivary gland function in patients with xerostomia using 99m TC-scintigraphy. *Nagoya Journal of Medical Science, 58*, 149–55.

Kahrilas, P. J. (1990). Esophageal motor activity and acid clearance. *Gastroenterology Clinics of North America, 19*, 537–50.

Kelemen, G., & Montgomery, W. W., (1958). Symmetrical, asymptomatic submaxillary-gland enlargement in older age groups. *New England Journal of Medicine, 258*, 188–9.

Kitamura, M., Kiyak, H. A., & Mulligan, K. (1986). Predictors of root caries in the elderly. *Community Dentistry and Oral Epidemiology, 14*, 34–8.

Kutta, H., Kampen, U., Sagowski, C., Brenner, W., Bohuslavizki, K.-H., & Paulsen F. (2005). Amifostine is a potent radioprotector of salivary glands in radioiodine therapy. *Strahlentherapie und Onkologie, 181*, 237–45.

Lagalla, G., Millevolte, M., Capecci, M., Provinciali L., & Ceravolo, M. G., (2000). Botulinum toxin type A for drooling in Parkinson's disease: A double blind, randomized, placebo-controlled study. *Movement Disorders, 21*, 704–7.

Layfield, L. J., Glasgow, B. J., Goldstein, N., & Lufkin, R. (1991). Lipomatous lesions of the parotid gland. *Acta Cytologica, 35*, 553–6.

Longman, L. P., Higham, S. M., Rai, K., Edgar, W. M., & Field, E. A. (1995). Salivary gland hypofunction in elderly patients attending a clinic. *Gerodontology, 12*, 67–72.

Lustmann, J., Regev, E., & Melemed, Y. (1990). Sialolithiasis: A survey on 245 patients and a review of the literature. *International Journal of Oral and Maxillofacial Surgery, 193*, 135–8.

Mandel, I.D. (1980). Sialochemistry in diseases and clinical situations affecting salivary glands. *Critical Reviews in Clinical Laboratory Sciences, 12*, 321–66.

Mandel, L., & Hatzis, G. (2000). The role of computerized tomography in the diagnosis and therapy of parotid stones: A case report. *JADA, 131*, 479–82.

Mandel, L., & Reich, R. (1992). HIV parotid gland lymphoepithelial cysts. *Oral Surgery Oral Medicine Oral Pathology, 74*, 273–8.

Mandel, S. J., & Mandel, L. (2003). Review: Radioactive iodine and the salivary glands. *Thyroid, 13*, 265–71.

Mandel, L., & Suratttanont, F. (2002). Regression of HIV parotid swellings after antiviral therapy: Case reports with computed tomographic scan evidence. *Oral Surgery Oral Medicine Oral Pathology Oral Radiology and Endodontics, 94*, 454–9.

Mandel, L., & Tamari K. (1995). Sialorrhea and gastroesophageal reflux. *JADA, 126*, 1537–41.

MacEntee, M. I., Clark, D. C., & Glick, N. (1993). Predictors of caries in old age. *Gerodontology, 10*, 90–7.

Meurman, J. H., Laine, P., Keinanen, S., Pyrhonen, S., Teerenhovi, L., & Lindquist C. (1997). Five-year follow-up of saliva in patients treated for lymphomas. *Oral Surgery Oral Medicine Oral Pathology Oral Radiology and Endodontics, 83*, 447–52.

Nagler, R. M. (2004). Salivary glands and the aging process *Biogerontology, 5*, 223–33.

Nagler, R. M., & Hershkovich, O. (2005). Age-related changes in unstimulated salivary function and composition and its relations to medications and oral sensorial complaints. *Aging Clinical and Experimental Research, 17*, 358–66.

Nagler, R., Marmary, Y., Golan, E., & Chevion, M. (1998). Novel protection strategy against Xray-induced damage to salivary glands. *Radiation Research, 149*, 271–6.

Nahlieli, O., Nakar, L. H., Nazarian, Y., & Turner, M. D. (2006). Sialendoscopy: A new approach to salivary gland obstructive pathology. *JADA, 137*, 1394–1400.

Nessan, V., & Jacoway, J. (1979). Biopsy of minor salivary glands in the diagnosis of sarcoidosis. *New England Journal of Medicine, 301*, 922–4.

Olewiecki, S., Kotecha R., Kingston, T., & Rothera, M. P. (1992). Sarcoidosis-lymphoma syndrome. *Journal of the Royal Society of Medicine, 85*, 176–7.

Persson, R. E., Izutsu, K. T., & Truelove E. L. (1991). Differences in salivary flow rates in elderly subjects using xerostomic medications. *Oral Surgery Oral Medicine Oral Pathology, 72*, 42–6.

Proctor, G. B., Shori, D. K. (1996). The effects of ethanol on salivary glands, in alcohol and the gastrointestinal tract. In V. R. Preedy & R. R. Watson (Eds.), (pp. 111–22). Boca Raton: CRC Press.

Prouix, M., de Courval, F. P., Wiseman, M. A., & Panisset, M. (2005). Salivary production in Parkinson's disease. *Movement Disorders, 20*, 204–7.

Rabinov, K., & Weber, A. (1985). *Radiology of the salivary glands* (pp. 26591). Boston: Hall.

Sadeghi, N., Black M. J., & Frenkiel, S. (1996). Parotidectomy for the treatment of chronic recurrent parotitis. *Journal of Otolaryngology, 25*, 305–7.

Saunders, R. H., & Handelsman, S. L. (1992). Effects of hyposalivary medications on salivary flow rates and dental caries in adults aged 65 and older. *Special Care in Dentistry, 12*, 116–21.

Schiodt, M. (1992). HIV-associated salivary gland disease: A review. *Oral Surgery Oral Medicine Oral Pathology, 73*, 164–7.

Schioldt, M., Greenspan, D., Daniels, T. E., Nelson, J., Legott, P. J., Warra, D. W., et al. (1989). Parotid gland enlargement with xerostomia associated labial sialadenitis in HIV-infected patients. *Journal of Autoimmunity, 2*, 415–25.

Scott, J. (1960). Prominence of the submandibular glands in the aged. *Journal of the American Geriatrics Society, 8*, 53–4.

Ship, J. A., DeCarli, C., Friedland, R. P., & Baum, B. J. (1990). Diminished submandibular salivary flow in dementia of the Alzheimer type. *Journals of Gerontology, 45*, M61–6.

Ship, J. A. & Fischer, D. J. (1997). The relationship between dehydration and parotid salivary gland function in young and older healthy adults. *Journals of Gerontology Series A-Biological Sciences and Medical Sciences, 52*, M 310–9.

Ship, J. A., Pillemer, S. R., & Baum, B. J. (2002). Xerostomia and the geriatric patient. *Journal of the American Geriatrics Society, 50*, 535–43.

Somerman, M. J. (1987). Dental implications of pharmacological management of Alzheimer's patient. *Gerodontology, 6*, 59–66.

Spiro, R. H. (1986). Salivary neoplasms: Overview of a 35-year experience with 2807 patients. *Head & Neck Surgery, 8*, 177–84.

Sreebny, L. M. (1989). Recognition and treatment of salivary induced conditions. *International Dental Journal, 39*, 197–204.

Sreebny, L. M., & Schwartz, S. S. (1997). A reference guide to drugs and dry mouth. *Gerodontology, 14*, 33–47.

Uccini, S., D'Offizi, G., Angelici, A., Prozzo, A., Riva, E., Antonelli, G., et al. (2000). Cystic lymphoepithelial lesions in the parotid gland in HIV-1 infection. *AIDS Patient Care STDS, 14*, 143–7.

Vissink, A. Spijkervet, F. K., & van nieuw Amerongen, A. (1996). Aging and saliva: a review of the literature. *Special Care in Dentistry, 16*, 95–103.

Vitali, C., Bombardieri, S., Jonsson, R., Moutsopoulos, H. M., Alexander, E. L., Carsons, S. E., et al. (2002). Classification criteria for Sjogren's syndrome: A revised version of the European criteria proposed by the American–European Consensus Group. *Annals of the Rheumatic Diseases, 61*, 554–58.

Wang, S. L., Zou, Z. J., Wu, Q. G., Sun, K. H. (1992). Sialographic changes related to clinical and pathologic finding in chronic obstructive parotitis. *International Journal Oral & Maxillofacial Surgery, 21*, 364–8.

Wang, S., Li, J., Zhu, X., Zhao, A., Sun, T., & Dong, H. (1998). Gland atrophy following retrograde injection of methyl violet as a treatment in chronic obstructive parotitis. *Oral Surgery Oral Medicine Oral Pathology Oral Radiology and Endodontics, 85*, 276–81.

Ward, M. J., & Levine P. A. (1998). Salivary gland tumors in essentials of head and neck oncology. In L. G. Close, D. L. Larson, & J. P. Shah (Eds.), (1st ed.). Thieme, New York, NY.

Younger, H., Harrison, T., & Streckfus, C. (1998). Relationship among stimulated whole, glandular flow rates, and root caries prevalence in an elderly population; a preliminary study. *Special Care in Dentistry, 18*, 156–63.

Chapter 16
Mastication, Nutrition, Oral Health and Health in Older Patients

Angus W.G. Walls

Introduction

The mouth is the portal of entry for all foods to enter the digestive tract and thereby be available for digestion and absorption to sustain life. It is not surprising therefore that there are clear and profound links between the health status of the oral environment and foods, and there are also reciprocal links between the foods that we eat and health of the teeth, their supporting tissues and the oral mucosa. The objective of this chapter is to discuss the evidence for the links between foods and the oral environment and to establish how the dental team can maximise health benefits for their patients.

The changes in population demography and the epidemiology of oral disease with reference to the aging population have been described previously in this book and will not be reviewed in detail. However, it is pertinent to reflect on the combination of both changes in demography and oral health status and how this interaction is likely to influence the numbers of people with different patterns of oral health status that will be seen. The outcome of this interaction appears to be country specific and depends on the relative rates of fall of edentulism and increase in age cohorts with population growth. Thus for the United States, it has been suggested that the numbers of people who are edentulous will remain high because of the relatively low rates of reduction in edentulism over the next 20 years compared with population growth in the age groups where edentulism remains prevalent (Douglass et al., 2002). Whereas in Europe the numbers of people who are edentulous are likely to fall as the rates of reduction in edentulism are higher in some European countries than they are in the United States (Mojon et al., 2004). It should be noted that this difference reflects the higher base rates for edentulism in some European countries than those seen in the United States, rather than differing standards of care (Zitzmann et al., 2007). On both continents, there will be an overall growth of both

A.W.G. Walls
Professor of Restorative Dentistry, School of Dental Sciences, Newcastle University, Framlington Place, Newcastle upon Tyne, NE2 4BW
e-mail: a.w.g.walls@ncl.ac.uk

I.B. Lamster, M.E. Northridge (eds.), *Improving Oral Health for the Elderly*,
© Springer Science+Business Media, LLC 2008

Table 16.1 Reported eating impacts, reported difficulty eating raw carrots and reported fruits and vegetables intake as a 4-day mean from the U.K. National Diet and Nutrition Survey for people aged 65 years and over (Steele et al., 1998)

	Edentate	Teeth Upper	Teeth Lower	Fewer than 17 teeth in both jaws	More than 17 teeth in both jaws
N	498	19	109	137	198
Eating impact	11%	26%	8%	11%	5%
Carrots	45%	47%	33%	37%	9%
F&V intake (4-day mean)	460 g	384 g	463 g	451 g	538 g

the aging population and the proportion of that population who are dentate. There are few data which show differences in rates of change in edentulism between social or ethnic groups, however it is likely that the social and ethnic disparities in oral health status will remain in this *improving* situation, and there is some suggestion that the magnitude of the disparities may increase with slower rates of decline in edentulism among the socially disadvantaged.

One of the key determinants in the relationship between oral health and nutrition is the number and distribution of any remaining teeth and complete denture use. To this end, it is again worth noting that a proportion of older dentate people are edentate in 1 arch (predominantly the upper). There are few data available on the prevalence of this pattern of oral health but rates of 2.7% for the adult population in Switzerland and 23% for the over 65s in the United Kingdom have been reported (Steele et al., 1998; Zitzmann et al., 2008). These individuals have similar functional patterns to those who have few teeth evenly distributed in both jaws and those who are edentulous. The small number of people who are edentulous in the lower jaw and function with a lower complete denture against a partial natural upper dentition reports more problems with chewing and swallowing foods than any other group (Table 16.1).

The Impact of The Oral Environment on Nutrition

Masticatory Efficiency

Our ability to chew foods is determined by the number and distribution of teeth in the mouth and the presence of dentures. Masticatory efficiency can be measured in a variety of different ways, but it is most commonly determined by measuring the efficiency with which some form of test food is broken up by a given number of chewing strokes or cycles. A wide range of test foods have been used from hard substances like raw carrot and almonds, through to pieces of silicone rubber, with efficiency of comminution being measured optically or with graded sieves (Feldman et al., 1980; Gunne, 1985; Akeel et al., 1992; van der Bilt et al., 1993; Mowlana et al., 1994) to coloured chewing gums (chewing efficiency is measured with the latter by assessing the quality of mixing of the colours within the gum). The use of these methodologies have demonstrated that masticatory efficiency decreases in individuals with fewer teeth, in those who rely on removable partial dentures and in those who use conventional complete dentures.

Whilst the numbers of teeth have been shown to influence chewing efficiency by these techniques, periodontal disease and increasing tooth mobility have also been shown to reduce maximum biting force, although the relationship between biting force and masticatory efficiency is unclear. This is particularly difficult to identify in subjects who have attachment loss as they also tend to have fewer teeth. The relative impact of the effect of numbers of and mobility of teeth has not as yet been clarified (Kleinfelder and Ludwigt, 2002; Alkan et al., 2006; Johansson et al., 2006).

There is a complex relationship between masticatory efficiency and professional measures to improve chewing function. Generally, the provision of extra functional units whether in the form of a removable or fixed prosthesis results in improvement in measured chewing efficiency. These improvements are greater for restorations that are more stable, so for example a fixed dental prosthesis will result in a greater improvement than a removable prosthesis for a given improvement in the number of functional units. Furthermore, the use of osseointegrated dental implants as over-denture abutments to support a removable prosthesis will also result in improved chewing function compared with patients without this extra support and retention. Not surprisingly, overdenture-supported fixed dental prostheses are significantly more efficient than complete removable dentures. One of the great paradoxes in this process is that change in perceived chewing function is often not accompanied by a concomitant change in diet. Subjects within studies often report that they can chew better and feel more confident when chewing, but when their diet is explored in detail, there is no evidence of change in dietary pattern. This holds true for complete dentures, removable partial dentures and implant-supported structures (Gunne, 1985; Garrett et al., 1997; Moynihan et al., 2000).

Chewing serves a number of functions: it allows the individual to break down foods into sufficiently small pieces that they can be agglomerated into a bolus for swallowing; it causes mixing of saliva with food to help to initiate foods digestion, the saliva also helps to bind the food bolus together; it results in breakdown of the structure of food again to facilitate digestion in the stomach and small bowel, and finally, it results in the release of the chemical components of food that are associated with taste. Impaired chewing function will affect all of these components. People with poorer masticatory function are less efficient at breaking food down to facilitate bolus formation. They tend to use fewer chewing strokes and "accept" larger food particle sizes in the food bolus prior to swallowing. Whilst there are no documented problems associated with this, there could be an increased risk of choking in people who chew their food less effectively and who also have impaired swallowing, for example, dysphagic people post stroke.

People with complete dentures often complain of impaired taste, which is usually attributed to coverage of the palatal vault with the acrylic denture base. This, however, is counter-intuitive as there are few if any taste buds on the hard palate.

Impaired taste is more likely to be associated with poorer release of tasteants from foods which are not chewed well.

There are few data available concerning the impact of chewing on foods digestion. The classical work by Farrell in the 1950s remains as one of the few pieces of research in this area. He showed that with a modern diet and modern methods of foods preparation, digestion was influenced by the type of food but not by how much that food was chewed. These data do need to be viewed with caution in relation to the older adult; the experimental work was undertaken using dental students as volunteers whose dentitions were grossly intact so their masticatory efficiency was high and would have resulted in relatively efficient break up of food for a given number of chewing strokes. Furthermore, their gastric motility and function would be significantly better than an older person.

The ability to chew foods also influences the way in which food is prepared. In their analysis of data from the Health Professional Survey, Hung and colleagues demonstrated that people who had more than five teeth extracted during an 8-year follow-up period were less likely to improve their diet in a "healthy" way and were more likely to change their foods choice, avoiding foods that were crunchy in texture or hard to chew (for example, they ate fewer raw carrots and crispy apples than those individuals who had fewer teeth removed). The "tooth loss" group was also more likely to change the pattern of foods preparation to accommodate their altered masticatory status. They were more likely to cook foods rather than eating them raw (Hung et al., 2005). The impact of this change on the bioavailability of nutrients will vary from food to food. For example, the bioavailability of carotene from carrots will be enhanced by cooking to a reasonable level, whereas removal of the skin from a potato will markedly lower the vitamin C level.

Masticatory Efficiency and Foods Choice

In addition to the effects outlined above, an individual's ability to chew foods will also affect the foods that they choose to eat; not surprisingly, people do not elect to buy foods that are difficult for them to chew, so foods that are perceived as difficult to chew like apples and raw carrot are either not purchased at all or cooked to make them more manageable. Similarly people do not choose to buy foods which may cause them discomfort while chewing. Thus, edentulous people tend not to buy raspberries; this fruit is not difficult to chew, but if a raspberry pip gets underneath the denture, the subject then bites onto it and it will cause marked discomfort. Other apparently "soft" foods are also consumed in limited quantities or not at all, for example, lettuce and other salad greens are a challenge for the edentulous, not because they are difficult to chew but because the leaf can become "stuck" to the surface of their denture during chewing. Putting a finger into your mouth to dislodge a lettuce leaf is simply not socially acceptable in many circumstances.

It is thought that these preferences in terms of foods choice are largely responsible for the variation in diet seen between dentate and edentulous individuals

Table 16.2 A comparison of dietary intakes between individuals with intact (20 or more), compromised (19 or fewer) and no teeth between the U.K. National Diet and Nutrition Survey for People Aged 65 years (Sheiham et al., 2001) and Older and the Department of Veterans Affairs Dental Longitudinal Study (Krall et al., 1998). The figures in parentheses are the Daily Reference Values (DRVs) or Reference Daily Intakes (RDIs) for the food group concerned (FDA, 2007)

	Intact		Compromised		Edentulous	
	UK	US	UK	US	UK	US
Protein g/day (50 g/day)	72.3	80.0	66.6	74.0	60.1	68.0
NSP g/day (25 g/day)	16.2	21.0	12.9	19.0	11.0	16.0
Calcium mg/day (1 g/day)	883	773	812	677	722	689
Niacin mg/day (20 mg/day)	33.8	32.0	31.0	28.0	27.0	34.0
Vitamin C mg/day (60 mg/day)	82	159	73	149	60	127

(Table 16.2). These differences are quite marked, particularly for example in the intake of non-starch polysaccharide (dietary fibre), where the daily intake for edentulous older people in the United Kingdom was less than half the recommended value (11 g/day compared with 25 g/day) the figures from the Veterans Administration study are not quite as bleak in terms of intake relative to RDA (recommended daily allowance), however the pattern remains the same with lower levels of dietary intake among the edentulous compared with the dentate. In their analysis of data from NHANES III, Nowjack-Ramer and Sheiham showed reduced monthly intake of carrots and salads and daily intake of dietary fibre (table 16.3). These data support similar data from previous studies which have shown altered dietary fibre intake in edentulous compared with dentate subjects (Moynihan et al., 1994; Joshipura et al., 1996; Petti and Scully, 2005)

Shinkai and co-workers have questioned some of the assumptions around edentulism as a variable influencing foods selection. As with any scientific study, there

Table 16.3 Mean intake of food items for complete-denture-wearers compared with the fully dentate among persons 25 years and older (NHANES III: United States, 1988–1994) from (Nowjack-Raymer and Sheiham, 2003)

Food Items and Dental Status Category (n)	Mean (SE)	Unadjusted p Values	Adjusted Mean (SE)a	Adjusted p Values a
Carrots				
Denture (1370)	7.1 (0.3)	<0.0001	2.7 (1.5)	<0.0001
Dentate (2420)	8.1 (0.3)	—	5.8 (1.1)	—
Tossed Salad				
Denture (1370)	8.1 (0.6)	<0.0001	6.9 (1.5)	<0.0001
Dentate (2419)	11.3 (0.4)	—	10.3 (1.2)	—
Dietary Fibre				
Denture (1365)	15.8 (0.3)	< 0.0001	15.1 (2.2)	0.04
Dentate (2421)	19.0 (0.4)	—	17.6 (1.3)	—

a Adjusted for age, gender, race/ethnicity, socio-economic status, smoking status, caloric intake and supplement use.

are a variety of ways of estimating dietary intake. The analyses above have shown changes in specific foods types, whereas Shinkai used the Healthy Eating Index (USDA, 2007) which is a measure of diet quality that assesses conformance to federal (US) dietary guidance. Using this broad measure of dietary quality, they found no association between oral health status and the HEI, with social variables as the key determinants of the HEI score. These studies pose serious questions about the relationship between oral functional status and dietary choice/intake. To explore this area further, we analysed the U.K. National Diet and Nutrition Survey data with specific reference to fruits and vegetables intake (the data were incomplete in relation to computing an HEI score; this was the "best" generic marker of dietary quality we could identify within the NDNS data). The distribution of intake data is shown in Fig. 16.1 with a markedly skewed pattern and a mean intake of 232.5 g/day (compared with the RDA of 450 g/day for the United Kingdom including up to 80 g of fruit juice); logistic regression modelling of these data showed that social background and educational attainment were important influences in relation to achieving the 450-g intake threshold as were age (with reduced likelihood with increasing age) and the number of pairs of contacting teeth (Steele et al., 1998). The influence of the numbers of teeth appears relatively small compared with social variables, although for these data, as the Odds Ratio is per contacting pair of teeth so would

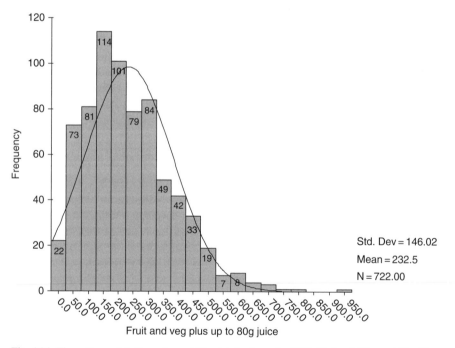

Fig. 16.1 The pattern of fruits and vegetables intake from the U.K. National Diet and Nutrition Survey for people aged 65 years and over (consumption of all fruits and vegetables plus up to 80 g/day of fruit juice) (Finch et al., 1998)

Table 16.4 The reported relationships between oral health status and biochemical markers of micronutrient status for dentate (20 or more teeth) and edentulous subjects from the U.K. National Diet and Nutrition Survey for People Aged 65 years (NDNS) (Sheiham et al., 2001) and The U.S. National Health and Nutrition Examination Series III (NHANES III) (Nowjack-Raymer and Sheiham, 2003)

		UK NDNS		NHANES III	
		Dentate	Edentate	Dentate	Edentate
Ascorbate	μmol/l	49.1	39.4		
Retinol	μmol/l	2.30	2.09		
Ascorbate	mg/dl			0.95(0.06)	0.87(0.09)
Folate	ng/dl			6.1(0.6)	4.7(0.9)
β carotene	μg/dl			16.6(2.4)	9.8(3.6)

be raised to the power 8 for an "intact" dentition with 28 teeth (giving an OR of 2.14) or to the power 4 for a shortened dental arch (giving an OR of 1.46). It is likely that discrepancy in results seen between these National cross-sectional data and the studies from Shinkai and others are simply a question of power within the study with relatively small large numbers of subjects in National data sets (Shinkai et al., 2001; Shinkai et al., 2002).

Oral Health Status and Biochemical Measures of Nutritional Status

There are two reports of relationships between oral functional status and biochemical measures of nutritional status, relating to the UK NDNS survey for people aged 65 years and over (Sheiham et al., 2001) and NHANES II (Nowjack-Raymer and Sheiham, 2003). Although different measures were used in these data, there is a consistent trend for individuals with poorer dentitions to demonstrate lower haematological levels of specific micronutrients. The micronutrients concerned are those that would be anticipated bearing in mind the reported patterns of dietary restriction and altered foods choice.(Table 16.4).

Implications for Health on the Basis of Dietary Change Between Dentate and Edentulous Subjects

The patterns of dietary change associated with having few or no teeth are in the direction that would be regarded as "unhealthy", for example, increase in cholesterol intake (Krall et al., 1998), reduced intake of fruits and vegetables(Sheiham et al., 2001), and reduced intake of dietary fibre (Moynihan et al., 1994; Joshipura et al., 1996). These dietary changes may elevate the risk of individuals to a wide variety of systemic diseases, for example, atherosclerosis leading to both stroke and cardiovascular risk, a variety of cancers and dietary control in diabetes to name but a few. There are very few data which look specifically at the links between oral health, nutrition and systemic disease risk (Ritchie et al., 2002); there are however associations between edentulism and significant weight loss (Ritchie et al., 2000; Sheiham et al., 2002) and indeed between edentulism and poor oral health with increased mortality (Hamalainen et al., 2003; Österberg et al., 2007). In addition, there are well-documented association between inflammatory oral disease associated with tooth loss and atherosclerosis on which some of the association may be explained by variations in diet associated with tooth loss rather than inflammatory change (Joshipura et al., 2000). The evidence is insufficient at this stage other than to say that there are associations between oral health status and dietary change which have an impact in addition to social variables on dietary intake. These changes are such that there may be an increased risk of life-threatening systemic disease associated with altered oral health status and/or chewing efficiency. Obviously this link is secondary to the dietary effects (i.e. it is not the tooth loss that results in increased risk of disease, rather the dietary change that is associated with tooth loss).

Can Oral Health Care Make a Difference?

The underlying premise to the discussion above is that oral health status, and specifically altered chewing ability, influences foods choices and hence diet, with change in a detrimental manner when oral health status deteriorates towards edentulism. The logical assumption therefore is that an improvement if oral health status through appropriate dental interventions will result in positive dietary change. Unfortunately, this is not the case. With the exception of the Health Professional Study in the U.S. dietary interventions designed to improve chewing efficiency, result in a self-perceived improvement in chewing but no alteration in diet. This has been shown for all forms of removable prosthetic intervention, including partial denture (RPD) provision, and both conventional and implant supported complete dentures (Gunne, 1985; Garrett et al., 1997; Moynihan et al., 2000). There is a consistent trend in all studies for professional intervention to be associated with perceived improvement if chewing ability, but no change in dietary selection. Intriguingly one study on patients with implant-supported restorations has shown a change in anthropometric measures of nutritional status without any apparent change in dietary intake (Morais et al., 2003).

Whilst direct oral health intervention appears to have little effect, a tailored dietary intervention, delivered during dental treatment has been shown to be highly effective in promoting a "healthy" diet with an increase in fruits and vegetables intake in excess of 200 g/day in subjects with conventional complete dentures (Moynihan et al., 2005), even more marked improvements are apparent when a similar intervention is delivered to people with implant-supported prostheses (El-Feky et al., 2006).

Change in dietary habits is something that will not occur unless people are challenged to change and helped with the change process.

Impact of Nutrition on Oral Disease

Nutrients and Oral Mucosal Health

The evidence for alterations in the oral mucosa with age is equivocal. There is some evidence for mucosal atrophy with reductions in the attachment apparatus between the mucosa and the dermis (the rette pegs) from specific areas of the mouth (for example, the lateral border of the tongue). The impact of these changes on the susceptibility of the mucosa to nutritional deficiencies is unclear. The oral mucosal lining has a very rapid rate of turnover like many other mucosal surfaces within the gastrointestinal tract. Consequently, reductions in micronutrients that are critical for mucosal turnover and integrity will manifest themselves with oral mucosal lesions at a relatively early stage.

Iron, Vitamin B_{12} and Folate

These micronutrients are critical for maintenance of oral mucosal integrity; deficiency states will result in mucosal change affecting both the tongue and the oral mucosal lining. The tongue tends to lose the irregularity on its surface, producing a smooth surface that is often also bright red in appearance rather than the pink of keratinised oral mucosa. Oral ulceration is more common, particularly minor oral ulcers (Porter et al., 1992), as are red lesions (erythroplasias) of the oral mucosa. The latter are regarded as pre-malignant lesions. Iron deficiency is also associated with burning mouth syndrome in older people (a condition where sufferers complain of a painful burning mouth particularly when eating some foods) (Hakeberg et al., 1997), angular cheilitis (sores at the angles of the mouth which may also be infected with either candida or staphylococci), and a mucosal stomatitis associated with the area beneath the plate of an upper denture, again candida are commonly involved (Sweeney et al., 1994; Chapple and Matthews, 2007).

Alcohol

Oral health is reduced in subjects with relatively high alcohol intake. The oral health changes include the following:

- Erosive pattern tooth wear in people who are professional wine tasters due to the acidity of many wines, and also in alcoholics due to a combination of pH of the drink itself plus chronic regurgitation of stomach contents into the oral environment as a consequence of alcohol-induced gastric mucosal irritation.
- Increased levels of dental caries both through the sugars and acid contents of drinks, as well as through generalised neglect in individuals who become addicted to alcohol. This is a particular problem currently in young people with

alcopops, which contain high levels of sugar as well as acids as flavouring agents.
- Increased risk of oral cancer, with some variation in risk associated with both the patterns of alcohol consumption and the type of alcohol consumed. It is thought that the concentration of some cancer preventing compounds like polyphenols in some forms of alcoholic beverage may moderate the interaction between the intake of alcoholic drinks and cancer risk (Petti and Scully, 2005).

Oral Cancer

There are some nutritional links to oral cancer, through the pre-malignant lesions associated with iron deficiency as well as high levels of alcohol intake, and specific problems associated with tobacco (either when smoked or in smokeless forms), betel quid and areca nut. The estimated relative risk of developing oral cancer in individuals who chew areca nut alone is 58.4 (95% confidence interval 7.6–447.6) (Lu et al., 1996). Chewing betel quid is endemic in the Indian subcontinent and increasing among Indian ex-patriots in the United Kingdom. This combination of tobacco leaf and slaked lime is particularly harmful, resulting initially in sub-mucous fibrosis and subsequently in overt squamous carcinoma (Zain et al., 1999; Warnakulasuriya, 2004).

Antioxidants and Periodontal Disease

Periodontal disease is the single most common chronic inflammatory disease in man. It results in very limited morbidity until the loss of bony attachment is sufficiently severe to cause mobility of the teeth and ultimately tooth loss. This can occur simply through shedding or as a consequence of a dentist extracting teeth.

The disease is susceptible to all of the normal influences on chronic inflammatory pathways, which will include the effects of nutritional antioxidants in moderating inflammatory change. There is a considerable body of evidence linking reactive oxygen species and antioxidant activity to periodontal disease and to disease progression (Chapple and Matthews, 2007), with some specific examples of nutritional deficiency having been identified that are associated with accelerated patterns of periodontal attachment loss (Amaliya et al., 2007). There have been some attempts to moderate the severity of this disease with both locally and systemically delivered antioxidant supplements, however, with the exception of instances where overt micronutrient deficiency are involved, for example, the management of scurvy with vitamin C, these have shown limited benefit. There are some promising results from experimental animal models using specific antioxidant enzymes, but these have yet to be translated into clinical practice (Chapple and Matthews, 2007)

Dental Caries

Dental caries is an environmental disease consequential to the interactions between bacteria in plaque on the surface of teeth and sugars in food. Mature plaque, which has a characteristic microbial flora, is capable of metabolising sugars to produce acid, once the pH of the plaque falls below the critical pH for demineralisation of tooth tissue the surface and sub-surface tissue begins to dissolve. This process is influenced by four variables: the nature of the substrate (dentine has a higher critical pH for demineralisation than enamel), an individual's oral hygiene (poor oral hygiene facilitates the formation of plaque), fluoride (this can enhance the remineralisation process and help to prevent ongoing change) and salivary function which is essential for remineralisation to occur. All of these are dealt with elsewhere in this text.

Sugars Consumption

Sugars are an important component of all diets and yet they are also responsible for being the source of acids that result in tooth decay. There is a considerable body of evidence linking caries to sugars intake in younger people, including national epidemiological studies. However, there are fewer data which link decay in older adults to sugars consumption. Vehkalahti was able to demonstrate a link between the use of sugars in tea and coffee and root caries in a Finnish population (Vehkalahti and Paunio, 1988), and Steele et al. (2001) found a 2-fold increase in risk of root caries in subjects with high frequency of sugars intake in their analysis of the U.K. National Diet and Nutrition Survey for people aged 65 years and over. One particular area of concern is the high level of untreated dental caries in institutionalised populations. This is the result of a combination of poor access to dental care and also a relatively cariogenic diet with a high frequency of sugars intake daily.

There are three variables that determine the impact of dietary sugars on the teeth: age, frequency and quantity.

Which Sugars are Important?

It is clear that the most cariogenic sugars are highly refined carbohydrates, particularly sucrose but also glucose. Natural sugars, like fructose and lactose, can also be metabolised in plaque to produce acids but the metabolic processes are less efficient and any metabolism results in the production of less acid. It is also relatively unusual for people to have diets that include high frequency of intake of such sugars. Finely ground starch can also be metabolised to produce acids by oral bacteria but again at lower levels than seen with sucrose.

Refined sugars are widely used in the food industry both as preservatives and sweetening agents, and are often described as hidden sugars particularly as many savoury foods contain substantial quantities of added sugar (prime examples would be tomato ketchup, chutney and baked beans, but there are many others).

Is Frequency or Quantity Important?

Demineralisation of tooth tissue occurs during the period when the plaque pH lies below the threshold level for the concerned tissue (about 5.4 for enamel and 6 for dentine). The pattern of pH change and recovery would suggest that for each episode of pH fall, dentine will be exposed to a longer period of demineralisation than enamel. Remineralisation occurs during times when plaque pH is above the demineralising threshold. Current evidence suggests that it is the frequency of sugars intake that is more important than the overall quantity in predicting the severity of caries. With low frequency of intake, the natural defence/repair mechanisms are at their most effective, however when frequencies are high demineralisation dominates, resulting in caries. There is no evidence on what frequency of sugars intakes might be regarded as *safe* for root caries; the evidence that is available relates to enamel caries in younger subjects where dentists would normally recommend no more than four episodes of sugar containing foods/drinks intake per day. It is of note that the mean number of sugars intakes daily for the "free-living" 65+ population in the United Kingdom was 5.1, rising to 7.9 for the "institution" sample in the 65+ NDNS programme (Steele et al. 1998).

One specific problem that relates to elderly infirm individuals is the use of energy supplements as part of their diet to try to maintain an adequate calorific intake. These supplements are often in liquid or syrup form and are drunk over long periods of time by their users resulting in demineralisation. The syrupy nature of these preparations is of particular relevance as their rate of oral clearance will be low, particularly in individuals with impaired salivary flow.

Sugars in Medicines

Sugars are used in medicines as preservatives in syrups and mixtures, and to hide the bitter flavour of drugs. There has been a long and successful campaign for the replacement of sugars in medicines for children with artificial sweeteners and other agents. Drugs delivered to adults are commonly taken in tablet or capsule form but there is increasing use of liquid preparations in older adults and also drugs which have prolonged oral clearance (tablets that are sucked or chewed for example rather than swallowed). Currently most of these drugs retain sugars as sweeteners or preservatives, which can pose a problem in relation to decay in susceptible individuals. Similarly, chewable preparations that have an intrinsically low pH (for example, vitamin C preparations) will add to the overall acid burden of the oral environment (Maguire and Baqir, 2000).

Summary

This chapter has given an overview of both the relationships between oral health status and nutrition and nutrition and oral health.

Foods choice is affected by the number and distribution of remaining teeth in the mouth. This in turn alters dietary patterns towards a "less healthy" diet, lower in fruits and vegetables intake and potentially higher in fats intake. These changes are reflected in some biochemical measures of nutritional status and in Body Mass Index. Oral health interventions alone do not influence dietary intake and must be associated with a dietary intervention to stimulate change in foods intake. When appropriate dietary and oral health interventions are given simultaneously, there is a marked and synergistic effect resulting in significant improvement in diet.

Diet can also affect oral health both through sugars as a key variable in the development of caries and through micronutrient intake in relation to oral mucosal integrity and disease. There is increasing interest in the role of antioxidant defence in relation to oral inflammatory disease, dietary supplementation or local delivery of antioxidants may have a future role in managing these common disease processes.

References

Akeel R, Nilner M, Nilner K (1992). Masticatory efficiency in individuals with natural dentition. Swed Dent J 16:191–198.

Alkan A, Keskiner I, Arici S, Sato S (2006). The effect of periodontal surgery on bite force, occlusal contact area and bite pressure. J Am Dent Assoc 137:978–983; quiz 1028.

Amaliya, Timmerman MF, Abbas F, Loos BG, Van der Weijden GA, Van Winkelhoff AJ, et al. (2007). Java project on periodontal diseases: the relationship between vitamin C and the severity of periodontitis. J Clin Periodontol 34:299–304.

Chapple IL, Matthews JB (2007). The role of reactive oxygen and antioxidant species in periodontal tissue destruction. Periodontol 2000 43:160–232.

Douglass CW, Shih A, Ostry L (2002). Will there be a need for complete dentures in the United States in 2020? J Prosthet Dent 87:5–8.

El-Feky AF, Thomason JM, Seal CJ, Ellis JS, Moynihan PJ (2006). Impact of Dietary Intervention following Prosthetic Rehabilitation with Implant-supported Dentures. Pan-European Federation of the IADR. Cardiff.

FDA (2007). 'Daily Values' Encourage Healthy Diet.

Feldman RS, Kapur KK, Alman JE, Chauncey HH (1980). Aging and mastication: changes in performance and in the swallowing threshold with natural dentition. J Am Geriatr Soc 28: 97–103.

Finch S, Doyle W, Lowe C, Bates CJ, Prentice A, Smithers G, et al. (1998). National diet and Nutrition survey: people aged 65 years or over. Vol 1: report of the diet and nutrition survey London: Stationary Office.

Garrett NR, Kapur KK, Hasse AL, Dent RJ (1997). Veterans Administration Cooperative Dental Implant Study—comparisons between fixed partial dentures supported by blade-vent implants and removable partial dentures. Part V: Comparisons of pretreatment and posttreatment dietary intakes. J Prosthet Dent 77:153–161.

Gunne HJ (1985). Masticatory efficiency and dental state. A comparison between two methods. Acta Odontologica Scandinavic 43:139–146.

Hakeberg M, Berggren U, Hagglin C, Ahlqwist M (1997). Reported burning mouth symptoms among middle-aged and elderly women. Eur J Oral Sci 105:539–543.

Hamalainen P, Meurman JH, Keskinen M, Heikkinen E (2003). Relationship between dental health and 10-year mortality in a cohort of community-dwelling elderly people. Eur J Oral Sci 111:291–296.

Hung HC, Colditz G, Joshipura KJ (2005). The association between tooth loss and the self-reported intake of selected CVD-related nutrients and foods among US women. Community Dent Oral Epidemiol 33:167–173.

Johansson AS, Svensson KG, Trulsson M (2006). Impaired masticatory behavior in subjects with reduced periodontal tissue support. J Periodontol 77:1491–1497.

Joshipura K, Ritchie C, Douglass C (2000). Strength of evidence linking oral conditions and systemic disease. Compend Contin Educ Dent Suppl:12–23; quiz 65.

Joshipura KJ, Willett WC, Douglass CW (1996). The impact of edentulousness on food and nutrient intake. J Am Dent Assoc 127:459–456.

Kleinfelder JW, Ludwigt K (2002). Maximal bite force in patients with reduced periodontal tissue support with and without splinting. J Periodontol 73:1184–1187.

Krall E, Hayes C, Garcia R (1998). How dentition status and masticatory function affect nutrient intake. J Am Dent Assoc 129:1261–1269.

Lu CT, Yen YY, Ho CS, Ko YC, Tsai CC, Hsieh CC, et al. (1996). A case-control study of oral cancer in Changhua County, Taiwan. J Oral Pathol Med 25:245–248.

Maguire A, Baqir W (2000). Prevalence of long-term use of medicines with prolonged oral clearance in the elderly: a survey in north east England. Br Dent J 189:267–272.

Mojon P, Thomason JM, Walls AW (2004). The impact of falling rates of edentulism. Int J Prosthodont 17:434–440.

Morais JA, Heydecke G, Pawliuk J, Lund JP, Feine JS (2003). The effects of mandibular two-implant overdentures on nutrition in elderly edentulous individuals. J Dent Res 82:53–58.

Mowlana F, Heath MR, Van der Bilt A, Van der Glas HW (1994). Assessment of chewing efficiency: a comparison of particle size distribution determined using optical scanning and sieving of almonds. J Oral Rehabil 21:545–551.

Moynihan PJ, Snow S, Jepson NJ, Butler TJ (1994). Intake of non-starch polysaccharide (dietary fibre) in edentulous and dentate persons: an observational study. British Dental Journal 177:243–247.

Moynihan PJ, Butler TJ, Thomason JM, Jepson NJ (2000). Nutrient intake in partially dentate patients: the effect of prosthetic rehabilitation. Journal of Dentistry 28:557–563.

Moynihan PJ, Bradbury J, Thomason JM, Walls AW, Allen PF (2005). Nutrition counseling increases fruit and vegetable intake in the edentulous. Journal of Dental Research:In Press.

Nowjack-Raymer RE, Sheiham A (2003). Association of edentulism and diet and nutrition in US adults. J Dent Res 82:123–126.

Österberg T, Carlsson G, Sundh V, Mellström D (2007). Number of teeth – a predictor of mortality in 70-year-old subjects. Community Dent Oral Epidemiol In Press.

Petti S, Scully C (2005). Oral cancer: The association between nation-based alcohol-drinking profiles and oral cancer mortality. Oral Oncol.

Porter S, Flint S, Scully C, Keith O (1992). Recurrent aphthous stomatitis: the efficacy of replacement therapy in patients with underlying hematinic deficiencies. Ann Dent 51:14–16.

Ritchie CS, Joshipura K, Silliman RA, Miller B, Douglas CW (2000). Oral health problems and significant weight loss among community-dwelling older adults. J Gerontol A Biol Sci Med Sci 55:M366–371.

Ritchie CS, Joshipura K, Hung HC, Douglass CW (2002). Nutrition as a mediator in the relation between oral and systemic disease: associations between specific measures of adult oral health and nutrition outcomes. Crit Rev Oral Biol Med 13:291–300.

Sheiham A, Steele JG, Marcenes W, Lowe C, Finch S, Bates CJ, et al. (2001). The relationship among dental status, nutrient intake, and nutritional status in older people. J Dent Res 80: 408–413.

Sheiham A, Steele JG, Marcenes W, Finch S, Walls AW (2002). The relationship between oral health status and Body Mass Index among older people: a national survey of older people in Great Britain. Br Dent J 192:703–706.

Shinkai RS, Hatch JP, Sakai S, Mobley CC, Saunders MJ, Rugh JD (2001). Oral function and diet quality in a community-based sample. J Dent Res 80:1625–1630.

Shinkai RS, Hatch JP, Rugh JD, Sakai S, Mobley CC, Saunders MJ (2002). Dietary intake in edentulous subjects with good and poor quality complete dentures. J Prosthet Dent 87:490–498.

Steele JG, Sheiham A, Marcenes W, Walls AWG (1998). National diet and nutrition survey: people aged 65 years or over. Vol 2: report of the oral health survey London: Stationary Office.

Steele JG, Sheiham A, Marcenes W, Fay N, Walls AW (2001). Clinical and behavioural risk indicators for root caries in older people. Gerodontology 18:95–101.

Sweeney MP, Bagg J, Fell GS, Yip B (1994). The relationship between micronutrient depletion and oral health in geriatrics. J Oral Pathol Med 23:168–171.

USDA (2007). Healthy Eating Index: Unites States Department of Agriculture.

van der Bilt A, van der Glas HW, Mowlana F, Heath MR (1993). A comparison between sieving and optical scanning for the determination of particle size distributions obtained by mastication in man. Arch Oral Biol 38:159–162

Vehkalahti MM, Paunio IK (1988). Occurrence of root caries in relation to dental health behavior. J Dent Res 67:911–914.

Warnakulasuriya S (2004). Smokeless tobacco and oral cancer. Oral Dis 10:1–4.

Zain RB, Ikeda N, Gupta PC, Warnakulasuriya S, van Wyk CW, Shrestha P, et al. (1999). Oral mucosal lesions associated with betel quid, areca nut and tobacco chewing habits: consensus from a workshop held in Kuala Lumpur, Malaysia, November 25–27, 1996. J Oral Pathol Med 28:1–4.

Zitzmann N, Hagmann E, Weiger R (2007). What is the prevalence of various types of prosthetic dental restorations in Europe? Clin Oral Implants Res.

Zitzmann NU, Staehelin K, Walls AWG, Menghini G, Weiger R, Stutz EZ (2008). Oral health and dental restorations in Switzerland. Community Dent Oral Epidemiol.

Chapter 17
Orofacial Pain and Neurological Disorders Affecting the Head and Neck

Ali Makki and Susan Roche

Musculoskeletal Conditions

Musculoskeletal disorders can affect any skeletal muscle including those of the head, neck, trunk, and the extremities. The focus of this section will be on the conditions affecting the muscles of mastication, which are comprised of the following: (1) masseter; (2) temporalis; (3) medial pterygoid; and (4) lateral pterygoid. Masticatory muscle disorders can occur at any age and may range from mild to incapacitating pain. When the pain is severe, it may interfere with the patient's ability to maintain a normal diet, resulting in significant weight loss and concomitant deterioration of the patient's physiological reserve. In addition, there may be an accompanying decrease in the range of mouth opening that could lead to pain and fatigue when talking. Severe musculoskeletal pain can significantly impact activities of daily living (ADL), lead to social isolation, and cause or exacerbate pre-existing anxiety and/or depression.

The ability of the healthcare provider to diagnose musculoskeletal pain conditions is critical in affording the elderly patient with comprehensive overall care. But many dentists and physicians have either not received the necessary training to perform an adequate musculoskeletal examination or lack the clinical experience to do muscle palpation properly. Travell and Simons (1983) have done groundbreaking research in this area and explain how to properly examine the patient, recognize referred pain patterns, diagnose, and treat these conditions. A thorough knowledge base of the referral patterns will aid the clinician in identifying the involved muscle that is the actual source of the pain disorder.

The clinician must also be knowledgeable enough to form an adequate differential diagnosis that includes conditions, which refer pain to the orofacial region, such as dental or sinus infections, inflammatory conditions involving the temporomandibular joint, disc displacement, salivary gland disorders, heart

A. Makki
Bureau of Health Professions, Faculty Training Fellow in Geriatric Medicine, David Geffen School of Medicine at UCLA, Lecturer & Clinical Faculty, Section of Oral Medicine and Orofacial Pain, UCLA School of Dentistry, Los Angeles, CA, USA

I.B. Lamster, M.E. Northridge (eds.), *Improving Oral Health for the Elderly*,
© Springer Science+Business Media, LLC 2008

attacks, neuropathies, tumors, and neurovascular disorders. Clark, Minakuchi, and Lotaif (2005) provide an excellent review of the prevalence of various orofacial pain disorders affecting the elderly. As discussed in this chapter, certain orofacial pain disorders are more common in the elderly, so a reasonable familiarity with the respective epidemiology should help prevent misdiagnosis, unnecessary treatments, and prolonged suffering.

The following musculoskeletal conditions will be discussed in this section: (1) myalgia; (2) myofascial pain; (3) myositis; (4) myospasm; and (5) myofibrotic contracture. Myalgia and myofascial pain are the most commonly encountered conditions, but the etiology of chronic musculoskeletal pain is still poorly understood; however, contributing mechanisms include: (1) inflammation; (2) sensitized nociceptors within the muscle; (3) endogenous chemical buildup; and (4) central sensitization (Lotaif, Mitrirattanakul, & Clark, 2006). It is also hypothesized that hypoperfusion of the muscle may be involved in myofascial pain and to a lesser extent in fibromyalgia (Maekawa, Clark, & Kuboki, 2002). Bruxism is not strongly correlated to stress, anger, physical activity, or sleep quality as was previously believed (Watanabe, Ichikawa, & Clark, 2003). The most important concept to remember is that masticatory muscle disorders and temporomandibular joint disorders should be treated conservatively, and irreversible dental treatments, such as performing occlusal equilibration by the removal of enamel in an attempt to obtain a "more stable bite", should be avoided.

Myalgia

By definition, non-referred muscle pain is called myalgia. The pain is typically local and the diagnosis of myalgia is made once other muscle disorders have been ruled out. Muscle pain may be attributed to bruxism, ischemia, metabolic conditions, fatigue, delayed-onset muscle soreness, autonomic nervous system effects, or protective splinting (Okeson, 1996).

Myofascial Pain

Myofascial pain (MFP) presents as a regional dull aching pain in the muscle and may or may not be worsened by jaw function. Localized tender sites, known as trigger points, characteristically present as tight, hyperirritable bands of muscle tissue or fascia, which produce an increase in pain and result in characteristic and consistent referral patterns on palpation. Travell and Simons (1983) have beautifully illustrated anatomic diagrams of each muscle, demonstrating the referral patterns and their associated symptoms.

It is important to remember that location of the pain may not necessarily be the source of the pain, particularly when trigger points are involved. This factor is probably the most common reason for misdiagnosis of pain in the oral and craniofacial region. Pain may be referred to particular teeth from a remote trigger point located in the following muscles: (1) temporalis; (2) masseter (superficial); and (3) anterior digastric. Therefore, it is crucial that the clinician perform a muscle palpation examination to determine if the patient's toothache or jaw pain complaint can be altered or reproduced, particularly when no obvious pathology exists. Pain may also be referred to the ear and the temporomandibular joint if a trigger point exists in any of the following muscles: (1) masseter (deep); (2) medial pterygoid; (3) lateral pterygoid; and (4) sternocleidomastoid (clavicular head). The variety of referral patterns in orofacial pain associated with the masticatory muscles can confuse a clinician who is unfamiliar with the trigger point referral patterns. In addition, a novice may mistake a "trigger zone" of trigeminal neuralgia (discussed later in the chapter) for a myofascial trigger point, or vice-versa, which can result in a misdiagnosis. The patient history outlining the pain quality, its temporal pattern, the aggravating factors, as well as its severity, duration, and frequency helps to differentiate the various orofacial pain disorders. The clinician's failure to spend the necessary time to review these components of the pain history is a major reason for misdiagnosis of MFP.

Myofascial pain disorder must be differentiated from fibromyalgia, myalgia, myositis, intermittent claudication, neoplasia, dental pathology, temporomandibular joint arthritides, and neuropathies. The presence of a trigger point as defined earlier, and reproducibility of the patient's pain complaint by palpation of the trigger point, is a hallmark of myofascial pain. The diagnostic criteria for myofascial pain must also include a pain reduction by $\geq$ 50% following the topical application of a vapocoolant spray or by the injection of a local anesthetic into the trigger point, followed by stretching of the involved muscle (Okeson, 1996). A patient with myofascial pain may also experience stiffness in the muscle, the perception that the teeth do no occlude properly, decreased ability to open the mouth, otic symptoms (i.e., fullness, pain, tinnitus, and vertigo), tooth pain, autonomic symptoms, and tension-type headache. Hyperalgesia may also be present in the site of referred pain.

Myositis

Myositis is a condition that presents as an acute, constant pain in the affected muscle. In the orofacial region, the associated inflammation results from trauma, strain or a spreading infection involving the masticatory muscles. The masseter and medial pterygoid muscles are most commonly involved. A condition known as a "sterile myositis" is associated with severe clenching and bruxing, which can cause swelling over the muscle without presence of any infection. Myositis is typically associated with diffuse tenderness over the entire muscle, significant limitation of mouth opening due to swelling and pain, and increased pain complaint with movements of the jaw. In addition to swelling, there may be redness and an increase in temperature over the affected muscle. It is crucial to treat the myositis to prevent it from progressing to myofibrotic contracture, which generally has long-term sequelae and a poor prognosis.

Myalgia, myofascial pain, intermittent claudication, and sialadenitis, particularly involving the parotid gland, should be included in the differential diagnoses for myositis.

Myospasm

A true case of myospasm involving the muscles of mastication is a very uncommon occurrence and presents clinically with significant limitation of mouth opening, which results from a continuous, involuntary contraction of one or more of the masticatory muscles. Other terminology used to describe a myospasm includes trismus or cramp. The clinical presentation of myospasm involves acute onset at rest as well as with jaw movements. It may be necessary to order an electromyography (EMG) study to differentiate if the limited mouth opening is the result of a myospasm, myofibrotic contracture, or to help rule out a non-reducing displaced disc occurring within the temporomandibular joint. If an EMG is performed, it will typically demonstrate a significant increase in muscle activity compared to the resting state. An inexpensive alternative to the EMG would be the use of a vapocoolant spray and/or muscle relaxants for diagnostic purposes to help differentiate these conditions (Ram, Kumar, & Clark, 2006). It should be noted that myospasm may result from trauma, acute overuse, strain, and overstretching. Although a very rare occurrence, inadvertent injection of local anesthetic into the medial pterygoid muscle by the dentist, administering an inferior alveolar nerve block, may result in myospasm. In addition, oral medications can also produce muscle spasms. This is well documented with some classes of antipsychotics and paradoxically with some tranquilizers.

Myospasm must be clinically differentiated from the following conditions: myofibrotic contracture, neoplasia, myalgia, myofascial pain, and anterior disc displacement without reduction.

Myofibrotic Contracture

Myofibrotic contracture is extremely rare in the orofacial pain population. Fibrotic changes and sometimes calcification in the muscle tissues are the cause of contracture. It involves painless contracture of one of the masticatory muscles with the masseter being the most commonly involved muscle. The sternocleidomastoid muscle may also be involved in patients who have received radiation therapy for head and neck cancer. The contracture results in a significant decreased range of motion, and usually passive stretching fails to increase the amount of movement. With respect to jaw movements, the maximum range of opening will have a "hard end-feel". Often, pain is absent or minimal, unless excessive force is applied in an attempt to gain an increased range of opening.

Myofibrotic contracture may be the sequela of trauma, infection, or myofibrosis secondary to radiation therapy. Prolonged limitation of mouth opening from interocclusal fixation (i.e., following fracture or post-orthognathic jaw surgery) can also result in myofibrotic contracture. The resulting fibrosis or scarring that occurs in the muscle makes this condition nearly impossible to reverse.

The differential diagnosis includes: myospasm, ankylosis of the temporo-mandibular joint, anterior disc displacement without reduction, and coronoid hyperplasia.

Treatment of myofibrotic contracture is primarily palliative. In some of the less advanced cases, depending on the particular muscle, the location, and the extent of the fibrosis or calcification, the injection of botulinum toxin A seems to afford some gain in the range of motion, but the overall prognosis for improvement is usually less than desirable.

Splint Therapy

With splint therapy the patient wears a removable, hard acrylic appliance, covering the entire dentition on either the maxillary or the mandibular arch. Other terms used for a splint include, nightguard, intraoral appliance, occlusal guard, ortho-pedic appliance, orthotic, bite guard, and bruxism appliance. Occlusal appliances have been shown to be very beneficial in the treatment of masticatory muscle pain and arthralgia (Kreiner, Betancor, & Clark, 2001). The exact mechanism of treat-ment response for splint therapy is poorly understood however, it is believed to decrease the loading forces placed on the masticatory muscles resulting in less trauma caused by bruxism. For patients with a nocturnal bruxism habit, splints are typically worn at nighttime during sleep and are intended for long-term use. The splint should not be worn more than approximately 8–12 hours per day. Long-term splint wear of extended duration (24 hours per day) can create malocclusions, which require orthodontic therapy to correct and may leave the dentist liable for treat-ment expenses or malpractice. The patient should always be warned not to wear the occlusal appliance in excess of 12 hours per day, and partial-coverage appliances are not recommended due to super-eruption of the teeth in the unsupported areas.

Psychological Support

Consultation with a specially trained pain psychologist should be an integral part of treatment planning in orofacial pain management. Specifically, it can be very beneficial in decreasing masticatory muscle symptoms, particularly when the pain is induced or exacerbated by generalized anxiety or anxiety-driven disorders or daytime parafunctional habits (i.e., clenching, bruxing, nail biting, cheek biting, and protrusion). Nocturnal bruxism, during sleep, is believed to be an unconscious habit, therefore, it is difficult, if not impossible to modify since there is no vol-untary component to the movements. However, biofeedback, stress management, behavior modification, relaxation therapy, implementation of consistent exercise regimens have been useful in providing decreased muscle tension and reduction of muscle pain.

Temporomandibular Joint Disorders

Temporomandibular joint disorders include the following: (1) developmental disorders: (2) disc derangement disorders; (3) dislocation; (4) inflammatory disorders; (5) arthritides; (6) ankylosis; and (7) fracture (Okeson, 1996). Developmental disorders will not be addressed in this section since they are generally diagnosed and treated at a young age.

Disc Displacement Disorders

Note: Another term used in the past to refer to disc displacement disorders was internal derangement, but it is less commonly applied today. Also, clinicians should refrain from perpetuating the lay term "TMJ" when referring to the pathological conditions of the temporomandibular joint (TMJ). Instead, healthcare providers should educate the public that TMJ only refers to the anatomical name of the joint, and the disorders of the joint and related structures are collectively called temporomandibular disorders (TMDs) or TMJ disorders.

In order to understand the disc displacement disorders, a reasonable working knowledge of the anatomy of the TMJ is essential. The TMJ is a synovial joint, which performs both gliding and hinging movements. It is composed of the mandibular fossa (part of the temporal bone), the condyle, and the articular disc. When referring to the TMJ, the term "disc" is preferred to "meniscus". The disc divides the TMJ space into superior and inferior joint compartments, and it is composed of dense fibrous connective tissue (not hyaline cartilage); therefore, it is capable of some degree of self-repair. The discs seat over the condyles, bilaterally, and accompany them during normal jaw movements in the absence of any displacement. The functions of the disc are to: (1) distribute the loading forces (acting as a shock absorber); (2) stabilize condylar movements; and (3) decrease wear and tear of the supporting tissues. The disc is biconcave in shape and is made up of the following: (1) anterior band; (2) intermediate zone; and (3) posterior band. The thickest portion of the posterior band should be positioned directly above the condyle at a 12 o'clock position. Approximately one-third of the general population has a disc, which is not in this position, and this is considered to be a normal variation of anatomical placement. Disc deformation is associated with disc displacement and the direction of the displacement is most commonly anteromedially (Solberg, Hansson, & Nordstrom, 1985). The disc may become displaced due to trauma and by chronic loading forces placed on the disc-condyle complex (e.g., due to bruxism). It is believed that the supporting ligaments attaching the discs to the condyles become torn or overstretched resulting in disc displacement. Once the disc is displaced, it typically does not return to its previous "normal" position due to overstretching and fibrosis of the retro-discal tissues and other supporting structures, particularly once the condition becomes long-standing.

Disc Displacement with Reduction

When the condyle moves forward within the TMJ and seats onto the anteriorly displaced disc, the disc *reduces* or improves its position with respect to the condyle. In anterior disc displacement *with* reduction (ADDR), when disc reduction occurs, a clicking or popping noise is heard. This noise is reproducible during opening and closing movements of the mandible. Soft tissue studies by magnetic resonance imaging (MRI) will reveal that the disc seats onto the condyle during mouth opening and often will reveal a lack of extensive degenerative change in the osseous structures. ADDR may or may not be accompanied by pain; however, mandibular movements will intensify the pain in the presence of inflammation or some degenerative structural changes. The jaw will *deviate* to the side of the disc displacement during mouth opening and then returns to the midline after the condyle seats onto the disc. Normally, a reciprocal clicking will be heard on closing. There is typically no limitation of jaw opening, however, the patient may report episodic catching of the mandible with mouth opening. Generally, jaw sounds without any functional limitation or pain do not warrant treatment, and it should be noted that benign jaw clicking or noises, in the absence of other factors, is not by itself prelude to degenerative joint disease.

Disc Displacement Without Reduction

Without reduction, the anteriorly displaced disc does not seat onto the condyle when moving forward from a closed mouth to an open mouth position. This condition is known as anterior disc displacement *without* reduction (ADDWR). When ADDWR is acute, there is limited mouth opening of ≤ 35 mm with sudden onset. It should be noted that the normal inter-incisal jaw opening range is from 40 to 60 mm. On mouth opening, the jaw *deflects* to the affected side and does not return to the midline at the maximum opening position. There is also limited lateral movement of the jaw to the contralateral side if the ADDWR is unilateral. Soft tissue imaging will reveal a disc that is not seated onto the condyle in an open position and the osseous structures usually reveal an absence of significant osteoarthritic changes. There may be accompanying pain brought on with forced mouth opening, and the patient will typically report that the previously heard "clicking noises" have suddenly ceased since the jaw has "locked". If the patient does not volunteer such information, the clinician should specifically inquire about such pattern or similar history, since it will help with the differential diagnosis. Palpation of the affected joint may produce pain and the patient may experience the sensation that the teeth contact too soon on the ipsilateral side. If the condition does not resolve, it may become chronic (present > 4months). With chronic ADDWR, the pain is typically less than it was in the acute stage and the range of mouth opening may improve but will not return to the previous baseline maximal opening values.

This condition may be confused with the following disorders: Myospasm, osteoarthritis, polyarthritis, fibrotic ankylosis, and neoplasia.

The most important concept for the clinician to remember is that a displacement of the disc does *n*ot require treatment unless one of the following conditions exists: (1) pain; (2) limited mouth opening that interferes with normal functioning; or (3) prolonged and repeated jaw locking episodes. The goal of treatment is to decrease the pain and to improve the range of motion and jaw function. It is important to understand that while the range of mouth opening may not return to the pre-displacement (baseline) position, the patient may be able to function comfortably with only a modest increase in mouth opening as a result of conservative treatment or due to adaptive changes in the disc-condyle complex over time.

Condylar Dislocation

When the condyle translates beyond the articular eminence during mouth opening and cannot return to the closed mouth position, the term dislocation (also "open lock" or subluxation) is used to describe this condition. This situation may occur when the patient yawns, opens maximally, or when prolonged mouth opening is required (e.g., during a dental procedure). The cause may be joint hypermobility with accompanying muscle hyperactivity, which causes the dislocation to be either momentary or prolonged. At the time of dislocation, there may be significant pain, which should subside once the dislocation reduces; however, some mild residual pain may occur.

Dislocation may necessitate intervention by a dentist or other qualified clinician, where gentle pressure is applied in a downward and posterior direction by placing one's thumbs on the patient's posterior molar teeth. If residual pain is present, analgesics will typically provide pain relief. In cases where the dislocation has persisted for hours, secondary muscle splinting can also contribute to the ongoing pain; therefore, muscle relaxants can be beneficial.

Inflammatory Disorders

Inflammation occurring within the TMJ commonly results from bruxism, trauma, systemic conditions (i.e., polyarthritides), and less commonly from infection. It is important to note that clinically one cannot reliably differentiate between synovitis and capsulitis. Inflammation typically presents as localized TMJ pain, which is worsened by jaw function particularly when the joint is loaded in a posterior-superior direction. The radiographs or computed tomography (CT) scan may not reveal extensive degenerative joint changes or arthrosis, except in osteoarthritic and rheumatic conditions. There may be pain at rest, restriction of mouth opening due to pain, and swelling over the TMJ, in the preauricular area. An MRI study may reveal the presence of joint effusion, which can result in a patient's inability to occlude the posterior molar teeth on the affected side.

Ear infection must be ruled out as a source of the localized TMJ pain as well as osteoarthritis, rheumatoid arthritis, psoriatic arthritis, and neoplasia.

Arthritides

Arthritis is a common cause of TMJ pain in elderly patients. Typically, there is pain with jaw movements and tenderness over the TMJ, especially on palpation during arthritic flare-ups. Evidence of degenerative changes (i.e., osteophytosis and erosion) and narrowing of the joint space will be revealed in imaging studies of the TMJ. There may also be crepitus or restricted range of jaw opening on examination.

Polyarthritides, capsulitis, synovitis, and neoplasia may have similar clinical presentations, and further investigation may be required to rule out rheumatic disorders.

Pain relief is typically achieved by the use of analgesics and splint therapy. In addition, the splint should be worn and monitored for changes on the occlusal surface of the appliance at follow-up visits. It is crucial that the dentist determines if stabilization of the condyles has occurred prior to performing expensive, irreversible dental therapies to correct any malocclusion caused by degenerative changes typically resulting in condylar erosion that lead to a loss in the height of the condyle. In the elderly patient, intra-articular steroidal joint injections, in the absence of contraindications, prove to be a safe treatment, but multiple injections in short intervals are contraindicated. In severe erosive conditions, intra-articular injection of hyaluronate sodium (Hyalgan®) may be beneficial in affording relief to the patient by accommodating function. Referral to a rheumatologist is recommended for the definitive diagnosis and management of rheumatoid arthritis, particularly if severe degenerative changes are present.

Ankylosis

Ankylosis is an uncommon condition; however, it can occur as a result of trauma or fracture. Fibrous ankylosis typically occurs when fibrous adhesions form within the superior joint compartment secondary to joint inflammation, trauma, or arthritides. With fibrous ankylosis, there will be limited range of jaw opening and limited lateral movement to the contralateral side, where the mandible will deflect to the affected side on opening. Imaging demonstrates a relatively normal joint space; however, the affected side does not have normal condylar translation. MRI may not always reveal the presence of fibrous ankylosis, therefore, arthroscopic examination of the TMJ may be necessary.

Bony ankylosis typically results from the proliferation of osteoblasts causing the union of the condylar head(s) to the temporal bone. The range of opening is extremely limited if both sides are affected. Unilateral bony ankylosis will also cause deflection to the affected side and limited lateral movement to the contralateral side. Imaging of osseous structures will reveal proliferation of bone, making the joint space indistinguishable, and will reveal the inability of the condyle to translate out of the mandibular fossa.

Ankylosis must be differentiated from ADDWR and myofibrotic contracture. This is usually accomplished by a radiographic study. However, currently only an MRI can reveal the disc itself and not any other type of imaging study. So, a panoramic screening X-ray is adequate to make the diagnosis of ankylosis. Treatment of ankylosis typically involves arthroscopic surgery and possibly open joint surgery followed by physical therapy.

Fracture

Fracture of the mandible, maxilla, temporal bone, or the zygoma may occur with significant facial trauma. The elderly are more prone to falls, and the most common locations of mandibular fractures are subcondylar (29%), followed by the angle (24.5%), and then the symphysis (22%) (Tucker, 1998). Mandibular symphyseal fractures may remain occult on routine imaging and therefore must be ruled out since studies indicate that elderly patients who sustain facial injuries are less likely to recall the event (Wade, Hoffman, & Brennan, 2004)

Myospasm, disc displacement, and ankylosis must be ruled out. At a minimum, diagnostic imaging must include a panoramic radiograph (Panorex) and more extensive radiographic imaging (CT, plain radiography) may be ordered depending on the location and extent of the trauma. The clinical presentation typically involves limitation of mouth opening, limited protrusion, and limited lateral movements to the contralateral side (if unilateral fracture). Surprisingly, the pain may only be mild and the main complaint by the patient may be difficulty in eating, especially hard and chewy foods.

Eagle's Syndrome

Eagle's syndrome (not to be confused with Eagle-Barrett syndrome) is a rare condition but can mimic facial neuralgias, headaches, earaches, and temporomandibular joint disorders (Mendelsohn, Berke, & Chhetri, 2006). The typical age of onset is 30–50 years with a female-to-male predominance of 3:1 and an incidence of 0.16%. The etiology of the elongation of the styloid process remains elusive and a history of recent neck trauma or surgery (i.e., tonsillectomy) may be present or absent. Many patients presenting with calcification or elongation of the stylohyoid process never experience any pain. Patients with Eagle's syndrome may present with dizziness, transient syncope, pain in the throat, dysphagia, headache, otalgia, glossodynia, or neck pain.

Eagle's syndrome has two classic presentations: (1) throat pain that radiates to the ear in a post-tonsillectomy patient; and (2) a constant, throbbing pain following the distribution of the carotid artery (Mendelsohn et al., 2006). Pain may result from stimulation of cranial nerves V, VII, IX, or X by the elongated styloid process thereby producing a broad range of referred pain and varied symptoms. If the styloid process growth deviates laterally and impinges on the external carotid artery, pain may radiate to the face up to the orbital region. When medial deviation and impingement of the internal carotid artery occur, the pain will radiate to the occiput. Head pain associated with Eagle's syndrome is typically a constant, throbbing pain, which must be differentiated from other headaches. The facial pain associated with Eagle's syndrome may present as throbbing or stabbing. Glossopharyngeal neuralgia, trigeminal neuralgia, otic disorders, headaches, TMD, myofascial pain disorder, and neoplasia must be considered in the differential diagnosis.

Rotation of the head, swallowing or yawning can trigger pain and should be tested in the clinical setting. Digital palpation of the tonsillar fossa will reveal a small, bony prominence, which may reproduce the pain. Additionally, a panoramic radiograph, plain X-rays or CT scan of the skull will reveal an elongated, calcified stylohyoid process, which will help to differentiate this condition from other disorders.

Headaches in the Elderly Patient

While primary headaches are less common in the elderly, headache as a symptom still represents a frequently encountered and challenging problem. There are many causes of new-onset headaches in the elderly, some of which can be particularly worrisome. The risk of serious secondary disorders in persons older than 65 years is much higher than in younger persons, and certain "red flags" associated with a headache should alert the clinician to carry out thorough investigation of the headache complaint (Solomon, Kunkel, & Frame, 1990). Such warning signs include a "first-" or "worst headache", paralysis, papilledema, drowsiness, confusion, memory impairment, and loss of consciousness.

The work-up should include the appropriate imaging and laboratory studies, and most importantly the clinician should keep in mind that when dealing with headaches in any patient, especially in the elderly, one should not become too comfortable with the notion of just "making the diagnosis" and selecting a quick "magic bullet". One must realize that the diminished physiological reserve in the older patient produces weakened compensatory mechanisms, which may otherwise allow a disease to present at an earlier and less severe stage. Likewise a weakened compensatory mechanism contributes to a weaker capacity to recover, which necessitates initiating a rapid diagnostic timeline.

Approximately 10–20% of the headaches, especially new-onset cases, seen in the elderly are due to secondary causes (Lipton, Stewart, Diamond, et al., 2001). In a survey of elderly patients over the age of 65 in a residential setting, 4.8% of the new-onset headaches were primary headaches and 66.7% were due to secondary causes (Lyness, Cox, Curry, et al., 1995). The International Headache Society (IHS) classification criteria for the diagnosis of headaches (Olesen, 2004) will be used throughout this chapter, and neuropathic pain disorders will be addressed in the next section.

Migraine

Though migraine seems to diminish in severity and frequency with aging, especially after menopause, a significant number of elderly patients continue to have migraine, and 1–3% of patients experience their first migraine headache after the age of 50 (Silberstein, Lipton, & Sliwinski, 1996). The female-to-male ratio for migraines decline from 3:1 to 2:1 after menopause, and migraine with aura tends to be less prevalent in the elderly. An aura is a transient, stereotypical, visual, or neurological episode usually lasting 4–60 minutes, and it does not occur in all migraine patients.

Migraine is usually, but not always, associated with headache and can be accompanied by systemic and autonomic symptoms. Interestingly, older patients who may have had migraine with aura in younger age may no longer have the headache and only continue to have auras (Cohen, Matharu, & Goadsby, 2004), which present as episodic focal neurological disturbances that often tend to be confused with transient ischemic attacks (TIAs). Though not uncommon, aura without headache in the elderly is usually referred to as a late-life migraine accompaniment and may take the form of the following recurrent symptoms: paresthesias (numbness, tingling, pins-and-needles sensation, or a heavy feeling of an extremity); visual disturbances (transient blindness, homonymous hemianopsia, and blurring of vision); brain stem and cerebellar dysfunction (ataxia, clumsiness, hearing loss, tinnitus, vertigo, and syncope); and disturbances of speech (dysarthria or dysphasia).

Features that help distinguish migraine accompaniments from TIAs include a gradual buildup of sensory symptoms, a march of sensory paresthesias, serial progression from one accompaniment to another, longer duration (most TIAs last for less than 15 minutes), and multiple stereotypical episodes. A careful evaluation is important before initiating treatment of migraine in the elderly. A detailed history of prior migraine attacks, especially during youth if such information is available, must be obtained. The incidence and prevalence of cerebrovascular disease increase with advanced age; therefore, managing the older migraineur requires adequate familiarity with the individual's general health status and the foresight to err on the side of caution. Special problems in the elderly, including various comorbidities may prohibit the use of some migraine medications, and as a general rule, the risk of falls should always be considered before prescribing drugs that produce somnolence, sedation, and dizziness.

Certain medications may exacerbate migraine in elderly patients. For example, vasodilating antihypertensive medications, such as nifedipine and methyldopa, can worsen migraine or lead to an increase in headache frequency. Similarly, nitrates may precipitate an attack of migraine in those who are predisposed. Prophylactic options are limited in the geriatric population because of the likelihood of contraindications and adverse effects, but if the episodes are frequent and the clinician decides to go forward with preventive treatment, the adage "start low and go slow" is particularly appropriate.

Beta-blockers (e.g., propranolol, nadolol, and timolol maleate) may be helpful but are contraindicated with concomitant hypotension, asthma, chronic obstructive pulmonary disease, congestive heart failure, and depression. They can also lead to unacceptable lethargy or confusion. Tricyclic antidepressants (TCAs) are contraindicated with concomitant cardiac dysrhythmia, urinary retention, closed-angle glaucoma, and prostatic enlargement and can result in intolerable sedation, confusion, urinary retention, conduction block, or orthostatic hypotension.

When considering a TCA, nortriptyline and desipramine have fewer anticholinergic properties and are preferable to amitriptyline, if no absolute contraindication exists. The anticonvulsants valproic acid, topiramate, and gabapentin may be useful but can have significant cognitive and other central nervous system side effects (e.g., sedation) and increase the risk of falls. Adjunctive therapy with antiemetics can be particularly helpful; however, the elderly are vulnerable to the sedative and extrapyramidal side effects of antiemetics.

Botulinum toxin (Botox®) type A is a controversial but emerging prophylactic therapy for migraine and may be particularly useful in the geriatric population because of the relative absence of systemic absorption and its safety profile. Nonprescription and herbal alternatives with purported modest efficacy include magnesium, riboflavin, feverfew, butterbur root (*Petasites hybridus*), and coenzyme Q10, but caution should be exercised to minimize drug interactions when recommending alternative remedies.

Tension-Type Headache

Tension-type headache (TTH) is the most common type of headache across all populations, and its prevalence over the lifetime is 69% in men and 88% in women (Rasmussen, 1992). As with other primary headaches, such as migraine, the prevalence of TTH also diminishes in the elderly but to a lesser extent than migraine. The associated pain is described as bilateral, dull aching, and non-throbbing, which can be temporal, frontal, fronto-temporal, occipital, or present in a combination of these locations.

Patients often use the terms "pressure", "tightness", "soreness", or "a tight band around the head" to describe their headache, and unlike migraine, the pain associated with TTH does not seem to be exacerbated by movement. There is usually no phonophobia, photophobia, nausea, or vomiting reported with TTH, but in severe episodes, the patient may experience any of these symptoms, but only one at a time with each headache episode and with milder presentation than those associated with migraines. TTH is divided into episodic and chronic type with each category further subdivided into TTH with- and without pericranial tenderness. As defined by the latest IHS criteria any headache that occurs more than 15 days per month is classified as a chronic headache. The relationship between temporomandibular joint parafunction, craniofacial muscle fatigue, and TTH is under debate. Although, there is not always a correlation between muscle tenderness and the degree of headache, TTH sufferers have more tenderness in their pericranial muscles than do non-sufferers (Langermark & Olesen, 1987).

Hypertension and Cerebrovascular-Associated Headaches

The elderly are prone to hypertension and cerebrovascular disease and both are common causes of new-onset headaches in this population. Headaches may accompany stroke, and patients with a history of recurrent throbbing headaches, especially women, are more likely to have headaches associated with stroke. The quality, onset, and duration of stroke-associated headaches vary widely, and they are equally likely to be abrupt and to be gradual in onset. In patients presenting with what they consider to be the worst headache of their lives, subarachnoid hemorrhage (SAH) should be ruled out. Stroke-associated headaches are usually unilateral, focal, and of mild to moderate severity, and usually less than one half of the patients report an incapacitating headache. The headache may be throbbing or non-throbbing, and in rare cases they may be stabbing. The headache is more often ipsilateral than contralateral to the side of the cerebral ischemia. Headache is more common in ischemia of the posterior circulation than of the anterior circulation. Also, headaches tend to be more commonly associated with cortical events than subcortical events. The headache of longest duration is associated with cardio-embolic and thrombotic infarcts. Usually the headache associated with lacunar infarction is of medium duration, and the shortest headache duration is seen in TIAs.

Temporal Arteritis

Also known as giant cell arteritis, temporal arteritis (TA) is a systemic panarteritis that selectively involves the medium and large arteries of the head and neck. Approximately half of the patients with TA have polymyalgia rheumatica. Headache is the most common symptom of TA, and frequently a throbbing pain is reported in the temporal region unilaterally, but it can also be bilateral. The pain may be intermittent or continuous and is more often severe than moderate or slight. For some patients, the pain may be worse at night when lying on a pillow or while combing the hair or when washing the face.

Typical findings on examination include tender, swollen branches of the external carotid artery (usually the superficial temporal artery). Decreased pulsation of the superficial temporal arteries is present on physical examination in about half of the patients and intermittent jaw claudication occurs in 38% of cases. With claudication, the patient typically reports jaw pain with function only. The diagnosis is based on clinical suspicion but is not always confirmed until further laboratory testing. The three common tests are the Westergren erythrocyte sedimentation rate (ESR), the C-reactive protein (CRP) level (an acute-phase plasma protein from the liver), and temporal artery biopsy. The ESR is usually a good indicator of an inflammatory process, but used alone it is not sensitive for the diagnosis of TA. It is usually necessary to order these tests in combination to make a definitive diagnosis, and the ESR is the first step in the diagnostic work-up. For elderly patients, the ESR range of normal may vary from less than 20 mm/hr–40 mm/hr, but it must be noted that elevation of the ESR is not specific for TA, since an elevated ESR can be seen in any infectious, inflammatory, or rheumatic disease. TA with a normal ESR has been reported in up to one-third of the patients. When abnormal, the ESR averages 70–80 mm/hr and may reach 120 or even 130 mm/hr.

The major concern with temporal arteritis is vision loss, although if allowed to progress, it may affect arteries in other areas of the body. This condition is potentially vision threatening; however, if promptly treated, permanent vision loss can be prevented. Vision is threatened when the inflamed arteries obstruct blood flow and oxygen to the retina and the optic nerve. In patients without any contraindications, treatment of TA is typically started with oral steroids, and the headache will often improve within 24 hours.

Neuropathic Pain Disorders

Neuropathic pain has been traditionally subdivided into three broad categories, which include neuralgias, peripheral neuropathic pain, and central neuropathic pain. In short, neuralgias are mostly due to demyelinating processes, and other neuropathies are due to ectopic discharges or neuroplastic changes that affect the central nervous system (CNS) at the cortical level. Neuropathic orofacial pain is continuous, constant, more persistent, and often presents as aching and/or burning, whereas neuralgias tend to be paroxysmal, lancinating, and electric-shock-like in quality. Theoretically, both peripheral and central neuropathic pain can occur anywhere in the distribution of the trigeminal nerve due to idiopathic causes with no identifiable etiology, such as in atypical odontalgia (a central pain disorder), but peripheral neuropathies, mostly tend to occur in association with orofacial nerve injuries or with post-oral surgical trauma. Given the number of dental procedures performed around the world each day, it is surprising that traumatically induced neuropathies are not more commonplace, perhaps determined by an individual's genetic make up, especially in response to the body's healing capacity and immune response.

In order to clarify any ambiguity, it should be noted that neuropathic conditions could be viewed as a spectrum, where neuralgias may be placed in between peripheral and central neuropathic pain. Furthermore, some conditions may start as peripheral pain but with continued sensitization they can advance to centralized pain disorders. Although not always a definitive test, one of the clinical ways to distinguish whether a chronic pain condition is peripheral or central in nature is to test the patient's response to local anesthetic blockade. If the pain is blockable, it is most likely indicative of a peripheral mechanism, and if the response is negative it is indicative of a centralized pain condition, in the absence of other pathology. The pathophysiology of central pain is attributed to neurophysiological changes in the CNS that will lead to the development of dynamic mechanical allodynia. Generally, centralized pain disorders do not respond to peripheral treatments, such as the application of topical medications, but they do respond to TCAs and anticonvulsant medications. Some peripheral neuropathies may also develop a central component, hence their response to peripheral blockade will not be complete, and the anesthetic test will be equivocal. This may sometimes be observed with a traumatic trigeminal nerve injury or a long-standing case of trigeminal neuralgia (TN), which adds to its already complex clinical presentation.

Trigeminal Neuralgia

Also known by its French name, *tic douloureux* ("painful tic"), as described by André in 1756, TN is a disabling facial pain disorder that was first recognized and reported by the renowned Iranian physician Avicenna (980–1037 C.E.) in Persia. It was not until over a century later that another well-respected Persian physician, Ismail Jurjani (1066–1136 C.E.) became the first to suggest the vascular compression theory of trigeminal neuralgia (Ameli, 1965). However, this excruciating neuropathic facial pain disorder remained virtually untreatable until the 1940s, when serendipitously a group of patients receiving anticonvulsant medications for various seizure disorders, who also suffered from TN, reported attenuation or complete resolution of their facial pain condition. This discovery was a momentous breakthrough in providing relief and hope to patients, who previously had to resort to suicide attempts to rid them of this devastating disease.

It is noteworthy that today the main challenge faced by clinicians in diagnosing TN remains not only the infrequency of encountering this illusive pain disorder, but also the misleading and complex patient history and expression of symptoms that mimic similar patterns seen in other pain conditions. In fact, TN may display characteristics of both acute and chronic pain disorders. Most patients suffering from TN will typically be seen by dentists, internists, otolaryngologists, neurologists, and oral surgeons before a proper diagnosis is reached. All too often before a correct diagnosis is made, the patient will have suffered many unnecessary treatments. Although dental pathology can activate an impending case of TN or exacerbate an existing condition, invariably, a subset of patients especially in the early stages of the disease will be misdiagnosed with dental disorders such as cracked-tooth syndrome (Cameron, 1964) and acute pulpal conditions as the primary cause of their pain, without further investigation or formulation of a reasonable list of differential diagnoses (Merrill & Graff-Radford, 1992) by the respective clinician.

Regrettably, one of the tragic consequences of misdiagnosing TN is serial root canal therapy and/or dental extractions without affording any tangible relief to the patient. Therefore, it is imperative that clinicians request consultations from the appropriate specialists to rule out other possibilities before contemplating heroic attempts that may lead to iatrogenic outcomes.

Another confounding factor that leads to a delayed diagnosis or a misdiagnosis is the phenomenon known as pre-trigeminal neuralgia (PTN), first delineated by Sir Charles Symonds (1949). Presently, there is no classification for PTN by the IHS or the International Association for the Study of Pain (IASP) due to disagreements about its pathophysiology, but it is of tremendous clinical value and of immense benefit to patients that clinicians remain pragmatic and recognize this empirical "intermediate" state. Based on clinical evidence it appears that PTN initially lacks the characteristic stabbing, electric-shock-like pain paroxysms of classical TN (Fromm, Graff-Radford, Terrence, et al., 1990). Whether PTN does not exist as some argue, or whether it is simply a variant of TN is immaterial, and the course of treatment remains the same. The pain responds to anticonvulsant medications and later develops into a definite form of TN. Typically PTN patients describe a dull aching pain that lasts for longer periods of time without presentation of a lancinating pain. Others may report a dull aching background pain with a superimposition of a sharper pain, which may be spontaneous and sometimes mimics the characteristics of referred myofascial pain.

Classical Trigeminal Neuralgia

According to the latest IHS definitions (Olesen, 2004), classical trigeminal neuralgia (IHS 13.1.1) cannot be attributed to a secondary cause or disorder, and the pain is produced by peripheral ephaptic transmissions in demyelinated segments of the trigeminal nerve (CN V). The demyelination is usually the result of vascular compression (Sindou, Howeidy, & Acevedo, 2002) of the nerve root at the dorsal root entry zone caused by the superior cerebellar artery. The causes of vascular compression remain idiopathic, but anatomical variations may predispose the patient to such impingement. There is usually no clinically evident neurological deficit noted, but some patients report subtle reduction in sensation to light touch. The pain onset is sudden, and commonly unilateral. It is described by most patients as brief electric-shock-like, stabbing, intermittent paroxysms of pain in the distribution of one or more branches of CN V. The paroxysms last from seconds up to 2 minutes, followed by a refractory period of a few minutes. These paroxysms can occur many times daily at intervals. Some patients, especially with the presence of frank trigger zones, report that talking, eating, brushing the teeth, washing the face, shaving, and even a light breeze on the face may induce the stabbing pain. Others may report spontaneous pain, and some patients may have both triggered and spontaneous attacks. Pain episodes typically occur for a few weeks to months, followed by a pain-free remission period of months to years. It is seen unilaterally in more than 95% of cases and commonly involves one or two branches with the following order of frequency: V2 > V3 > V1. In rare bilateral cases, the pain is not synchronous with the contralateral side, and it is of relatively rare prevalence. The prevalence of TN in the United States is 3:5 (male-to-female) per 100,000 per year. Age of onset is after the fourth decade, and the peak onset is between the fifth and seventh decades. Onset prior to age 30 is uncommon, and secondary etiologies, such as neoplasia or multiple sclerosis should be suspected, especially in younger females. Diagnosis of TN is by history, signs, symptoms, and by excluding other pathology. A history of recent dental concerns and treatments should be evaluated very closely and communication with other managing clinicians is imperative. Each patient with a diagnosis of TN should undergo magnetic resonance imaging (MRI) with and without contrast, preferably using 3D reconstruction techniques to rule out secondary causes.

Symptomatic Trigeminal Neuralgia

The pain of secondary or symptomatic trigeminal neuralgia (IHS 13.1.2) is indistinguishable from classical TN, but the causative lesion is other than vascular compression and may include neoplastic compression (i.e., acoustic neuroma or cholesteatoma), an aneurysm, or a vascular malformation (Edwards, Clarke, Renowden, et al., 2002). In contrast to classical TN, there may be sensory impairment in the distribution of the affected trigeminal division and other neurological deficits in other cranial nerves may be observed, depending on the location and extent of the causative lesion. Also, unlike the classical form, symptomatic TN does not demonstrate a refractory period between paroxysms.

Trigeminal neuralgia mimics a wide variety of orofacial pain disorders and must be differentiated from other local causes of pain such as dental conditions, sinus disorders, and head and neck neoplasia. After ruling out dental infections and endodontic causes, it is diagnostically useful to try local anesthetic blockade. As in most peripheral pain processes, TN pain is blockable in most cases. Although not an exhaustive list, the differential diagnosis, especially in the elderly should include intracranial lesions (neoplasms and aneurysms), glossopharyngeal neuralgia, jabs and jolts syndrome, nervus intermedius neuralgia, short-lasting unilateral neuralgiform headache attacks with conjunctival injection and tearing (SUNCT), cracked-tooth syndrome, reversible/irreversible pulpitis, trigeminal post-herpetic neuralgia, and giant cell arteritis. The reader must keep in mind not to confuse the terms "trigeminal neuralgia" with "trigeminal nerve disorder", which differ in etiology and pathophysiology. It has become a common mistake to generically take liberty with the term "neuralgia" and to loosely refer to any trigeminal-related pain as "trigeminal neuralgia".

TN is one of the very few chronic neuropathic pain disorders, for which a variety of excellent treatment options are available. As with any other disorder, before choosing a therapeutic method, the goal should be to tailor the treatment to each patient's individual needs, preferences, health status, age, and assessment of the risk-versus-benefits of each option. Of particular interest to the geriatric patient is the general operability, degree of interference of the disease with the individual's activities of daily living (ADL), and the existence of advance directives in patients suffering from dementia.

The pharmacological management of TN is usually the first step in treatment, and anticonvulsants are the drugs of choice. Carbamazepine is commonly used as the first-line medication and remains the only drug that has been subjected to several placebo-controlled trials in large populations (Campbell, Graham, & Zilkha, 1966) over the past few decades. However, other medications are also gaining popularity, especially those that do not routinely require periodic blood tests to monitor for any possible blood dyscrasia as is the case with the use of carbamazepine.

Currently, the most definitive treatment for classical TN is the use of microvascular decompression (MVD) surgical techniques popularized by Jannetta (1997). Studies show that at 1–2 year post-MVD, 75–80% and at 8–10 years, 58–64% of patients remain pain-free, and 4–12% suffer minor recurrences (Barker, Jannetta, Bissonette, et al., 1996). Elderly patients tolerate MVD well, provided there is no contraindication to general anesthesia and the patient is in reasonable health (Javadpour, Eldridge, Varma, et al., 2003). The present view is to operate earlier in the process, once a definitive diagnosis of classical TN has been made. This recommendation differs from the past when surgery was only used as last resort due to failure of pharmacological management (Nurmikko & Jensen, 2006). It is believed that unless there is an absolute contraindication to a patient undergoing surgery, depending on the individual's health condition and age-related risk factors, surgery should be attempted after a relatively short pharmacological treatment. The current argument is based on findings that indicate delaying surgery can increase the risk of developing other neuropathies that can become refractory to treatment (Nurmikko, 2003).

Another fairly successful and viable alternative to MVD for high-risk patients, and those who prefer a non-invasive approach, is the gamma knife radiosurgery, which is gaining more popularity as stereotactic techniques improve and the success rates increase. However, current studies demonstrate a higher success rate with MVD than with the gamma knife procedure (Brisman, 2006). Other treatment options include neurodestructive techniques, such as cryosurgery, neurectomy, gangliolysis, and radiofrequency ablation. In general, the aforementioned procedures should be used on a case-by-case basis since they provide only temporary relief, and in most cases pain recurs within a few years, where 40–50% of patients experience a recurrence in 36 months (Lopez, Hamlyn, & Zakrzewska, 2004). These procedures are also associated with the risk of post-treatment dysesthesias (Peters & Nurmikko, 2002), such as the development of *anesthesia dolorosa*, which is defined as a central pain condition characterized by persistent pain and dysesthesia in an area of nerve deafferentation that is simultaneously anesthetic.

Glossopharyngeal Neuralgia

Similar in characteristics to TN, glossopharyngeal neuralgia is a disorder present in the distribution of the ninth cranial nerve (CN IX) and may be present in the distribution of the auricular and pharyngeal branches of the tenth cranial nerve (CN X). Patients experience transient severe stabbing pain in the ear (otic variety), in the base of the tongue, in the tonsillar fossa, or beneath the angle of the mandible.

Swallowing, stimulation of the back of the throat, coughing, and talking are the most common triggers, with periods of remission and relapse similar to TN. In addition to sharp pains, clicking and scratching, or a foreign body sensation in the throat are reported. The pain is strictly unilateral, extremely intense, stabbing, or burning, which interferes with eating. It has also been reported that syncope may be associated with attacks of pain in 2% of the patients (Bruyn, 1983). This phenomenon may be explained by the fact that CN IX is a mixed nerve containing motor, somatosensory, visceral sensory, and parasympathetic fibers. It also communicates with the sympathetic trunk of CN X. Consequently, the connections between somatic and autonomic medullary nuclei and between visceral afferents of the two nerves may provide the anatomical explanation for the syncopal episodes observed in some patients. Glossopharyngeal neuralgia is an uncommon disorder with an incidence of 0.5 persons per 100,000 per year in the United States. It is more commonly seen in people 50 years or older (57%), but oddly 43% of the cases are reported in patients between the ages of 18 and 50 (Olesen, 2004).

Also like TN, glossopharyngeal neuralgia is subclassified into classical (13.2.1) and symptomatic (13.2.2) forms. The list of pathologic conditions affecting CN IX, including vascular compression is similar to those affecting CN V. An additional disease that needs to be ruled out is sino-oropharyngeal carcinoma, which may produce similar pain in the same region. Therefore, consultation with an otolaryngologist is necessary. As with TN, the diagnosis of glossopharyngeal neuralgia is primarily based on history. When formulating a differential diagnosis, it must be borne in mind that communication between CN IX and CN X can cause severe bradycardia, sick sinus syndrome, or asystole; therefore, glossopharyngeal neuralgia must be differentiated from primary dysrhythmias and carotid sinus syndrome, which is also marked by asystole (Merrill, 2006). Generally, if the syncopal episodes consistently follow the neuralgic episodes, then it is more likely that the etiology of the vasomotor activity is due to neural convergence of glossopharyngeal neuralgia rather than other primary vasomotor phenomena. One must also rule out TN of the third division and Eagle's Syndrome, which is similarly characterized by pain on swallowing, secondary to impingement of a calcified stylohyoid ligament.

Nervus Intermedius Neuralgia

Characterized by neuralgic-type paroxysms of sudden, severe, momentary stabbing pain felt in the auditory canal, nervus intermedius neuralgia is a rare nerve disorder with an onset between the fifth and seventh decades, with a prevalence of 0.03 per 100,000 per year in the United States. The male-to-female ratio is equal. Referred pain to deep facial structures and posterior pharynx may accompany the paroxysms. Other reported symptoms during attacks include rhinorrhea, salivation, tinnitus, and vertigo. It should be noted that the intermedius nerve forms a small sensory branch of the seventh cranial nerve (CN VII), and both visceral afferents and somatic sensory fibers travel proximally to reach the trigeminal nucleus and *nucleus solitarius*. The cell bodies of the sensory afferents are located in the geniculate ganglion, and their peripheral axons reach the skin in the external auditory meatus, but there is no direct evidence implicating either the intermedius nerve or the geniculate ganglion as the causative source of this neuralgia. Therefore, some controversy surrounds the actual origin of this neuralgic pain disorder. Compression of the eighth cranial nerve (CN VIII) has also been associated with nervus intermedius neuralgia, and some have even suggested that nervus intermedius neuralgia may be an otic variant of glossopharyngeal neuralgia (Bruyn, 1983), or associated with herpetic inflammation (Hunt, 1907).

The clinical diagnosis of nervus intermedius neuralgia is almost entirely based on the pain description and by ruling out otolaryngological and other neurological disorders, such as glossopharyngeal neuralgia, TN, and geniculate neuralgia (Ramsay Hunt syndrome). The current IHS classification has set out diagnostic criteria for nervus intermedius neuralgia, which require the presence of both paroxysmal pain and a trigger area in the posterior wall of the auditory canal. This pain should also be differentiated from the ice-pick-like pain of migraine, which similarly manifests as repetitive lancinating deep ear pain, as reported by some migraineurs (Raskin & Schwartz, 1980). Because of the presence of autonomic features, such as rhinorrhea in some patients, cluster headache should also be considered in the differential diagnosis.

Pharmacotherapy, similar to treating other neuralgias is recommended, and based on the controversies that exist as to the exact etiology of nervus intermedius neuralgia, surgical management should be considered as a last option. It is noteworthy that based on the original hypotheses about the pathophysiology of this rare neuralgic disorder, some surgeons have performed neurodestructive procedures with only moderate success, and argue that due to significant overlap in sensory innervation in the region, single nerve approaches have not yielded good results (Lovely & Jannetta, 1997).

Post-herpetic Neuralgia

Acute herpes zoster (HZ) is a neurocutaneous reactivation disease, occurring only in those previously infected with the varicella-zoster virus (VZV). Viral inflammation of the root ganglion that preferentially destroys large myelinated nerve fibers in the respective distribution of the infected nerve (Scadding, 1994) is responsible for the pain sequelae of HZ. The pain of acute HZ precedes the onset of herpetic eruption by a few days (preherpetic neuralgia), and the acute state may be marked by general malaise, fever, and sometimes headaches. For poorly understood reasons, long after the vesicular eruption of acute HZ has healed, neuralgic pain continues in a condition known as post-herpetic neuralgia (PHN) in the affected dermatome with variations in the pain quality, which somewhat differs from that in HZ. Thirteen percent of the cases involve the trigeminal nerve and 80% of the trigeminal cases involve the ophthalmic division. The disease affects between one and three people per 1000 population per year and can affect any age group, but it is more frequently seen in the elderly and the immunocompromised individuals. Almost all persons older than 65 years of age have been previously infected with VZV. About 16% of patients continue to have pain at 6 months after the acute onset of HZ, and between 5 and 10% of patients still have pain at 12 months (Johnson, 2001). More than 60% of patients over the age of 60 develop pain, and approximately 50% suffer pain lasting 1 year or more (Watson, Evans, Watt, 1988).

The appearance of the herpetic vesicular eruptions in the distribution of the trigeminal branch (usually ophthalmic), history of burning pain in the perieruptive stage, and elevated protein level and pleocytosis in the spinal fluid are pathognomonic of HZ. Although the diagnosis of acute HZ and PHN is fairly straightforward and characteristic, there are subtle differences in pain quality between the two. In HZ the pain is usually reported as burning and tingling with occasional lancinating components felt in the skin. In PHN, pain persists after 3 months and the pain quality is typical of neuralgic disorders. It is characterized by constant burning and aching with frank superimposition of jabs of shooting or lancinating pain. There may be lacrimation (when involving the ophthalmic branch of CN V), itching and crawling dysesthesias in the skin of the affected dermatome. The area may be hypoesthetic but may involve zones of hyperesthesia characterized by attacks of pain, triggered by light mechanical contact.

In elderly patients, the clinician should consider the possibility of immunosuppression as a precipitating factor in the occurrence of this disease and take the necessary precautions when initiating care. The mainstay of treatment of HZ has become the administration of oral antiviral agents such as acyclovir, famciclovir, and valacyclovir within the first 72 hours after the onset of rash. The duration of the PHN is decreased by as much as 50% with antiviral therapy. Although steroids may improve acute pain, they do not decrease the incidence of PHN. A newer agent, brivudine has proved superior to acyclovir in reducing the period of new blister formation and shortening the period of acute pain (Rabasseda, 2003), but it is not currently available in the United States. Traditionally, for the treatment of PHN, tricyclic antidepressants (TCA) have been most widely used, but unfortunately this class of drugs may be contraindicated in the treatment of many geriatric patients due to numerous anticholinergic adverse effects. Gabapentin has emerged as an effective agent (Rice & Maton, 2001), which is now favored for use as the first-line pharmacotherapeutic agent in the elderly. In younger patients a combination of TCAs and gabapentin may also be used. Topical capsaicin provides improvement in pain in 15–30% of the patients and the odds ratio for pain relief is 0.29 (Volmink, Lancaster Gray, et al., 1996).

References

Ameli, N. O. (1965). Avicenna and trigeminal neuralgia. *Journal of Neurological Sciences, 2*(2), 105–107.

Barker F. G., Jannetta P. J., Bissonette D. J., Larkins, M. V., Jho, H. D. (1996). The long-term outcome of microvascular decompression for trigeminal neuralgia. *New England Journal of Medicine, 334*(17), 1077–1083.

Brisman, R. (2006). Microvascular decompression vs. gamma knife radiosurgery for typical trigeminal neuralgia: Preliminary findings. *Stereotactic Functional Neurosurgery, 85*(2–3), 94–98.

Bruyn, G. W. (1983). Glossopharyngeal neuralgia. *Cephalalgia, 3*(3), 143–157.

Cameron, C. (1964). Cracked tooth syndrome. *Journal of the American Dental Association, 68*, 405–411.

Campbell, F. G., Graham, J. G., & Zilkha, K. J. (1966). Clinical trial of carbamazepine (Tegretol) in trigeminal neuralgia. *Journal of Neurology, Neurosurgery and Psychiatry, 29*(3), 265–267.

Clark, G. T., Minakuchi, H., & Lotaif, A. C. (2005). Orofacial pain and sensory disorders in the elderly. *Dental Clinics of North America, 49*(2), 343–362.

Cohen, A. S., Matharu, M. S., Goadsby, P. J. (2004). SUNCT syndrome in the elderly. *Cephalalgia, 24*, 508–509.

Edwards, R. J., Clarke, Y., Renowden, S. A., Coakham, H. B., et al. (2002). Trigeminal neuralgia caused by microarteriovenous malformations of the trigeminal nerve root entry zone. *Journal of Neurosurgery, 97*(4), 874–880.

Fromm, G. H., Graff-Radford, S. B., Terrence, C. F., Sweet, W. H., et al. (1990). Pre-trigeminal neuralgia. *Neurology, 40*(10), 1493–1495.

Hunt, J. R. (1907). On herpetic inflammations of the geniculate ganglion: A new syndrome and its complications. *Journal of Nervous and Mental Disorders, 34*, 73–96.

Jannetta, P. J. (1997). Outcome after microvascular decompression for typical trigeminal neuralgia, hemifacial spasm, tinnitus, disabling vertigo and glossopharyngeal neuralgia. *Clinical Neurosurgery, 43*, 331–383.

Javadpour, M., Eldridge, P. R., Varma, T. R. K., Miles, J. B., Nurmikko, T. J., et al. (2003). Microvascular decompression for trigeminal neuralgia in patients over 70 years of age. *Neurology, 60*(3), 520.

Johnson, R. W. (2001). Herpes zoster—predicting and minimizing the impact of post-herpetic neuralgia. *Journal of Antimicrobial Chemotherapy, 47*(Topic T1), 1–8.

Kreiner, M., Betancor, E., & Clark, G.T. (2001). Occlusal stabilization appliances: Evidence of their efficacy. *Journal of the American Dental Association, 132*, 770–777.

Langermark, M., & Olesen, J. (1987). Pericranial tenderness in tension-type headache. *Cephalalgia, 7*, 249–255.

Lipton, R.B., Stewart, W.F., Diamond, S., & Reed, M. (2001). Prevalence and burden of migraine in the United States: Data from the American Migraine Study II. *Headache, 41*, 646–657.

Lopez, B. C., Hamlyn, P. J., & Zakrzewska, J. M. (2004). Systematic review of ablative neurosurgical techniques for the treatment of trigeminal neuralgia. *Neurosurgery, 54*, 973–983.

Lotaif, A. C., Mitrirattanakul, S., & Clark, G. T. (2006). Orofacial muscle pain: New advances in concept and therapy. *Journal of the California Dental Association, 34*(8), 625–630.

Lovely, T., & Jannetta, P. J. (1997). Surgical management of geniculate neuralgia. *American Journal of Otolaryngology, 18*(4), 512–517.

Lyness, J. M., Cox, C., Curry, J., Conwell, Y., King, D. A., Caine, E. D., et al. (1995). Older age and the underreporting of depressive symptoms. *Journal of the American Geriatric Society, 43*, 216–221.

Maekawa, K., Clark, G.T., & Kuboki, T. (2002). Intramuscular hypoperfusion, adrenergic receptors, and chronic muscle pain. *Journal of Pain, 3*(4), 251–260.

Mendelsohn, A.H., Berke, G.S., & Chhetri, D.K. (2006). Heterogeneity in the clinical presentation of Eagle's Syndrome. *Otolaryngology – Head and Neck Surgery, 134*(3), 389–393.

Merrill, R. L. (2006). Differential diagnosis of orofacial pain. In D. M. Laskin, S. C. Green, & W. L. Hylander (Eds.), *TMDs: An evidence based approach to diagnosis and treatment* (pp. 299–317). Chicago, IL: Quintessence Publishing Company.

Merrill, R. L., & Graff-Radford, S. B. (1992). Trigeminal neuralgia: How to rule out the wrong treatment. *Journal of the American Dental Association, 123*(2), 63–68.

Nurmikko, T. J. (2003). Recent advances in the diagnosis and treatment of trigeminal neuralgia. *International Journal of Pain Medicine and Palliative Care, 3*, 2–11.

Nurmikko, T. J., & Jensen, T. S. (2006). Trigeminal neuralgia and other facial neuralgias. In J. Olesen, P. J. Goadsby, & N. M. Ramadan (Eds.), *The Headaches* (3rd ed. pp. 1053–1062). Philadelphia, PA: Lippincott, Williams, & Wilkins.

Okeson, J. P. (Ed.). (1996). *Orofacial pain: Guidelines for assessment, diagnosis, and management* (pp. 128–184). Carol Stream, IL: Quintessence Publishing Company.

Olesen, J. (Ed.). (2004). The international classification of headache disorders, 2nd ed. *Cephalalgia, 24*(Suppl. 1), 1–150.

Peters, G., Nurmikko, T. J. (2002). Peripheral and gasserian ganglion-level procedures for the treatment of trigeminal neuralgia. *Clinical Journal of Pain, 18*(1), 28–34.

Rabasseda, X. (2003). Brivudine: A herpes virostatic with rapid antiviral activity and once-daily dosing. *Drugs Today* (Barcelona), *39*(5), 359–371.

Ram, S., Kumar, S. K. S., & Clark, G. T. (2006). Using oral medications, infusions and injections for differential diagnosis of orofacial pain. *Journal of the California Dental Association, 34*(8), 645–654.

Raskin, N. H., & Schwartz, R. K. (1980). Ice-pick-like pain. *Neurology, 30*(2), 203–205.

Rasmussen, B. K. (1992). Migraine and tension-type headache in a general population: Psychosocial factors. *International Journal of Epidemiology, 21*(6), 1138–1143.

Rice, A. S., & Maton, A. (2001). Gabapentin in postherpetic neuralgia: A randomized, double-blind, placebo controlled study. *Pain, 94*(2), 215–224.

Scadding, J. W. (1994). Peripheral neuropathies. In P. D. Wall, & R. Melzak (Eds.), *Textbook of Pain* (pp. 667–683). New York: Churchill Livingstone.

Silberstein, S. D., Lipton, R. B., & Sliwinski, M. (1996).Classification of daily and near-daily headaches: Field trial of revised IHS criteria. *Neurology, 47*(4), 871–875.

Sindou, M., Howeidy, T., & Acevedo, G. (2002). Anatomical observations during microvascular decompression for idiopathic trigeminal neuralgia. *Acta Neurochirugica* (Wien), *144*(1), 1–12.

Solberg, W. K., Hansson, T. L., & Nordstrom, B. (1985). The temporomandibular joint in young adults at autopsy: A morphologic classification and evaluation. *Journal of Oral Rehabilitation, 12*(4), 303–321.

Solomon, G.D., Kunkel, R.S., & Frame, J. (1990). Demographics of headaches in elderly patients. *Headache, 30*, 273–276.

Symonds, S. C. (1949). Facial pain. *Annals of the Royal College of Surgeons of England, 4*, 206–212.

Tucker, M. R. (1998). Management of facial fractures. In L. J. Peterson, E. Ellis, J. R. Hupp, et al. (Eds.), *Contemporary oral & maxillofacial surgery* (pp.587–611). St. Louis, MO: Mosby.

Travell, J. G., & Simons, D. G. (1983). *Myofascial pain and dysfunction: The trigger point manual; the upper extremities* (Vol. 1). Baltimore, MD: Williams & Wilkins.

Volmink, J., Lancaster T., Gray, S., Silagy, C., et al. (1996). Treatments for postherpetic neuralgia—a systematic review of randomized controlled trial.*Family Practice, 13*(1), 84–91.

Wade, C. V., Hoffman, G. R., Brennan, P. A. (2004). Falls in the elderly people that result in facial injuries. *British Journal of Oral and Maxillofacial Surgery, 42*(2), 138–141.

Watanabe, T., Ichikawa, K., & Clark, G. T. (2003). Bruxism levels and daily behaviors: 3 weeks of measurement and correlation. *Journal of Orofacial Pain, 17*(1), 65–73.

Watson, C. P., Evans, R. J., Watt, & V. R. (1988). Post-herpetic neuralgia and topical capsaicin. *Pain, 33*(3), 333–340.

Chapter 18
Oral Pathology Affecting Older Adults

David J. Zegarelli, Victoria L. Woo, and Angela J. Yoon

Preface to Chapter on Oral Pathology and Oral Cancer

For many, the primary concern regarding oral health care does not reach further than their dentition. However, in this chapter we will omit the dentition and we will focus instead on the oral soft tissues, the mucosa and submucosa. These soft tissues, unlike teeth, are quite cellular and disturbances in cells can give rise to very serious disease. Two of the illnesses described in this chapter are potentially fatal (squamous cell carcinoma and pemphigus vulgaris). Other illnesses are painful, chronic, benign but "incurable", and thus worrisome to those patients who are afflicted.

Prior to a discussion of oral mucosal disease in older patients, it is necessary to review the clinical appearance of a normal healthy mouth. Afterward, we will be able to understand disease better for we have a basis to compare with the norm. Healthy oral soft tissues are pink in color. Some dark-skinned individuals will have irregularly sized and shaped asymptomatic flat brown patches reflecting racial pigmentation. These melanotic spots are normal and do not reflect pathology. Most people have bilateral blue lines on the ventral tongue surface, this being a reflection of normal anatomy: the lingual veins. Many healthy people have a slightly white palate, which is normally flat and symptom-free, reflecting a slightly thickened keratotic surface that effectively blocks out the underlying vasculature. Some people present with multiple tiny ectopic skin sebaceous glands referred to as Fordyce spots; they are yellow-orange in color and are commonly found on the buccal mucosae. Of course, normal mouths are wet. They may even appear to the patient as being mucusy or "slimey", simply a manifestation of normal saliva production and secretion. Unfortunately, some patients think one or more of these phenomena as being abnormal, a form of pathology. Also, a normal healthy mouth is symptom-free, the patient should not feel pain and or paresthesia. Lastly, what is a mucosal surface? The authors use a definition that a mucosal surface is a

D.J. Zegarelli
Columbia University College of Dental Medicine, Department of Pathology, 630 West 168th Street, New York, 10032, USA, Tel: 212-305-4599, Fax: 212-305-5958
e-mail: djz1@columbia.edu

I.B. Lamster, M.E. Northridge (eds.), *Improving Oral Health for the Elderly*,
© Springer Science+Business Media, LLC 2008

normal anatomic site that leads from the inside of the body to the external body surface. Thus, all anatomic internal surfaces from the mouth to the rectum have a mucosal surface. These include the inner surfaces of the esophagus, stomach, small intestine, large intestine, appendix, as well as the internal linings of the urinary bladder, ureters, and urethra. An important point is that all oral anatomic sites are covered by a mucosal surface whether they be tongue, buccal mucosa, palate, mouth floor, or gingiva. Finally, anatomically the oral mucosa is covered everywhere by stratified squamous epithelium. Thus, the diseases covered in this chapter are simply alterations of this epithelium or, stated differently, alterations of the mucosal surface.

With this background information, we will cover the most important illnesses that occur in mouths of older patients. There are many oral diseases found in this population, but there is a subgroup of seven that encompasses approximately 90% of patients commonly encountered in a clinical oral pathology practice. They include the malignancy squamous cell carcinoma and its precursor epithelial dysplasia, the superficial fungal infection candidiasis, three dermatoses – lichen planus, mucosal pemphigoid, and pemphigus vulgaris, a symptom complex known as burning mouth syndrome, and a dry mouth having the synonym "xerostomia". This chapter concludes with laboratory testing. And since the biopsy procedure is frequently advocated in this chapter, it will be described in detail at that time.

Squamous Cell Carcinoma

Squamous cell carcinoma (SCC) is the most common oral malignancy. It accounts, varying from one investigative study to another, for between 70% and 90% of all oral cancers (Neville et al., 2002a; Neville and Day, 2002). It should be relatively easy to detect and diagnose, for it occurs on the mouth surface in plain view of the examining clinician. A routine oral examination with mouth mirror and gauze should be sufficient for its detection. In a mucosal surface location, it is unnecessary to utilize sophisticated internal imaging (CT scans, MRI) for its detection. There are characteristic background features that frequently accompany this potentially fatal disease (Choi and Kahyo, 1991; Cowan et al., 2001; Gupta et al., 1980; McDowell, 2006; Neville et al., 2002a; Neville and Day, 2002). First, most oral SCC patients are over 50 years of age. Secondly, there is a male predilection. Thirdly, many patients with this illness are or had been smokers, possibly heavy alcohol consumers as well. Lastly, although SCC can be found on any surface site, there is a definite predilection for lateral tongue surfaces and anterior mouth floor. In its early premalignant phases (known as epithelial dysplasia and graded microscopically as being mild, moderate, severe, and carcinoma in situ), it is usually red or white or red and white in color (Fig. 18.1). Experienced clinicians often describe it then as having a red/white dotted pebbly appearance. Often it is flat or only slightly raised. Besides color changes from normal pink to red and white, there are certain

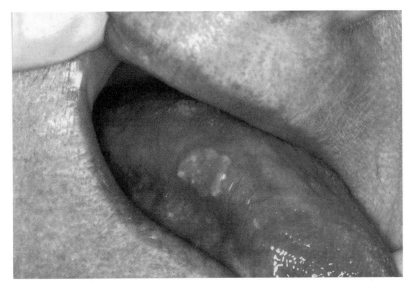

Fig. 18.1 This is a 65-year-old white female with a one-pack-per-day cigarette habit for more than 40 years. She has this adherent flat white patch of the lateral tongue surface. It was firm and tender upon palpation. Biopsy revealed carcinoma in situ (*See* Color Plate 13)

subjective changes as well. With digital pressure, the patient will usually complain of some discomfort or frank pain, and the clinician will feel that the lesion is firmer than adjacent normal tissues (Neville et al., 2002a; Sciubba, 2000; Sciubba, 2001). However, if the SCC is detected in an advanced stage, the tumor presents as a mass. Then, there is obvious bulky tissue protruding from the mucosal surface (Fig. 18.2). Here, the tumor is not difficult for either the patient or the doctor to detect. Most likely, it would be indurated and painful, particularly when palpated. Treatment commences (Neville et al., 2002a; Sciubba, 2000) with biopsy confirmation. Prior to definitive ablative procedures, a biopsy must be performed to verify that the suspicious lesion is indeed SCC. Although it is not this article's intention to deliver a treatise on squamous cell cancer therapy, suffice it to say that most tumors are treated surgically, and often there is a requirement for radiation therapy and/or chemotherapy as well. These treatment options are determined by an oncologist. Overall 5-year survival rates average 50% (Howaldt et al., 1999; Sciubba, 2001). If detected at a very early stage when the tumor is less than 2.0 cm in greatest dimension and there is no evidence of regional or distant metastases, the survival rate may be as high as 90%. On the other hand, if detected at a much later stage, the primary lesion being very large orally with distant metastases, the survival rate can be as low as 10%. There is a final important concept. If a patient presents with a visually and symptomatic suspicious lesion and the background data do not conform to established SCC data (the patient is female, less than 50 years old, a non-smoker), do not assume the lesion is not cancer. Perform a biopsy for definitive diagnosis.

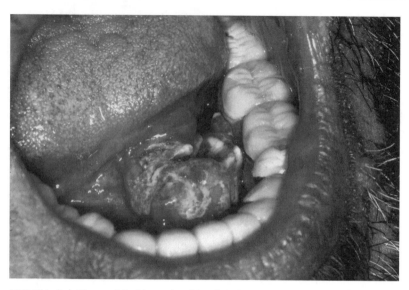

Fig. 18.2 This is a 48-year-old white male with a five-cigar-per-day tobacco habit. He presented initially with this large firm-fixed painful mass of the anterior floor of mouth. Biopsy revealed squamous cell carcinoma. Despite treatment, he died of disease 6 months after initial biopsy procedures (*See* Color Plate 14)

Other Oral Malignancies

As mentioned in the previous paragraph, most but not all oral cancers are surface squamous cell carcinomas. The malignant tumors comprising the remaining 10%–30% will be either primary oral cancers or metastatic tumors originating in non-oral sites (Neville et al., 2002a). These latter tumors manifest orally when they metastasize to the mouth from a non-oral site such as prostate, breast, lung, or skin. They do so by piercing the body's lymph and venous vessels at the primary organ site. When spreading to oral tissues, these metastatic tumors are frequently deposited in the posterior mandible (Neville et al., 2002a). Within a relatively short time period, the tumor cells proliferate to form an intraosseous mass that eventually causes jaw expansion, pain, and/or paresthesia.

The metastasis can so destroy adjacent bone and tooth structures to cause tooth mobility and malocclusion. When metastasizing to oral soft tissue sites, metastatic oral cancers prefer the gingival mucosa overlying jawbone. Whether metastasizing to gingiva or mandible, long-term prognosis is generally dismal since the tumor has already pierced the vasculature and spread internally. Additional primary oral malignancies include fibrosarcoma, leiomyosarcoma, liposarcoma, chondrosarcoma, and osteosarcoma. The large variety of tumor types simply reflects the normal cellular composition of oral mucosa, submucosa, and the jaws; all normal anatomic cell types have a potential to become malignant. Normal oral anatomy also includes salivary glands. Malignant salivary gland tumors can form as well, particularly in the palate and buccal mucosa. The more common salivary malignancies in the palate, buccal mucosa, and the major salivary glands include the malignant-mixed tumor, the mucoepidermoid carcinoma, the adenoid cystic carcinoma, and the polymorphous low-grade adenocarcinoma. All of these primary and metastatic tumors unlike the surface SCC are subsurface in origin. They can present anywhere orally as a rapidly growing subsurface nodule that eventually ulcerates, becomes painful, and subsequently fixed to adjacent normal tissues. Regardless of tissue type, anatomic location, or prevailing clinical pattern, biopsy confirmation is necessary prior to definitive treatment.

Candidiasis

This surface fungal infection has a variety of synonyms used simultaneously by health professionals and the lay public. It is called moniliasis, thrush, and perleche. When occurring at mouth corners, it is referred to as angular cheilitis, if on the mid-dorsal tongue surface, it is called median rhomboid glossitis. The most common candidal pathogen causing this mucosal infection is *Candida albicans* (Fotos et al., 1992). Its relatively high infectivity rate within the much larger candidal microbe group is most likely a reflection of its ability to adhere to oral mucosa. Presently, candidiasis is one of the most common diseases in an oral medicine and clinical oral pathology practice, hence its placement immediately after oral cancer. This microbe is ubiquitous, but as a pathogen has low virulence. It causes oral infection in those individuals who are systemically or locally compromised (Epstein and Polsky, 1998; Sherman et al., 2002). Compromises can be obvious as in uncontrolled diabetes mellitus, severe anemic conditions, generalized debilitation from malignant disease, HIV infection or as subtle as steroid rinses for canker sores, affected mucosa beneath a removable denture, or habitual use of xerostomic agents such as lithium (for depression). Patients receiving antibacterial antibiotic therapy for seemingly unrelated illnesses such as cystitis have been known to acquire oral candidiasis when oral bacterial microbes have also been affected by the antibiotic. Although candidiasis can be found at any age, it is generally senior citizens who are infected because they are more likely to have one or more of the many possible systemic and local compromising factors. In summary, acquiring infection can be as simple as a medical compromise combined with the microbe's ubiquitous nature. Clinically (Fotos and Lilly, 1996; Sherman et al., 2002), candidiasis presents with characteristic features. The oral mucosa will have one or more soft flat red patchy sites, each site often several square centimeters in size. In severe cases, the entire mouth may be red. When affecting the dorsal tongue, the filiform papillae can be destroyed leaving a flat bald red appearance (Fig. 18.3). Simultaneously, the microbes may aggregate as small moveable white plaques known as "milk curds" (Fig. 18.4). There are oral anatomic sites of candidal preference. They include the dorsal tongue and palate. The dorsal tongue prevails due to its irregular papillary surface allowing the candidal microbes a multitude of places to lodge. The palate predominates due to its resting status against the tongue dorsum and due

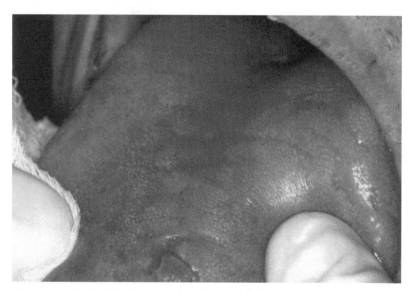

Fig. 18.3 This is a 73-year-old white male complaining of a burning tongue. Note the atrophic red dorsal tongue surface with an ulcerative lesion at the inferior margin. A fungal culture was vividly positive in one week's time (candidiasis). The tongue appearance reversed itself to normal after one week of antifungal therapy (*See* Color Plate 15)

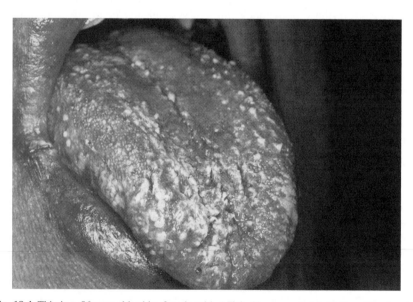

Fig. 18.4 This is a 56-year-old white female with AIDS. She presented initially with a burning mouth and these moveable white "milk curds" of candidal microbes. A fungal culture was very positive in one week's time (candidiasis), and she improved dramatically with antifungal therapy (*See* Color Plate 16)

to its frequent use as a surface beneath an upper denture where again the microbe can lodge and be protected. A variety of clinical names have been applied to these candidal forms. If a mouth is infected in red patchy sites only, it is referred to as acute atrophic candidiasis. If infected in a red patchy pattern having white milk curds, it is called acute pseudomembranous candidiasis. Red patches of candida beneath an upper denture are referred to as chronic atrophic candidiasis (denture stomatitis). If chronic candidal infections yield a white adherent lesion, a form of leucoplakia, it is called chronic hypertrophic candidiasis. Infection at mouth corners is known as angular cheilitis, and a symmetric candidal infection of the mid-tongue dorsum is referred to as median rhomboid glossitis. Symptomatically, some patients are completely pain-free. However, candidal-infected patients frequently complain of oral burning or mouth sensitivity. Further questioning usually leads the patient to state that with consumption of warm or spicy foods their mouths feel as if they were "hot", "scorched", or "burned". Candidal laboratory corroboration (Fotos and Lilly, 1996; Sherman et al., 2002) is managed in several ways. First, many clinicians do not use laboratory testing; they simply diagnose and treat on the basis of clinical appearance, symptoms, and medical history. Some doctors swab an infected site and attempt fungal growth on Sabouraud's medium. Since the microbe grows slowly in culture, this procedure may take 14 days. It is also important to note that since the candidal microbe is ubiquitous, merely finding it on culture may not verify disease. Many normal mouths carry the microbe as well. Microscopic corroboration can be done in three ways. Dermatologists frequently use the KOH prep. Here, a live smear of the suspected infection is studied immediately via the use of an office microscope. Secondly, a smear can be taken, fixed in alcohol, and stained with PAS (Periodic Acid Schiff). The stained smear is then scanned for fungal microbes. Lastly, some candidal-infected mouths are biopsied, particularly the leucoplakic-appearing lesions of chronic hypertrophic candidiasis. When the microbe is detected on mucosal biopsy and seen to be invading the squamous epithelium, disease is verified. This is a very sensitive diagnostic test for it captures the microbe invading the patient. Since the leucoplakic pattern of candidiasis is rather infrequent relative to the other candidal forms, biopsy corroboration is not used very often. Therapeutically (Allen, 1992; Blomgren et al., 1998), there are numerous antifungal agents available. Most patients are treated with mycostatin (nystatin) or an azole antifungal. Nystatin is effective and safe. However, patient compliance may be compromised due to its inconvenience. Oral nystatin is a bottled liquid to be used 4–5 times a day. The patient is directed to rinse and expectorate one teaspoon, after each meal and at bedtime, 2 minutes each time. The azole antifungal medications include clotrimazole (mycelex), ketoconazole (nizoral), and fluconazole (diflucan). Mycelex is a topical medication in lozenge form. Nizoral and diflucan are swallowed. The azoles are more effective than nystatin, but their use may be complicated by potential liver toxicity and drug interactions. This is particularly true for ketoconazole and fluconazole. Most investigators state that oral candidiasis should be treated for a minimum of two to three weeks (Blomgren et al., 1998). Lastly, candidal infections can be problematic regarding recurrence. Many patients who are severely medically compromised have new infections occur soon after the antifungal agent is discontinued.

It is not unusual for many elderly patients to take medications that so alter the oral environment as to make candidal re-infection inevitable. When these medications cannot be discontinued, combined with the microbe's ubiquitous character, new infections occur. Consequently, for these patients, long-term use (usually on a monthly basis) of antifungal agents is recommended. The medication is taken for several days every month (10, 14, or 20 days) beginning with the first day of each month.

Oral Dermatoses

The oral mucosa can be affected by dermatologic disease. This phenomenon occurs for skin and oral mucosa have a very similar anatomy; both are covered by stratified squamous epithelium. Consequently, some illnesses that occur on the skin can occur orally and vice versa. The most common and most important oral dermatoses include lichen planus, mucosal pemphigoid, and pemphigus vulgaris. Lichen planus and mucosal pemphigoid are included due to their prevalence in the general population. Pemphigus vulgaris is actually quite rare. However, it is included due to its similar clinical appearance to lichen planus and mucosal pemphigoid and due to it being potentially lethal. Although clinically and microscopically benign, this disease is potentially fatal and it is important on that basis alone. Each of these three diseases presents with an identical diagnostic problem. Since physicians and dentists have been taught these illnesses are primarily skin diseases; many feel uncomfortable in making a diagnosis of them orally when the patient does not have concurrent skin lesions. The clinician should remember that a patient with lichen planus, mucosal pemphigoid, or pemphigus vulgaris may have oral lesions only and thus may present first to the dentist.

Lichen Planus

Lichen planus (LP) is the most common of these three dermatoses. At the CUCDM clinical oral pathology service, more than 70 new patients are seen annually with this illness. Its cause is unknown but thought to be related in part to an altered cell-mediated immune response to specific chemicals in the affected patient's environment (Agarwal and Saraswat, 2002; Lozada-Nur and Miranda, 1997a; Scully et al., 2000). These chemicals may be as seemingly harmless as cinnamon (Agarwal and Saraswat, 2002; Neville et al., 2002a), a common confectionary item, or as apparently helpful as medications used to control various illnesses such as hypertension, arthritis, and gout. It is not possible in all patients to detect a specific causal substance. Some patients have lichen planus-like lesions as a manifestation of graft versus host disease. Others have claimed that the lesions are exacerbated during stressful periods. Due to this varied etiologic background, it is not surprising that a variety of terms have been applied to those afflicted, such as lichen planus, lichen planus-like drug reactions, lichenoid lesions, and graft versus host disease. Although several chemical substances have been implicated in its genesis, when these same chemicals are pharmacologic agents used to control other more serious illnesses, they usually cannot be eliminated. To complicate this matter further, cessation of the offending agent does not guarantee immediate or even long-term LP elimination. Orally, lichen planus truly has a "multiforme" appearance. There are six basic disease patterns (Eisen et al., 2005; Setterfield et al., 2000; Thron et al., 1988). They consist of white papules, white laces, white plaques, red erosive lesions, beige white frequently painful ulcers, and vesicles and bullae (Fig. 18.5 and 18.6).

When combining these varied forms with a concept that any and all may exist simultaneously at various oral sites, the disease is truly multiforme. This may cause diagnostic difficulty. However, two of the patterns are very characteristic; white papules and white laces are considered highly diagnostic of LP and should not be ignored. When symptomatic, the oral LP patient will invariably complain of pain, not burning pain or sensitivity. Although pain may be encountered in a variety of these six lichenoid lesions, it is more often encountered in the ulcerated, erosive, and vesiculo-bullous patterns and less often in the white papular, lacey, and plaquey forms. The papular, lacey, and plaquey forms have intact epithelial surfaces, whereas ulcerated lesions are associated with epithelial denudation and intense inflammation. Vesiculo-bullous lesions readily collapse into ulcers and in that manner become painful. Erosive forms are red and may or may not be painful. One should also recall the subjective component of pain. In some cases, patients with large lichenoid

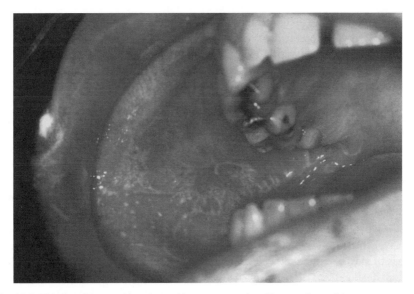

Fig. 18.5 This is a 57-year-old patient with asymptomatic white papules and laces upon several oral mucosal sites as demonstrated here involving the buccal mucosa. A biopsy confirmed lichen planus and since the patient was symptom-free, no medications were prescribed initially (*See* Color Plate 17)

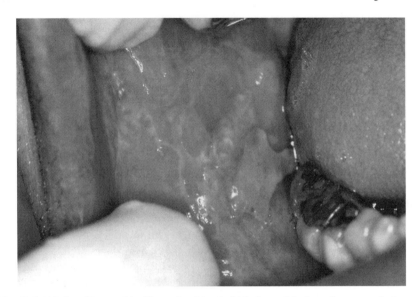

Fig. 18.6 This is a 68-year-old white male with painful lesions of the buccal mucosa. Oral examination revealed painless white lacey lines and painful beige ulcers of lichen planus. Biopsy confirmed LP and the patient was given sublesional steroid injections which eliminated the painful ulcers (*See* Color Plate 18)

ulcers do not have pain. In other patients having only one or two tiny LP ulcers, there is a complaint of significant pain. Regardless of patients' symptoms, there is another very important consideration in the management of lichen planus, its relationship to oral squamous cell carcinoma. For more than 40 years, there have been published studies stating, suggesting, or implying a relationship of oral lichen planus patients eventually developing oral SCC (McCreary and McCarten, 1999; Mignogna et al., 2004; Silverman et al., 1991). Although a variety of statistics have been reported, those that suggest this relationship generally quote a 1%–2% association of LP with oral cancer. That is, over a period of time, 1%–2% of all oral lichen planus patients develop oral SCC. For a number of valid scientific reasons, this oral dermatosis is almost universally accepted as not being precancerous. One important reason rests with its microscopic appearance (Neville et al., 2002a). A characteristic microscopic pattern of lichen planus will not have cellular atypia identified with malignancy or premalignancy (epithelial dysplasia). Instead, there will be overlying keratin, a band-like layer of chronic inflammatory cells, and destruction of the basal cell layer (liquefaction degeneration). It is this destroyed basal cell layer that leads to loss of surface epithelial adhesion that eventually leads to vesicle and ulcer formation. In all clinical LP patterns, there is a band-like layer of chronic inflammatory cells. Thus, there is always a potential for pain or at least some discomfort. Note that when lichen planus lesions evolve toward SCC, cellular epithelial atypia forms first in the lower epithelial layers. If the evolving lesion is then biopsied, it will be read as lichenoid dysplasia and not lichen planus. Treatment of lichen planus (Chainani-Wu et al., 2001; Silverman et al., 1991; Sugerman and Savage, 2002) is as varied as its clinical presentation. First, since lichenoid lesions may be caused by specific chemical agents, questioning the patient with this in mind is mandatory. It may be possible to eliminate an offending agent and achieve considerable if not complete resolution of lichenoid lesions without having to prescribe even more medications. Secondly, since oral lichen planus is associated with oral cancer, there should be follow-up of all LP patients. This is done at least annually, for suspicious LP lesions even more frequently. Third, if the affected patient has classic and painless white papules, laces, and plaques, the authors suggest no medication, for the lesions are neither cosmetic nor painful problems. This approach takes into account that there is presently no cure for this dermatosis. Treatment becomes more complex when the patient is symptomatic. It is important to eliminate painful lesions even if a cure is not possible. Immunosuppressant agents such as steroids are helpful in the management of these patients. These effective medications (Chainani-Wu et al., 2001; Lozada-Nur and Miranda, 1997b; Silverman et al., 1991; Sugerman and Savage, 2002) come in topical (low dose), injectable (moderate dose), and systemic (high dose) forms. There is always an attempt to control the lesions and eliminate pain with the lowest possible dose. Therefore, in most cases, the patient commences treatment with topical steroids (Lozada-Nur and Miranda, 1997b; Silverman et al., 1991) such as liquid forms (dexamethasone) used as a rinse and expectorant or aerosol forms such as beclomethasone dipropionate (Q Var inhalation aerosol) used as a spray. Generally, each is delivered four times per day, once after each meal and once at bedtime. This regimen is employed with the assumption that the patient will neither eat nor drink for at least a half hour and the topical medication will have a chance to linger. Most painful lesions improve significantly with topical steroid medication only. However, if these topical agents are insufficient in eliminating symptoms, the clinician can use injectable or systemic steroids. Injectable steroids (Xia and Hong et al., 2006) have the negative features of being painful to administer (even if preceded by a local anesthetic injection); they must be administered in a doctor's office, and they cannot be used at gingival or palatal sites. Gingival and hard palate lesions are thin and taut making it almost impossible to inject a therapeutic volume. However, high-dose steroid side effects can be minimized when using injectable steroids. Simply use the relatively insoluble depot steroids that linger in tissues longer than non-depot forms, thus creating maximal local benefit to the painful lesion while causing minimal systemic side effects. Systemic steroids (Lozada-Nur and Miranda, 1997b; Silverman et al., 1991), particularly prednisone in 5 mg tablets, can be very effective and easy to administer. The patient may use the following 22-day regime: 50 mg the first day, 30 mg/day the next 7 days, then 15 mg/day the following 7 days, and finally 5 mg/day for another 7 days. One must understand the possible adverse side effects of systemic steroids including this possibility even at low dosages when used long term. Furthermore, there is the potential benefit of having a topical steroid improvement simultaneously with a systemic one via the use of a single steroid medication. Dexamethasone elixir 0.5 mg/5.0 ml can first be rinsed as a topical agent and subsequently be swallowed for its systemic effects. Often, lesions are not eliminated with steroid medications. Instead, pain improvement appears with a change in LP pattern, from a painful ulcerative form to a painless white lacey form. There is a potential complication (Chainani-Wu et al., 2001; Neville et al., 2002a) involving LP patients being treated with steroids. It is possible to induce candidiasis (see appropriate preceding section). One should suspect this complication when a lichen planus patient complains of oral burning and angular cheilitis following steroid use. To combat this mucosal infection, or to help prevent it, the patient should be treated with one of the antifungal medications such as nystatin or an azole such as clotrimazole or fluconazole. Lastly, other medications have been used in treating painful lichenoid lesions. They include but are not limited to immune enhancers, immune suppressants, valium, vitamin A as a topical or systemic medication, griseofulvin, and many more. Steroid therapy is emphasized due to its effectiveness at low dosages.

Mucosal Pemphigoid

Mucosal pemphigoid (MP) has a number of synonyms. They include the terms mucus membrane pemphigoid and cicatricial pemphigoid, the latter a term in frequent use by dermatologists. This dermatosis has a preference for women, at a ratio of 2.5:1, female to male, (Dayan et al., 1999). Most patients are middle aged and older (Dayan et al., 1999). In the general population, this disease is not as common as lichen planus but it is a clinically important problem. Its etiology is unknown but autoimmune factors are involved (Dayan et al., 1999). Intraorally, the gingiva is the primary site of occurrence (Casiglia et al., 2001). Maxillary and mandibular gingival soft tissues are involved with a slight preference for the maxilla. The buccal gingival surfaces are usually more involved than the lingual surfaces. Unlike the other diseases covered in this chapter, there is a very predictable simple repetitive clinical appearance found in almost all affected individuals. They present with a perfectly flat and band-like pattern of intense erythema (Casiglia et al., 2001), involving the maxillary and mandibular gingiva (Fig. 18.7). This red gingival band may vary in width from 4.0 to 10.0 mm. There may be small skip zones of intervening pink healthy gingiva, but this red band is easy to detect by both patient and doctor. A second characteristic feature is the ability of these affected oral sites, and at times seemingly unaffected normal gingival sites as well, to desquamate or slough away with only minimal digital pressure (Mutasim, 2003). This second feature is especially evident when pressure is delivered not at a vertical right angle to the gingival surface but at a much more acute glancing angle. It is as if the clinician can push away the surface squamous epithelium by merely applying slight digital pressure to the affected tissues. In doing so, an ulcer that ultimately may become painful is created. This feature of sloughing, or more frequently referred to as desquamation, may be problematic when attempting to biopsy an MP site. This desquamating feature is dramatic enough to have some refer to MP as "desquamative gingivitis" (Casiglia et al., 2001). However, most investigators use this term in a generic sense. It refers simply to the clinical phenomenon of sloughing gingiva that can be detected in several disease entities including but not limited to lichen planus, mucosal pemphigoid, and pemphigus vulgaris (Casiglia et al., 2001). Although gingival involvement is so

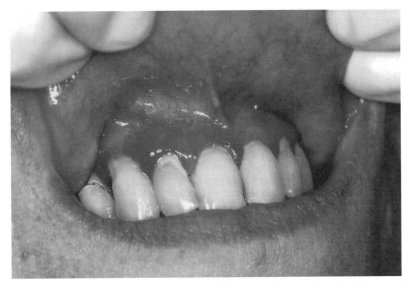

Fig. 18.7 This is a 67-year-old white female with mildly uncomfortable "sloughing" lesions of the maxillary and mandibular gingival soft tissues. Examination revealed flat red lesions that dislodged with minimal pressure. Biopsy confirmed mucosal pemphigoid (*See* Color Plate 19)

characteristic of this disease to have the term desquamative gingivitis applied, other oral sites may be involved as well. When involved, they may present as red surface areas as previously described. They can also present as beige white ulcerations. This latter appearance can occur anywhere in the oral cavity (Darling and Daley, 2005; Dayan et al., 1999), for as previously mentioned there is a proclivity for surface tissues to slough and leave an ulcer. As in lichen planus, blisters can form in MP. They tend to rupture quickly leaving an ulcerated base. Like so many other illnesses, symptoms will vary. Some patients have no pain. Others will complain of pain particularly when beige white ulcers are present. Some will state that their gingival tissues peel and shed (slough). Confirmation of the disease is based on its characteristic microscopic appearance. Thus, a biopsy is required. In fact, two biopsy specimens should be collected, one to be processed and read in the standard fashion and the other to be processed via direct immunofluorescence. The standard biopsy is taken from an actual lesion and is placed in regular 10% formalin solution. It is read by a pathologist following routine processing. Microscopically, the squamous epithelium is usually devoid of rete pegs with discreet separation of the epithelium from the underlying vascularized fibrous tissue (Casiglia et al., 2001; Darling and Daley, 2005). A mild non-specific inflammatory infiltrate will be present. As noted, there can be a problem during the biopsy procedure as a result of the tissues tending to slough. If sloughing occurs while performing the biopsy, the surface epithelium will be lost and the pathologist will be forced to diagnose the specimen as non-specific ulceration and inflammation with no mention of MP (Chan et al., 2002). The second biopsy is done to diagnose the illness via direct immunofluorescence (DIF)

(Chan, 2001). Generally, normal soft tissues are removed from a perilesional area (i.e., uninvolved gingiva). This specimen is carefully secured without desquamation and placed in Michel's solution. The procedure of DIF microscopy is reserved for only a handful of dermatologic illnesses, MP being one of them. Although it is usually considered ancillary to the standard biopsy procedure it is still important. There are other testing procedures that can be used to diagnose MP as well. One is the Nikolsky sign. This is a non-specific somewhat crude clinical test that simply involves digital pressure being applied to uninvolved normal tissues in a patient suspected of having MP. If while doing this a lesion is created, the resulting lesion would be termed a (+) Nikolsky sign and thus highly indicative of this dermatosis. A more specific test using laboratory procedures is one termed indirect immunofluorescence (Dayan et al., 1999). Here, antibody testing is performed as in the DIF test, but the specimen is a blood sample instead of a biopsy specimen. Mucosal pemphigoid and lichen planus are very similar to one another. Therefore, it is understandable that treatment for one is often similar if not identical to the other. Steroids (Mutasim, 2003) can be used as in lichen planus, in topical, injectable, and systemic forms. Diaminodiphenylsulfone (Dapsone) (Ciarrocca and Greenberg, 1999; Kirtschig and Murrell et al., 2002) is also used therapeutically, and the patient should be evaluated beforehand for specific blood dyscrasias. Per surface area of involvement, MP lesions are more resistant to medication control than LP lesions, but fortunately, MP patients are more often asymptomatic. Lastly, MP patients may have non-oral involvement as well. Since ophthalmic (Chan et al., 2002; Higgins et al., 2006) and vaginal lesions (Chan, 2001) may occur, referral to appropriate internists, ophthalmologists, and gynecologists may be indicated. Skin lesions may occur as in the disease known as bullous pemphigoid (Mutasim, 2003). Lastly, as in lichen planus, there is currently no cure.

Pemphigus Vulgaris

Pemphigus vulgaris (PV) is the least common of the three dermatoses covered in this chapter. In fact, this illness is very rare. Its importance lies in the knowledge that it is frequently confused with lichen planus and mucosal pemphigoid and that this illness is potentially fatal (Bystryn and Rudolph, 2005) although clinically and microscopically benign. PV occurs rather evenly between the genders (Iamaroon et al., 2006) and generally occurs in the fourth–sixth decades of life (Bystryn and Rudolph, 2005). As for lichen planus and mucosal pemphigoid, its exact cause is unknown. There are autoimmune features (Patel et al., 1983), but other causal factors appear to be involved as well. Thus, we see a similarity in both PV and MP, and the main difference between the two is the location of the immune reaction. In MP, the reactive site is at the basement membrane immediately below the squamous epithelium. In PV, the reactive site lies between affected squamous epithelial cells (Darling and Daley, 2006). Clinically, any oral soft tissue site may be involved. Commonly, the patient presents with multiple, variable-sized flat red/white irregularly shaped painful ulcers. An important factor in differentiating PV from other oral ulcerative illnesses lies in the presentation of the PV beige white ulcers with little or no surrounding erythema (Fig. 18.8). At times, diagnostic work-ups are inconclusive and patients remain undiagnosed or misdiagnosed for weeks and even months. As these oral lesions gradually worsen, the throat may be involved (Bystryn and Rudolph, 2005) leading to pain so severe that the patient is unable to eat properly leading to a weight loss (Zegarelli and Zegarelli, 1977). In the past, there was mention of a broad-based genetic predisposition for this disease, since it was found more frequently in certain ethnic groups such as Ashkenazi Jews and southern Europeans (Mediterranean countries), e.g., Italians and Greeks (Ahmed et al., 1990; Bystryn and Rudolph, 2005; Darling and Daley, 2006). This disease is also best corroborated microscopically. As in MP, two biopsies are required for a complete PV work-up. One is processed and read in the standard fashion and the other is processed for DIF. The standard biopsy is removed from an actual lesion and the DIF biopsy is removed from a normal perilesional site such as unaffected gingiva. Microscopically, there is a highly specific appearance. One sees an intraepithelial cleft, often directly above the basal layer of the surface squamous epithelium, and, separation of squamous cells from one another referred to as acantholysis (Darling and Daley, 2006). Once again as in MP, ancillary testing via a blood sample is encouraged (indirect immunofluorescence), and a (+) Nikolsky sign may be apparent if uninvolved tissues are lightly rubbed or tapped. Years ago, death due to this

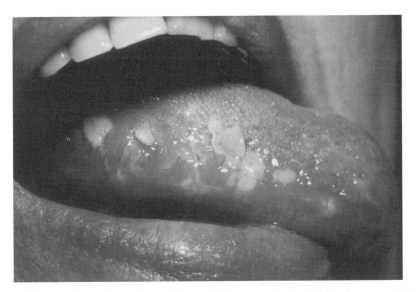

Fig. 18.8 This is a 54-year-old white female with several months of painful oral mucosal lesions that began in her throat and " spread to my mouth". She lost 17 pounds due to an inability to eat. Although these white lesions appear leucoplakic, they were in fact classic painful focally ulcerated lesions of pemphigus vulgaris. A biopsy confirmed PV demonstrating intraepithelial clefting and acantholysis (*See* Color Plate 20)

disease was usually secondary to widespread open skin sores with secondary infection and electrolyte imbalance. This was particularly true before the modern era of antibiotics. Today, many more patients are salvaged and the threat lies with the dosage levels of immunosuppressive medications required to control the disease (Dick and Werth, 2006). As in LP and MP, there is no definitive cure. This disease is controlled with the use of potent immunosuppressants such as steroids (Yeh et al., 2005). Usually systemic steroids are first used at high doses. When control is achieved, the dosage levels are reduced until new lesions develop. The higher the final dose needed for control, the more likely steroid side effects will occur. Consequently, other immunosuppressants are used either solely or in combination with the systemic steroids. They include cytoxan, methyltrexate, and mycophenolate mofetil (Bystryn and Rudolph, 2005; Enk and Knop, 1997;Yeh et al., 2005).

Burning Mouth Syndrome and Burning Mouth Symptoms

Patients may present to their physicians and dentists with a chief complaint of a burning mouth. There are seven major causes of oral burning and they include but are not limited to anemia (particularly pernicious anemia), diabetes mellitus, gastroesophageal reflux disease (GERD), geographic tongue, trauma, candidiasis, and burning mouth syndrome (BMS) (Eli et al., 1994; Zegarelli, 1997). Occasionally, some patients present with multiple causes. The initial identification of BMS occurred more than 50 years ago (Ziskin and Moulton, 1946). The etiology of BMS remains an enigma, but over the years there has been an emphasis on emotional factors, stress, depression, psychology, and post-menopausal symptoms. (Eli et al., 1994;Zakrzewska et al., 2003). A typical patient with BMS has no visible oral lesions but complains of a burning discomfort, often confined to the anterior tongue (tip), anterior palate, and lips (Zegarelli, 1984) (Fig. 18.9). There is a pronounced female predilection and the patients are usually older than 40 years (Bergdahl and Bergdahl, 1999). Often, the burning symptoms commence following a particularly stressful event. Many patients complain that the symptoms began after a routine dental visit (Grushka et al., 2002) or after a dinner out when spicy food was consumed. Prior to establishing a diagnosis of BMS with its background of stress, every attempt should be made to rule in or rule out causes related to the first six entities mentioned in this section. Anemia, diabetes mellitus, GERD, geographic tongue, trauma, candidiasis, and any other background medical data peculiar to that patient should be ruled in or out before the diagnosis of BMS is made (Zegarelli, 1997). Thus, a BMS diagnosis is made in part via the exclusion of other causal factors. Patients with burning symptoms related to the first six causes should have visible lesions and/or abnormal laboratory tests (pernicious anemia, diabetes mellitus). Most burning mouth symptom patients having either BMS or candidiasis as a cause. The next most common cause is geographic tongue. Lastly, a limited number of patients have oral burning due to uncontrolled anemia, diabetes mellitus, GERD, or trauma. Trauma-related oral burning is recognized easily by the patient or primary

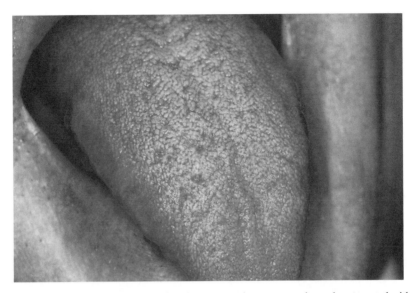

Fig. 18.9 This is an 82-year-old white female concentration camp survivor who presented with an otherwise negative medical history, a normal appearing oral mucosa, and a several months history of a burning mouth. In part via the process of exclusion, the final diagnosis was recorded as burning mouth syndrome (*See* Color Plate 21)

care doctor. In this situation, there is no need for an oral pathologist. As noted, some patients may have multiple factors causing their burning mouth symptoms. For example, pernicious anemia may induce a secondary candidiasis and such a patient may have oral burning due to both illnesses. In summary, the typical BMS patient is a female more than 40 years presenting with a chief complaint of oral burning confined to the anterior tongue and palate (Eli et al., 1994) and having no visible lesions at these sites (Savage et al., 2006). Further questioning eliminates other medical conditions contributing to these symptoms, and the patient relates a particularly stressful event that immediately preceded the onset of symptoms. BMS patients differ widely regarding symptom duration. Following reassurance, some BMS patients became asymptomatic within 1–2 months' time. As examples, one patient developed tongue burning the day after her husband was diagnosed with tongue cancer 35 years before. Other BMS patients mention being treated badly by physicians and dentists. Some were ejected from the doctor's office when burning symptoms persisted despite the doctor's best efforts. In contrast, some patients improve dramatically when simply reassured that there is no physical evidence of disease and that oral cancer is not present. When reassured, some leave the office immediately and either improve substantially or learn to live with these symptoms. Other patients are skeptical about psychogenic factors as being causal, frequently interrupt the doctor, and endlessly pose negative questions that become impossible to answer. This BMS group of patients often see many practitioners, one patient having visited more than 300 doctors over a 10-year span. When reassurance does not alleviate the symptoms, a variety of psychomimetic agents are commonly used. These include but are not limited to clonazepam (klonopin) (Grushka et al., 1998), lorazepam (ativan), amitriptyline (elavil), and sertraline (zoloft) (Zakrzewska et al., 2003). Even agents such as capsaicin (Spice and Hagen, 2004) have been used with varied success. Lastly, in more recent years, BMS has been expanded to include other symptoms as well (Zegarelli, 1997). Patients have been labeled with BMS who present with dysgeusia (a bad taste) or a complaint of xerostomia when a normal amount of saliva is present. (Soares et al., 2005).

Xerostomia

Xerostomia is not a specific disease. Instead, it is the condition of having a dry mouth (Hochberg et al., 1998). This is a very common problem in a senior citizen population (Ship et al., 2002). The most common causes include medications (Astor et al., 1999) and Sjogren's syndrome (Al-Hashimi, 2005). Numerous medications have the side effect of causing a dry mouth. These include medications used for hypertension (i.e., hydrochlorothiazide) (Ship et al., 2002), for depression such as lithium (Ship et al., 2002), for urinary incontinence (Kripke, 2006) such as tolterodine tartrate (detrol), and others, which are commonly used by older adults. While use of these medications has improved quality of life and longevity, many medications have side effects that manifest in the oral cavity, modifying the environment from moist to dry (Fig. 18.10). A second and less common cause of xerostomia is Sjogren's syndrome. This illness has a predilection for adult white females. There are two forms, primary and secondary. Primary Sjogren's has two components, dry mouth and dry eyes. Secondary Sjogren's has three features: dry eyes, dry mouth, and an autoimmune illness such as lupus erythematosus, rheumatoid arthritis, or Hashimoto's thyroiditis (Neville et al., 2002b). Regardless of the cause, the patient presents with a complaint of dry mouth. The dryness may be accompanied by other symptoms as well, including discomfort or frank pain with observable soft tissue lesions, a burning mouth, or even a sudden increase in the caries rate (Cassolato and Turnbull, 2003; Ship et al., 2002). Complaints of soreness or discomfort are usually secondary to the relative dryness (a lack of oral lubrication), with the cheeks and lateral tongue surfaces being irritated by the adjacent teeth. All should recall that the hardest and sharpest objects in the body are teeth. And if the mouth is less moist, the lateral tongue surfaces and cheek surfaces may be irritated (Astor et al., 1999) by rubbing against the dentition during everyday oral movements related to speaking, eating, and swallowing. If the dryness and irritations become intense, visible lesions will develop on the cheek and lateral tongue surfaces. These punctate, well-delineated, and benign-appearing ulcers have a beige white and/or red surface. They may be intensely painful even if only a few millimeters in diameter. A third side effect related to xerostomia is candidiasis (Ship et al., 2002) (see the preceding section). Candida is ubiquitous and a change in the oral environment from moist to dry can predispose to candidal infection. The patient then presents with

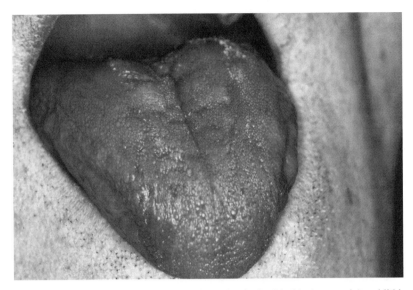

Fig. 18.10 This is a 72-year-old female on desipramine hydrochloride (norpramin) and lithium – leading to a dry mouth (xerostomia). Gloved fingers would adhere slightly to the tongue mucosa and peel away when moved slowly off the affected oral soft tissues

features of oral dryness and candidiasis, such as having an erythematous mouth, angular cheilitis, frank colonies of Candida (milk curds), and oral burning. Another important effect of xerostomia is an increase in caries susceptibility. The increase in caries can be sudden and severe. This leads to additional patient health and financial burdens. To offset these deleterious effects, the patient and the clinician can do one or more of the following. First, speak to the primary care physician to see if the causal medications can be replaced or eliminated (Cassolato and Turnbull, 2003; Ship et al., 2002). Secondly, the patient should be encouraged to stimulate saliva-tion via the use of sugar-free foods such as carrots, celery, and lozenges. Third, the patient should be directed to keep the mouth moist by consuming frequent sips of water. Fourth, to reduce and eliminate oral ulcers, topical medications such as triam-cinolone acetonide/nystatin cream (Mycolog II) may be helpful. In conjunction with topical medications, the dentist may choose to smooth sharp cusps of adjacent teeth to further eliminate the possibility of irritation. Next, if these ulcers persist, consid-eration should be given to their surgical removal, but healing may be delayed when the mouth is dry. Cevimeline hydrochloride (Evoxac) and pilocarpine hydrochloride (Salagen) (Chainani-Wu et al., 2006) have been used successfully to reduce xeros-tomia. These medications have side effects as well. Antifungal agents may also be needed. Lastly, the patient should be counseled regarding xerostomia-induced caries. A thorough review of proper home care and the need for increased dental visits should be discussed. Additionally, the topical use of fluoride compounds is encouraged with or without the use of specially constructed dental trays.

Laboratory Testing

The lesions and illnesses that have been reviewed (squamous cell carcinoma, candidiasis, lichen planus, mucosal pemphigoid, and pemphigus vulgaris) are confirmed via appropriate laboratory testing. Even burning mouth syndrome is diagnosed in part via laboratory testing when blood analysis eliminates anemia and diabetes mellitus as being causal. Blood tests can easily be ordered in the dental office. A dentist can simply use his/her prescription pad letterhead to order the appropriate tests. The patient is directed to a local medical laboratory or hospital laboratory, the bloods are drawn, and the reports are sent via fax and mail. Fungal cultures are also easy to perform. Simply swab a sterile Q tip over the suspected oral site and plate it immediately upon a Sabouraud's agar slant. The slant may remain in the clinician's office and viewed daily. Since fungal microbes grow slowly in culture, 14 days are allowed to establish growth on Sabouraud's medium. However, if there is heavy colonization, creamy white colonies are observed 2–4 days following inoculation. Fungal and epithelial smears are also easy to perform. For suspected candidal infections, a dental spatula is stroked firmly over the suspected site and gently smeared on a glass microscopic slide. It is fixed immediately with either a liquid or spray-on commercial alcohol fixative and then sent to the pathology laboratory with the appropriate instructions. It is stained with PAS and read and reported by the pathologist. For epithelial cytology, the smear is performed in the same manner. It is stained in hematoxylin and eosin or Papanicolaou stain instead of PAS. Usually, collection of these samples is painless. Occasionally, some discomfort may result when scraping a tender oral lesion. Therefore, a local anesthetic prior to any instrumentation should be considered. Note that the use of a topical anesthetic gel may interfere with smear fixation and staining. The final laboratory technique described in this section is the intraoral mucosal biopsy. In general, a biopsy should be performed for definitive diagnosis. A biopsy specimen provides cellular architecture, a feature generally necessary for a definitive diagnosis and unavailable in the smear/cytology technique. A mucosal biopsy may be incisional or excisional. An incisional biopsy is a sampling that provides the appropriate diagnosis prior to definitive therapy. An excisional biopsy serves two purposes: it provides a diagnosis and accomplishes complete surgical removal of the lesion. Details regarding the choice of an incisional biopsy versus an excisional biopsy are extensive and are outside the scope of this chapter. Patient preparation for incisional and excisional biopsies is the same. A topical anesthetic is used prior to injection with a local anesthetic. Vasoconstrictor use is encouraged as it improves anesthetic duration and promotes vasoconstriction. Following anesthesia, the appropriate soft tissue specimen is removed and placed in formalin. Traditional scalpels and punch biopsy instruments are generally used. The common #15 scalpel blade is preferred and can be used in conjunction with a punch biopsy instrument. The skin or mucosal punch is a circular cutting instrument available in various sizes (2.0, 2.5, 3.0, 3.5, 4.0, 5.0, 6.0, and 8.0 mm). Being circular cutting instruments, they provide simultaneously length and width cuts where a regular scalpel blade requires more than one surgical entry. Whether a #15 scalpel blade or punch is used for length and width, a traditional scalpel blade is necessary to free the inferior margin. The 3.5, 4.0, and 5.0 mm punch sizes are most helpful in oral biopsy procedures. The use of cautery instruments in mucosal biopsies is not recommended, as the excised margins following such a procedure are inadequate for microscopic analysis. When suturing is necessary following the surgical procedure, 4-0 and 5-0 black silk sutures are preferred. There is no attempt to suture gingival and most hard palatal biopsy sites. Instead, stasis is achieved with firm gauze pressure or silver nitrate application. The formalin-fixed specimen along with the biopsy requisition form is then sent to the pathology laboratory. Once received in the laboratory, the specimen is accessioned, grossed, cut, and stained. These technical and other processing steps require approximately 24 hours, and the prepared slides are read by the pathologist the next day. At times, additional cuts and special stains are required to finalize the definitive diagnosis. These steps will require more time. New York State protocol provides that the clinician receives the pathology report and the patient (or his/her representative, an insurance company) receives the bill. Most pathology laboratories supply necessary biopsy materials including formalin bottles, requisition forms, mailers with postage included.

References

Agarwal, R., & Saraswat, A. (2002). Oral lichen planus: an update. Drugs Today, 38: 533–537.

Ahmed, A.R., Yunis, E.J., Khatri, K., Wagner, R., Notani, G., Awdeh, Z., & Alper, C.A. (1990). Major histocompatibility complex haplotype studies in Ashkenazi Jewish patients with pemphigus vulgaris. Proceedings of the National Academy of Sciences of the United States of America, 87(19): 7658–7662.

Al-Hashimi, I. (2005). Xerostomia secondary to Sjogren's syndrome in the elderly: recognition and management. Drugs and Aging, 22(11): 887–899.

Allen, C.M. (1992). Diagnosing and managing oral candidiasis. Journal of American Dental Association, 123: 77–82.

Astor, F.C., Hanft, K.L., & Ciocon, J.O. (1999). Xerostomia: a prevalent condition in the elderly. Ear, Nose, & Throat Journal, 78(7): 476–479.

Bergdahl, M. & Bergdahl, J. (1999) Burning mouth syndrome: prevalence and associated factors. Journal of Oral Pathology & Medicine, 28(8): 350–354.

Blomgren, J., Berggren, U., & Jontell, M. (1998). Fluconazole versus nystatin in the treatment of oral candidiasis. Acta Odontologica Scandinavica, 56: 202–205.

Bystryn, J.C. & Rudolph, J.L. (2005). Pemphigus. Lancet, 366(9479): 61–73.

Casiglia, J., Woo, S. B., & Ahmed, A. R. (2001). Oral involvement in autoimmune blistering diseases. Clinics in Dermatology, 19(6): 737–741.

Cassolato, S.F., & Turnbull, R.S. (2003). Xerostomia: clinical aspects and treatment. Gerodontology, 20(2): 64–77.

Chainani-Wu, N., Gorsky, M., Mayer, P., Bostrom, A., Epstein, J. B., & Silverman, S. (2006). Assessment of the use of sialogogues in the clinical management of patients with xerostomia. Special Care in Dentistry, 26(4): 164–170

Chainani-Wu, N., Silverman, S., Lozada-Nur, F., Mayer, P., & Watson, J.J. (2001). Oral lichen planus: patient profile, disease progression and treatment responses. Journal of American Dental Association, 132: 901–909.

Chan, L.S. (2001). Mucous membrane pemphigoid. Clinics in Dermatology, 19(6): 703–711.

Chan, L.S., Ahmed, A.R., Anhalt, G.J., Bernauer, W., Cooper, K. D., Elder, M.J., Fine, J. D., Foster, C., Ghohestani, R., Hashimoto, T., Hoang-Xuan, T., Kirtschig, G., Korman, N.J., Lightman, S., Lozada-Nur, F., Marinkovich, M.P., Mondino, B. J., Prost-Squarcioni, C., Rogers, R.S., Setterfield, J.F., West, D.P., Wojnarowska, F., Woodley, D. T., Yancey, K. B., Zillikens, D., & Zone, J.J. (2002). The first international consensus on mucous membrane pemphigoid: definition, diagnostic criteria, pathogenic factors, medical treatment, and prognostic indicators. Archives of Dermatology, 138(3): 370–379.

Choi, S.Y., & Kahyo, H. (1991). Effect of cigarette smoking and alcohol consumption in the aetiology of cancer of the oral cavity, pharynx and larynx. International Journal of Epidemiology, 20: 878–885.

Ciarrocca, K.N., & Greenberg, M.S. (1999). A retrospective study of the management of oral mucous membrane pemphigoid with dapsone. Oral Surgery Oral Medicine Oral Pathology Oral Radiolology & Endodontics, 88(2): 159–163.

Cowan, C.G., Gregg, T.A., Napier, S.S., McKenna, S.M., & Kee, F. (2001). Potentially malignant oral lesions in Northern Ireland: a 20 year population based perspective of malignant transformation. Oral Diseases, 7: 18–24.

Darling, M.R., & Daley, T. (2005). Blistering mucocutaneous diseases of the oral mucosa-a review: part 1. Mucous membrane pemphigoid. Journal of the Canadian Dental Association, 71(11): 851–854.

Darling, M.R., & Daley, T. (2006). Blistering mucocutaneous diseases of the oral mucosa-a review: part 2. Pemphigus vulgaris. Journal of the Canadian Dental Association, 72(1): 63–66.

Dayan, S., Simmons, R.K., & Ahmed, A.R. (1999). Contemporary issues in the diagnosis of oral pemphigoid: a selective review of the literature. Oral Surgery Oral Medicine Oral Pathology Oral Radiology & Endodontics, 88(4): 424–430.

Dick, S.E., & Werth, V.P. (2006). Pemphigus: a treatment update. Autoimmunity, 39(7): 591–599.

Eisen, D., Carrozzo, M., Bagan Sebastian, J.V., & Thongprasom, K. (2005). Number V oral lichen planus: clinical features and management. Oral Disease, 11: 338–349.

Eli, I., Baht, R., Littner, M.M., & Kleinhauz, M. (1994). Detection of psychopathologic trends in glossodynia patients. Psychosomatic Medicine, 56(5): 389–394.

Enk, A.H., & Knop, J. (1997). Treatment of pemphigus vulgaris with mycophenolate mofetil. Lancet, 350: 494

Epstein, J.B., & Polsky, B. (1998). Oropharyngeal candidiasis: a review of its clinical spectrum and current therapies. Clinical Therapeutics, 20: 40–57.

Fotos, P.G., & Lilly, J.P. (1996). Clinical management of oral and perioral candidosis. Dermatologic Clinics, 14: 273–280.

Fotos, P.G., Vincent, S.D., & Hellstein, J.W. (1992). Oral candidosis: clinical, historical and therapeutic features of 100 cases. Oral Surgery Oral Medicine Oral Pathology Oral Radiology & Endodontics, 74: 41–49.

Grushka, M., Epstein, J.B., & Gorsky, M. (2002). Burning mouth syndrome. American Family Physician, 65(4): 615–620.

Grushka, M., Epstein, J., & Mott, A. (1998). An open-label, dose escalation pilot study of the effect of clonazepam in burning mouth syndrome. Oral Surgery Oral Medicine Oral Pathology Oral Radiology & Endodontics, 86(5): 557–561.

Gupta, P.C., Mehta, F.S., Daftary, D.K., Pindborg, J.J., Bhonsle, R.B., Jalnawalla, P.N., Sinor, P.N., Pitkar, V.K., Murti, P.R., Irani, R.R., Shah, H.T., Kadam, P.M., Iyer, K.S., Iyer, H.M., Hegde, A.K., Chandrashekar, G.K., Shiroff, B.C., Sahiar, B.E., & Mehta, M.N. (1980). Incidence rates of oral cancer and natural history of oral precancerous lesions in a 10 year follow-up study of Indian villagers. Community Dentistry and Oral Epidemiology, 8: 283–333.

Higgins, G.T., Allan, R.B., Hall, R., Field, E.A., & Kaye, S.B. (2006). Development of ocular disease in patients with mucous membrane pemphigoid involving the oral mucosa. British Journal of Ophthalmology, 90(8): 964–967.

Hochberg, M.C., Tielsch, J., Munoz, B., Bandeen-Roche, K., West, S.K., & Schein, O.D. (1998). Prevalence of symptoms of dry mouth and their relationship to saliva production in community dwelling elderly: the SEE project. Salisbury Eye Evaluation. Journal of Rheumatology, 25(3): 486–491.

Howaldt, H.P., Kainz, M., & Euler, B. (1999). Proposal for modification of the TNM staging classification for cancer of the oral cavity. Journal of Craniomaxillofac surgery, 27: 275–288.

Iamaroon, A., Boonyawong, P., Klanrit, P., Prasongtunskul, S., & Thongprasom, K. (2006). Characterization of oral pemphigus vulgaris in Thai patients. Journal of Oral Science, 48(1): 43–46.

Kirtschig, G., Murrell, D., Wojnarowska, F., & Khumalo, N. (2002). Interventions for mucous membrane pemphigoid/cicatricial pemphigoid and epidermolysis bullosa acquisita: a systemic literature review. Archives of Dermatology, 138(3): 380–384.

Kripke, C. (2006). Anticholinergic drugs for overactive bladder. American Family Physician, 73(1): 66.

Lozada-Nur, F., & Miranda, C. (1997a). Oral lichen planus: epidemiology, clinical characteristics, and associated diseases. Seminars in cutaneous medicine and surgery, 16: 273–277.

Lozada-Nur, F., & Miranda, C. (1997b). Oral lichen planus: topical and systemic therapy. Seminars in cutaneous medicine and surgery,16: 295–300.

McCreary, C.E., & McCarten, B.E. (1999). Clinical management of oral lichen planus. The British journal of oral & maxillofacial surgery, 37: 338–343.

McDowell, J.D. (2006). An overview of epidemiology and common risk factors for oral squamous cell carcinoma. Otolaryngologic clinics of North America. 39: 277–294.

Mignogna, M.D., Fedele, S., Russo, L.L., Muzio, L.L., & Bucci, E. (2004). Immune activation and chronic inflammation as the cause of malignancy in oral lichen planus: is there any evidence? Oral Oncology, 40: 120–130.

Mutasim, D.F. (2003). Autoimmune bullous dermatoses in the elderly: diagnosis and management. Drugs & Aging, 20(9): 663–681.

Neville, B.W., Damm, D.D., Allen, C.M., & Bouquot, J.E. (2002a). Epithelial pathology. Oral & Maxillofacial Pathology. Second Edition. Saunders. Philadelphia, Pa. 315–388.

Neville, B.W., Damm, D.D., Allen, C.M., & Bouquot, J.E. (2002b). Salivary gland pathology. Oral & Maxillofacial Pathology. Second Edition. Saunders. Philadelphia, Pa. 401–404.

Neville, B.W., & Day, T.A. (2002). Oral cancer and precancerous lesions. Cancer journal for clinicians, 52: 195–215.

Patel, H.P., Anhalt, G.J., & Diaz, L.A. (1983). Bullous pemphigoid and pemphigus vulgaris. Annals of Allergy, 50(3): 144–150.

Savage, N.W. Boras, V.V., & Barker, K. (2006). Burning mouth syndrome: clinical presentation, diagnosis and treatment. Australasian Journal of Dermatology, 47(2): 77–81.

Sciubba, J.J. (2000). Oral precancer and cancer: etiology, clinical presentation, diagnosis, and management. Compen Continuing Education Dental, 21: 892–898.

Sciubba, J.J. (2001). Oral cancer. The importance of early diagnosis and treatment. American Journal of Clinicians Dermatology, 2: 239–251.

Scully, C., Eisen, D., & Carrozzo, M. (2000). Management of oral lichen planus. American Journal of Clinicians Dermatology, 1: 287–306.

Setterfield, J.F., Black. M.M., & Challacombe, S.J. (2000). The management of oral lichen planus. Clinicians Experimental Dermatology, 25: 176–182.

Sherman, R.G., Prusinski, L., Ravenel, M.C. & Joralmon, R.A. (2002). Oral candidosis. Quintessence International, 33: 521–532.

Ship, J.A., Pillemer, S.R. & Baum, B.J. (2002). Xerostomia and the geriatric patient. Journal of American Geriatrics Society, 50(3): 535–543.

Silverman, S., Gorsky, M., & Lozada-Nur. (1991). A prospective study of findings and management in 214 patients with oral lichen planus. Oral Surgery Oral Medicine Oral Pathology Oral Radiology & Endodontics, 72: 665–670.

Soares, M.S., Chimenos-Kustner, E., Subira-Pifarre, C., Rodriguez de Rivera- Campillo, M.E., & Lopez-Lopez, J. (2005). Association of burning mouth syndrome with xerostomia and medicines. Medicina Oral, Patologia Oral Cirugia Bucal, 10(4): 301–308.

Spice, R., & Hagen, N.A. (2004). Capsaicin in burning mouth syndrome: titration strategies. Journal Of Otolaryngology, 3(1): 53–54.

Sugerman, P.B., & Savage, N.W. (2002). Oral lichen planus: causes, diagnosis and management. Australian Dental Journal, 47: 290–297.

Thron, J.J., Holmstrup, P., & Rindum, J. (1988). Course of various clinical forms of oral lichen planus: a prospective follow-up study of 611 patients. Journal of Oral Pathology, 17: 213–218.

Xia, J., Hong,Y.,Yang, L., Huang,Y., & Cheng, B. (2006). Short-term clinical evaluation of intralesional triamcinolone acetonide injection for ulcerative oral lichen planus. Journal of Oral Pathology & Medicine, 35: 327–331.

Yeh, S.W., Sami, N., & Ahmed, R.A. (2005). Treatment of pemphigus vulgaris: current and emerging options. American Journal of Clinical Dermatology, 6(5): 327–342.

Zakrzewska, J.M., Forssell, H., & Glenny, A.M. (2003). Interventions for the treatment of burning mouth syndrome: a systematic review. Journal of Orofacial Pain, 17(4): 293–300.

Zegarelli, D.J. (1984). Burning mouth: an analysis of 57 patients. Oral Surgery Oral Medicine Oral Pathology Oral Radiology & Endodontics, 58(1): 34–38.

Zegarelli, D.J. (1997). Diseases of the oral mucosa. Avery's Drug Treatment. Fourth Edition. Barcelona, Spain, 625–627.

Zegarelli, D.J., & Zegarelli, E.V. (1977). Intraoral pemphigus vulgaris. Oral Surgery Oral Medicine Oral Pathology Oral Radiology & Endodontics, 44(3): 384–393.

Ziskin, D.E., & Moulton, R. (1946). Glossodynia: a study of idiopathic orolingual pain. Journal of the American Dental Association, 33: 1422–1432.

Part IV
Professional Recommendations and Future Needs

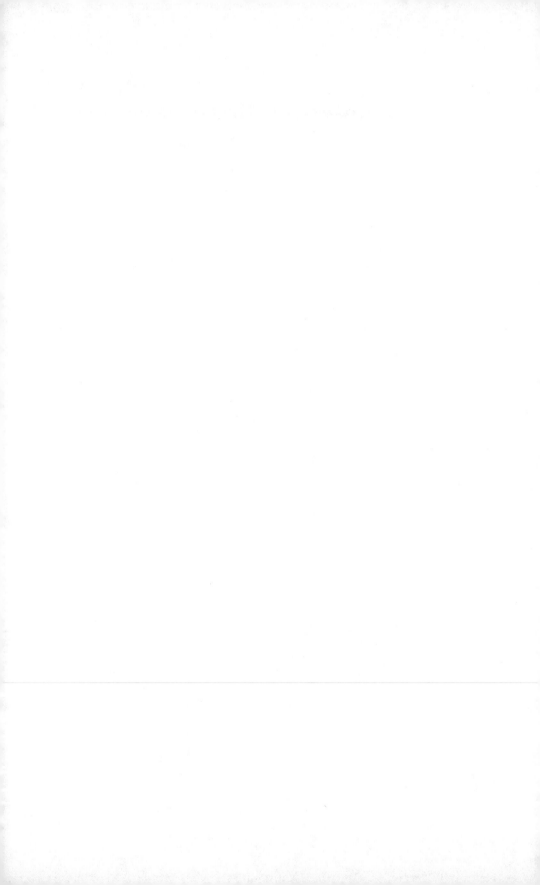

Chapter 19
Educating the Dental Profession

Lynn M. Tepper

Background

The beginning of the twenty-first century has witnessed a tremendous growth in the population of individuals over sixty-five. By 2030, 20% of the US population will be 65 or over, as compared to 12.4%, in 2000 (Federal Interagency Forum on Aging Related Statistics, 2004). Oral health demographics have also changed. The Third National Health and Nutrition Examination Survey (NHANES) found that 72% of adults aged 65–75 had some or all of their natural teeth (Brown, Winn, & White, 1996). Therefore, they remain at least as much at risk for dental disease as younger age groups. A lifetime of dental disease, tooth loss, complex medical conditions, and medications adds to the complexity involved in treating these patients. A notable change is the trend toward increased tooth retention as individuals age (Tepper, 1999). With increased tooth retention, this population will be at increased risk for caries and periodontal disease, as well as the modifying effect of oral inflammation and infection on certain systemic illnesses and conditions such as cardiovascular diseases, cerebrovascular diseases, diabetes mellitus, and respiratory disorders (Lamster, 2004). In addition, these patients often face several barriers impeding access to dental care including cultural and linguistic miscommunication, financial hardship, physical disability, and health care provider attitudes (Dolan, Atchison, & Huynh, 2005). Lack of perceived need has also been described as a barrier to dental care for this population (Surgeon General, 2000). Improving the oral health status of our older population has become a major role of academic dental institutions (American Dental Education Association, 2003), and needs to be included in both medical and public health education as well.

Maintaining good health is a feature of this new generation of older people, and with this brings a heightened quality of life compared to past generations. Good oral health is a critical factor in maintaining general health in older people (Berkey & Berg, 2001). Oral health was identified as one of the 22 priority areas in the *Healthy People, 2010*, the comprehensive, nationwide health promotion and disease

L.M. Tepper
630 West 168 St, NY, NY 10032, Tel: 212-305-3126
e-mail: LMT1@columbia.edu

I.B. Lamster, M.E. Northridge (eds.), *Improving Oral Health for the Elderly*,
© Springer Science+Business Media, LLC 2008

prevention agenda. Quantifiable targets were set for improvements in health status, risk reduction, and service delivery. Objectives related to improved oral health status for older people were established, including goals for increases in the utilization of oral health care services by older adults and long-term care residents. Several major themes emerged including the disparity in oral health among population subgroups, the oral health needs of the institutionalized elderly, and the need to train more dental personnel in geriatric dentistry (U.S. Department of Health and Human Services, 1990).

Dental, medical, and public health educational agendas must address these important disparities. As a result, there has been an increase in educational initiatives in response to this demographic change in all of the public health, social and behavioral science, and medical health professions, including dentistry. Geriatric dental educational programs have been developed for this reason, as well as because of the increasing percentage of those who maintain all or some of their natural teeth, the increase in the numbers of medically complex older patients, and the need for a greater understanding of the skills required to provide effective dental care for older adults (Mohammad, Preshaw, & Ettinger, 2003).

This chapter is designed to provide students and health care practitioners with a better understanding of the scope and content of geriatric dental education, to review the history of what was has been accomplished to date, to examine examples of current programs, and to make some recommendations for the future education of dental, medical, and public health professionals regarding care for older adults. Geriatric dental education and competencies at all levels will be defined, along with requisite subject matter, and the need for interdisciplinary training and collaboration necessary to provide coordinated, comprehensive, and quality care for older adults.

Geriatric Dental Education Defined

Geriatric dental education was originally defined as "that portion of the predoctoral dental curriculum that deals with special knowledge, attitudes, and technical skills required in the provision of oral health care to older adults" (Ettinger & Beck, 1984). This definition, however, has expanded over the past 20 years to include education at the postgraduate and continuing educational levels. Although there has been a recognized need to train dental students in care for the older, medically complex adult, geriatric dentistry is not a recognized dental specialty. Care for this population has been referred to as "Special Care Dentistry" by the Commission on Dental Accreditation, which has adopted new standards for dental and dental hygiene education to better prepare them to care for individuals with particular and extraordinary requirements (Waldman et al., 2005). Special Care Dentistry has been described as "an approach to oral health management tailored to the individual needs of people with a variety of medical conditions or limitations that require more than routine delivery of care." It "encompasses preventive, diagnostic, and treatment services for these patients" (Commission on Dental Accreditation, 2004). The need to recognize geriatric dentistry as a dental specialty has been acknowledged, but has not presently achieved this status. When geriatric dentistry is recognized as a specialty, support could then be established to fund training programs in hospitals and other health care institutions.

For the purposes of this discussion, it includes all pertinent gerontological and clinical topics related to the care of older adults. The growth in the numbers of older adults who present with one or more chronic, debilitating, physical or mental illnesses with associated medications or psychological problems have compounded the need for this specialized, multidisciplinary training. Categorically, elders seen in dental settings include the well elderly, the frail elderly, the functionally dependent elderly, and the severely disabled, medically complex elderly (Yellowitz & Saunders, 1989). There is no doubt that dental professionals need to develop both the special behavioral and clinical skills required to treat this population. Educational experiences should result in competent management skills, as well as a concerned and caring attitude toward older adults.

Historical Perspectives

Historically, as with medical and public health education, the 1970s saw the first growth of geriatrics content in dental education, but it was not until the 1980s that a sharp increase in formal geriatric education programs were documented. From 1975 to 1985, the number of dental schools reporting geriatric dentistry as part of their academic curricula had risen from 52% to 100% (Moshman et al., 1985). In addition to the realization of the above demographic factors, another reason for this sharp increase was the national funding of geriatric dental programs in American dental schools, such as the Geriatric Dental Education Program at Columbia University College of Dental Medicine in 1982. Many didactic and outpatient training programs with innovative approaches were developed and implemented during this period (Tepper, 1990). Since then, awareness of the need for geriatrics and gerontology content in the undergraduate dental curriculum has increased substantially. Examples of the most current innovative educational approaches will be discussed in a subsequent section of this chapter.

Gerontology and geriatric dentistry content in U.S. dental schools has increased substantially over the past 20 years. However, there still remains a general lack of clinical training, particularly in community-based clinics and in non-traditional care settings such as patients' homes or long-term care facilities. There have been several national initiatives to develop curricula in this area. The American Association of Dental Schools has organized the Geriatric Dentistry Curriculum Project intended to enhance predoctoral geriatric curricula. Curriculum Guidelines for Geriatric Dentistry (1989) were developed by the Section on Community and Preventive Dentistry of the AADS, and serve as an important curriculum development aid for dental educators (American Association of Dental Schools, 1989). Revised since its inception in 1982, these guidelines were the first to identify the special knowledge, attitudes, and technical skills required to provide oral health care to older adults. More recently, the American Dental Education Association (ADEA) has refined and

updated predoctoral dental education guidelines with extensive recommendations
for curriculum development (ADEA, 2006).

Dental and allied dental health curricula should be characterized in terms of
their impact on students, expressed as competencies or skills essential to beginning
the practice of dentistry and allied dental practice (U.S. Department of Health and
Human Services, 1990). Many dental schools still lack intensive geriatric clinical
training experiences with specially trained geriatric dentists in a variety of clinical settings. Those with model programs, however, will be discussed later in this
chapter.

Current State of Geriatric Dental Education

As stated above, the need for dental education with greater emphasis on care for the
older patient has received increased attention over the past 25 years. Calls for curricular changes in geriatric dental education in the 1980s included the expansion of
the predoctoral, graduate, and continuing dental education levels (Saunders, 1985;
Kress & Vidmar, 1985). As mentioned previously, "Curriculum Guidelines for Geriatric Dentistry" was published in the Journal of Dental Education in 1989, and
widely distributed. This initiative provided universities with specific guidelines for
developing and implementing core courses and material related to the care and management of the older patient (American Association of Dental Schools, 1989).

The most recent contribution to geriatric dentistry curriculum development was a
Resource Guide developed in CD-ROM format by the American Dental Education
Association (ADEA, 2006). The purpose of this publication was an acknowledge-
ment of the need to further understand the important aspects of the actual deliver
of dental services and maintenance of care for older patients as being essential to
preparing future dentists to meet their oral health needs. This Resource Guide was
intended to support predoctoral dental education, highlighting the importance of
comprehensive patient evaluation, the impact of basic science principles on aging,
the impact of chronic disease and its treatment, and some of the socio-demographic
factors that affect an older person's quality of life (ADEA, 2006). It recognized the
fact that dental schools organize curricula in unique ways, and hence designed the
Guide to assist faculty in achieving specific educational outcomes, with suggested
content topics and resources. Six themes were suggested, including: Demographic
Aspects of Aging, Aging Process and Common Systemic Conditions, Normal Aging
of the Oral Complex, Common Oral Conditions of Older Adults, Social Aspects
of Care in Older Adults, and Delivery and Maintenance of Care for Older Adults.
Patient case studies complement the six concepts, and reflect issues likely to be
experienced when treating the independent older adult. Innovative practices by peers
were included to demonstrate some of the excellent and innovative approaches being
used to educate dental students in geriatric dentistry.

With guidelines in place, efforts are currently being put forth to determine what
motivates a student to pursue geriatric dentistry. Baumeister reported a higher number of weeks spent in extramural clinical rotations, socially conscious attitudes,

and the dental school's demographic and dental market context correlated to a student's interest in treating special care patients (Baumeister et al., 2007). MacEntee utilized a self-reporting journal model to ascertain dental students' reactions to a clinical rotation through a long-term care facility. Over the 2-year period, students reported the experience positively and acknowledged its importance in their professional maturation (MacEntee, Prukscapong, & Wyatt, 2005). Teasdale and Shaikh reported successful outcomes with undergraduate dental students with the use of a self-instruction CD-ROM-based educational tool (Teasdale & Shaikh, 2006).

A recent (2003) study of all 54 American dental schools revealed that: (1) 100% teach at least some aspects of geriatric dentistry; (2) 98% have curricula containing required didactic material; (3) 67% have a clinical component of geriatric dental teaching, and 77% of these require it; (4) 63% have a geriatric program director or a chair of a geriatric section; (5) 30% have a specific geriatric dentistry clinic within the dental school; (6) 11% have a remote geriatric dentistry clinic; and (7) 37% plan to extend the geriatric education in the future (Mohammad, Preshaw, & Ettinger, 2003). Only 41% include clinical experience in geriatric dentistry. Clearly, more must be done to provide students with this necessary experience.

Curricular Competencies Defined

Before developing educational interventions in any area of study, it is of prime importance to fully understand and establish the outcomes and competencies required as a result of instruction (Tepper, 1980). To do this, one needs to completely understand how the subject to be taught is integrated into practice. Geriatric dentistry differs from general dentistry for other age groups in many ways. Mohammad (2001) has described six of the major aspects which differ:

1. Geriatric dentistry is concerned with providing dental care to a population aged 65 or greater.
2. Eighty-six percent of people aged 65 or more have at least one major chronic disorder such as arthritis, osteoporosis, respiratory disease, cardiovascular disease, cancer, and neurological disorders.
3. Many suffer from physical disabilities such as hearing loss, poor vision, and taste disorders which may impact on their ability to comply with a dentist's instructions.
4. Many of the elderly utilize polypharmacy (five or more medications taken concurrently), with oral side effects such as xerostomia (dry mouth).
5. Significant numbers also suffer from cognitive dysfunction such as dementia, which may negatively influence impact compliance with oral health care.
6. The combined effects of physical, psychological, and mental disorders may conspire to make treatment planning and execution a major challenge for the dentist. Furthermore, the practice of geriatric dentistry challenges the ingenuity of the dentist in synchronizing demanding technical procedures with the normal and pathological effects of aging on the oral hard and soft tissues.

Using the health characteristics of older adults described above, curriculum guidelines which result in practice competencies can then be developed.

It is clear to see from these practice differences that the domains of knowledge in geriatric dentistry must include competencies which are clinical, behavioral, and attitudinal. They must reflect the knowledge-based competencies, the behavioral outcomes, and the attitudinal change competencies which are necessary for working with this age group (Tepper, 1980; Glista & Petersons, 2003; Dorfman et al., 2007).

Educational Needs: The Scope of Practice

Who Provides Care?

The types of providers of care for older people reflect similar categories in medicine, dentistry, and public health in general. There are essentially four groups of dental professionals that serve older patients: (1) private general dentists in the community who treat older people as part of their general private practices; (2) public oral health care providers who practice in neighborhood community and public health center clinics; (3) dental personnel who practice in non-traditional settings such as in patients' homes and residential facilities, often in addition to their community-based offices; and (4) academic geriatric dentists based at universities and/or teaching hospitals who teach, conduct research, provide leadership and consultation, and treat more clinically challenging older patients.

General Dentists in Private Practice Settings

As it is with medical providers, private practice dentists, hygienists, and dental assistants provide the majority of geriatric dental services in this country. They treat older people in mixed-age practices, and are among the most in need of continuing education in gerontology and geriatric dentistry. Many were trained before these subjects were incorporated into their dental education, and before the demand for these skills were so necessary. This care is provided primarily to older adults living independently who require little if any assistance in their daily activities. They access dental care as would younger individuals. Dental professionals providing services to them require education and clinical training in gerontology and geriatrics which provides them with an understanding of the normal physical, psychological, and social changes that occur with age, and their potential impact on the delivery of dental services. They also require clinical training about the aging oral cavity, and the preventive, restorative, and rehabilitative approaches to dental therapy that are most appropriate and effective for these elders (U.S. Department of Health and Human Services, 1990).

Community-Based Public Health Settings

Community-based dental care providers employed by public health centers and clinics provide a sizable amount of oral health care to those on public assistance and those that cannot afford private dental care. They include dentists, dental hygienists, and dental assistants, working together in small clinical settings, or larger public health centers, along with other medical and social service providers. These professionals are similar to practitioners in private practice in terms of their need for continuing geriatric dental education and training, for the reasons elaborated upon above.

Non-traditional Practice Settings

The more frail, functionally dependent, and debilitated older population who reside either at home with full-time assistance, or in long-term care facilities require a slightly different skill set. They need to be treated by dental professionals with more extensive skills, sensitivity, and clinical experiences in geriatrics. A thorough understanding of these patients' extensive medical conditions, drug histories, and complicating psychosocial issues in addition to any specific oral conditions is required to treat them effectively. Geriatric dental academicians are desperately needed to guide, inspire, and mentor dental professionals in training. Training for this needed population has been slow to develop, with only very limited educational opportunities available.

Academic Geriatric Dental Settings

Training programs for geriatric dental academicians needs to be based at dental schools located within large university medical centers, which can provide training with a strong public health component, multidisciplinary faculty, and an interdisciplinary approach. The lack of funding for training programs needs to be addressed, as it lies at the core of this unmet need. Career opportunities, however, are flourishing, with increased demand in universities and teaching hospitals.

The Subject Matter of Geriatric Dentistry

Predoctoral Education

The information that dental professionals will need to have in order to care for this aging population represents a spectrum of topics relevant to the etiology, diagnosis, prevention, and management of oral diseases in older adults. It should ideally be divided into three parts: an overview of various perspectives on aging, clinical care of the older patient, and practice considerations which influence the kinds of care they are able to provide. These topics include but are not limited to:

I Overview of Aging

- Demographics of the Older Population;
- Myths and Realities of Aging;
- Psychological Aspects of Aging;

- Multicultural Aspects of Aging;
- The Biology of Aging;
- The Effects of Aging on Drug Therapy;
- Oral Physiology;
- Disease-Related Changes in Older Adults; and
- Care Options for the Older Adult.

II Clinical Care of the Older Adult

- Assessment of the Older Adult;
- Nutrition and Oral Health;
- Modifications of Treatment Planning for the Older Adult:

  - Restorative Considerations;
  - Periodontic Considerations;
  - Prosthetic Considerations;
  - Endodontic Considerations; and
  - Oral and Maxillofacial Surgical Considerations.

III Oral Health Delivery for Older Adults

- Organizing and Delivering Oral Health Care;
- Treatment for the Confined Individual;
- Treatment to the Dentally Underserved;
- Treatment to the Medically Compromised;
- Preventive Dentistry for the Older Adult;
- Financing Oral Health; and
- Marketing Oral Health Care to the Older Adult Population.

Goals for Predoctoral Geriatric Education

As a result of having taken a geriatric dentistry course, students should be able to:

- Understand the many factors influencing the aging process;
- Maintain or improve the quality of life for their patients by providing them with optimal oral health care;
- Appreciate the multidisciplinary needs of the older patient;
- Expel some of the myths and stereotypes about aging and the aged which exist in Western society;
- Understand what is included in the subject area of geriatric dentistry; and
- Integrate their previous coursework and apply it to diagnosis and treatment planning for their older patients (Tepper, 2006).

These goals are basic to an understanding of the multidisciplinary nature of the needs of our older population, as well as a structure by which the curriculum needs to be organized in terms of content, resources, and requirements. Similar goals have been recently developed by the American Dental Education Association, and distributed to dental schools throughout the United States (ADEA, 2006).

The scopes of practice for general dentists and dental specialists are defined by the accreditation standards for their respective educational programs, by the ADA Principles of Ethics and Code of Conduct, and by the definitions of dentistry and the definitions of individual specialties as approved by the ADA. These are reflected in predoctoral course content, as developed by dental school faculty. Since the above list of geriatric dentistry course content is so wide in scope, it is suggested that other means of education besides the traditional didactic approach, be utilized. This includes approaches cited by the American Dental Education Association such as CD-ROM Case Studies, Web Resources, and community outreach experiences (ADEA, 2006).

Currently, schools and colleges of dental medicine offer a variety of educational experiences, with general suggestions and guidelines having been provided by the American Dental Education Association at various times (ADEA, 1989; ADEA 2006). The content of these courses should reflect the intended outcomes, as with education in all disciplines. The nature of the curriculum is multidisciplinary, and should reflect a variety of experiences that represent the interdisciplinary nature of treating the older adult. In consideration of the limited time often offered for these courses, it is usually an introductory overview of the processes of aging and the concerns of the older patient that are presented, in addition to the central focus which is the subject of providing the most appropriate oral health care for their older patients.

The multidisciplinary nature of gerontology and geriatric dentistry necessitates a perspective that integrates biological, psychological, and social aspects of aging along with oral health care. Many geriatric dentistry courses are presented toward the end of the students' didactic exposure, and require the student to draw upon information presented previously in the basic biological sciences, behavioral sciences, pathophysiology, oral diagnosis, and clinical dental coursework introduced earlier. Treating the older patient includes many considerations, including but not limited to immunity in the older patient, physiologic changes in all systems of the body, medication management and side effects, as well as oral pathologic changes seen in an aging individual. Psychological and social matters are related to the often complex changes including family relationships, self-confidence, self-esteem; personal skill losses related to one's ability to perform activities of daily living; sensory changes that affect function; communication barriers, cognitive changes, coping with losses and depression; and financial issues may add to the complexity of addressing oral health problems. Many geriatric dentistry courses use lectures by specialized dental practitioners, as well as medical, public health, and mental health professionals. Case studies and case analyses, as well as assigned readings to assist students in integrating and synthesizing knowledge around the subjects of gerontology and geriatric dentistry are often provided. Computerized case studies which require students to make clinical decisions based on multidisciplinary patient informational data are often used to drive home the multidimensional aspects of treatment planning for their older dental patients.

Innovative Models of Geriatric Dental Education

Currently there are several innovative models that utilize unique strategies, approaches, programs, processes, and systems to educate predoctoral students in geriatric dentistry. All programs acknowledge that this rapidly growing older population has complex dental, medical, and psychosocial needs that require oral care by competent dental clinicians with a unique set of attitudes, knowledge, and skills. They also advocate the need for an interdisciplinary team approach to provide optimal care.

Marquette University

Marquette University, as part of a school-wide curricular revision and renewal, developed a 4-year integrated geriatric dentistry curriculum and implemented during the 2003–2004 academic year. Geriatric concepts were woven into existing didactic material, rather than creating separate discipline-based courses. The key features of the curriculum employ a general dentistry approach, provide clinical experiences with older adults during all 4 years of instruction, facilitate progressive reinforcement of basic and behavioral sciences, and emphasize principles of preventive dentistry, public health, and ethics. The curriculum uses different teaching methods, including dental rounds, computer-assisted independent learning, small group discussions, and case-based instruction, to emphasize problem-solving skills, critical thinking, and lifelong learning. The curriculum emphasizes early clinical and community-based training, exposing students to the role of the dentist as a member of an interdisciplinary team caring for older adults (ADEA, 2006). Their Interdisciplinary Geriatric Oral Health Website was developed to provide an electronic learning environment for practicing health professionals and health professions students nationwide. It has been used in undergraduate and graduate teaching programs, as well as for continuing education purposes. The website represents a unique partnership between the Marquette University School of Dentistry and the Wisconsin Geriatric Education Center. This is a consortium of universities, health professions schools, health care systems, and community organizations nationally recognized for its excellence in interdisciplinary health professions education and training) (www.marquette.edu/dentistry; www.cuph.org.oralhealth/index.htm).

The University of Colorado

The University of Colorado School of Dentistry has developed "An Interdisciplinary Model for Community-Based Geriatric Dental Education: The Colorado Total Long-term Care Dental Program," which is based on the philosophy of the need to repay a portion of their educational indebtedness by practicing in an underserved area of Colorado or by donating dental services to high-need or indigent populations. As a result of this, they have implemented a program to involve students in community service which has also significantly developed their clinical skills by treating older adults who are part of a community-based long-term care program.

Students attend interdisciplinary team meetings and are provided the opportunity to work closely with geriatric health care providers (e.g., geriatricians, nurses, social workers, physical and occupational therapists, nutritionists, and mental health professionals) to improve their assessment, diagnostic, treatment planning, and geriatric patient management capacities (http://www.uchsc.edu/coa/index).

The University of Iowa

The University of Iowa College of Dentistry Geriatric and Special Needs Program is one of the longest-running community outreach programs in the College of Dentistry and The University of Iowa. It is composed of the Geriatric Mobile Unit (GMU) and the Special Care Clinic (SCC). First established in the early 1980s, the GMU provides comprehensive dental care for 10 nursing homes within a 40-mile radius of Iowa City. The GMU has a 30-foot motor home that is used to transport portable dental equipment to the nursing home, which is then set up in one or two rooms at the nursing home for several weeks. The use of portable dental units with high-speed handpieces enables the four dental students and supervising faculty to provide high-level comprehensive dental care for residents. The SCC was established in the late 1980s to support the GMU. The SCC has eight dental chairs and provides emergency and comprehensive dental care for frail and dependent patients with special dental needs, including those adults and older adults with complex medical conditions, physical and intellectual disabilities, and psychiatric conditions. Dental students spend a 5-week full-time rotation in the GMU and the SCC. A coordinated GMU dental hygiene nursing home program also visits all the nursing homes on a 6-monthly recall program. The GMU and SCC also provide a hands-on interdisciplinary clinical educational experience for geriatric dental fellows and geriatric medical fellows, in addition to dental hygiene, dental assisting, and pharmacy students (www.dentistry.uiowa.edu).

The University of Pittsburgh

The University of Pittsburgh School of Dental Medicine offers a unique Certificate in Geriatric Dentistry in response to the current and anticipated educational needs in the area of gerontology (ADEA, 2006). Members of the University of Pittsburgh Council on Aging collaborated to create a university-wide Graduate Certificate in Gerontology which is designed to serve professionals in diverse disciplines who are interested in acquiring basic knowledge about gerontology and geriatrics and gaining specialized knowledge of aging and aging processes in their particular fields of practice. Led by the School of Dental Medicine's Liaison to the Council on Aging, the Graduate Certificate in Geriatric Dentistry was developed by a working group of dental faculty and the Co-Director of the Geriatric Education Center of Pennsylvania, a component of the University Center for Social and Urban Research. Support to create the curriculum for the Graduate Certificate in Geriatric Dentistry was provided in part by a grant from the Health Services and Resources Administration (www.dental.pitt.edu/students/collaborative_ program.php#Geriatric_ Dentistry).

Columbia University

Columbia University College of Dental Medicine developed a Geriatric Dentistry Education Program in 1982 as a result of an award from the National Institute of Health, National Institute of Dental Research. Since that time, geriatric dentistry has been featured as a year-long senior didactic course, with CD-ROM multidisciplinary patient case studies. Students in all 4 years are involved in the ElderSmile Program, which was announced in 2004, and provides oral health education and screening to community elders living in underserved areas of New York City. This program represents the further development and expansion of the geriatric dentistry program which began in 1982. The College operates a Geriatric Dental Clinic once a week which is staffed by a multidisciplinary group of faculty and selected senior students. There is a monthly Geriatric Dentistry Symposia for students and faculty which provides informative round-table discussions concerning contemporary issues involved in treating older, medically compromised patients. Continuing education courses in gerontology and geriatric dentistry are offered to practicing dentists and dental hygienists on a yearly basis. The College's Advanced Education in General Dentistry (AEGD) offers a specialized program in geriatric dentistry which involves students and faculty rotating through a long-term care facility in the community (www.dental.columbia.edu/aegd).

Postdoctoral Clinical Training in Geriatric Dentistry

The development of specialized geriatric dentistry clinicians needs to be placed upon expanding postdoctoral training opportunities, as well as for practicing clinicians, clinical faculty, and geriatric academicians. This is occurring internationally. In Holland, a specialty in Geriatric Dentistry has been established. Schaub proposed an educational curriculum that includes seven learning modules. They are: affinity; somatic and mental disabilities; communicative skills and coping with behavioral disturbances; emergency medical care; history taking, assessment, prevention, treatments and evaluation; organization and legislation; and scientific training (Schaub & de Baat, 2006). In Yad Sarah, Israel, a 3-year Geriatric Dentistry program was established, including training in didactic, clinical, and home care settings (Zini & Pierrokovsky, 2006). Dentists participate on a voluntary basis and are awarded a diploma upon completion of the 3-year program.

In the United States, the older adult dental patient should receive even greater emphasis in General Practice Residency (GPR) and Advanced Education in General Dentistry (AEGD) programs. These are ideal programs in which to have students specialize in the care of older patients, or simply include older patients in different settings (community, institutions, and home care) in their clinical training programs. Since most of them will work primarily in private practice settings, they should be trained to competently care for older patients with complex medical, psychosocial, and dental care needs. For general practitioners who are in need of advanced skills in managing the growing number of older patients in their practices, continuing education is a real need. Universities and local dental associations should take the lead in providing this type of education. Advanced education for the practitioner can also be accomplished through intensive mini-courses at dental schools and through dental seminars and online courses.

Academic Geriatric Dentists: Clinical, Didactic, and Research Training

Postdoctoral faculty training programs in geriatric dentistry would train dental professionals who have mastered not only the technical procedures of dentistry, but the biological, psychological, and social science and research applicable to clinical geriatric dental practice. The Veteran's Administration was the first to initiate fellowship-training programs in geriatric medicine (1978), and geriatric dentistry (1982). Since the closure of these programs in 1992, the Health Resources and Services Administration (HRSA) has promoted joint fellowships in medicine and dentistry (Ettinger, Chalmers, & Frenkel, 2004), which continued until 1998, when the Health Professions Education Partnerships Act amended the Public Health Service Act to authorize funding for the purpose of providing support for geriatric training projects to train physicians, dentists, and behavioral and mental health professionals who plan to teach geriatric medicine, geriatric dentistry, or geriatric behavioral or mental health (www.hrsa.gov/grants). Dentists trained in programs such as these are intended to become leaders in geriatric dentistry training programs, serving as experts, role models, and initiators of further training programs within academic dentistry (U.S. Department of Health and Human Services, 1990). These programs are, however, headed up by medical schools, which may have directly influenced the small number of dental school faculty members with this needed training, resulting in the special interests and competencies in geriatric dentistry necessary to train dental students being presently far from adequate.

Geriatric dentists in academic settings must possess a variety of skills and attributes which include proficiency in scientific inquiry and methods, and grant writing. This calls for additional training in research methodology and grantsmanship, which can be accomplished by universities with public health schools, preferably in conjunction with dental schools which can offer specialized dental research opportunities. The focus can be on basic biological research, clinical research, educational research, behavioral science research, or health services research. The National Institute of Dental Research (NIDR), in collaboration with the National Institute on Aging, began offering geriatric dentistry research initiatives in 1986. The Veteran's Administration had a major role in this initiative, providing training sites for clinical research programs. Two years later, the NIDR Research and Action Program to Improve the Oral Health of Older Americans and Older Adults at High Risk was launched to expand further research programs targeting older adults (U.S. Department of Health and Human Services, 1990). The objectives of these programs are to develop highly qualified clinical researchers who are committed to a career pathway in oral health research.

Most recently, the National Institutes of Health, National Center for Research Resources has created a national consortium that will transform how clinical and translational research is conducted, ultimately enabling researchers to provide new treatments more efficiently and quickly to patients (National Center for Research Resources, 2007). These programs, known as Clinical and Translational Science Awards (CTSA), will eventually link 60 institutions together to energize the discipline of clinical and translational science. Academic dentists interested in clinical geriatric research may participate in these programs, thereby enhancing their knowledge and skills in geriatrics (http://www.ncrr.nih.gov/clinicaldiscipline.asp).

There is a need to expand these programs to support additional geriatric dentistry researchers in order to increase the knowledge base in oral health and aging. This in turn will serve as a foundation to develop additional education and training programs in geriatric dentistry, as well as educating practitioners in the care of their older patients.

Dental Hygiene and Dental Assisting Training

The education and training of dental hygienists and auxiliary health care workers in geriatric dentistry has not been well documented in the literature. A 1985 study estimated that about 7% of hygienists practice in non-traditional clinical setting which provide care to special patient groups, including physically, mentally or emotionally challenged, geriatric, or medically compromised patients (Cohen, LaBelle, & Singer, 1985). However, the training of dental hygienists for the purpose of identifying and reporting elder abuse has been documented (Murphree et al., 2002), as well as caring for people with disabilities (Johnson, 2000). The use of computer-based simulated geriatric patients has been used in training dental auxiliary staff (Johnson et al., 1997). However, there has been little documented in the way of formal geriatric dental education for these professional groups. Although core competencies for hygienists have been established (American Dental Education Association, 2004), none deal specifically with the care of the older dental patient. The nearest competencies referring to care of this population are competencies related to the referral of patients who may have a physiologic, psychological, and or social problem for comprehensive evaluation, as well as identifying individual and population risk factors and developing strategies that promote health related quality of life. For these reasons alone, a specialized curriculum in the treatment of the older dental patient needs to be specifically incorporated into the training of dental hygienists and dental assistants, as well as emphasized in continuing education programs for these practitioners. These dental auxiliaries trained in geriatric dentistry, working as part of the dental team, would be assuming a larger role in the care of this population, than those working in dental practices without this specialized training. Several states allow hygienists to work in long-term care settings under indirect supervision. Dental assistants are assuming more integral roles in restoration placement, impression taking, and simple prosthodontic procedures (U.S. Department of Health and Human Services, 1990). Managed dental care, in order to be cost-effective, may promote and increased need for an expanded role of dental auxiliaries. Competency-based evaluation and standards of care should be proactively defined for each level of dental provider in order to facilitate the best oral health outcomes possible for the older population.

Continuing Education in Geriatric Dentistry

The growth of subject matter and advances in treating older adults has resulted in the need for dentists, dental hygienists, and dental assistants to keep up with the latest technological advances in dentistry, as well as the expanding knowledge base about the diverse needs of this population. This includes general clinical care, improving their skills in diagnosis, treatment planning, and the medical and psychosocial management of their older patients. This type of training opportunity would be central in teaching oral health professionals how to work effectively with members of the interdisciplinary geriatric health care team. It would also assist them in expanding their responsibilities for primary health care using expanded function dental assistants and hygienists.

Interpersonal Communication and Ageism

Modern medical and dental education has recently placed more emphasis on the psychosocial and multicultural aspects of patient care. Behavioral science is now represented as a department or division in most schools of dentistry and medicine. It is within these courses that the principles of good doctor–patient relationships and communication styles are learned (Hannah, Millichamp, & Ayers, 2004). An emphasis on eliminating the negative stereotyping that often influences the practitioner–patient relationship needs to be part of the curriculum. Educational interventions at every level have helped reduced racism and sexism, but have been lagging in addressing *ageism*, the third "ism" that plagues relationships at every level. Addressing ageism in the dental curriculum is an important requisite to insure patient relationships foster the rapport necessary to provide optimal care and compliance (Waldrop et al., 2006). Negative stereotyping of older people needs to be addressed directly, not only at the cognitive level (i.e. knowledge-based), but also at the affective and behavioral levels.

The Interdisciplinary Nature of Care

Definitions and Rationale

The terms *multidisciplinary* and *interdisciplinary* are often used interchangeably. Multidisciplinary care refers to the many specialties, often working within the same organization or institution, that frequently plan goals and interventions for their patients independently of other specialties. In contrast, an interdisciplinary team approach assumes joint responsibility for treatment outcomes by setting goals and making treatment decisions together (Miller, 2004). The frequent collaboration among interdisciplinary teams (formally or informally) is what explicitly differentiates interdisciplinary team approaches from multidisciplinary team approaches.

The multidisciplinary nature of geriatrics and gerontology necessitates the need for an interdisciplinary training and teamwork approach to education and training. One discipline alone cannot meet the often complex and multiple needs that the elderly confront.

Interdisciplinary Care Models

Perhaps much could be gained by examining the interdisciplinary geriatric care models presented in the disciplines of medicine, psychology, social work, and nursing. The Columbia Cooperative Aging Program is one such program developed in response to the lack of dedicated resources to finance a comprehensive residency in geriatrics (Maurer et al., 2006). Residents complete a comprehensive assessment of older patients under the supervision of social workers, physicians, psychiatrists, geriatric nurses, and public health educators. Narrative assignments were implemented to stimulate reflection upon the reasoning processes utilized throughout the assessment. Positive effects were reported regarding knowledge of and attitudes toward older patients.

Interdisciplinary approaches have even grown to encompass cooperation between entire learning institutions. The Consortium of E-Learning in Geriatrics Instruction (CELGI) was formed in 2003, and now contains participants from 40 different schools from different fields of geriatric care (Ruiz et al., 2007). CELGI concentrates on providing a coordinated approach to formulating and adapting specifications, standards, and guidelines; developing education and training in e-learning competencies; evaluating the effect of e-learning materials; and disseminating these materials. No dental education institution is currently listed as a member of the consortium.

There have been several models of interdisciplinary training and service provision which have been supported by the Hartford Foundation. Geriatric interdisciplinary team training (GITT) is an initiative funded by the John A. Hartford Foundation since 1995. Building from the substantial knowledge gained from the Veteran's Administration project in interdisciplinary team training and lessons from the Pew Foundation initiative, GITT was reconceived by the Foundation to address the need for teams in the care of older adults in the new era of managed care and health care cost containment. This training program has served to help us understand attitudes toward teams, how teams function, and how teams should be trained (Fulmer, Flaherty, & Hyer, 2003). The Jahnigen Scholars program offers 2-year career development awards that support 10 junior medical faculty each year to promote medical specialties to train in multiple medical disciplines, with the purpose of sustaining a career in research and education in geriatric medicine (www.americangeriatrics.org/hartford/jahnigen).

Interdisciplinary training for nurses in geriatrics has addressed the care of the frail, medically compromised older adult. Their belief is that because one health care professional can not possibly have all of the specialized skills required to implement such a model of health care delivery, interdisciplinary team care must evolve in both training and practice (Dyer & Hyer, 2003). Interdisciplinary gerontology training programs for psychologists ("geropsychology") are small in number, but the need for specially trained psychologists is increasing, both in the community, and in long-term care facilities. There are several training models that prepare students in this specialty, which emphasize training with other disciplines and the domains of knowledge required for work with this population (Hinrichsen & Zweig, 2005). Similarly, social work education and practice have recognized the need for teamwork in addressing the complex needs of older adults. Wesley (2005) identified the need to increase awareness of the complex needs of older adults in social work education, and to integrate content and practical with other disciplines (Wesley, 2005). Social workers, along with psychologists, psychiatrists, general practitioners, nurses, and nurse practitioners have identified the need to break from the traditional paradigm of health care which emphasized disease and cure, and offer a more realistic model of care of health care delivery in which the interdisciplinary team care has evolved to include palliative care. They also have identified the many challenges that occur when Geriatric Interdisciplinary Teams are involved in providing care to frail older patients (Dyer et al., 2003). Dental involvement in interdisciplinary geriatric care efforts have not been extensively described in the literature. Currently, there are several dental programs that take part in interdisciplinary care teams. The University of the Pacific School of Dentistry has reported such work with the provision of routine care at a senior health center. Undergraduate dental students are called upon to present patients to an interdisciplinary team and also help educate senior health center staff on issues in oral health (Chavez & LaBarre, 2004). The dental education programs at Marquette University, the University of Iowa, and the University of Pittsburg offer training experiences with other disciplines at the predoctoral level, and the American Dental Education Association has recommended guidelines for interdisciplinary training and practice at all levels (ADEA, 2006).

Interdisciplinary teamwork is essential to meet the multiple, complex needs of older adults. The sooner practitioners learn to work collaboratively and interdependently, the more likely it will be to insure that comprehensive and coordinated care will take place for this growing population.

Conclusion

Oral health care for older adults which is comprehensive in nature requires an understanding of both the biomedical and psychosocial concerns of this population. Dental providers are members of a multidisciplinary health care team. In this role, they share the responsibility of understanding the older patient as a person and not just a "clinical case." The process of educating dental care professionals provides educators with a significant opportunity for helping both students and practitioners develop an awareness of how their older patients' bio-psycho-social concerns influence the practice of their profession, and how they directly influence the quality of life for them.

Oral health care should be part of the training of all health care providers. It should be integrated into curricula at all levels. In practice settings, medical decision-making should take into account the oral health needs of the individual. Treatment which does not consider oral health is incomplete and incompetent.

Interdisciplinary education and training along with other medical, public health, and social service specialties needs to become a regular part of geriatric dental education. These specialties also need to include geriatric dentistry as part of their educational and training experiences. This can be accomplished in team-like settings, emphasizing cooperative problem-solving with multifactorial issues related to the comprehensive care of older people.

Developing educational interventions that promote geriatric dental education should be among the major academic goals of this decade. These programs will provide dental practitioners with increased knowledge of aging and the skills to both assess and respond to their oral as well as their general medical and social concerns. Geriatric dentistry needs to be recognized as a dental specialty, as other dental specialties, which require special training and accreditation. However, at present, it is not, which has directly influenced the numbers of dentists who limit their practice to care of the elderly. At the root of this problem is the need to address funding which would enable this specialized training to take place, not only for the dental profession, but for the other medical and mental health professionals who treat the growing numbers of older, medically complex individuals in our society.

References

American Association of Dental Schools (1989). Curriculum guidelines for geriatric dentistry, *Journal of Dental Education, 5*, 313–316.

American Dental Education Association (2003). Improving the oral health status of all Americans: Roles and responsibilities of academic dental institutions. Washington, D.C.

American Dental Education Association (2004). Competencies for entry into the profession of dental hygiene: (As approved by the 2003 House of Delegates). *Journal of Dental Education, 68*, 745–749.

American Dental Education Association (2006). Oral health for independent adults: ADEA/GSK pre-doctoral resource curriculum guide (CD Rom).

Baumeister, S.E., Davidson, P.L., Carreon, D.C., Nakazono, T.T., Gutierrez, J.J, & Anderson, R.M. (2007). What influences dental students to serve special care patients? *Special Care Dentistry, 27*, 15–22.

Berkey, D., & Berg, R. (2001). Geriatric oral health issues in the United States. *International Dental Journal, 6*, 254–264.

Brown, L.J., Winn, D.M., & White, B.A. (1996). Dental caries, restoration and tooth conditions in the U.S. adults, 1988–1991. *Journal of the American Dental Association, 127*, 1315–1325.

Chavez, E.M., & LaBarre, E.E. (2004). A predoctoral clinical geriatric dentistry rotation at the University of the Pacific School of Dentistry. *Journal of Dental Education, 68*, 454–459.

Cohen, L., LaBelle, A., & Singer, J (1985). Educational preparation of hygienists working with special populations in nontraditional settings. *Journal of Dental Education, 49*, 592–595.

Commission on Dental Accreditation (2004). Accreditation standards for dental education programs. Chicago: American Dental Association, June 30, 2004.

Dolan, T.A., Atchison, K., & Huynh, T.N. (2005). Access to dental care among older adults in the United States. *Journal of Dental Education, 69*, 961–974.

Dorfman, L.T., Murty, S.A., Ingram, J.G., & Li, H. (2007). Evaluating the outcomes of gerontological curriculum enrichment: A multi-method approach. *Gerontology and Geriatrics Education, 27*, 1–21.

Dyer, C.D., & Hyer, K. (2003). Frail older patient care by interdisciplinary teams: A primer for generalists. *Gerontology and Geriatrics Education, 24*(2), 63–74.

Dyer, C.B., Hyer, K., Feldt, K.S., Lindemann, D.A., Busby-Whitehead, J., Greenberg, S., Kennedy, R.D., & Flaherty, E. (2003). Frail older patient care by interdisciplinary teams: A primer for generalists. *Gerontology and Geriatrics Education, 24*, 51–62.

Ettinger, R., & Beck, J. (1984). Geriatric dental education curriculum and the needs of the elderly. *Special Care Dentistry, 4*, 207–213.

Ettinger, R., Chalmers, J., & Frenkel, H. (2004). Dentistry for persons with special needs: How should it be recognized? *Journal of Dental Education, 68*, 803–806.

Federal Interagency Forum on Aging Related Statistics (2004). Older Americans 2004: Key indicators of well-being; http://www.agingstats.gov/.

Fulmer, T., Flaherty, E., & Hyer, K. (2003). Geriatric interdisciplinary team training (GITT) initiatives. *Gerontology and Geriatrics Education, 24*, 3–12.

Glista, S., & Petersons, M. (2003). A model curriculum for interdisciplinary allied health gerontology education. *Gerontology and Geriatrics Education, 23*, 27–40.

Hannah, A., Millichamp, C.J., & Ayers, K. (2004). A communication skills course for undergraduate dental students. *Journal of Dental Education, 68*, 970–977.

Healthy People, 2010. Washington, DC: National Center for Health Statistics, U.S. Department of Health and Human Services; http://www.healthypeople.gov/.

Hinrichsen, G.A., & Zweig, R.A. (2005). Models of training in clinical geropsychology. *Gerontology and Geriatrics Education, 25*, 1–4.

Johnson, L.A., Cunningham, M.A., Finkelstein, M.W., & Hand, J.S. (1997). Geriatric patient simulations for dental hygiene. *Journal of Dental Education, 61*, 667–677.

Johnson, T.L. (2000). Pilot study of dental hygienists' comfort and confidence levels and care planning for patients with disabilities. *Journal of Dental Education, 64*, 839–846.

Kress, G.C., & Vidmar, G. (1985). A compendium of objectives for geriatric dentistry. *Journal of Dental Education, 49*, 627–635.

Lamster, I.B. (2004). Oral health care services for older adults: A looming crisis. *American Journal of Public Health, 94*, 699–702.

MacEntee, M.I., Prukscapong, M., & Wyatt, C.C. (2005). Insights from students following an educational rotation through dental geriatrics. *Journal of Dental Education, 69*, 1268–1376.

Maurer, M.S., Costley, A.W., Miller, P.A., McCabe, S., Dubin, S., Cheng, H., Varela-Burstei, E., Lam, B., Irvine, C., Page, K.P., Ridge, G., & Gurland, B. (2006). The Columbia Cooperative Aging Program: An interdisciplinary and interdepartmental approach to geriatric education for medical interns. *Journal of the American Geriatrics Society, 54*, 520–526.

Miller, P.A. (2004). Interdisciplinary teamwork: The key to quality care for older adults. In Tepper, L.M., & Cassedy, T.M. (Eds.), *Multidisciplinary perspectives on aging* (pp. 259–276). New York: Springer.

Mohammad, A.R. (2001). *Geriatric dentistry: a clinical guidebook*, 2nd ed. Columbus: Ohio State University.

Mohammad, A.R., Preshaw, P.M., & Ettinger, R.L. (2003). Current status of predoctoral geriatric education in U.S. dental schools. *Journal of Dental Education, 5*, 509–514.

Moshman, J., Warren, G.B., Blandford, D.H., & Aumack, L. (1985). Geriatric dentistry in the predoctoral curriculum. *Journal of Dental Education, 4*, 689–695.

Murphree, K.R., Campbell, P.R., Gutmann, M., Plichta, S.B., Nunn, M., McCann, A.L., & Gibson, G. (2002). How well prepared are Texas dental hygienists to recognize and report elderly abuse? *Journal of Dental Education, 66*, 1274–1280.

National Center for Research Resources, National Institutes of Health (2007). Washington, D.C. (May 27, 2007) http://www.ncrr.nih.gov/clinicaldiscipline.asp

Oral health in America: A report of the surgeon general (2000). Rockville, MD: U.S. Department of Health and Human Services, National Institute of Dental and Craniofacial Research, National Institutes of Health.

Ruiz, J.G., Teasdale, T.A., Hajjar, I., Shaughnessy, M., & Mintzer, M.J. (2007). The consortium of e-learning in geriatrics instruction. *Journal of the American Geriatrics Society, 55*, 458–463.

Saunders, R.H. (1985). Graduate education in geriatric dentistry. *Gerondontology, 4*, 53–57.

Schaub R.M., & de Baat, C. (2006). Specialties in dentistry, 4: Post-academic specialization in geriatric dentistry. *Nederlands tijdschrift voor tandheelkunde, 113*, 496–501.

Teasdale, T.A., & Shaikh, M. (2006). Efficacy of a geriatric oral health CD as a learning tool. *Journal of Dental Education, 70*, 1366–1369.

Tepper, L.M. (1980). *Gerontology in higher education: The development of competency-based curricula.* (Doctoral Dissertation, 1980).

Tepper, L.M. (1990). Outpatient programs from the training point of view: Geriatric dentistry training at Columbia University. In Bennett, R., & Killeffer, E. (Eds.), *Successful models of community long term care services for the elderly* (pp. 85–90). New York: The Haworth Press.

Tepper, L.M. (1999). Paying attention to oral health. *City health information, 20*, 7–8.

Tepper, L.M. (2006). Gerontology and Geriatric Dentistry: A Course Syllabus. New York: Columbia University College of Dental medicine.

U.S. Department of Health and Human Services, Public Health Service, Bureau of Health Professions (1990). *A National Agenda for Geriatric Education, 1*, 125–152.

Waldman, H.B., Fenton, S.J., Perlman, S.P., & Cinotti, D.A. (2005). Preparing dental graduates to provide care to individuals with special needs. *Journal of Dental Education, 69*, 249–254.

Waldrop, D.P., Fabiano, J.A., Nochajski, T.H., Zittel-Palamara, K.M., Davis, E.L., & Goldberg, L.J. (2006). More than a set of teeth: Assessing and enhancing dental students' perceptions of older adults. *Gerontology and Geriatrics Education, 27*, 37–56.

Wesley, S. C. (2005). Enticing students to Careers in gerontology: Faculty and student perspectives. *Gerontology and Geriatrics Education, 25*(3), 13–29.

Yellowitz, J., & Saunders, M. (1989). The need for geriatric dental education. *Dental Clinics of North America, 33*, 8–11.

Zini, A., & Pierrokovsky, J. (2006). Gerodontology teaching program at the geriatric dental clinic in Yad Sarah. *Refuat Hapeh Vehashinayim, 24*, 31–34.

Chapter 20
Dental Services Among Elderly Americans: Utilization, Expenditures, and Their Determinants

L. Jackson Brown

Introduction

For the large majority of the U.S. population, access to dental care is excellent. The percentage of the population who utilize dental services has increased markedly and steadily since World War II (Brown, 2005a; Brown & Lazar, 1998; U.S. Department of Health and Human Services, 1972, 1999, 2002, 2004, 2006). In 2005, 65% of those 2 years old and older visited a dentist within the last year; 78% visited within 2 years. Moreover, millions of middle-class Americans with family incomes greater than $50,000 did not visit a dentist within that time period, but certainly had the resources to access dental care. The nation's overall oral health is improving (Johnson, Kelly, & Van Kirk, 1965; Kelly, Van Kirk, & Garst, 1967a; Kelly, Van Kirk, & Garst, 1967b; Baird & Kelly, 1970; Kelly & Harvey, 1974; Kelly & Harvey, 1979; Brown, 2005a; Dye et al., 2007). Near-term and long-term outlooks for the affordability and accessibility of dental care for the majority of Americans remain excellent, a situation that owes in no small part to dentistry's outstanding record of prevention, efficiency, and cost-control.

However, access to dental services in the United States exhibits marked variation among different segments of the population (Jack & Bloom, 1988; Bloom, Gift, & Jack, 1992; Brown & Lazar, 1999; Hughes, Duderstadt, Soobader, & Newacheck, 2005). Individuals, who want dental care, who have the financial resources to pay it, who live in areas with abundant dental personnel, and who can get to a dentist without undue difficulty demonstrate the greatest use of dental services in the United States (Aday, 1993; Brown, 2005a; Shi & Stevenss, 2005).

Amidst an abundance of dental services for the huge majority of Americans, pockets of our citizens do not access dental services commensurate with the overall population (Brown, 2005a; U.S. Department of Health and Human Services, 2000). For individuals with meager incomes, especially those who live in areas with few dental personnel, access is more difficult. For individuals who are not ambulatory or have severe disease, disabilities, or other special problems, harsh barriers to dental care are facts of life.

L.J. Brown
President of L. Jackson Brown Consulting

I.B. Lamster, M.E. Northridge (eds.), *Improving Oral Health for the Elderly*,
© Springer Science+Business Media, LLC 2008

When examining remedies to limited access to dental care in the United States, attention primarily has focused on our children – with good reason. They represent the future. Among children, if oral disease can be prevented or treated early, that entire generation will reap a lifetime of benefit. Moreover, the nation reaps generations of improved oral health and the need to commit fewer resources to maintain adult oral health (Brown, Beazoglou, & Heffley, 1994).

The results of this attention to our children are remarkable. Caries has been reduced by over 70% from post-World War II levels (Brown & Lazar, 1999; Dye et al., 2007). More teeth are retained and untreated caries in those teeth has been greatly reduced. All segments of the child population have benefited, including disadvantaged children. Moreover, these improvements from early prevention and more access have been observed in adults, especially those aged 45 or younger (Brown & Swango, 1993; Brown, Wall, & Lazar, 2002).

Despite overall improvement in oral health, disparities in utilization of dental care between disadvantaged children and the remainder of children are among the largest in all health care (U.S. Department of Health and Human Services, 2000; Kelly, Binkley, Neace, & Gale, 2005; Kenney, McFeeters, & Yee, 2005; Kim, 2005). Thus, it is not surprising that children have been the primary beneficiaries of the meager public funds that are available for dental services from all levels of government in the United States.

Too often, dental services for the elderly have not engaged the nation's attention, but rather have been an afterthought. This is in contrast to the provision of medical services for the elderly which has been a major focus to public policy (Drake, 1994). The attention to the medical needs of seniors is understandable since the elderly years, like childhood, can be a period of dependency. It is frequently also a period that requires extensive and complicated management of chronic diseases and disabilities. The nation's expenditures on health care for the elderly are enormous and growing apace (Lubitz, Beebe, & Baker, 1995; Rettenmaier & Saving, 2007).

The senior years can also be a period of need for extensive and complicated oral health care. Today's elderly missed the greatest benefits of modern oral health prevention because their dentitions developed and their childhood years passed before the modern era of prevention began. Their caries experience, periodontal disease, and tooth loss were greater as children and young adults than later generations. As a consequence, today's elderly have extensive and complicated oral health needs (Dolan & Atchison, 1993). It should be remembered that the Surgeon General's Report on Oral Health emphasized that an individual should not be considered in good health unless he/she is also in good oral health (U.S. Department of Health and Human Services, 2000).

For purposes of this discussion, the elderly will be defined as those individuals 65 years of age or older. This, of course, is largely an arbitrary cutoff, due in no small part to the original age of eligibility for social security benefits. Nevertheless, for many persons, age 65 has represented a major life transition. A large proportion retired around that age and lived on reduced incomes the remainder of their lives. Among previous generations of elderly, the large majority never had private dental insurance coverage during their working years. For the minority who received dental insurance through their employment, most lost the coverage when they retired

(U.S. Department of Health and Human Services, 1999, 2002). As the elderly aged into their seventies or older, they frequently developed one or more chronic diseases. Some had difficulty undertaking activities of daily living, including attending a dentist. As a result, the elderly, and especially the older elderly (aged 80+), too often disappeared from the dental offices of our country (Dolan, Atchison, & Huynh, 2005; Dolan, Corey, & Freeman, 1988).

Over the last couple of generations, there has been a small revolution in the lifestyle and economic circumstances of the U.S. elderly. The elderly of the late twentieth and early twenty-first centuries have more economic resources, are more ambulatory, and have improved functional capacity compared to their predecessors (He, Sengupta, Velkoff, & DeBarros, 2005). In addition, today's elderly, although they missed the greatest benefits of prevention, have on average better oral health than previous generations of elderly. A smaller percentage is edentulous and the dentate elderly has retained more of their teeth (Brown, 2005b; Dye et al., 2007).

This progress in the oral health of the elderly deserves celebration. However, the edentulous elderly should still receive regular dental check-ups and indicated therapy. The dentate elderly remain at risk for the traditional oral diseases, including caries and periodontal diseases. It is not uncommon for elderly individuals to lose a substantial portion of the bony mass in their mandibles, rendering replacement therapy more complicated and expensive (Eiseman, Johnson, & Coll, 2005). Xerostomia can be a problem for some elderly (Astor, Hanft, & Ciocon, 1999). Perhaps most important, oral cancer, a disease that increases in incidence with age, impacts the elderly more frequently. All elderly should receive periodic examinations for all oral conditions and especially for the early detection of oral cancer (U.S. Department of Health and Human Services, 2000).

With many changes occurring in the social, economic, and health circumstances of the U.S. elderly, now is a propitious time to revisit their oral health conditions and their access to dental services. A survey of utilization among the elderly should document past trends and take a glimpse at what the future may hold. It is appropriate that this assessment be undertaken, not only for today's elderly, but for the generations of Americans who will join their ranks as we progress deeper into the new century.

The American Elderly

Size and Projected Growth

The U.S. population has grown continuously throughout its history. Population growth accelerated during the immediate post-World War II years (U.S. Census Bureau, 2002). In fact, U.S. Census Bureau intercensus projections underestimated the size of the U.S. population documented during the 2000 census (U.S. Census Bureau, 2004d). The U.S. population will continue to grow. The Census Bureau projects that the U.S. population will reach 363.6 million by 2030 and 419.9 million by 2050 (U.S. Census Bureau, 2004c). This growth rate will result in 51 million

Table 20.1 U.S. population and elderly population 1900–2030

	Year	Total Population	65+ as Percent of total	Elderly population			
				65+	65–74	75–84	85+
	1900	76.2	4.1	3.1	2.2	0.8	0.1
	1910	92.2	4.3	3.9	2.8	1.0	0.2
	1920	106.0	4.7	4.9	3.5	1.3	0.2
	1930	123.2	5.4	6.6	4.7	1.6	0.3
	1940	132.2	6.8	9.0	6.4	2.3	0.4
	1950	151.3	8.1	12.3	8.4	3.3	0.6
	1960	179.3	9.2	16.6	11.0	4.6	0.9
	1970	203.3	9.9	20.1	12.4	6.1	1.5
	1980	226.5	11.3	25.6	15.6	7.7	2.2
	1990	248.7	12.6	31.2	18.1	10.1	3.1
	2000	281.4	12.4	35.0	18.4	12.4	4.2
	2010	308.9	13.0	40.2	21.3	12.9	6.1
Projections	2020	335.8	16.3	54.6	31.8	15.6	7.3
	2030	363.6	19.5	71.5	37.9	23.9	9.6

Source: 65+ in the United States, 2005, U.S. Depts. of HHS & Commerce

more Americans, over an 18% increase in just 30 years. By mid-century, the population increase will expand to almost 140 million more Americans, a near 50% increase and approximately equivalent to the entire U.S. population in 1950 (see Table 20.1).

Even more astounding, the elderly portion of the population will increase disproportionately faster than the total population (U.S. Census Bureau, 2004c). In 1900, the elderly comprised about 4% of the total U.S. population. By 1950, the percentage had increased to 8%. In 2000, the percentage had grown to 12.4%. By 2030, the elderly are projected to represent almost 20% of the U.S. population (see Table 20.1) (He et al., 2005).

Absolute numbers are more relevant for assessing the resources that will be required to address the elderly demand for dental services. In 1900, there were only 3.1 million Americans of age 65 or older. By mid-century their number had increased to 12.3 million, and by 2000, the elderly had increased to 35.0 million. Census projections estimate the elderly will number over 71 million by 2030. This would represent a doubling of the elderly population in 30 years at an annual growth rate of almost 2.4%. Some demographers believe that these projections are underestimates (Ahlburg, 1993; Camarota, 2001).

Age Composition

The age distribution of the elderly will also change. In 1950, there were 8.4 million elderly 65–74 years old. Individuals in this age range are frequently called the young elderly. Then as now, a large percentage of individuals in this age range remained robust and were fully ambulatory. A majority were self-sufficient whether living with their spouses or alone. That same year, 3.3 million elderly were 75–84 years old and slightly more than one-half million were 85 years of age or older. The latter two age groups are frequently referred to as the old elderly (He et al., 2005). Then as now, many of those individuals had developed multiple chronic diseases, had limited mobility, and required assistance with activities of daily living. A substantial percentage no longer could live independently.

In the 2000 census, the number of elderly was documented at 35 million, of which 18.4 million were between 65 and 74 years of age, another 12.4 were between 75 and 84 years, and the 85+ group had grown to 4.2 million. Census projections for 2030 estimate 37.9 million elderly aged 65–74, another 23.9 million aged 75–84 and 9.6 million aged 85 and older will be alive. Every elderly age group is expected to double in the next 30 years (U.S. Census Bureau, 2004c). Even at today's utilization rates, the elderly in 30 years will represent a substantial proportion of the demand for dental services. For reasons explained later, utilization among future generations of elderly is very likely to increase.

Gender Composition

Over the last century, a larger number of women compared to men lived to advanced age. Table 20.2 displays the number of elderly population in 2000 and the projected elderly population out to 2030, by age and gender (He et al., 2005; U.S. Census Bureau, 2004a, 2004b, 2004c). In 2000, over 4 million more women compared to men aged 65–84 were alive. For those 85 years or older, women outnumbered men 3 million to 1.2 million. By 2030, the number of women aged 65–84 is projected

Table 20.2 Sociodemographic characteristics projected to 2030

Sociodemographic characteristics	2000		2030	
	Number	Percent	Number	Percent
Total elderly	39.2	100	81.0	100
Total 65–84	30.8	78.6	61.8	76.3
Male	13.2	33.7	28.0	34.6
Female	17.6	44.9	33.8	41.7
Total 85+	4.2	10.7	9.6	11.9
Male	1.2	3.1	3.3	4.1
Female	3.0	7.7	6.3	7.8
White-NH	29.3	74.7	51.7	63.8
Other	0.4	1.0	6.8	8.4
Black-NH	2.8	7.1	1.4	1.7
Asian	0.8	2.0	3.7	4.6
Hispanic (any race)	1.8	4.6	7.8	9.6

Source: U.S. Census Bureau

to double to 33.8 million while the number of men will more than double to 28.0 million. For those aged 85+, women will double to 6.3 million and men will triple to 3.3 million. In 2030, elderly women will remain more numerous than men but the ratio will narrow. As will be discussed later, the narrowing ratio could have significant implications for the economic status of elderly women and for the living arrangements of both genders. The elderly in 2030 will be predominately baby-boomers and post baby-boomers. Fewer of them will be edentulous and the dentate will retain more teeth.

Racial/Ethnic Composition

The racial/ethnic composition of the United States is changing rather rapidly. Table 20.2 also displays the racial/ethnic composition of the elderly population in 2000 and its projected composition in 2030 (U.S. Census Bureau, 2004d). The data indicate that diversity among the elderly will increase but markedly less than the diversity of the total U.S. population. Elderly are now and will remain predominately non-Hispanic Whites, at least through the 2030 timeframe. In 2000, non-Hispanic Whites comprised 68.7% of the total population but 83.5% of the elderly. By 2030, the percentage of non-Hispanic Whites is predicted to decrease to about 57% of the overall population; however, that group will still comprise nearly three-fourths of the elderly. Hispanics of any race are projected to register the greatest growth both in the overall population and among the elderly. Elderly non-Hispanic Blacks and Asians are predicted to increase, but both will remain a relatively small percentage of the elderly over the next 30 years.

The implications for the demand for dental services of these racial/ethnic changes could be substantial. As mentioned, among the elderly, non-Hispanic Whites will remain the huge majority. Historically, that group has had a lower rate of edentulism, has retained more teeth, and utilized dental services at a greater intensity than other segments of the population (Brown, 2005b; Dye et al., 2007). Whether or not these historical trends will persist will be an important factor in predicting the future demand for dental services among the elderly.

Economic Status

As a group, the economic circumstances of the elderly have been improving. Far from the past vision of the elderly as almost universally destitute, today's elderly have accumulated more financial resources than ever before (He et al., 2005; Employee Benefit Research Institute, 2006). A majority have sufficient income and assets to live independently and enjoy their senior years. However, by focusing on the group as a whole, one overlooks the breathtakingly huge variation in material well-being that exists among segments of the elderly.

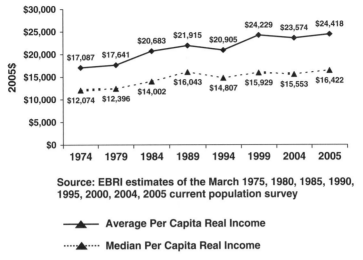

Source: EBRI estimates of the March 1975, 1980, 1985, 1990, 1995, 2000, 2004, 2005 current population survey

Fig. 20.1 Real average and median income of the elderly, selected Years 1974–2005
Source: EBRI estimates of the March 1975, 1980, 1985, 1990, 1995, 2000, 2004, 2005 current population survey

Figure 20.1 shows that the average per capita real income from all sources for the elderly for selected years since 1974. Average per capita real income (measured in 2005 in dollars) increased from approximately $17,000 in 1974 to about $24,500 in 2005 – over a $7,000 (43%) increase in per capita income in 31 years (Employee Benefit Research Institute, 2006). The median income among elderly exhibited a similar trend but with a less rapid increase. In fact, median income leveled off around 1989 and has been essentially stable since then.

The relationship between the two trend lines indicates something about the change in the distribution of income among elderly. First, the median income, throughout the time period, was substantially below the average per capita income. This indicates that the income distribution of the elderly is skewed upwards, i.e., a minority of the elderly has a relatively high income which raises the average income of the entire group. This obscures the fact that a majority of the elderly are concentrated in the lower income range. In addition the spread between the average and the median has widened over the period. The median income leveled off before the average income, suggesting that the skew of the income distribution has become more pronounced recently. This trend bears careful monitoring because it is an indicator of income inequality and illustrates the limitations of using averages when assessing the number of elderly who have financial difficulty accessing dental care.

While the income stream to the elderly as a group has improved, elderly income remains the lowest of any age group (He et al., 2005; Employee Benefit Research Institute, 2006). In 2003 median household income among the elderly was $23,787, almost $20,000 below the overall median household income. (The reader is alerted to the difference between household and per capita income – the latter measures the income stream of the entire household.) It was even below the median income of young people just starting the careers ($27,000). The young, however, can look forward to an increase of income and an accumulation of assets as their careers progress. In contrast, it is rare that the income of the elderly increase as they age, and their assets sometimes dissipate as they cope with the loss of the income stream of a deceased spouse or the expense of failing health and supervised care.

Overall, the elderly receive 39% of their income from social security. Another 24% derives from earnings – many elderly still work, at least part-time (He et al., 2005). Eighteen percent is derived from pensions acquired through their working years. Sixteen percent derives from income from assets. Combined, these sources provide a fairly broad range of income streams; no one source, not even social security, completely dominates. This is a pattern that should provide comfort. Overall the elderly do not have to depend totally on one source of income. For many, if they decide to quit a part-time job, they may be pinched but can probably get by. If they cannot rent the house they own or the stock market drops, many have other income upon which to rely.

Figure 20.2 provides a harsher picture and displays the "have nots" and "haves" among the elderly (He et al., 2005; Employee Benefit Research Institute, 2006). These data illustrate the huge variation in the economic circumstances of the elderly that exists. The pie chart on the right is for the quintile with the highest income – greater than $32,000 annually in 2005. Social security plays a moderate role in their income stream. Close to 40% of the income for this quintile came from earnings. This group stills works; one cannot know from these data the reasons why they work: Some may be the young elderly still robust enough to work and find the activity enjoyable. Some may be in occupations that allow them to continue part-time. Others may have to work because of large family expenses. For whatever reason, over 80% of their income is derived from sources other than social security. These individuals have sufficient income to live a fairly comfortable life. Their medical expenses are largely covered by Medicare. Many also carry supplemental health insurance, and sometimes long-term care insurance. These elderly should have enough discretionary income to access the private dental delivery system if they do not have severe medical co-morbidities and are reasonably ambulatory.

The left pie chart provides a stark contrast. The median income of the lowest quintile of elderly is $7,900 or less annually. This is a grinding, subsistence level of poverty. These individuals are almost completely dependent on social security; they simply could not make it without it. Little money is left after paying for food, shelter, and possibly some medical expenses. These individuals are unlikely to have the discretionary income for dental care, and many do not seek care except when they are in pain or have some other emergency condition.

Several factors are associated with the large variation in income among the elderly. Age is an associated factor – on average, the older the senior the smaller the income stream. Gender is also a factor – single women have lower incomes than single men and both are much lower than married couples. Race/ethnicity is also a factor – African Americans and Hispanics have lower incomes than Whites and Asians, even after controlling for age and gender. Of course, these factors are likely

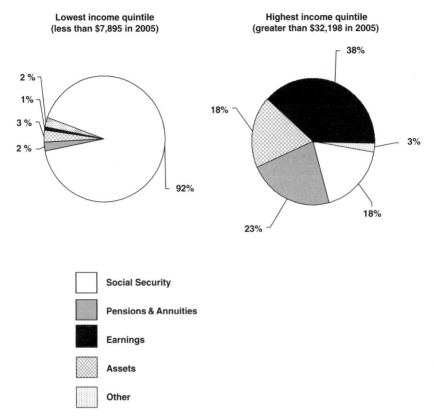

Fig. 20.2 Income sources of the elderly, lowest and highest quintiles, 2005
Source: EBRI estimates of the March 2006 current population survey

not to be truly causal. Instead, they are likely proxies for more basic drivers, such as education, occupation, health problems, and need for assisted living (He et al., 2005; Andersen & Benham, 1970).

Table 20.3 shows the impact of age, gender, and living single or as a couple on elderly incomes, controlling for the other two factors. Clearly, income goes down with age. Median household income among married couples aged 65–69 was over $45,000 in 2003. This is an income that is sufficient for a comfortable, but not luxurious lifestyle. However, the median income of married couples declined to less than $30,000 among those aged 75 and older. Of course, many married couples lose a spouse and join the ranks of single elderly as they grow older. It is difficult to explain married couples' decline in income with age, except as a slow erosion of financial resources due to declining health as a couple progresses through their senior years. Single men enjoy a smaller income advantage over single women but both of the groups demonstrate fewer declines in income with age. Of course, their incomes were not as high at the beginning of their senior years.

Table 20.3 Elderly Income by Age, Living Arrangements, and Race/Ethnicity, 2005

	65–69($)	70–74($)	75+($)
Married couple	45,305	36,055	29,280
Men living alone	17,842	18,298	16,937
Women living alone	16,474	14,332	13,172
Non-Hispanic White	35,798	28,451	20,298
Asian	32,652	24,084	15,649
African American	20,503	18,200	13,903
Hispanic (any race)	19,962	17,971	15,685

Source: 65+ in the United States, 2005, U.S. Depts. of HHS & Commerce

Median household income by age and race/ethnicity is also displayed in Table 20.3. Older seniors, as a group, have less income. Non-Hispanic Whites and Asians have higher incomes than Hispanics and African Americans by a sizable amount. The former two groups exhibit greater income decline with age. This may be related to the higher starting incomes for non-Hispanic Whites and Asians.

According to He et al. (2005), 1,720,500 elderly lived at or below the federal poverty level (FPL). The number of elderly living below FPL declined slightly from 1,772,031 who were in that state in 1990. Since the elderly population grew over the decade, the percent of elderly living below the FPL also declined. In 1990, 5.7% of the elderly were living in poverty, compared to 4.9% in 2000.

Table 20.4 shows how poverty rates and types of poverty among the elderly compared to other age groups. A smaller percentage of elderly experience episodic poverty (a temporary state of poverty due to some life event such as loss of job, divorce, time-limited illness, or disability). Individuals generally recover from this type of poverty; that is why it is called episodic. Teenagers are much more likely

Table 20.4 Poverty indicators and poverty by gender and race/ethnicity among the Elderly 1996, 1999

Poverty Indicators			
	Age		
Types of poverty	65+	18–64	<18
Exit from poverty	32.4	53.9	47.9
Entry into poverty	3.3	3.1	4.5
Chronic poverty	3.8	1.4	2.6
Episodic poverty	15.4	17.2	26.8
Percent FPL or below			
Race/ethnicity	Gender		
	Men	Women	
Hispanic (any race)	16.6	21.7	
Asian	12.3	16.0	
Black	17.7	27.4	
White-NH	5.4	10.0	
Total	7.3	12.5	

Source: 65+ in the United States, 2005, U.S. Depts. of HHS & Commerce than elderly to experience episodic poverty, even working-age individuals experience a slightly higher rate.

Chronic poverty is less common than the episodic type (He et al., 2005). Individuals remain in this type of poverty for extended periods due to the absence of employable skills, permanent disability, family breakup, and perhaps personal behavior habits. Elderly persons are more likely to experience chronic poverty because they may be too old to work. They may have expended their financial resources as a result of severe life events. Disabling disease, for example, frequently comes with two expenses – managing the disease and securing care-taking services. Taking both types of poverty together, about 20% of the elderly are in a poverty status, compared to close to 30% of teenagers and 18.5% of the working-age group. Not much difference by age group was observed regarding the likelihood of entering poverty of either type, but the elderly were much less likely to exit poverty once there.

Table 20.4 also shows that 12.5% of the elderly women and 7.3% of elderly men were below the federal poverty level of the year 2003 (He et al., 2005). These estimates exclude those who experience short episodes of poverty, which accounts for the difference with the previous percentage. A higher percentage of elderly women were living below the FPL than men, regardless of their race/ethnicity

Race/ethnicity is a rather strong predictor of poverty. As displayed in Table 20.4, over 27% of African American women were below the FPL in 2005 while only 10% NH White women were in that category (He et al., 2005). One possible explanation which cannot be discerned from these data alone is that African American elderly women may be more likely to be living alone than their NH White counterparts. However, other factors are also likely in play. Hispanics show the second highest percentage below poverty. There is a smaller difference between male and female poverty among Hispanics.

Some elderly have accumulated assets throughout their lives; these individuals can rely on more financial resources than contemporary income (U.S. Census Bureau, 2004e). Table 20.5 describes the median net worth by age of all elderly and by quintile of net worth. Overall, the median net worth of elderly persons was slightly over $100,000 in 2000. It does not show much decline with advancing age. Over 76% of the elderly's net worth resides in their home equity. When home equity is excluded, the median elderly person starts his/her senior years with about $27,000 in financial or personal property assets. Those around the overall median net worth are able to maintain their financial assets until they reach 75 years and older. Then, those assets decline by about one-third to $19,000. Taking the difference between total net worth and financial holding gives home equity, which is about $86,000 for the young elderly and is nearly as much at $81,000 for those 75 and older.

The reader may examine the table for all five quintiles. Here only the bottom and top quintiles will be compared. The median net worth among the top net worth quintile of youngest elderly was around $450,000 and increased to $569,000 among those 75 years and older. Financial assets increase with age also, from $238,000 to $414,300. These are probably the individuals that had multiple sources of income,

Table 20.5 Median household income of elderly, by age and quintile of income, 2000

		65–69($)	70–74($)	75+($)
	Median net worth	$114,050	$120,000	$100,100
All elderly				
	Excluding home equity	$27,588	$31,400	$19,025
	Median net worth	$32,000	$43,230	$46,266
Bottom quintile				
	Excluding home equity	$2,900	$2,885	$4,000
	Median net worth	$104,800	$113,893	$116,166
Second quintile				
	Excluding home equity	$22,332	$31,513	$31,269
	Median net worth	$155,319	$201,563	$226,263
Third quintile				
	Excluding home equity	$52,550	$84,900	$226,263
	Median net worth	$222,918	$312,877	$322,785
Fourth quintile				
	Excluding home equity	$2,900	$2,885	$4,000
	Median net worth	$449,800	$452,992	$569,000
Top quintile				
	Excluding home equity	$237,925	$272,681	$414,369

Source: 65+ in the United States, 2005, U.S. Depts. of HHS & Commerce

the right pie chart in Fig. 20.2. They are the "haves"; they start with assets and maintain a strong income stream. Their assets grow instead of dwindling.

The bottom quintile presents a very different picture. Median net worth among those aged 65–74 is $32,000 of which $29,000 is home equity. Home equity does seem to increase slightly among the older elderly in this quintile. This is likely because of the secular increase in real estate values that have been the norm over the last 30 years. It is also probable that these elderly with small assets are also the ones represented by the left pie chart in Fig. 20.2. Little is gained by asking them to spend assets they do not have. Taking equity out of their homes through reverse mortgages does not have much potential and could leave them in difficult circumstances as regards to housing.

Again, a picture of "haves" and "have nots" emerges. A good portion of the elderly has accumulated some assets they can fall back on in times of need, but a significant number of elderly are without that asset cushion. If the latter are going to access dentistry, as well as other services they need, they will require public assistance. Thus, it seems the issue of public support for dental services is more related to lack of financial resources rather than to age alone.

Health and Mobility Barriers to Access

Besides the economic and cultural issues found among the elderly that may limit their access to dental services, several other life circumstances, relatively common among the elderly, create additional difficulties in receiving dental services (Fitzpatrick, Powe, Cooper, Ives, & Robbins, 2004).

Institutionalized and non-ambulatory elderly have obvious difficulties accessing dental care from private community-based dental practices (Lester, Ashley, & Gibbons, 1998; Kinsey & Winstanley, 1998). These people need assistance either in getting to the source of dental care or by having dental care brought to them. This group will grow in the future because the elderly infirm, a major constituent of this group, will increase. These individuals are no longer able to live independently and/or have limited mobility.

The percentage of elderly in nursing homes increases dramatically with age. Only 1% of men and women aged 65–74 are nursing home residents (He et al., 2005). The percentage increases in the 75–84 age range to 5.1% of women and 3.1% of men. Among those 85 and older, 21.1% of women and 11.7% of men are in nursing homes (Table 20.6). In addition, a substantial number reside in assisted-living facilities.

African Americans are more likely to live in nursing homes than Whites, and they arrive there younger. For example, 7.5% of African American women aged 75–84 are in nursing homes compared to 4.9% of White women that age. Among women aged 85 and older the percentage of African American and White women in nursing homes is about the same. Both African American and White men are less likely than women to live in nursing homes regardless of age; they are also more likely to have a younger, living spouse to care for them.

Twenty-nine percent of the elderly have a physical disability (He et al., 2005; Waldrop & Stern, 2003). The prevalence of disability increases significantly with age. Of elderly women with disability only 10% were aged 65–74, 33.7% were aged 75–84, and 56% were aged 85 and older. Elderly men develop disabilities earlier than women. Twenty-two percent of men aged 65–74, nearly 40% of those aged 75–84, and 38% of those 85 and older exhibited disability. These data suggest, but do not prove, that disability in men is more closely related to survival than it is with women (see Table 20.7).

The prevalence of elderly with total disability is declining (He et al., 2005) (see Table 20.7). Of the 29% with disability only about 20% were categorized as totally disabled. Those who are both disabled and institutionalized represented 4.2% of the elderly and this percentage has also declined in recent years. Activity limitations are also prevalent among the elderly. According to a recent study, over 20% of those over age 65 had difficulty going outside the home. About 12% of elderly men and 22% of women had difficulty climbing 10 steps without resting. The limitations

Table 20.6 Percent of elderly living in nursing homes, by age, gender, and race – 1999

		65–74	75–84	85+
	Total	1.0	3.1	11.7
Men	White	0.9	2.9	11.5
	Black	2.1	5.2	12.8
	Total	1.1	5.1	21.1
Women	White	1.1	4.9	21.0
	Black	1.6	7.5	20.6

Source: 65+ in the United States, 2005, U.S. Depts. of HHS & Commerce

Table 20.7 Selected statistics on disability and chronic diseases among the elderly

Trends in the prevalence of disability by type

	1982	1989	1999
IADL only	5.7	4.8	3.2
1–2 ADLs	6.9	6.7	6.0
3+ ADLs	6.7	6.7	6.4
Disabled and Institutionalized	6.8	6.1	4.2
Totally Disabled	26.2	24.4	19.7

Prevalence of any disability by age and gender, 2000

	Men	Women
65–74	22.3	10.1
75–84	39.6	33.7
85+	38.2	56.1

Prevalence of chronic diseases by gender, 2000

	Men	Women
Coronary heart disease	24.3	15.4
Hypertension	42.9	50.2
Stroke	8.9	7.6
Cancer	22.8	18.0
Diabetes	15.1	13.0
Arthritis	30.6	38.5

in mobility can lead to difficulty in the ability to perform activities of daily living (ADL), such as taking a bath or shower, dressing oneself, or cooking a meal. About 10% of the elderly have self-care disability which limits their ability to perform activities of daily living. Figure 20.8 shows the trends in ADL and IADL (instrumental activities of daily living) such as going to the supermarket or to the dentist. If one cannot perform ADL, it is reasonable to assume they are unable to perform IADL (National Center for Health Statistics, 2002).

All of the individuals described above need assistance and/or special transportation to visit a dental office. Those with neither have extreme difficulty attending a dentist. As a result, most do not go to the dentist very often. An option is to bring dental care to them; sometimes it is the only option. In the United States, dental delivery systems are not widely available that can accommodate the needs of these people.

The U.S. Census Bureau publication, *65+ in United States: 2005,* estimates that 80% of the elderly have one chronic disease and 50% have two or more chronic diseases (He et al., 2005) (see Table 20.7). Depending on the severity of these medical conditions, elderly with chronic diseases can experience difficulty attending a dentist in a community office. Not infrequently, these individuals require care provided by specially trained dental personnel using special facilities. Sometimes, a hospital setting is necessary, where appropriate medical equipment including emergency equipment is available and medical personnel are close by. The trained dental personnel and delivery programs to provide care for those with severe medical co-morbidities are not widely available.

Fortunately, the number of elderly with chronic disease severe enough that they truly cannot attend a private community-based dentist is a small fraction of the number of elderly with chronic diseases. Most elderly with chronic diseases can safely receive their dental care from private dental offices in the community. Therefore the 50% estimate should be viewed an upper limit and a large overestimate of the number of elderly who require special provisions and facilities for the oral health care.

Because of the barriers to access caused by disability, limited mobility, and disease, the living arrangements of community-living elderly can have a profound influence on their ability to access dental care. If they are living with a spouse, relatives, or even with close friends, those individuals can help the elderly get to a dentist. When they live alone and family is not close, the ability to get to a dentist is more limited. It is women who more frequently live alone because more of them outlive their spouses. Nearly 42% of elderly White women live alone, compared to only 19% of White men (see' Table 20.8). Among African Americans, 39% of women and just fewer than 30% of men live alone. Asians are far more likely to live with a spouse or relatives. Only 19% of elderly Asian women and 8% of Asian men live alone (He et al., 2005).

Approximately 1.9 million elderly lived in a non-metro county with an urban population less than 2,500 and not contiguous to a metro county (Wall & Brown, 2007). These individuals were considered to be living in remote locations. Of those, around 380,000 elderly were both economically disadvantaged and remote.

While these sparsely populated and isolated counties are located throughout the United States, they are concentrated in the South and Midwest regions. In the West, counties are larger. One must look below the county level to define remote living. This analysis has been done and shows that vast regions of the West are remote. In the West, especially, very few people live in these remote areas.

In many cases, the combination of population and income in some sparsely populated counties and sub-county areas has not been and will never be able to support private dental practices. The demand base is simply not sufficient. As a result, some remote areas have experienced extended periods without any dentists and with little chance that a dentist will locate there in the future (Wall & Brown, 2007).

It is important to make a distinction between two types of remote areas. Some remote areas are populated primarily with economically self-sufficient populations. Others are remote, sparsely populated, and are comprised primarily of economically

Table 20.8 Living Arrangements of the Elderly Population, by Gender and Race/Ethnicity

		Spouse	Relatives	Non-Relatives	Alone
Men	Hispanic	68.7%	14.4%	4.7%	12.0%
	Asian	68.5%	22.5%	0.5%	8.3%
	Black	56.6%	9.5%	4.3%	29.5%
	Non-Hispanic White	72.9%	5.7%	2.7%	18.7%
Women	Hispanic	39.9%	36.0%	2.2%	21.9%
	Asian	42.6%	35.8%	2.2%	19.4%
	Black	25.4%	33.5%	2.1%	39.0%
	Non-Hispanic White	42.9%	13.6%	1.7%	41.8%

disadvantaged residents. The former have more options to get care through the private community-based delivery system than the latter, who face both geographic and economic barriers to access (Brown, 2005a).

In areas with relatively small populations of people and dentists, a few dentists, one way or another, can create a temporary shortfall or a temporary surplus. A small subtraction or infusion of workforce into a region with a relatively small population can quickly trade a workforce imbalance in one direction for an imbalance in the opposite direction.

Barriers to Dental Care: Elderly and the Total Population

Conditions which can create barriers to accessing dental care from the current private practice community-based delivery system have just been reviewed. To understand why these barriers are particularly pertinent when assessing the elderly population, it is useful to compare the overall and the elderly populations along the dimensions displayed in Fig. 20.3. The total population is on the left of the chart and the elderly population on the right.

The data for Fig. 20.3 are largely from the year 2000. The population estimates for the unshaded boxes are underestimates and probably larger underestimates for the total population than for the elderly. Data from various sources were used to estimate the sizes of the various subpopulations in Fig. 20.3. Most of the data

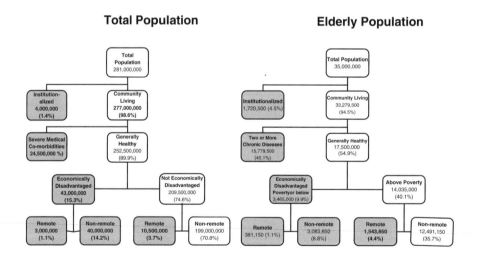

Note: The percentages are of the total population

Fig. 20.3 Populations of U.S. total and elderly populations with significant barriers to care are in the gray boxes, 2000
Note: The percentages are of the total population

come from U.S. Census Bureau (2001, 2005); Sanford (1996); U.S. Department of Health and Human Services (1990); Wall and Brown (2007). Estimates of the populations and their percent of the total are shown in the boxes. In constructing these charts, the total U.S. population and the total elderly population are shown at the top of the pyramid. Then each population with life circumstances likely to cause carriers to access to estimated from various sources and subtracted from the total. For each subpopulation of the total U.S. population, the elderly were separated from the total population to yield estimates for elderly in each of the boxes. The data for the elderly on disability, ambulation, chronic disease, and living arrangements have already been discussed in detail. Each topic was sourced when it was discussed.

Individuals represented by the unshaded boxes in Fig. 20.3 were ambulatory, not economically disadvantaged, community-living at non-remote locations, and generally healthy. These individuals can most easily access the current community-based private dental care delivery system. Individuals represented by the shaded boxes have one or more life circumstances (previously reviewed) that are significant barriers to their access to care (Phillips, Mayer, & Aday, 2000; Kiyak & Reichmuth, 2005). Figure 20.3 shows that, compared to the total population, a higher percentage of the elderly who exhibit life circumstances experience potential barriers to access. In 2000, the U.S. census counted 281 million Americans (U.S. Census Bureau, 2003). Of that total, according to our estimation, 191 million were ambulatory, not economically disadvantaged, community-living in non-remote locations, and generally healthy (i.e., the unshaded boxes on the left side of Fig. 20.3). For the overall population approximately 68% are represented by unshaded boxes and 32% by shaded boxes. In 2000, the elderly population was 35 million. Of that total, approximately 16.6 million (47.7% of all elderly) are represented by unshaded boxes, leaving 18.4 million (52.6%) with one or more potential barriers to access.

The prevalence of various types of potential barriers differs between the overall population and the elderly. The largest barrier to access dental care for both the overall and the elderly populations is economic disadvantage (U.S. Census Bureau, 2001). It is also the easiest barrier to address when it is the only barrier present. Among the non-elderly, most economically disadvantaged individuals are ambulatory, generally healthy, and living in non-remote communities. In contrast, higher percentages of the elderly are institutionalized, frail, and have severe medical co-morbidities, or functional limitations. Thus, among the elderly, economic disadvantage occurs more frequently in combination with other barriers to access.

It cannot be overstressed that the presence of barriers to care does not mean these individuals did not utilize dental services. In fact, millions in the shaded boxes did visit a dentist and receive care for oral needs. Nevertheless, the presence of one of these barriers indicates that for many, accessing dental care is more difficult. For those with more severe and/or multiple barriers, accessing care from community dentists is extremely difficult or impossible.

Demand and Need for Dental Care Among the Elderly

It may seem that a large amount of background information on the elderly has been presented before the topics of demand for care, need for care, and actual use of care are addressed; however, this information is vital for understanding the coming topics. All of the characteristics of the elderly population previously described, as well as behavioral and attitudinal characteristics that were not be addressed, play vital roles in determining the demand for dental care.

In the United States, almost all dental services are delivered through private markets that respond to the economic forces of supply and demand (Brown, 2005b; Centers for Medicare & Medicaid Services, 2007). The huge majority of this care is provided by dentists and their staff who are in private practice in local communities. In the short term, and even the rather long term, this is the existing delivery system that can provide care for a large population, such as the 35 million (and increasing) elderly Americans.

Under a market system, dental services are provided to those who are willing and able to pay the dentist's fee for the services. This makes an assessment of demand for dental services essential for understanding the actual delivery of care. Under traditional demand theory, consumers are the primary determinant of the use of dental services. The level of demand is influenced by many factors such as education, income, values, knowledge about and attitudes towards the importance of dental care (Brown, 2004b; Conrad, 1983; Feldstein, 1973; Grossman, 1972; Hay, Bailit & Chiriboga, 1982; Holtmann & Olsen, 1976; Hu, 1981; Manning, Bailit, Benjamin, & Newhouse, 1984; Phelps & Newhouse, 1974; Tuominen, 1994; Upton & Silverman, 1972, Yule & Parkin, 1985).

The prices of dental care (the fees dentists charge) play a special role in demand. They are the information system which indicates how much dental care will be demanded, by whom, in what parts of the country (Brown, 2005b). The demand for dental care reflects the amount of care desired by patients at alternative prices, given all of the other factors that influence the desire for care. These other factors may actually have more impact on demand than price, but price is the equilibrating information system which permits the coordination of many individuals' decisions regarding demand. The quantity of dental services desired is negatively related to price, and changes in the quantity of care demanded are significantly responsive to changes in dental fees.

The entire dental segment of the economy is a series of inter-related markets for dental services, dental equipment and materials, and dental personnel. The latter two markets, demand for dental education and equipment and supplies, are derived from the demand for dental services and generate the physical and human resources necessary to provide the care demanded (Brown & Meskin, 2004).

The concept of need for care is different from demand, and a clear distinction must be drawn between the two in order to understand how future access to care is likely to evolve and what interventions are likely to be effective in altering access to care for some subpopulations in the future (Brown, 2005b). The level of unmet need in a population is usually determined from health level measurements based on epidemiological foundations or other research identifying untreated dental disease. Normative judgments by health professionals are required regarding the amount and kind of services needed by an individual in order to attain or maintain some level of health. The underlying assumption is that those in need should receive appropriate care.

The fundamental and critical distinction between need for care and demand for care is the following: Once the level of need is determined, the quantity of dental services that "*should*" be provided can be determined, by matching normative value judgment, unmet need, and appropriate care. It is frequently difficult for health professionals to reach consensus on the appropriate values to apply and in the assessment of the appropriate care needed for existing clinical conditions. Realized demand, on the other hand, is the care that "*will*" be provided.

Not all dental care is provided in response to overt biological need. A substantial amount of care is demanded by individuals with little or no current need for care, based on the desire to prevent future dental problems. Essentially, they are buying information about their current oral state. Esthetic issues, unrelated to disease, also play a role. Nevertheless, disease levels and trends are important to obtain a complete view of the conditions influencing the demand for care.

While need and demand are distinct, they are related to one another in a reciprocal fashion. Need for care is one factor in demand for care. Demand, if it is expressed in a visit to a dentist, leads to provision of dental services which reduces unmet need. Dentists provide almost as much unreimbursed care as is funded by all levels of government (American Dental Association, 2001). Nevertheless, in a market system, dentists provide a huge majority of care to those who are willing and able to pay the market price. These three factors, need, demand, and use of care, can interact to create either a positive cycle or a negative cycle of utilization and oral health.

Let us start with the most positive utilization cycle. It starts with an individual who is not sure that unmet need for care exists in his/her oral cavity. The individual has the financial resources to see a dentist and values the information and services that oral health professionals provide. That individual is likely to visit a dentist regularly to have a trained health professional diagnose his/her oral condition, to treat any need discovered, and to provide appropriate preventive services. Any disease that develops is likely to be discovered early and treated with minimal interventions. Initiation of new disease or progression of chronic disease should be minimized. To a greater extent than any previous generation, more of today's elderly have followed this positive cycle.

A negative cycle occurs when an individual does recognize, does not value, cannot get to a dentist, or does not have the financial resources necessary for dental services. Disease may develop and progress, unbeknownst to the individual. If unattended, these needs can accumulate and become more severe. When an acute episode does occur, treatment usually requires more invasive and complex intervention. Over time, teeth are likely to require extraction and the entire periodontium can be compromised to the extent it can no longer support the dentition. The end-result can be the complete loss of the entire dentition. Despite the overall improvement in oral health among the elderly, many elderly have followed the negative cycle to various stages of oral compromise, including edentulism.

Measures of Need for Care

Caries Among the Elderly: Prevalence and Trends

The oral disease burden of the elderly is addressed in detail in another chapter. Here, the prevalence of and trends in caries and edentulism will be briefly surveyed to provide a basis to assess need for care among the elderly and how the distribution of need corresponds to the distribution of use of care. Need for periodontal services, oral surgery due to trauma, and other orofacial diseases, such as oropharyngeal cancers, are not addressed.

Dental caries, which creates a biological need for care, has been the primary foundation of the demand for dental services in modern times (Brown, 1989; Brown, 2005b). The prevention and treatment of caries and its sequela are large components of demand. Among adults, and especially the elderly, primary caries does not usually create the most need for care; rather it is sequela of caries, and their management, that creates a large demand for tertiary care, such as replacement of missing teeth with fixed and removal prostheses, oral surgery, endodontic therapy. Periodontal services also are widely needed by the elderly.

Elderly individuals have experienced a lifetime of disease attacks and progression. This can lead to a rather high prevalence of dysfunction and disability among the elderly. At the same time, their immune defenses slowly erode, leaving them more vulnerable to further deterioration of their health status. This is a classical model for medicine in general and it certainly applies to the oral cavity.

The first thing to know is, like the rest of the U.S. population, the elderly's caries and edentulism rates have improved over time. The caries improvement can be seen in Figs. 20.4 and 20.5 (U.S. Department of Commerce, 1979b; U.S. Department of Health and Human Services, 2005). Since today's elderly were born before 1943, they missed the effective preventive programs that emerged after World War II. They also did not receive as much oral health promotion and dietary information as later generations. The result was that the elderly experienced a high rate of caries attack during their childhood and early adult years. This led to numerous restorations and loss of teeth. Unattended disease progressed, sometimes becoming acute. Over time, the need for more complicated and expensive therapy developed. For those who wanted and could afford that treatment, complex restorations, crowns, bridges, and removable prostheses were provided. For those that did not visit a dentist or visited a dentist only on the occasion of an acute episode, teeth were mostly extracted and oral tissue damage progressed. This slowly led to the oral and masticatory dysfunction. This is the epidemiologic and treatment needs picture presented by today's elderly.

The DMF (decayed, missing, and filled) score is an imperfect measure of total caries experience in the elderly. Nevertheless, it is the best epidemiologic measure available for national representative data. Figures 20.4 and 20.5 demonstrate that

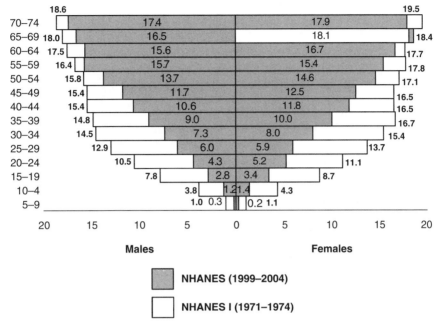

Fig. 20.4 Change in DMFT by age and gender, 1971–1974 and 1999–2004
Source: NHANES I (1972–1974) and NHANES (1999–2004)

the elderly experienced the most caries and the least improvement in total caries over time. The DMF is a cumulative index. Within an individual, it never declines. The average DMF never declines in a stable population. Average DMF can only change if individuals enter and leave the group, which is exactly what happens with the elderly population and specific age groups within the elderly population over time. As elderly individuals with higher DMF are replaced by individuals with lower DMF, the average DMF can decline.

The inner, shaded portion of the bars in Fig. 20.4 displays DMFT scores for the 1999–2004 period. For this recent time period, the men's average DMFT scores were 16.5 and 17.4 for 65–69 and 70–74 year olds, respectively. For women, the average DMFT scores were 18.4 and 17.9, respectively. DMF surfaces would be several folds larger than the DMF teeth for each of those comparisons.

Figure 20.5 displays the percentage change in DMFT by age over the time period. In general, the percentage improvements in DMFT decrease with age. The bar chart demonstrates that compared to the caries experience for younger age groups, the elderly have shown only slight improvement over the generation of elderly living 30 years ago. As mentioned this is partially explained by the differential exposure to modern prevention, especially community water fluoridation, by different birth cohorts. Decreases of at least 24% were experienced by the younger birth cohort in each age group to the age of 50 years. A clear improvement advantage is noticeable among older women compared to men. The seeming increase over time for 65 to

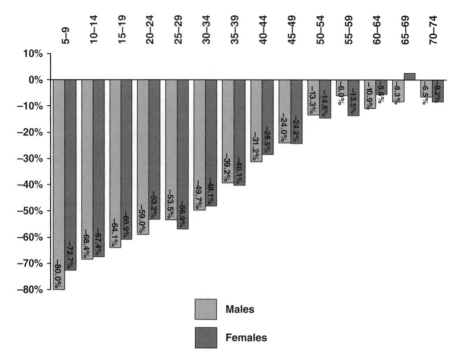

Fig. 20.5 Percentage change in DMFT, by age and gender, 1971–1974 and 1999–2004
Source: NHANES I (1972–1974) and NHANES (1999–2004)

74-year-old women could well be a statistical artifact of small sample size. The large declines in caries experience among younger birth cohorts portents well for a future reduction of need for care due to caries and its sequela for future generations of elderly.

Each component of the DMF index can be assessed separately. The filled component measures the number of filled teeth and is an indicator (albeit imperfect) of the amount of utilization because existing restorations were placed by dentists. The missing component measures the number of teeth lost for any reason. It is a gross indicator of utilization because most missing teeth were extracted by dentists. However, the two components provide clues to different types of treatment provided. Filled teeth suggest treatment at an earlier stage of disease and possibly more expensive treatment if the restoration is gold. Alternatively, missing teeth suggest disease has advanced to a more severe state, and either the required extraction or the alternative to extraction was too expensive for the patient. The decayed component measures the amount of untreated caries. Untreated caries accumulates during periods between visits to dentists. The larger number of untreated teeth is frequently associated with less regular utilization of dental services. These individual components "D", "M", "F" will be discussed for dentate elderly only. The edentate elderly all have the same DMFT score and the index is composed entirely of missing teeth.

The individual components show substantial variation among dentate elderly by income, education, and race/ethnicity. According to a recent report using National

Health and Nutrition Survey (HANES) data from 1999 to 2004, the prevalence of any untreated caries among dentate seniors 65 and older by poverty status was 21% for those elderly whose incomes were greater than 200% FPL; it increased to 37% for those from 100% to 199% of the FPL and increased further to 46.6% among those at less than 100% of FPL (Dye et al., 2007). Along the education dimension, the percentages were 20.7%, 24.4%, and 36.5% for those with more than high school, high school graduates, and less than high school, respectively. The prevalence of untreated caries in non-Hispanic Whites was 25.0%, non-Hispanic Blacks 53.9% and Mexican Americans 49.1%.

The average of decayed surfaces (DS) was 0.72 for those greater than 200% of the FPL, 1.42 for those 100%–199% of FPL, and 2.15 for those at less than FPL. Looking at education, average DS was 0.66 for elderly with more than a high school education, 0.98 for high school graduates, and 2.15 for those with less than high school. Finally, the average DS was 0.95 for non-Hispanic Whites, 2.64 for non-Hispanic Blacks, and 3.08 for Mexican Americans.

The "M" component is also higher among low-income dentate elderly compared to higher income counterparts, suggesting either more severe disease or different treatment choices. By poverty status, average MS was 36.3 for those greater than 200% FPL, 54.1 for those 100%–199% of FPL, and 57.5 for those less than FPL. For education, average MS was 32.1 for those with more than high school, 45.7 for high school graduates, and 55.5 for those with less than high school. Non-Hispanic Whites registered an average MS of 39.5, non-Hispanic Blacks 59.5, and Mexican Americans 46.1.

In contrast, the "F" component exhibits a positive relation with income and education – the higher the income or education, the more the filled teeth. As mentioned, this suggests more treatment of caries and hence more utilization of conservative dental care. By poverty status, the average FS was 34.6 for those greater than 200% FPL, 21.4 for those 100%–199% of FPL, and 12.2 for those less than FPL. The average filled surfaces (FS) was 37.3 for those with more than a high school education, 26.8 for high school graduates, and 14.8 for those with less than high school. Finally, the average FS was 31.9 for non-Hispanic Whites, 8.8 for non-Hispanic Blacks, and 13.0 for Mexican Americans.

The separate dimensions of the DMF index are highly correlated along the dimensions of education, income, and race/ethnicity. Bivariate analyses of these socioeconomic dimensions cannot explicate the separate contributions of each dimension. A multivariate analysis of the DMF and its components is indicated with the various socioeconomic and racial/ethnic factors as independent variables. This analysis is beyond the scope of the present effort.

Edentulism Among the Elderly: Prevalence and Trends

For the total population and among all age groups, total loss of teeth (edentulism) has declined steadily since 1960 (see Fig. 20.6). Unlike caries experience the percentage reduction is directly related to age. Among those 65–74, the

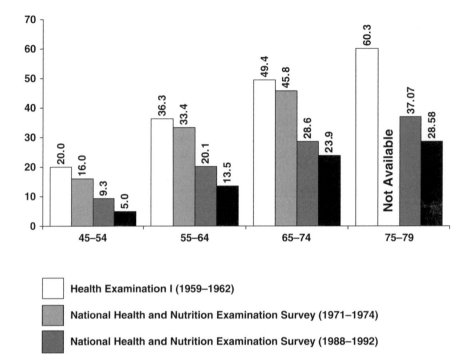

Fig. 20.6 Percent edentulous among U.S. adults, by age group: 1960–2002
Note: NCHS, National Health and Nutrition Examination Surveys

percent edentulous declined from nearly one-half of that age group in 1960 to about 24% in 1999–2002, a 50% decrease in prevalence (U.S. Department of Commerce, 1979a, 1979b; U.S. Department of Health and Human Services, 1997, 2007). Among those aged 75–79, the decline was from 60% to about 29%, another 50% decrease. These data provide enormously good news on several fronts. Edentulism is associated with several oral problems and results in reduced masticatory function. As will be shown later edentulism is a potent predictor of lack of utilization. The large declines between birth cohorts for younger age groups provide strong support to believe that edentulism among future generations of elderly will decline markedly. As a result, utilization can be expected to increase among future elderly.

Table 20.9 shows the percentage edentulous by poverty level, education, and race/ethnicity. The percent of elderly, who are edentulous, declines extraordinarily with increasing income. Among elderly with income below the FPL, 45.3% (almost one-half) have lost all of their teeth. Among those whose income is 400% or more than the FPL, the percent edentulous is only 8.8%. The difference between highest and lowest income elderly is 36.5%. This huge difference suggests a combination of (1) a lifetime of different caries and periodontal disease prevalence and severity and (2) and a lifetime of different utilization patterns and treatment choices.

Table 20.9 Prevalence of edentulism by income, education, race/ethnicty, 1999–2004

	Percent
<100% FPL	45.3
100–199% FPL	36.6
200–399% FPL	22.0
400 + % FPL	8.8
<High school	41.9
High school grad	29.3
>High school	12.7
Hisp (excluding mexicans)	41.0
Other race	39.5
Black-NH	32.9
White-NH	25.5
Mexican	22.1

NCHS, National Health and Nutrition Examination Surveys

In summary, these data paint a picture of improvement over time in edentulism, but only a moderate decline in DMFT. The decline in edentulism is very likely to continue with future generations of elderly. The decline in DMFT is very likely to accelerate in the future, especially when birth cohorts who experienced more preventive dentistry and more regular utilization during their younger years reach their senior years. Among the current elderly population, huge differences in edentulism and untreated caries are apparent.

Utilization of Care

Trends over Time

Figure 20.7 displays the percent of the population and percent of the elderly who visited a dentist during the previous year for the period from 1950 to 2003 (U.S. Department of Health and Human Services, 1972, 1999, 2002, 2004, 2006).

The chart shows that total visits to a dentist increased from a little over 200 million in 1950 to about 550 million in 2003, roughly a 2.5-fold increase. Part of the increase is due to the growth in population over the period. However, there has been a large secular increase in access to care which also played an important role in the increase in visits. Looking to the right-side axis for the scale, one sees that about 35% of the U.S. population visited a dentist in 1950; the percentage increased to about 65% in 2003. This is almost a doubling in an important measure of utilization of dental care.

The elderly have exhibited an even greater increase in utilization. Less than 15% of the elderly visited a dentist in 1950, a rate of utilization less than one-half the utilization of the overall population. Throughout the time period, utilization among the elderly increased steadily and rapidly, compared to the overall population. This

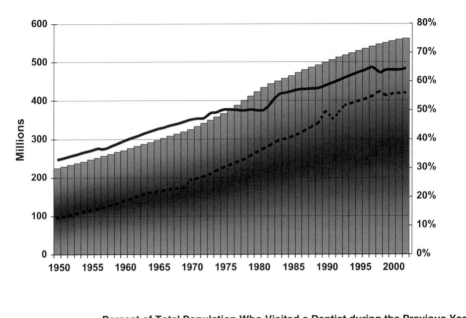

Fig. 20.7 Dental patient visits and percent of the population who visited the dentist, 1950–2003
Source: Centers for Disease Control and Prevention

has resulted in a narrowing of the difference between the two utilization rates. By 2003, about 55% of the elderly had a dental visit during the previous year, only about 10 percentage points below that of the overall population. Clearly, utilization of dental care among the elderly is converging on that of the overall population. Notice also that both utilization rates have leveled off in recent years. This bears monitoring to understand whether this is temporary or represents a more permanent circumstance.

Factors Associated with Variation in Utilization

Utilizations rates decline with age among the elderly (U.S. Department of Health and Human Services, 1972, 1999, 2002, 2005, 2006). For the youngest elderly (aged 65–69), 65% visited a dentist during the previous year in 2005. This is equivalent to the rate for the overall population. For elderly aged 85 and older, the percentage was about 46%, 20 percentage points below the youngest elderly. Barriers to access, such as illness, frailty, limited mobility, and institutionalization are more prevalent among older elderly and may explain a portion of the decline. More of the older elderly are edentulous which is likely to be the cause of another portion of the decline. Nevertheless in 2005, the oldest old utilized at a higher rate than the overall population did in 1950 – a rather remarkable demonstration of the increase in utilization of care over time.

Table 20.10 demonstrates enormous variation in utilization (percent that went to a dentist during the previous year) in the elderly population. With regard to age, elderly utilization declines steadily with age from a high of 59.3% utilization among all elderly aged 65–74 to 45.9% among those aged 85+. For gender, both male and female utilizations decline with age. Females utilize at a marginally higher rate during their younger senior years.

The striking features of these data are the stark gradients of utilization on the socioeconomic and the race/ethnicity variables (U.S. Department of Health and Human Services, 1972, 1999, 2002, 2004, 2006). Whites exhibit strong advantage in utilization over Blacks. While Whites maintain a reasonable utilization rate, even among those 85+, Black utilization plummets, eroding to only 15% among those Blacks aged 85 and older. The other racial category includes several races. These individuals also demonstrate significantly less utilization among their older seniors. Hispanics utilize at about two-thirds the rate of non-Hispanics, and their utilization rates also decline markedly with advancing age.

The most extreme gradient in utilization is by poverty level (U.S. Department of Health and Human Services, 1972, 1999, 2002, 2004, 2006). Those living at 400+% or more, utilize to a great extent, out utilizing most of the population in the non-elderly age categories. Although their utilization rate declines in older age

Table 20.10 Percent utilization by age, gender, race, ethncity, and poverty level, 1999–2004

	55–64	65–74	75–84	85+
All elderly	65.0	59.3	55.2	45.9
Gender				
Female	68.2	61.3	54.8	45.1
Male	61.5	56.9	55.7	47.4
Race				
White	66.8	61.4	57.4	48.6
Black	50.0	41.7	28.4	15.3
Other	63.5	53.0	63.3	30.7
Ethnicity				
Non-Hispanic	66.6	60.1	56.6	46.6
Hispanic	45.4	49.3	27.8	32.3
Poverty Level				
400+% FPL	80.6	79.2	81.8	61.8
200–399% FPL	56.5	60.0	56.4	48.8
100–199% FPL	41.1	39.9	42.3	36.4
<FPL	37.2	36.0	29.8	37.8

NCHS, National Health Interview Surveys

groups, even those 85+ utilize at about the national average. Those living below 200% of the FPL utilize at less than one-half the rate of the highest income group.

A decline in utilization with age is observed in all socioeconomic breakouts except for individuals living at less than 200% FPL. These lower income elderly do not exhibit much decline in utilization with age. A possible explanation is that their utilization has been low for so long that they continue to experience severe dental conditions and acute emergencies as they grow older. These conditions can almost force utilization.

Multivariate Analysis of Factors Which Affect Utilization

The data in Table 20.10 clearly indicate that income, race/ethnicity, and education are highly correlated. Bivariate analysis does not yield conclusions about the relative importance of income, education, race, etc. This section will provide some information regarding how the factors inter-relate in multivariate analysis.

We estimated a logit regression from the 1999 National Health Interview Survey. The dependent variable was utilization during the previous year (yes or no). Explanatory variables included the following:

Dental Insurance	Yes	No		
Gender	Male	Female		
Income	Poor	Low	Medium	High
Education	<High School	Some High School	High School Grad	Some College
Race	White-NH	Black-NH	Hispanic	Other
Dentate	Yes	No		

There were over 50,000 observations to estimate this equation. The results are considered good for cross-sectional data with incomplete specification (i.e., missing variables that could help explain utilization). Several interaction terms were included in the regressions, including age*income, race*income, dentate*income. An interaction of income and education was tried but the two variables were too correlated to permit the inclusion of that interaction. Interested readers may request more information on the technical aspects of the regression from the author.

The power of the model is the ability to compare sociodemographic profiles. All variables can be varied simultaneously. Alternatively, all variables can be held at specified values, except the variables of interest. This permits specified variables to be compared with the remaining sociodemographic profile held identical for both groups.

The predicted value of the logit equation is the predicted percent utilization for a particular profile of variables. Space does not permit an exhaustive presentation of all possible permutations in the specification of the explanatory variables; instead six examples are provided to demonstrate the huge variation in expected utilization of elderly with different profiles of the explanatory variables.

In the examples that follow, a logit model to predict visits to physician's office (not hospital visits) is included for perspective. Health care coverage for the elderly is universal for physician visits through Medicare. Thus, in the physician equation, individuals were assumed to have Medicare coverage. In contrast, most elderly are without any type of dental insurance coverage. Dental services are only sparsely covered by Medicare. Medicaid for adults is also very limited. Private dental insurance is not common among the elderly. Since most did not have private dental insurance, the examples are for those without dental insurance. If younger populations were being examined, dental insurance would play a larger role.

The first example, shown in Fig. 20.8, compares high income, well-educated dentate males 75–84 years old. The results of the logit predictions of physician and dentist utilization for the above population are displayed on the left side of the figure. The only difference in the populations is that the first dentist group (DDS1) and the first physician group (MD1) are non-Hispanic Black (B-NH) while the second

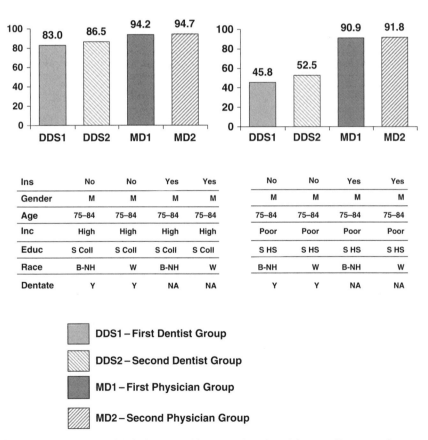

Fig. 20.8 Percent with a visit during the previous year, by selected factors – **first example**
Source: Multivariate Logit Model, using data from the 1999 NCHS Health Interview Survey

dental group (DDS2) and the second physician group (MD2) are non-Hispanic White (W-NH).

With this first sociodemographic profile, utilization rates of both physician and dentist services are high. The model predicts physician visits during the previous year for MD1 and MD2 at over 94% of that population. Dental utilization is almost as high; the percent of B-NH with a dental visit was a predicted 83.0%, for W-NH 86.5%. Race does not make a large difference in utilization if the populations have income, are well educated, and dentate.

A second example is for poor, some high school, dentate, males 75–84 years old who attended but did not graduate from high school. These results are displayed on the right side of Fig. 20.8. Again, the only difference is the DDS1 and MD1 group are B-NH and DDS2 and MD2 are W-NH. Hardly any falloff from the first example in the percent with a physician visit is predicted between the two physician visit groups (MD1 and MD2). In contrast, there is considerable decline from the first example in the predicted percent with a dentist visit for both dentist groups. The decline in predicted utilization between the two examples is largely due to income and education. Race has a slightly larger effect in the second example, but still is not a strong independent factor, once education and income are controlled. The greater impact of income and education on dentist visits, compared to physician visits, is likely partly due to safety net Medicare provides for everyone, including the economically disadvantaged, which is not present for dentist visits.

In a third example, high income, well-educated males are contrasted with poor males who did not attend high school. Both groups are from 75 to 84 years old. The results shown on the left side of Fig. 20.9 are for B-NH males. DDS1 are edentulous, while DDS2 are dentate. The physician models have the same characteristics, except dentate status is assumed irrelevant. In this example, race is controlled.

For the edentate, low-income, less well-educated group of B-NH males, their predicted dentist utilization is 4.5%. Among dentate, high-income, well-educated B-NH males, their predicted utilization is 83%. Compared to an opposite socioeconomic profile, an enormous decline is predicted by the model when low income, limited education, and edentate status are all present. In contrast, the two socioeconomic profiles exhibited only a minor difference in predicted physician utilization. The low-income group (MD1) had a predicted utilization of 90.2% while the high-income group (MD2) had a predicted utilization of 94.2%.

One might think that racial differences in perception and attitudes could lead edentate W-NH males to seek dental care more frequently. Example four shows this is not so. The right side of Fig. 20.9a shows the results for populations identical to the previous example, except these groups are W-NH. The dentist utilization rate for poor, less-educated edentulous W-NH males is 5.9%, very close to the edentate B-NH rate. The dentate, high-income W-MH males with some college were very similar to their B-NH counterparts with a dentist utilization rate of 86.5%.

A fifth example compares dentate and edentate high-income, well-educated W-NH males from 75 through 84 years old. This example is not accompanied by a figure. The only difference between the groups is that the DDS1 group is edentate and DDS2 is dentate. Again, that factor is assumed immaterial for physician visits.

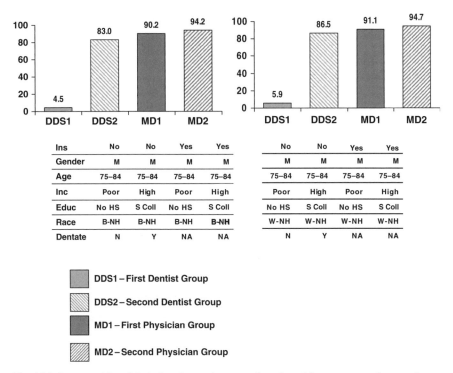

Fig. 20.9 Percent with a visit during the previous year, by selected factors – **second example**
Source: Multivariate Logit Model, using data from the 1999 NCHS Health Interview Survey

The dentists groups do not have private dental insurance while the physician groups have Medicare. For the edentulous group, their predicted dentist utilization is 38%; for the dentate group, their predicted utilization is 89%. Both physician groups, since they had identical characteristics, utilized at 94%.

A final example compares dentate and edentate, poor males aged 75–84 with some high school. Again, there is no accompanying figure. The major difference between this and the previous example is that these groups are poor and did not graduate from high school. DDS1 group is edentulous and DDS2 is dentate. Again, that factor is immaterial for physician visits. Neither dentist group had private dental insurance while the physician groups had Medicare. For the edentulous group, their predicted dentist utilization is 9.6%; for the dentate group, their predicted utilization is 58%. Both physician groups had high predicted utilization at 90.4%.

These examples demonstrate the well-known fact that edentulism is the one most potent predictor of lack of dental utilization available. It seems that once individuals become edentulous, most do not utilize dental services or do so very infrequently. This may be due to the misperception among the edentate that they no longer require dental services. It is a dangerous misperception; oral cancer and complications from wearing dentures are serious and relatively common conditions among the edentate elderly. When edentulism is present among individuals with low income and limited education, the combination is devastating for dental utilization.

Types of Services Received by the Elderly

The elderly received approximately 14% of the total number of dental services delivered during 2005 and 2006 (American Dental Association, 2007). In 2000, the elderly represented about 12.5% of the total population. Overall, the elderly are

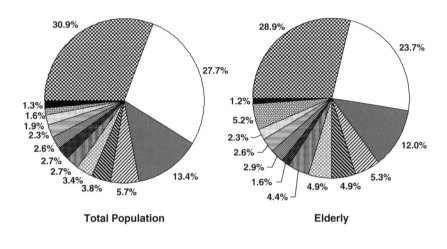

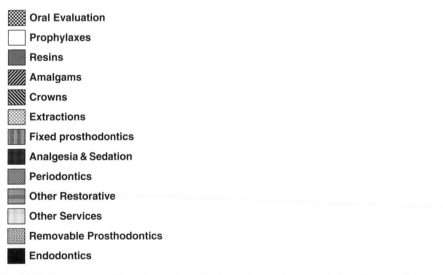

Fig. 20.10 Percentages of Dental procedures for the total and elderly populations, by type of procedure, 2005–2996
Source: ADA Survey of Dental Services Render, 2005–2006

using their proportionate share of dental services and perhaps a little more. However, it must be remembered that, on average, the elderly have more dental disease and need more expensive treatment.

Excluding a number of services that are not relevant for the elderly, such as orthodontics and excluding radiographs, Fig. 20.10 displays the percentage of various services received by the elderly, compared to the overall population. About 52% of elderly services are examinations and prophylaxes, compared to 58.8% for the overall population. Another 17% of services went to amalgams and resins, compared to about 19% for the overall population. Replacement services such as crowns, removal and fixed prosthodontics represent a higher percentage of services for the elderly, compared to the overall population. Removal prosthetics, especially, are more common, representing 5.2% of elderly case load compared to only 1.6% of the case load of the total population.

Figure 20.11 displays the previous data differently. It shows the percentage of the total of each type of service received by the elderly. The dotted line in the graph is the elderly proportion of all services. As mentioned, it is 14%. The bars that extend above the dotted line are services which are provided to the elderly at higher percentages than the overall to the overall population. For most types of services, the elderly percentage is close to the dotted line, indicating they are using a share of services proportionate to their size in the overall population. This is consistent with the similar distribution of services demonstrated in Fig. 20.10. Fixed bridges, extractions, and endodontics bars are all above the dotted line, indicating the elderly receive these services at a greater rate than their share of the population. The largest

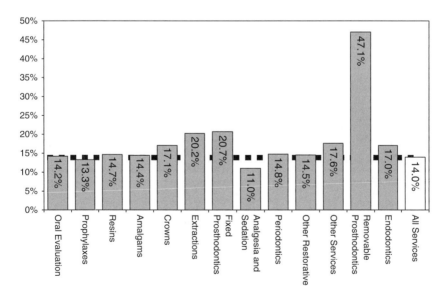

Fig. 20.11 Percentage of various services received by elderly, Aged 65+, 2005–2006
Source: ADA Survey of Dental Services Render, 2005–2006

outlier is removable prosthodontics (dentures). The elderly receive nearly half of all of these services.

Because of the predominance of the expensive types of services among the elderly, expenditures by type of services are different for the elderly, compared to the overall population. A higher proportion of expenditures for the elderly goes for prosthetic services and extractions. Socioeconomic gradients also influence the types of services the elderly receive. High-income elderly have more diagnostic and preventive services, compared to low-income elderly. They receive slightly fewer restorative services and slightly more prosthetic services than their low-income counterparts. The high-income elderly require only half as much oral surgery as the low-income elderly.

Interpretation and a Look to the Future

The preceding material has told a tale of two elderly. One group has income, lives in the community, is dentate, maybe lives with a spouse, and uses dental care to a greater extent than any previous generation of elderly. The other group is impoverished and probably did not get extended education. Almost one-half of the latter group is edentulous; others are frail with illness; still others are institutionalized. The latter group utilizes dental services at a remarkably lower rate than the former group. The contrast is much starker than similar comparisons of medical utilization.

It may be tempting to blame the private market system for not caring for those who need care. That would be a grievous mistake and a misinterpretation of what markets can do and what they cannot do. Markets, as they always have, respond to demand, not need. This is, at once, their weakness and their strength. It is a weakness because some who need it do not get even the basics, while others spend their time and money on what may seem to some as luxuries.

Resources in a market system are not allocated according to some ethical formula. The strength of market allocation is that it provides a decentralized method for individuals to follow their own preferences and pursue their own goals. Equally important, markets provide incentives to patients to husband their resources and to providers to be efficient. Over the longer term, market signals align the amount of supply with demand for services in roughly efficient geographic location. Markets distribute resources according to the basic financial stratification of a society (Stiglitz & Walsh, 2006; Tuominen, 1994).

This creates a special issue regarding dental services for the elderly because, in addition to present stratification, past social and financial stratification have influenced the oral health of the elderly. Dental diseases and the damage they cause are largely irreversible, except in their very early stages. They accumulate over time. When the elderly were children, effective preventive programs had not emerged. The oral health conditions of the today's elderly embed the social and biological circumstances of half a century and more ago. Treatment options made long ago, as well as lack of access to dental care, has left indelible imprints on the oral conditions of today's elderly.

It took a lifetime of unattended oral disease for the oral health of some of the elderly to get to where it is today. For most elderly living in poverty today, that condition did not spring suddenly out of nowhere, when those individuals reached 65. Many of those individuals endured deprivation and lack of opportunity for most of their lives. Those factors are the true underlying conditions that explain the two elderly populations, the "haves" and the "have nots" that we observe today. Much of the difference in utilization between the two elderly populations could be narrowed. With more equivalent utilization rates, oral health disparities should narrow, given sufficient time. Yet many of the "have not" elderly do not have the financial resources to begin redressing those disparities in utilization.

Society does not have to completely accept an extremely unequal allocation of dental services that results from an unequal distribution of financial resources. Society can decide to change that allocation. Understanding the behavior of markets provides policy guidelines to address these inequalities, if we can call forth the political will that is necessary. If more is wanted for the "have nots", markets offer at least the start of a solution. Change the distribution of demand; support through public policy and philanthropy those who cannot express their demand. The market will respond and its response can be facilitated with wise and timely supply-side initiatives. However, when designing policy remedies, care must to be taken not to endanger the functioning of markets and its vital incentive structure that permits markets to conserve resources through efficiencies on both sides of the market while empowering as much individual discretion as possible.

A Look at the Future

Approaches to policy remedies can take the long view or a shorter view. The long view offers much optimism to future generations of elderly, but it does little to address the need of today's elderly. Nevertheless, it is useful to review the long-run forces at work before we turn our attention to what can be done in the present.

The single most important way to help future generations with their oral health, as well as with myriad of their other needs, is to maintain a robust, growing economy. Moving people out of poverty by giving them the skills they need for future job markets is one of the most precious gifts a person can receive. While we are growing our economy, we must continue to battle economic disadvantage that can occur due to no fault of the individuals affected.

Future generations of elderly will be better able to fend for themselves if they receive good education during their formative years. If we grow the economy, seniors will have more financial resources. Defined contribution retirement accounts have turned the United States into a nation of capital owners. Perhaps some form of medical or dental savings accounts will emerge and provide the means for working individuals to accumulate funds for health care to be used during senior years.

Specific to oral health, our younger generations should continue to receive outstanding preventive interventions. Efforts at health promotion and education should continue apace. There are already several forces at work that will change oral health for future elderly. The prevalences of traditional dental diseases are declining. Edentulism, that most potent dissipater of utilization, is on the decline. The future elderly will be predominately dentate. Those individuals now in their thirties and forties will retain not only more teeth, but more sound teeth, when they are seniors. They will also be in better periodontal health. Combined with more skills, improved general health, and better financial security, the future bodes well for future generations of elderly.

Disadvantaged Elderly

The future trends carry high hopes, but they will be too late to help today's elderly. We must look to more immediate remedies for them. By far the largest subpopulation of elderly who experience difficulties in accessing dental care is the economically disadvantaged. As a group, these individuals do not access dental care with the regularity of the majority of the population. To the extent they get care, the majority of these individuals receive dental care from private community-based dentists, but a significant percentage utilize emergency rooms or community health centers.

Limited utilization is one of the factors that have led to disparities in oral health among disadvantaged populations (Hughes et al., 2005; Kelly et al., 2005; Kenney et al., 2005; Kim, 2005). These disparities have narrowed dramatically over the past generation among younger population and hopefully will continue to do so (Brown, 2005b). This is very good news and deserves to be celebrated. For reasons previous discussed, elderly oral health is an accumulation over many years. Disparities among seniors have not narrowed to the extent they have in younger cohorts, but as mentioned, they should in the future.

The fundamental cause of lack of access among disadvantaged populations is lack of effective demand (Brown, 2005a). In turn, the basis for that lack of demand is multifaceted. Limited knowledge of the need for and benefits derived from dental care can contribute. Cultural isolation or estrangement can also be a factor. In some cases, personally destructive behavior and unstable family structure can play a role. Especially among the elderly, illness and infirmity play significant roles. Policy options with good chances for success cannot ignore any of these factors. However, the fundamental condition, whether cause or effect, common to all of these circumstances is economic disadvantage.

As a result, access to care for disadvantaged populations cannot be long maintained without adequate funding that supports the demand for care among these populations. Moreover, because of the complexity of the underlying causes and the amount of the resources needed to address the problem, the dental profession alone cannot solve this problem (Brown, 2005a; Guay, 2004). Redressing these disparities requires the commitment and the support of the entire nation. Programs will be necessary to empower the disadvantaged to express their demand for dental services, hopefully with the individual discretion that the rest of our society enjoys. The following policy initiatives are vital:

- Support the demand for dental services among disadvantaged populations through increased public funding.
- Medicaid should be replaced with a more empowering method of finance that provides discretion to the disadvantaged and also provides incentive for them to husband the financial resources they receive.
- If Medicaid cannot be replaced, adequate Medicaid reimbursement rates and sufficient overall funding should be given to sufficiently permit the program to provide more real benefits it promises.
- Patient education and health promotion focusing on the importance of good oral health should be expanded.

Frail and Institutionalized Elderly

The private practice community-based delivery system is not designed to provide care for severely sick, frail, or institutionalized elderly. New, innovative approaches to the delivery of their care are required (Dolan, Peek, Stuck, & Beck, 1998; Heaton, Smith, & Raybould, 2004; Jones, Fedele, Bolden, & Bloom, 1994; Kiyak, 1989; Mai & Eng, 2007; Matear & Barbaro, 2006; Robbertz, Lauf, Rupp, & Alexander, 2006; Strayer, 1999). Institutionalized individuals lack the mobility to access dental services from the private, community-based dentists either because it is not physically possible for them to reach these dentists or because society has decided it may not be desirable for them to access community services. In some cases, special provision for their care is available. Dental care is frequently available within penal institutions and the military. It is sometimes available for long-term hospital patients. It is less frequently available for nursing home residents and the homebound.

Non-ambulatory individuals have obvious difficulties accessing dental care from private community-based dental practices. These people need assistance either in getting to the source of dental care or by having dental care brought to them. This group will grow in the future because the elderly infirm, a major constituent of this group, will increase. These individuals are no longer able to live independently and have limited mobility. If their general health is sufficiently impaired, individuals may require care provided by specially trained dental personnel using special facilities. Not infrequently, a hospital setting is necessary. Special programs are needed to provide dental services to this segment of the population. Frequently, these programs are not available (Yellowitz & Saunders, 1989).

In conclusion, because of the larger number of economically disadvantaged individuals, addressing their needs will require the most resources. Total cost to society for providing dental care to economically disadvantaged individual without other complicating health or mobility factors will depend on the scope of the dental procedures provided, price structure (market-determined vs. administered), as well as the cost-sharing features and the utilization rate of the program. Once their backlog of needs is addressed, the per capita cost of the program is not likely to be greatly higher than a similarly structured program for the overall population.

The cost of providing dental care for those individuals who are institutionalized, non-ambulatory, or sick and frail is difficult to estimate. It depends on the range of services that are offered and that can be medically tolerated. The latter is determined by the physical condition of the individual. Comprehensive dental care for those where it is appropriate is likely to involve high per capita cost. Emergency and limited maintenance care for those individuals where that option is more appropriate will cost less. Fortunately, the number of individuals in the above populations who truly cannot get to a private community-based dentist is a small fraction of the total population. Compared to the total resources going to dental care, providing dental care for these groups is not likely to require a huge addition to the dental workforce, but will likely require different types of care delivery and oral health personnel with special training. To facilitate the provision of dental services to the frail, disabled, severely ill, and institutionalized, non-market programs will be necessary to supplement market forces. Without doubt, more public and/or philanthropic funding are required to improve their access.

While solutions to the elderly's oral health needs are daunting, important progress is clearly within reach. There is no magic bullet that will secure any of the desirable goals for the elderly without renewed commitment by American society.

References

Aday, L. A. (1993). Equity, accessibility, and ethical issues: Is the U.S. health care reform debate asking the right questions? *American Behavioral Scientist,* 36(6), 724–40.

Ahlburg, D. A. (1993, March). The Census Bureau's New Projections of the US Population. *Population and Development Review,* (Vol. 19, No. 1), pp. 159–174.

American Dental Association (2001). *Future of dentistry.* Chicago: American Dental Association, Health Policy Resources Center.

American Dental Association. (2007). *2005–2006 Survey of dental services rendered.* Chicago: American Dental Association, Survey Center.

Andersen, R., & Benham, L. (1970). Factors affecting the relationship between family income and medical care consumption. In H. Klarman (Ed.), *Empirical studies in health economics.* Baltimore: John Hopkins Press.

Astor, F. C., Hanft, K. L., & Ciocon, J. O. (1999). Xerostomia: A prevalent condition in the elderly. *Ear Nose & Throat Journal,* 78, 476–479.

Baird, J. T. Jr., Kelly, J. E. (1970). Need for dental care among adults: United States, 1960–1962. March, 1970. 1000. PB88-228986. PC A03 MF A01. Accessed at http://www.cdc.gov/nchs/products/pubs/pubd/series/sr11/100-1/100-1.htm

Bloom, B., Gift, H. C., & Jack, S. S. (1992). *Dental Services and Oral Health: United States, 1989.* Vital Health Stat 10(183). National Center for Health Statistics. Washington, DC: U.S. Government Printing Office.

Brown, L. J. (1989, Summer). Contrasting the economic outlook for dentistry and medicine. *Journal of Medical Practice Management,* 5(1), 8–17.

Brown, L. J. (2005a). *Adequacy of current and future dental workforce: Theory and analysis.* Chicago: American Dental Association, Health Policy Resources Center.

Brown, L. J. (2005b). *Adequacy of current and future dental workforce: Theory and analysis.* Chicago: American Dental Association, Health Policy Resources Center.

Brown, L. J., & Lazar, V. (1998). The economic state of dentistry: Demand-side trends. *Journal of the American Dental Association,* 129, 1685–91.

Brown, L. J., & Lazar, V. (1999). Dental care utilization: How saturated is the patient market? *Journal of the American Dental Association,* 130, 573–80.

Brown, L. J., & Meskin, L. H. (Eds.). (2004). *The economics of dental education.* Chicago: American Dental Association, Health Policy Resources Center.

Brown, L. J., & Swango, P. A. (1993). Trends in caries experience in U.S. employed adults from 1971–74 to 1985: Cross-sectional comparisons. *Advances in Dental Research,* 7(1), 52–60.

Brown, L. J., Wall, T. P., & Lazar, V. (1999). Trends in untreated caries in permanent teeth of children 6 to 18 years old. *Journal of the American Dental Association, 130,* 1637–44.

Brown, L. J., Wall, T. P., & Lazar, V. (2002). Trends in caries among adults 18–45 years old. *Journal of the American Dental Association, 133,* 827–34.

Brown, L. J., Beazoglou, T. F., & Heffley, D. (1994, Mar–Apr). Estimated savings in dental expenditures from 1979 through 1989. *Public Health Reports, 9,* 195–203.

Camarota, S. (2001, August 2). *The impact of immigration on U.S. population growth.* Testimony prepared for the U.S. House of Representatives Committee on the Judiciary Subcommittee on Immigration, Border Security, and Claims. http://www.cis.org/articles/2001/ sactestimony701.html Accessed July 10, 2007.

Centers for Medicare & Medicaid Services. (2007). *National health expenditures.* Available at: http://www.cms.hhs.gov/statistics/nhe/historical/t2.asp. Accessed March, 2007.

Conrad, D. A. (1983). Dental care demand: Age-specific estimates for the population 65 years of age and over. *Health Care Finance Review, 4,* 47–57.

Dolan, T. A., & Atchison, K. A. (1993, December). Implications of access, utilization and need for oral health care by the non-institutionalized and institutionalized elderly on the dental delivery system. *Journal of Dental Education,* 57(12), 876–87.

Dolan, T. A., Atchison, K., & Huynh, T. N. (2005, September). Access to dental care among older adults in the United States. *Journal of Dental Education, 69*(9), 961–74.

Dolan, T. A., Corey, C. R., & Freeman, H. E. (1988, November). Older Americans' access to oral health care. *Journal of Dental Education, 52*(11), 637–42.

Dolan, T. A., Peek, C. W., Stuck, A. E., & Beck, J. C. (1998). Functional health and dental service use among older adults. *Journals of Gerontology. Series A, Biological Sciences and Medical Sciences, 53*(6), M413–8.

Drake, D. F. (1994). *Reforming the health care market: An interpretive economic history.* Washington, DC: Georgetown University Press.

Dye, B. A., Tan, S., Smith, V., Lewis, B. G., Barker, L. K., Thornton-Evans, G., et al. (2007). Trends in oral health status: United States, 1988–1994 and 1999–2004. National Center for Health Statistics. *Vital and Health Statistics* 11, 248. http://www.cdc.gov/nchs/data/ series/sr_11/sr11_248.pdf

Eiseman, L., Johnson, J., & Coll, J. (2005, January). Ultrasound measurement of mandibular arterial blood supply: Techniques for defining ischemia in the pathogenesis of alveolar ridge atrophy and tooth loss in the elderly? *Journal of Oral Maxillofacial Surgery, 63*(1), 28–35.

Employee Benefit Research Institute. (2006, May). *Notes Income of the Elderly Population Age 65 and Over,* 28(5), 1–12, – http://www.ebri.org/pdf/notespdf/EBRI_Notes_05-2007.pdf

Feldstein, P. J. (1973). *Financing dental care: An economic analysis.* Lexington, Massachusetts: DC Heath.

Fitzpatrick, A. L., Powe, N. R., Cooper, L. S., Ives, D. G., & Robbins, J. A. (2004, October). Barriers to health care access among the elderly and who perceives them. *American Journal of Pubic Health, 94*(10), 1788–94.

Grossman, M. (1972). *The Demand for health: A theoretical and empirical investigation.* New York: National Bureau of Economic Research.

Guay, A. H. (2004, November). Access to dental care: Solving the problem for underserved populations. *Journal of the American Dental Association, 135*(11), 1599–605.

Hay, J. W., Bailit, H., & Chiriboga, D. A. (1982). The demand for dental health. *Social Science and Medicine,* 16(13), 1285–89.

He, W., Sengupta, M., Velkoff, V. A., & DeBarros, K. A. (2005). U.S. Census Bureau, Current Population Reports *(Special Studies)*, P23-209, 65+in the United States. Washington, DC: U.S. Government Printing Office.

Heaton, L. J., Smith, T. A., & Raybould, T. P. (2004, October). Factors influencing use of dental services in rural and urban communities: Considerations for practitioners in underserved areas. *Journal of Dental Education,* 68(10), 1081–89.

Holtmann, A. G., & Olsen, E. O. (1976). The demand for dental care: A study of consumption and household production. *Journal of Human Resources, 11*, 546–60.

Hu, T. W. (1981). The demand for dental care services, by income and insurance status. *Advances in Health Economics and Health Services Research,* 2, 143–95.

Hughes, D. C., Duderstadt, K. G., Soobader, M. P., & Newacheck, P. W. (2005). Disparities in children's use of oral health services. *Public Health Reports,* 120(4), 455–62.

Jack, S. S., & Bloom, B. (1988). *Use of dental services and dental health: United States, 1986.* Vital Health Stat 10(165). National Center for Health Statistics. Washington, DC: U.S. Government Printing Office.

Johnson, E. S., Kelly, J. E., & Van Kirk, L. E. (1965). Selected dental findings in Adults by Age, race, and sex: United States, 1960–1962. Reprinted November 1965. 41 pp. (PHS) 1000. PB-267173. PC A03 MF A01. Accessed at http://www.cdc.gov/nchs/products/pubs/pubd/series/sr11/100-1/100-1.htm

Jones, J. A., Fedele, D. J., Bolden, A. J., & Bloom, B. (1994, Winter). Gains in dental care use not shared by minority elders. *Journal of Public Health Dentistry,* 54(1), 39–46.

Kelly, J. E., & Harvey, C. R. (1974). Decayed, missing, and filled teeth among youths 12–17 Years: United States. October 1974. 40 pp. (HRA) 75-1626. PB88-228044. PC A03 MF A01. Accessed at http://www.cdc.gov/nchs/products/pubs/pubd/series/sr11/100-1/100-1.htm

Kelly, J. E., & Harvey, C. R. (1979). May basic data on dental examination findings of persons 1–74 Years: United States, 1971–1974. 40 pp. (PHS) 79-1662. PB91-223800. PC A03 MF A01. Accessed at http://www.cdc.gov/nchs/products/pubs/pubd/series/sr11/100-1/100-1.htm

Kelly, J. E., Van Kirk, L. E., & Garst, C. (1967a). Total loss of teeth in adults: United States, 1960–1962. October 1967. 29 pp. (PHS) 1000. PB-262958. PC A03 MF A01. Accessed at http://www.cdc.gov/nchs/products/pubs/pubd/series/sr11/100-1/100-1.htm

Kelly, J. E., Van Kirk, L. E., & Garst C. C. (1967b). Decayed, missing, and filled teeth in adults: United States, 1960–1962. February 1967. 54 pp. PB-267323. PC A03 MF A01. Accessed at http://www.cdc.gov/nchs/products/pubs/pubd/series/sr11/100-1/100-1.htm

Kelly, S. E., Binkley, C. J., Neace, W. P., & Gale, B. S. (2005). Barriers to care-seeking for children's oral health among low-income caregivers. *American Journal of Pubic Health,* 95(8), 1345–51.

Kenney, G. M., McFeeters, J. R., & Yee, J. Y. (2005). Preventive dental care and unmet dental needs among low-income children. *American Journal of Pubic Health,* 95(8), 1360–66.

Kim, Y. O. (2005). Reducing disparities in dental care for low-income Hispanic children. *Journal of Health Care Poor Underserved, 16*(3), 431–43.

Kinsey, J. G., & Winstanley, R. B. (1998). Utilisation of domiciliary dental services. *Gerodontology, 15*(2), 107–12.

Kiyak, H. A. (1989, June). Reducing barriers to older persons' use of dental services. *International Dental Journal, 39*(2), 95–102.

Kiyak, H. A., & Reichmuth, M. (2005, September). Barriers to and enablers of older adults' use of dental services. *Journal of Dental Education, 69*(9), 975–86.

Lubitz, J., Beebe, B. A., & Baker, C. (1995). Longevity and medicare expenditures. *New England Journal of Medicine,* 332(15), 999–1003.

Lester, V., Ashley, F. P., & Gibbons, D. E. (1998, March). Reported dental attendance and perceived barriers to care in frail and functionally dependent older adults. *British Dental Journal, 184*(6), 285–89.

Mai, L., & Eng, J. (2007). Community-based elder care: A model for working with the marginally housed elderly. *Care Management Journals, 8*(2), 96–99.

Manning, W. G., Bailit, H., Benjamin, B., & Newhouse, J. P. (1984). *The demand for dental care: Evidence from a randomized trial in health insurance*. The Rand Corporation, Santa Monica, CA.

Manning, W. G., & Phelps, C. E. (1978, March). *Dental care demand: Point estimates and implications for national health insurance*. The Rand Corporation (R-2157-HEW ed.)

Matear, D., & Barbaro, J. (2006, January). Caregiver perspectives in oral healthcare in an institutionalised elderly population without access to dental services: A pilot study. *Journal of the Royal Society of Health, 126*(1), 28–32.

National Center for Health Statistics. (2002). *National vital statistics report*, Vol. 51(3), In passim.

Phelps, C. E., & Newhouse, J. P. (1974, October). *Coinsurance and the demand for medical services*. The Rand Corporation (R-964-1-OEO/NC ed.).

Phillips, K. A., Mayer, M. L., & Aday, L. A. (2000). Barriers to care among racial/ethnic groups under managed care. *Health Affairs (Millwood), 19*(4), 65–75.

Rettenmaier, A. J., & Saving, T. R. (2007). *The diagnosis & treatment of medicare*. Washington, DC: The AEI Press.

Robbertz, A. A., Lauf, R. C., Jr., Rupp, R. L., & Alexander, D. C. (2006, Sep–Oct). A qualitative assessment of dental care access and utilization among the older adult population in the United States. *General Dentistry, 54*(5), 361–65.

Sanford, J. A. (1996). A review of technical requirements for ramps: Final report – January 31, 1996. Access Board Research, Available at: http://www.access-board.gov/research/Ramps/report.htm. Accessed Oct. 25, 2005.

Shi, L., & Stevens, G. D. (2005). Disparities in access to care and satisfaction among U.S. children: The roles of race/ethnicity and poverty status. *Public Health Reports, 120*(4), 431–41.

Stiglitz, J. E., & Walsh, C. E. (2006). *Economics: 4th Edition*. New York: W.W. Norton & Co.

Strayer, M. (1999, September). Oral health care for homebound and institutional elderly. *Journal of the California Dental Association, 27*(9), 703–08.

Tuominen, R. (1994). *Health economics in dentistry*. 1st ed. Malinu, CA: MedEd.

U.S. Census Bureau. (2001). *Statistical Abstract of the United States: 2001*. 121st ed. Washington, DC: U.S. Government Printing Office.

U.S. Census Bureau. (2002). *United States – Race and Hispanic origin: 1790 to 1990*. Internet Release Date: September 13, 2002. http://www.census.gov/population/documentation/twps0056/tab01.xls

U.S. Census Bureau. (2003). *Population Change and Distribution: 1990–2000* (C2KBR/01-2) [PDF 523k] Available at http://www.census.gov/population/www/cen2000/briefs.html

U.S. Census Bureau. (2004a). *International data base*. Total Midyear Population. Available at: http://www.census.gov/ipc/www/idbsprd.html. Accessed October 18, 2004.

U.S. Census Bureau. (2004b). *Population Division, International Programs Center*. Available at: http://www.census.gov/ipc/www/idbprint.html. Accessed May 17, 2005.

U.S. Census Bureau. (2004c). *Projected population of the United States, by age and sex: 2000 to 2050*. As of July 1. Resident population. Internet Release Date: March 18, 2004, http://www.census.gov/ipc/www/usinterimproj/natprojtab02a.xls

U.S. Census Bureau. (2004d). *U.S. Interim projections by age, sex, race, and Hispanic origin*. Internet Release Date: March 18, 2004. http://www.census.gov/ipc/www/usinterimproj/natprojtab01a.xls, Accessed July 5, 2007.

U.S. Census Bureau. (2004e). *Current population survey. Annual social and economic supplement, detailed tables*.

U.S. Department of Commerce. (1979a). National Technical Information Service, Division of Health Examination Statistics. *National Health Examination Survey* (NHES I) 1959–1962. Hyattsville, MD: National Technical Information Service; 1979. Dental Findings 1 Data Tape Catalog Number 1006.

U.S. Department of Commerce. (1979b). National Technical Information Service, Division of Health Examination Statistics. *National Health and Nutrition Examination Survey*

(NHANES I) 1971–1974. Hyattsville, MD: National Technical Information Service; 1979. Dental Data Tape Catalog Number 4235.

U.S. Department of Health and Human Services. (1972). Centers for Disease Control, National Center for Health Statistics. *Dental visits: Volume and interval since last visit*. Washington, DC: U.S. Government Printing Office.

U.S. Department of Health and Human Services. (1997). National Center for Health Statistics. *Third National Health and Nutritional Examination Survey, 1988–1994*, NHANES III Examination Data File (database on CD-ROM: Series 11, No. 1A, ASCII Version). Hyattsville, MD: National Center for Health Statistics.

U.S. Department of Health and Human Services. (1999). Centers for Disease Control, National Center for Health Statistics. *National Health Interview Surveys* (various years before 2000). Hyattsville, Maryland: National Center for Health Statistics.

U.S. Department of Health and Human Services. (2000). *Oral health in America: A report of the surgeon general*. Rockville, MD: National Institute of Dental and Craniofacial Research, National Institutes of Health.

U. S. Department of Health and Human Services. (2002). Centers for Disease Control and Prevention, National Center for Health Statistics. *Data File Documentation, National Health Interview Survey, 2002* (machine readable data file and documentation). National Center for Health Statistics, Hyattsville, Maryland. Available at: http://www.cdc.gov/nchs/nhcs. Accessed April, 2007.

U.S. Department of Health and Human Services. (2004). National Center for Health Statistics. *National Health and Nutritional Examination Survey, 1999–2000*. Public-use data file and documentation. Available at: http://www.cdc.gov/nchs/about/major/nhanes/nhanes99_00.htm. Accessed June, 2004.

U.S. Department of Health and Human Services. (2005). National Center for Health Statistics. *National Health and Nutritional Examination Survey, 2001–2002*. Public-use data file and documentation. Available at: http://www.cdc.gov/nchs/about/major/nhanes/nhanes01_02.htm. Accessed March, 2005.

U. S. Department of Health and Human Services. (2006). Centers for Disease Control and Prevention, National Center for Health Statistics. *Data File Documentation, National Health Interview Survey, 2005* (machine readable data file and documentation). National Center for Health Statistics, Hyattsville, Maryland. Available at: http://www.cdc.gov/nchs/nhcs. Accessed April, 2007.

U.S. Department of Health and Human Services. (2007). National Center for Health Statistics. *National Health and Nutritional Examination Survey, 2003–2004*. Public-use data file and documentation. Available at: http://www.cdc.gov/nchs/about/major/nhanes/nhanes03_04.htm. Accessed June, 2007.

Upton, C., & Silverman, W. (1972). The demand for dental services. *Journal of Human Resource, 7*, 250–61.

Waldrop, J., & Stern, S. (2003). *Disability status: 2000*, U.S. Census Bureau, Census 2000 Brief Series. C2KBR-17, U.S. Department of Commerce.

Wall, T. P., & Brown, L. J. (2007). The urban & rural distribution of dentists. *Journal of the American Dental Association, 138*, 1003–1011.

Yellowitz, J., & Saunders, M. J. (1989, January). The need for geriatric dental education. *Dental Clinics of North America, 33*(1), 11–8.

Yule, B. F., Parkin, D. (1985). The demand for dental care: An assessment. *Social Science and Medicine, 21*, 753–60.

Chapter 21
Conclusion: Interdisciplinary Planning to Meet the Oral Health Care Needs of Older Adults

Mary E. Northridge and Ira B. Lamster

This volume may usefully be viewed as one effort in an ongoing initiative to answer the question, "How can the oral health care needs of older adults effectively be met?" As might be evident from the title of this final chapter and the assembled authors in this volume, we believe that an interdisciplinary approach is essential. Here we argue that there is a range of interdisciplinary science and scholarship that may be applied to answering a range of different questions. Further, we propose that the collection of chapters in the present volume constitutes what Lattuca (2003) has termed *informed disciplinary*, in that outreach to disciplines other than dentistry was critical in achieving the desired level of quality and comprehensiveness needed to advance the field. Finally, we outline key challenges that will require enhanced interdisciplinary collaboration if we are to be successful in meeting the oral health care needs of burgeoning numbers of older adults in the United States and throughout the world.

A Useful Typology of Interdisciplinary Science and Scholarship

It is important to emphasize that calls for interdisciplinary research to answer complex societal problems are not new. Klein (1996) suggests that the first use of the term *interdisciplinary* may have been by members of the Social Science Research Council (SSRC) in New York City in the mid-1920s, where it originated as bureaucratic shorthand for research that involved two or more of the several professional societies that comprised the SSRC (Lattuca, 2003). Lynch (2006) searched the Web of Science and reported that the first paper using the term "interdisciplinary" was published in 1944 on research in experimental biology by Brozak and Keys (1944). In scanning through the interdisciplinary citations over the ensuing decades, he noted that much of the earlier material, i.e., through the early 1980s, "focuses on better solutions to very applied problems, especially with regard to the need for

M.E. Northridge, Professor of Clinical Sociomedical Sciences, Dept. Sociomedical Sciences, Mailman School of Public Health, Columbia University, New York, NY, USA, Tel.: 212-305-1744
e-mail: men11@columbia.edu

I.B. Lamster, M.E. Northridge (eds.), *Improving Oral Health for the Elderly*,
© Springer Science+Business Media, LLC 2008

'multidisciplinary teams' for case management and treatment, in psychiatry, aging, and disability" (Lynch, 2006, p. 1119).

Likewise, a recent search by us of the PubMed database compiled by the National Library of Medicine and the National Institutes of Health of the United States (see www.ncbi.nlm.nih.gov) revealed scores of papers invoking interdisciplinary approaches and treatments for specific dental conditions, e.g., treatment planning in implant dentistry (Jivraj, Corrado, & Chee, 2007) and endodontic therapy for behavior-challenged children (Soares, Britto, Vertucci, & Guelman, 2006). In terms of broader interdisciplinary undertakings in dentistry, Pyle and Stoller (2003) wrote an especially thoughtful paper on interdisciplinary challenges in addressing oral health disparities among the elderly. With regard to empirical interdisciplinary research in dentistry, we have previously collaborated across schools at Columbia University in utilizing a spatial approach for investigating oral health disparities and planning oral health care services in New York City (Borrell, Northridge, Miller, Golembeski, Spielman, Sclar, & Lamster, 2006).

Although different definitions of interdisciplinary science and scholarship have been invoked over time and across locales to denote the general phenomenon of research and practice that embraces different disciplines (Lynch, 2006), we believe a typology derived by Lattuca (2003) is useful in categorizing our own interdisciplinary work, including this volume. It was motivated by her research with tenured faculty in traditional liberal arts and science fields, although she suggested that it might be transferable to faculty in applied and/or professional schools, such as our own (Mailman School of Public Health and Columbia University College of Dental Medicine). She found that narrow definitions of the term "interdisciplinary" that invoked integration as the litmus test failed to capture the range of interdisciplinary teaching and research engaged in by participating faculty.

Instead, Lattuca (2003) proposed a typology consisting of four categories of interdisciplinary scholarship, namely: (1) *informed disciplinary*, that is, teaching disciplinary courses informed by other disciplines and conducting research that asks disciplinary questions requiring outreach to other disciplines; (2) *synthetic disciplinarity*, that is, teaching courses that link disciplines and conducting research that asks questions that link disciplines; (3) *transdisciplinarity*, that is, teaching courses that cross disciplines and conducting research that asks questions that cross disciplines; and (4) *conceptual interdisciplinarity*, that is, teaching courses without a compelling disciplinary basis and conducting research that asks questions without a compelling disciplinary basis. Elaboration of these distinctions is provided by Lattuca (2003) and is invoked where apt in the remainder of this chapter.

While allowing that some refinement of this typology may prove useful in other settings, it nonetheless had the exhilarating consequence of freeing us up from debating whether or not the activities we are engaged in to provide oral health care to seniors are interdisciplinary or not. In addition, there is no hierarchy intended by this typology. Instead, it suggests that interdisciplinarity exists on a continuum, and different kinds of questions lead to different kinds of interdisciplinarity.

In thinking through this typology, we believe that this volume is an example of informed interdisciplinary, as discussed below. Nonetheless, other initiatives we are concurrently engaged in and envision in the course of providing oral health care to older adults fall into other categories. Along with Janz and Seiler (2003), we prefer to approach interdisciplinarity from the ground up through the use of specific examples and experiences to understand and draw conclusions about our own "work at the borders."

An Informed Disciplinary Approach to this Volume

Lattuca (2003) further explains that in informed disciplinary research, disciplinary questions may be informed by concepts or theories from another discipline or may rely upon methods from other disciplines, but these contributions are made in the service of a disciplinary question. For this volume, we believe that we have indeed borrowed methods, theories, concepts, and other disciplinary components from other fields motivated by our interdisciplinary question, "How can the oral health care needs of older adults be realistically met?" In doing so, we sought contributions from experts both outside of and within dentistry in order to shed light on the complex dimensions of this critical undertaking. For every chapter, our aim was to recruit an outstanding author on a given topic regardless of her/his discipline or profession and make the link to oral health care for seniors.

In her Foreword, Jeanette Takamura—with leadership in social work and aging—argues that this volume fills a gap too long ignored in the larger discourse on aging, not only in the United States, but throughout our graying world. Section 1 on *Population Health and Well-Being* articulates four overlapping perspectives on the volume theme which emphasize in turn; (a) shifting demographics ("The Aging U.S. Population," by Steven Albert); (b) clinical epidemiology ("The Oral Disease Burden Faced by Older Adults," by Ira Lamster and Natalic Crawford); (c) social disparities ("Social Disparities in Oral Health and Health Care for Older Adults," by Luisa Borrell); and (d) access to care ("Access, Place of Residence and Interdisciplinary Opportunities," by Janet Yellowitz).

Section 2 on *Health and Medical Considerations* is likely the most original section of this volume. Here we recruited leading physicians and scientists—several of whom had never appreciated the links between their areas of expertise and the provision of oral health care for older adults prior to joining us in this collaboration—who rose to the challenge and made these vital connections. Several of the included chapters have motivated continued interdisciplinary research and scholarship focused on questions prompted by this undertaking. While by no means exhaustive of the potential contributions, we believe the major health conditions of concern to those providing oral health care to older adults are represented in this section. They include (a) movement disorders ("Movement Disorders in Dental Practice," by Nina Browner and Steven Frucht); (b) cognitive impairment ("Cognitive Impairment," by James Noble and Nikolaos Scarmeas); (c) musculoskeletal conditions ("Musculoskeletal Conditions," by Jennifer Kelsey); (d) medical comorbidities ("Cardiovascular, Cerebrovascular Diseases and Diabetes Mellitus: Co-morbidities that Affect Dental Care for the Older Patient," by Neerja Bhardwaj, Shelly Dubin, Huai

Chang, Matthew Maurer, and Evelyn Granieri); (e) pharmacology ("Geriatric Pharmacology: Principles and Implications for Oral Health," by Brian Scanlon); (f) and tobacco and alcohol use ("Management of Alcohol and Tobacco Dependence in Older Adults," by David Albert).

Section 3 on *Oral Health and Dental Considerations* is the most comprehensive yet in-depth compilation available at the time this volume was finalized regarding state-of-the-art dental care for seniors written by the leading experts in dentistry worldwide. These contributions include (a) oral changes associated with aging ("Normal Oral Mucosal, Dental, Periodontal, and Alveolar Bone Changes Associated with Aging," by Stefanie Russell and Jonathan Ship); (b) periodontal disease as a determinant of systemic disease ("The Relationship between Periodontal Disease and Systemic Disease in the Elderly," by Dana Wolf and Panos Papapanou); (c) conventional tooth replacement ("Caries, Tooth Loss, and Conventional Tooth Replacement for Older Patients," by Ejvind Budtz-Jorgensen and Frauke Müller); (d) dental implantology ("Implant Dentistry as an Approach to Tooth Replacement for Older Adults," by Hans-Peter Weber); (e) salivary function in older adults ("Saliva and the Salivary Glands in the Elderly," by Louis Mandel); (f) mastication and nutrition ("Mastication, Nutrition, Oral Health and Health in Older Patients," by Angus Walls); (g) orofacial pain and neurological disorders ("Orofacial Pain and Neurological Disorders Affecting the Head and Neck," by Ali Makki and Susan Roche); and (h) mucosal disorders ("Oral Pathology Affecting Older Adults," by David Zegarelli, Victoria Woo, and Angela Yoon).

Finally, Section 4 on *Professional Recommendations and Future Needs* contains two chapters devoted to what we believe are the major barriers that must be overcome if we are to effectively meet the oral health care needs of burgeoning numbers of older adults, namely: (a) educating dentists to provide care for seniors ("Educating the Dental Profession," by Lynn Tepper) and (b) professional reimbursement for services ("Dental Services Among Elderly Americans: Utilization, Expenditures, and Their Determinants," by L. Jackson Brown). Further, we identified cultural competency and oral health care delivery models as two topics in need of future interdisciplinary engagement to better ensure that diverse groups of seniors across a variety of settings receive preventive care and treatment services throughout their lives. Because these topics are insufficiently developed at present, they are not covered as separate chapters in this volume.

Interdisciplinary Planning to Meet Future Needs

The magnitude and complexity of the looming crisis of oral health care needs for older adults led us to initiate an interdisciplinary program that is centered at the Columbia University College of Dental Medicine which we have titled *ElderSmile*. For each of its four components—clinical care, research, education, and policy—we have identified salient questions, such as those articulated next, that may lead to different kinds of interdisciplinarity. For clinical care, "What forms of delivery models will be needed to meet the diverse needs of increasing numbers of seniors across place and over time?" For research, "What are the mechanistic explanations for the connections between systemic conditions and oral disease burdens as people age?" For education, "How do we train sufficient numbers of dentists to care for older adults with complex medical and dental needs?" And for policy, "How do we create sustainable programs that provide seniors with prevention of and treatment for oral health conditions regardless of their ability to pay for needed services?"

To meet the challenge of providing oral health care to older adults, we now work in interdisciplinary teams. This approach clearly represents the model for the future. When the readers of this volume require oral health care services as seniors, we will all be in a better position to assess whether or not we were successful in implementing the advice offered in these pages.

References

Borrell, L. N., Northridge, M. E., Miller, D. B., Golembeski, C. A., Spielman, S. E., Sclar, E. D., & Lamster, I. B. (2006). *Special Care in Dentistry, 26*, 252–256.

Brozak, J., & Keys, A. (1944). General aspects of interdisciplinary research in experimental biology. *Science, 100*, 507–512.

Janz, B. & Seiler, T. (2003). Introduction to free space: reconsidering interdisciplinary theory and practice. *History of Intellectual Culture, 3*, 1–7.

Jivraj, S., Corrado, P., & Chee, W. (2007). An interdisciplinary approach to treatment planning in implant dentistry. *British Journal of Dentistry, 202*, 11–17.

Klein, J. T. (1996). *Crossing boundaries: Knowledge, disciplinarities, and interdisciplinarities.* Charlottesville, VA: UP of Virginia.

Lattuca, L. R. (2003). Creating interdisciplinarity: Grounded definitions from college and university faculty. *History of Intellectual Culture, 3*, 1–20.

Lynch, J. (2006). It's not easy being interdisciplinary. *International Journal of Epidemiology, 35*, 1119–1122.

Pyle, M. A., & Stoller, E. P. (2003). Oral health disparities among the elderly: interdisciplinary challenges for the future. *Journal of Dental Education, 67*, 1327–1334.

Soares, F., Britto, L. R., Vertucci, F. J., & Guelman, M. (2006). Interdisciplinary approach to endodontic therapy for uncooperative children in a dental school environment. *Journal of Dental Education, 70*, 1362–1365.

Index